THERAPY FOR
DIABETES
MELLITUS
AND RELATED DISORDERS

FIFTH EDITION

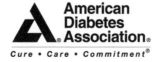

**American
Diabetes
Association®**

Cure • Care • Commitment®

Director, Book Publishing, Robert Anthony; *Managing Editor,* Abe Ogden; *Acquisitions Editor, Professional Books,* Victor Van Beuren; *Editor,* Greg Guthrie; *Production Manager,* Melissa Sprott; *Composition,* ADA; *Cover Design,* Koncept, Inc.; *Printer,* R.R. Donnelley.

Expert Reviewers: M. Sue Kirkman, MD; Mary Korytkowski, MD; and Andrew Ahmann, MD.

Printed in the United States of America
1 3 5 7 9 10 8 6 4 2

The suggestions and information contained in this publication are generally consistent with the *Clinical Practice Recommendations* and other policies of the American Diabetes Association, but they do not represent the policy or position of the Association or any of its boards or committees. Reasonable steps have been taken to ensure the accuracy of the information presented. However, the American Diabetes Association cannot ensure the safety or efficacy of any product or service described in this publication. Individuals are advised to consult a physician or other appropriate health care professional before undertaking any diet or exercise program or taking any medication referred to in this publication. Professionals must use and apply their own professional judgment, experience, and training and should not rely solely on the information contained in this publication before prescribing any diet, exercise, or medication. The American Diabetes Association—its officers, directors, employees, volunteers, and members—assumes no responsibility or liability for personal or other injury, loss, or damage that may result from the suggestions or information in this publication.

⊗ The paper in this publication meets the requirements of the ANSI Standard Z39.48-1992 (permanence of paper).

ADA titles may be purchased for business or promotional use or for special sales. To purchase more than 50 copies of this book at a discount, or for custom editions of this book with your logo, contact the American Diabetes Association at the address below, at booksales@diabetes.org, or by calling 703-299-2046.

American Diabetes Association
1701 North Beauregard Street
Alexandria, Virginia 22311

DOI: 10.2337/9781580403047

Library of Congress Cataloging-in-Publication Data

Therapy for diabetes mellitus and related disorders / Harold E. Lebovitz, editor. -- 5th ed.
    p. ; cm.
Includes bibliographical references and index.
ISBN 978-1-58040-304-7 (alk. paper)
1. Diabetes--Treatment. 2. Diabetes--Complications--Treatment. I. Lebovitz, Harold E., 1931- II. American Diabetes Association. III. Title: Diabetes mellitus and related disorders.
    [DNLM: 1. Diabetes Mellitus--therapy. 2. Diabetes Complications. WK 815 T398 2009]
    RC660.T476 2009
    616.4'6206--dc22
                            2009002172

Contents

Introduction: Goals of Treatment

Harold E. Lebovitz, MD

Diabetes mellitus is one of the major public health issues facing the world in the 21st century. The prevalence of type 1 diabetes is slowly increasing, whereas that of type 2 diabetes is increasing explosively. Changing lifestyles, longer life expectancy, and rapid growth of ethnic and racial populations that have high prevalence rates of type 2 diabetes are likely to double the worldwide prevalence of diabetes by the year 2025. The human toll of diabetes can be estimated not only by medical statistics—which show it to be the leading cause of end-stage renal disease and new cases of vision loss in individuals <65 years old and a major cause of macrovascular disease—but also by the quantity of health care resources that are consumed to care for patients with diabetes. Table 1 tabulates the estimated medical costs for diabetes in the U.S. in 2007. The average cost of caring for a patient with diabetes is greater than twice that of other patients receiving care in the health care system. Much of the disability and costs associated with diabetes are related to the care of individuals afflicted with its chronic complications. The major tasks of the health care establishment today are to implement current treatments that we know will prevent or minimize diabetes complications and to further define and implement the new strategies that we know will prevent or delay the development of type 2 diabetes and its complications in individuals with genetic predispositions.

Since the publication of the first edition of this manual in 1991, remarkable advances in understanding and treating diabetes mellitus and its related disorders have occurred. Data from many studies have proven the importance of glycemic control in preventing or delaying microvascular and neuropathic complications of both type 1 and type 2 diabetes. The importance of blood pressure control and the unique benefits of angiotensin-converting enzyme (ACE) inhibitors and angiotensin II receptor blockers (ARBs) in preventing microvascular and cardiovascular disease are now well established. The effect of statin drugs in reducing coronary artery disease events and mortality in patients with diabetes has been documented by many clinical trials. The rapid development of new types of therapeutic agents that aid in the management of all aspects of diabetes is truly remarkable. The ideal management of the individual with diabetes should ensure the following:

- no symptoms attributable to diabetes
- prevention of acute complications
- prevention of microvascular and neuropathic disease

• reduction in macrovascular disease risk to that of nondiabetic patients
• life expectancy equal to that of nondiabetic individuals

Recent data from the National Center for Chronic Disease Prevention and Health Promotion (NCCDPHP) highlights both the successes and failures that have been achieved in diabetes care in the U.S. in the last decade. There appears to be some progress in decreasing microvascular complications. The age-adjusted rate of visual impairment has decreased slightly from 22.5 per 100 diabetic patients in the 1997–1999 interval to 18.4 in the 2003–2005 interval. From 1996 to 2002, the incidence of end-stage renal disease related to diabetes significantly decreased in white men (337.3 cases per 100,000 diabetic patients to 222.7) and white women (212.4 to 165.8), stopped increasing among black men and women (470.2 and 344.5, respectively), and remained level in Hispanic men and women (322.2 and 259.6, respectively). Age-adjusted lower-extremity amputation rates have decreased from 7.6 and 8.1 per 1,000 diabetic patients in 1996 and 1997, respectively, to 4.8 and 4.4 in 2002 and 2003, respectively. Age-adjusted rates for any cardiovascular disease did not significantly change between 1997 and 2003.

The modest results achieved in reducing complications, coupled with the marked increase in the number of new cases of diabetes presenting each year and the earlier age of onset of diabetes (47.2% of cases of diabetes diagnosed in 2005 were in patients aged 45–59 years), highlights the importance of preventing or delaying the onset of diabetes and more effectively managing diabetes control in 2009.

Studies such as Steno-2, which showed remarkable reductions in both microvascular (risk reduction ~60%) and macrovascular (risk reduction 53%) complications in patients with type 2 diabetes by a strategy of intensive treatment of glycemia, blood pressure, lipids, and the procoagulant state, indicate that we can achieve great reduction in diabetes complications by a multifactorial approach to the management of all risk factors. The 5-year follow-up of the Steno-2 study showed that the benefits of early multifactorial treatment persist and are magnified for many years after the interval of the intensive therapy (hazard ratio for mortality 0.54 and for cardiovascular events 0.41). Fig. 1 depicts the metabolic

---

Table 1 Direct and Indirect Costs of Diabetes in the U.S. in 2007

■ Direct medical costs	$116 billion
Treating diabetes	$ 27 billion
Treating diabetes-related complications	$ 58 billion
Excess general medical costs	$ 31 billion

■ Per capita annual costs of health care for people with diabetes is $11,744 a year, of which $6,649 (57%) is attributed to diabetes.
■ One of every five health care dollars is spent caring for someone with diagnosed diabetes, and half of that is attributed to the diabetes component of their health care.
■ Diabetes-related hospitalizations totaled 24.3 million days in 2007, with a cost of $1,853 per day for diabetes care and $2,281 per day for diabetes-related chronic complications.
■ Physician's office visits directly attributed to diabetes care cost $9.9 billion.
■ Indirect costs (increased absenteeism, decreased productivity, disability, and early mortality) were $58 billion.

targets that were set for the Steno-2 study and the percentage of intensively treated and conventionally treated type 2 diabetic patients who achieved those goals during the 7 1/2-year study.

Tables 2 and 3 summarize the American Diabetes Association's suggested levels of glycemic control and lipoprotein levels that have been shown to significantly decrease the risk of micro- and macrovascular complications in both type 1 and type 2 diabetic patients.

Glycemic control that maintains plasma glucose values at <200 mg/dl (<11.1 mmol/l) will generally eliminate the symptoms of polydipsia, polyuria, polyphagia, weight loss, and increased fatigue. Maintaining plasma glucose levels at 150–165 mg/dl (8.3–9.2 mmol/l) is usually associated with a sense of well-being and good health. Preventing chronic microvascular and neuropathic complications and eliminating diabetes complications associated with pregnancy probably require normoglycemic or near-normoglycemic regulation. Minimizing macrovascular disease requires addressing all of the risk factors (e.g., smoking, hypertension, plasma triglycerides, and serum LDL and HDL cholesterol) as well as blood glucose control.

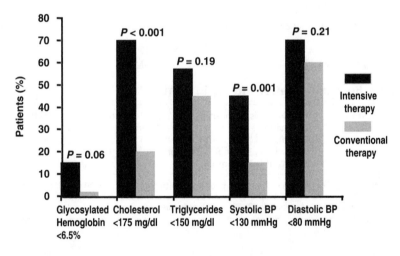

Figure 1 Percentage of patients in each group who reached the intensive treatment goals at a mean of 7.8 years. A total of 160 type 2 diabetic patients with microalbuminuria were randomized to intensive metabolic control or the ordinary control recommended by the Danish Diabetes Society. The intensive targets are listed below each column, and the percentage of each group attaining those values for the 7.5 years of the study is provided for each column. The risk reductions for micro- and macrovascular disease are given in the text. Reproduced with permission from Gaede et al. Copyright ©2003 Massachusetts Medical Society. All rights reserved.

Table 2 Recommendations for Glycemic Control

A1C	<7.0%*
Preprandial capillary plasma glucose	90–130 mg/dl
Peak postprandial capillary plasma glucose	180 mg/dl
(postprandial glucose measurements should be made 1–2 h after the beginning of the meal)	

Key concepts in setting glycemic goals are as follows:
- ■A1C is the primary target for glycemic control.
- ■Goals should be individualized based on:
  - –duration of diabetes
  - –age/life expectancy
  - –comorbid conditions
  - –known cardiovascular disease or advanced microvascular complications
  - –hypoglycemia unawareness
  - –individual patient considerations
- ■ Certain populations (children, pregnant women, and elderly) require special considerations.
- ■ More or less stringent glycemic goals may be appropriate for individual patients.
- ■ Postprandial glucose may be targeted if A1C goals are not met despite reaching preprandial glucose goals.

*Referenced to a nondiabetic range of 4.0–6.0% using a Diabetes Control and Complications Trial–based assay.

Table 3 Recommendations for Lipid Control

LDL cholesterol	For individuals without overt CVD: <100 mg/dl (<2.6 mmol/l)
	For individuals with overt CVD: <70 mg/dl (<1.8 mmol/l) is an option
HDL cholesterol	>40 mg/dl (>1.1 mmol/l) for men
	>50 mg/dl (>1.3 mmol/l) for women
Triglycerides	<150 mg/dl (<1.7 mmol/l)

Current NCEP/ATP III guidelines suggest that in patients with triglycerides ≥200 mg/dl, the "non-HDL cholesterol" (total cholesterol – HDL cholesterol) be utilized. The goal is ≤130 mg/dl (≤1.45 mmol/l). From American Diabetes Association (2009). CVD, cardiovascular disease.

In defining glycemic treatment goals, alleviating symptoms and increasing the sense of well-being are realistic goals for all individuals with diabetes. Striving for goals to prevent chronic complications requires that

- the patient's life expectancy is at least 10–15 years more
- the patient does not already have significant chronic complications
- the patient does not have an illness that contraindicates intensive treatment
- the patient is willing and able to follow a regimen for intensive treatment

Blood pressure control and regulation of serum lipids in diabetic patients require somewhat different goals than in nondiabetic patients and are discussed in great detail in subsequent specific chapters.

BIBLIOGRAPHY

American Diabetes Association: Economic costs of diabetes in the U.S. in 2007. *Diabetes Care* 31:596–615, 2008

American Diabetes Association: Standards of medical care in diabetes—2009 (Position Statement). *Diabetes Care* 32 (Suppl. 1):S13–S61, 2009

Centers for Disease Control and Prevention: Diabetes data & trends. Accessed 12 January 2009. Available online at http://apps.nccd.cdc.gov/DDTSTRS/default.aspx

Gaede P, Vedel P, Larsen N, Jensen GV, Parving HH, Pedersen O: Multifactorial intervention and cardiovascular disease in patients with type 2 diabetes. *N Engl J Med* 348:383–393, 2003

Gaede P, Lund-Andersen H, Parving H-H, Pedersen O: Effects of a multifactorial intervention on mortality in type 2 diabetes. *N Engl J Med* 358:580–591, 2008

1. Diagnosis and Classification of Diabetes Mellitus

Harold E. Lebovitz, MD

A cardinal feature in preventing the complications of diabetes is early diagnosis and treatment. This is particularly important in type 2 or late-onset autoimmune type 1 diabetes because these disorders start with a relatively asymptomatic period that lasts as long as several years. According to the Centers for Disease Control and Prevention, diabetes now affects nearly 24 million people in the U.S. This is an increase of >3 million in ~2 years according to new 2007 prevalence data. Another 57 million people are estimated to have pre-diabetes. Currently, ~25% of people with type 2 diabetes in the U.S. are undiagnosed. Unfortunately, this relatively symptom-free undiagnosed period is not benign; ~50% of newly diagnosed patients with type 2 diabetes already have evidence of early chronic complications.

Diabetes is a group of metabolic disorders characterized by inappropriate hyperglycemia that results in chronic microvascular, neuropathic, and/or macrovascular disease. The difficult task is to define inappropriate hyperglycemia. Several task forces have struggled with this issue and have concluded that an inappropriate blood glucose level is one that will lead to diabetic microvascular complications. Retinopathy was chosen as the primary complication because it is unique to diabetes, easy to quantify, and the most common chronic complication. Numerous studies have shown that a plasma glucose level ≥200 mg/dl (≥11.1 mmol/l) 2 h after a glucose challenge is associated with the development of diabetic retinopathy within 5–10 years. In 1979, it was proposed (but not measured) that this corresponded to a fasting plasma glucose (FPG) of 140 mg/dl (7.8 mmol/l). This value has since been shown to be wrong. Several recent studies show that FPG levels between 120 and 130 mg/dl (6.7 and 7.2 mmol/l) are comparable to the 2-h post–glucose challenge level of 200 mg/dl (11.1 mmol/l) and are associated with the subsequent development of retinopathy.

These data led to a new set of criteria for the diagnosis of diabetes (Table 1.1). Criteria 2 and 3 should be confirmed by repeat testing on a separate day. In redefining the criteria for the diagnosis of diabetes, it became necessary to define intermediate grades of glucose intolerance. Table 1.2 defines categories of glucose tolerance in terms of either FPG or 2-h post–glucose challenge levels. The reason for defining impaired fasting glucose (IFG) or impaired glucose tolerance (IGT) is that both degrees of glucose intolerance predict future development of diabetes, and both are associated with the metabolic syndrome and an increase in clinical cardiovascular disease. Individuals with either IFG or IGT are consid-

Table 1.1 Criteria for the Diagnosis of Diabetes Mellitus

1. Symptoms of diabetes plus casual plasma glucose concentration ≥200 mg/dl (≥11.1 mmol/l): casual is defined as any time of day without regard to time since last meal. The classic symptoms of diabetes include
   - polyuria
   - polydipsia
   - unexplained weight loss
   or
2. FPG ≥126 mg/dl (≥7.0 mmol/l): fasting is defined as no calorie intake for at least 8 h.
   or
3. 2-h plasma glucose ≥200 mg/dl (≥11.1 mmol/l) during an oral glucose tolerance test: the test should be performed as described by the World Health Organization with a glucose load containing the equivalent of 75 g anhydrous glucose dissolved in water.

Criteria 2 and 3 should be confirmed by repeat testing on a separate day. From American Diabetes Association, 2009.

ered to have pre-diabetes. Very recent studies have added a degree of complexity concerning the criteria that separate pre-diabetes from diabetes that has yet to be resolved. The Diabetes Prevention Program reported that its patient population with pre-diabetes had a 7.9% prevalence of diabetic retinopathy. The significance of such findings and their impact on the definition of diabetes need to be assessed.

Several studies have shown that the development of type 2 diabetes can be delayed by several years or more by identifying individuals with pre-diabetes and treating them with intensive lifestyle modification or pharmacological agents (see Chapter 17). The IFG category has been recently extended to include those individuals with FPG levels ≥100 mg/dl (≥5.6 mmol/l), and the normal range for FPG has been redefined as <100 mg/dl (<5.6 mmol/l).

The new diagnostic criteria for diabetes did not create more diagnoses of diabetes, but rather made it easier to diagnose the large pool of undiagnosed individuals with diabetes by FPG rather than by requiring an oral glucose tolerance test (OGTT). This reduced the percentage of diabetic patients who were undiagnosed from ~50 to 30%.

Table 1.2 Categories of Glucose Tolerance

FPG	2-h postload plasma glucose (oral glucose tolerance test)
Normal: <100 mg/dl (<5.6 mmol/l)	Normal: <140 mg/dl (<7.8 mmol/l)
IFG: ≥100 mg/dl (≥5.6 mmol/l) and <126 mg/dl (<7.0 mmol/l)	IGT: ≥140 mg/dl (≥7.8 mmol/l) and <200 mg/dl (<11.1 mmol/l)
Diabetes: ≥126 mg/dl (≥7.0 mmol/l)	Diabetes: ≥200 mg/dl (≥11.1 mmol/l)

From American Diabetes Association, 2009.

Table 1.3 Classification of Diabetes Mellitus

Type 1 diabetes	Other specific types
■ Immune mediated ■ Idiopathic	■ Genetic defects of β-cell function ■ Genetic defects in insulin action ■ Diseases of exocrine pancreas ■ Endocrinopathies
Type 2 diabetes	
■ May range from predominantly insulin resistant to predominantly insulin deficient	■ Drug- or chemical-induced diabetes ■ Infections ■ Uncommon forms of immune-mediated diabetes
Gestational diabetes	■ Other genetic syndromes sometimes associated with diabetes

From American Diabetes Association, 2009.

The new classification of patients with diabetes is based on etiology (Table 1.3). The classification system eliminates the terms "insulin-dependent" (IDDM) and "non–insulin-dependent" (NIDDM) and replaces them with "type 1" and "type 2" diabetes, respectively.

Type 1 diabetes is characterized by absolute insulin deficiency. Most of these patients have immune-mediated destruction of their β-cells, but a few have an unknown or idiopathic process that leads to β-cell loss.

Type 2 diabetes is the classic form of the disease, with varying degrees of insulin resistance and relative insulin secretory deficiency. The etiology is unknown. It is now recognized that type 2 diabetes is a heterogeneous disorder. It can occur in both children and adults and is frequently associated with obesity. Known causes of diabetes fall into the "other specific types" category, which includes the various forms of maturity-onset diabetes of the young (MODY). Gestational diabetes (GDM) remains the fourth category and is defined as any degree of glucose intolerance with onset or first recognition during pregnancy. GDM occurs in ~4% of U.S. pregnancies (135,000 cases annually). Diagnosis of GDM is based on an OGTT (Table 1.4). Diagnostic criteria for the 100-g OGTT

Table 1.4 Diagnosis of GDM with a 100- or 75-g glucose load

	mg/dl	mmol/l
100-g glucose load		
Fasting	95	5.3
1-h	180	10.0
2-h	155	8.6
3-h	140	7.8
75-g glucose load		
Fasting	95	5.3
1-h	180	10.0
2-h	155	8.6

Two or more of the venous plasma concentrations must be met or exceeded for a positive diagnosis.

are derived from the original work of O'Sullivan and Mahan, modified by Carpenter and Coustan. The results of the recent HAPO (Hyperglycemia and Adverse Pregnancy Outcomes) study may lead to a reconsideration and future modifications of the criteria for GDM.

BIBLIOGRAPHY

American Diabetes Association: Diagnosis and classification of diabetes mellitus (Position Statement). *Diabetes Care* 32 (Suppl. 1):S62–S67, 2009

DPP Research Group: The prevalence of retinopathy in impaired glucose tolerance and recent-onset diabetes in the Diabetes Prevention Program. *Diabet Med* 24:137–144, 2007

Centers for Disease Control and Prevention (CDC): Number of people with diabetes increases to 24 million [Press release]. 24 June 2008

HAPO Study Cooperative Group: Hyperglycemia and adverse pregnancy outcomes. *N Engl J Med* 358:1991–2002, 2008

Dr. Lebovitz is Professor of Medicine at the State University of New York Health Science Center at Brooklyn, Brooklyn, New York.

2. Genetic Counseling for Autoimmune Type 1 Diabetes

Jennifer M. Barker, MD, and George S. Eisenbarth, MD

DIAGNOSIS

Diabetes is diagnosed based on the presence of hyperglycemia and is often diagnosed in the setting of symptoms that includes polyuria, polydipsia, and weight loss. Once the diagnosis of diabetes is made, identifying the underlying cause is important for optimizing treatment and screening for associated conditions. The major forms of the disease are type 1 and type 2 diabetes. There are multiple other forms of diabetes that are rarer and often associated with single gene mutations.

Autoimmune type 1 diabetes can occur at any age. Approximately 50% of individuals develop the disorder before age 40 years, but another 50%, including relatives of patients, develop the disease as adults. The oldest anti-islet autoantibody (AIAA)-positive patient we have followed to diabetes was aged 69 years at diabetes onset. It is generally thought that most children developing type 1 diabetes have the immune-mediated form of diabetes (type 1A). With recent improvements in the ability to diagnose autoimmune diabetes and advances in genetic analysis of diabetes, it is clear that autoimmunity as the cause of childhood diabetes can vary from a major to a minor factor, depending on ethnicity, associated diseases, and, obviously, family history.

Whereas the majority of diabetes cases in childhood can be attributed to type 1 diabetes, there are subgroups of patients whose etiology of diabetes is different. As the rates of obesity have increased over the last several decades, there has been a parallel increase in type 2 diabetes. It has been recognized that as many as 50% of newly diagnosed adolescents of high-risk ethnic groups have type 2 diabetes (Table 2.1). These individuals usually lack a series of AIAAs, they often have BMI >25 kg/m^2, many have the most protective DQB1 HLA allele (~20% DQB1*0602), and many have insulin-resistant syndromes. Recently, genetic variants within the gene encoding for TCF7L2 (transcription factor-7-like 2) have been associated with type 2 diabetes in multiple populations. These variants can provide population-based association data but not individual diagnostic information at this time.

Diabetes that presents in the neonatal period (<3 months of age) can be largely attributed to single gene mutations. Immunodysregulation polyendocrinopathy enteropathy X-linked syndrome (IPEX) is an X-linked disorder caused by mutations of the FOXP-3 gene. The FOXP-3 gene is important for the development of regulatory T-cells. Male subjects with this disorder generally present with

Table 2.1 Differential Diagnosis of Autoimmune Diabetes in Childhood

Characteristics	Likely Diagnosis	Diagnostic Tests
Non-Hispanic Caucasian	90% autoimmune DM	Autoantibody positive, high-risk HLA
Hispanic American	50% not autoimmune DM, diabetes etiology unknown	Autoantibody negative
African American	50% not autoimmune DM, diabetes etiology unknown	Autoantibody negative
Transient hyperglycemia	"Stress" hyperglycemia	Autoantibody negative, normal IVGTT
DM + deafness/maternal inheritance	Mitochondrial DM	Autoantibody negative, mitochondrial gene analysis
MODY family history	MODY-2, MODY-3, etc.	Autoantibody negative, glucokinase, HNF gene sequence
DM + diabetes insipidus	DIDMOAD syndrome	Autoantibody negative, characteristic syndrome

DIDMOAD, diabetes insipidus, diabetes mellitus, optic atrophy, deafness; DM, diabetes mellitus.

severe enteropathy and AIAA-positive diabetes diagnosed within the first several weeks of life. This disorder is generally fatal; however, treatment with bone marrow transplant and immunosuppression with sirolimus has been reported to be successful. Mutations of the KCNJ11 gene have recently been recognized as a cause of both permanent and transient neonatal diabetes. This gene encodes Kir6.2, which is the pore-forming subunit of the ATP-sensitive K^+ channel. This is found in β-cells (among others) and plays a central role in the secretion of insulin. Heterozygous mutations in the channel, resulting in a decreased sensitivity to ATP, are associated with decreased insulin secretion and diabetes. Depending on the location of the mutation within the gene, the diabetes may also be associated with development delay and epilepsy (DEND syndrome). Other causes of neonatal diabetes include pancreatic aplasia (associated with homozygous IPF [insulin promoter factor] mutations), homozygous glucokinase mutations, and abnormalities of imprinting on 6p24 (resulting in transient neonatal diabetes).

The best-characterized nonautoimmune forms of diabetes in childhood are maturity-onset diabetes of the young (MODY)-2, -1, and-3. MODY-2 is often a mild form of diabetes with normal fasting blood glucose. MODY-2 results from a mutation in the glucokinase gene. MODY-3 can be confused with type 1 diabetes, is inherited as an autosomal-dominant trait, and is caused by mutations in the hepatic nuclear factor (HNF)-1α gene. MODY-1 results from a mutation in HNF-4α. MODY-3 is currently the most frequently defined form of MODY, but

Table 2.2 Type 1A–Associated Autoimmune Disorders

Disorder	Patients (%)	Relative of Patient with Type 1 Diabetes (%)	Screening Test
Celiac disease	5.4	2.6	Transglutaminase autoantibody
Graves' disease	0.5–2.0	?	Sensitive TSH assay
Hypothyroidism	1.4–5.0	?	Sensitive TSH assay
Addison's disease	0.5	?	Anti–21-hydroxylase autoantibody
Pernicious anemia	1.4	?	Serum B12
Type 1 diabetes	NA	5	AIAAs

patients develop this disorder as both children and adults. The most common forms of nonautoimmune diabetes in children are probably caused by none of the currently identified mutations, but rather are probably variants of type 2 diabetes and are polygenic in origin.

ASSOCIATED AUTOIMMUNE DISORDERS

The most important genetic counseling information that can be currently offered to families with type 1A diabetes is that individuals with autoimmune diabetes and their relatives are at increased risk for a series of organ-specific autoimmune disorders. Most of these disorders can be effectively treated. Table 2.2 lists several of the most common associated diseases, the diseases most important to diagnose, and screening tests. Over the past several years, genes involved in the development of multiple autoimmune diseases have been identified. The PTPN22 gene encodes the lymphoid-specific tyrosine phosphatase. A single nucleotide polymorphism at position 1858 (C > T) is associated with an amino acid change (Arg620-Trp). The T-allele has been associated with type 1 diabetes, Addison's disease, autoimmune thyroid disease, and rheumatoid arthritis, suggesting that the gene is important for the development of autoimmunity. Additional genes that have been associated with multiple autoimmune processes include cytotoxic T-cell–associated antigen (CTLA)-4 and the interleukin-2 receptor, and most importantly, alleles of HLA genes (e.g., DR3 and DR4 associated with type 1 diabetes, Addison's disease, and celiac disease).

Celiac Disease

Celiac disease is one of the most common associated diseases and is often asymptomatic in patients with type 1A diabetes. Celiac disease is primarily associated with the high-risk HLA alleles DR3, DQA1*0501, and DQB1*0201. Tests for transglutaminase (TTG) autoantibodies are both highly specific and sensitive. Recently, antibodies against deamidated gliadin peptide (DGP) have been strongly associated with celiac disease, whereas the older assay for antibodies reacting with gliadin lack both specificity and sensitivity. In a prospective study of children at risk for celiac disease, the levels of DGP antibodies closely paralleled those of TTG antibodies and decreased more quickly than TTG antibodies after the institution of a gluten-free diet.

Given the finding of high-titer TTG autoantibodies, follow-up intestinal biopsy usually confirms the diagnosis of celiac disease. With avoidance of gluten, the intestinal mucosa heals and autoantibodies disappear. When celiac disease is asymptomatic, the decision to screen and ultimately to treat the disease often relates to the long-term consequences of the disorder, which can include both osteoporosis and intestinal malignancies (both of which have been reported to be prevented by dietary therapy). Because the levels of TTG autoantibodies fluctuate, it is important to biopsy individuals close to the time of confirmation of high levels of autoantibodies. A test for TTG autoantibodies on the day of biopsy is recommended to aid evaluation.

Autoimmune Thyroid Disease and Addison's Disease

Addison's disease can develop in the absence of adrenal autoimmunity. In the absence of 21-hydroxylase autoantibodies, the diagnosis of X-linked adrenoleukodystrophy should be considered and plasma level of very-long-chain fatty acids obtained. X-linked adrenoleukodystrophy has associated neurologic compromise and variable age of presentation.

Autoimmune thyroid disease and Addison's disease are both also highly associated with HLA DR3. In patients with type 1A diabetes, Addison's disease is most often found in individuals with the highest-risk HLA genotypes: HLA DR3 and DR4. Of patients with type 1A diabetes, 2% have autoantibodies reacting with the enzyme 21-hydroxylase, a major adrenal autoantigen. Approximately 25% of 21-hydroxylase autoantibody–positive patients have Addison's disease on initial testing, and more progress to overt disease during follow-up. Because of the rarity of Addison's disease, it is often a missed diagnosis. In a patient with type 1A diabetes, a distinctive sign of Addison's disease is decreasing insulin dosage and recurrent hypoglycemia. Increasing insulin sensitivity can precede hyperpigmentation. If untreated, Addison's disease is fatal. The therapy is relatively simple, with oral replacement of gluco- and mineralocorticoids.

Abnormalities of thyroid function are common in people with type 1 diabetes. As many as 20% of patients with type 1 diabetes have autoantibodies associated with autoimmune thyroid disease, and over prolonged follow-up ~80% develop overt thyroid disease. To detect both autoimmune thyroid disease and hypothyroidism, we determine serum thyrotropin (thyroid-stimulating hormone [TSH]) with a sensitive assay to detect both high (hypothyroidism) and low (autoimmune thyroid disease) levels of TSH. In patients with type 1 diabetes, antithyroid autoantibodies appear to be more frequent than progression to overt thyroid disease, and a subset of patients with type 1 diabetes lack the autoantibodies yet progress to hypothyroidism. With hypothyroidism and type 1 diabetes, Addison's disease should be excluded before thyroid hormone replacement, for fear of exacerbating the Addison's disease.

Table 2.3 Empiric Risk of Type 1A Diabetes

Relative with Type 1 Diabetes (%)	Modifying Factor	Risk of Diabetes
Identical twin	Age at onset in first twin: if >25 yr of age, risk is <5%	50
Father	HLA DR3/DR4(DQ8): risk is ~25%	6
Mother	HLA DR3/DR4(DQ8): risk is ~25%	2
Sibling	HLA DR3/DR4(DQ8): risk is ~50%	5
First-degree relatives	HLA DR3 and DR4(DQ8)	20
	HLA DR3 or DR4(DQ8)	5
	HLA DR2 with DQB1*0502	5
	HLA DR2 with DQB1*0602	<0.2

Pernicious Anemia

Pernicious anemia is usually diagnosed late in life (often beyond the sixth decade). In patients with type 1A diabetes, pernicious anemia appears earlier in life. The major irreversible effect of pernicious anemia is loss of proprioception and vibratory sensation, which can occur in the absence of anemia (especially in patients receiving vitamin supplements). Screening for serum B12 followed by a Schilling test is usually adequate for diagnosis, although serum B12 levels can be low-normal with disease. Therapy for pernicious anemia consists of injections of vitamin B12.

Autoimmune Syndromes

There are three autoimmune syndromes associated with type 1A diabetes: IPEX and APS (autoimmune polyendocrine syndrome) types I and II. Diagnosis of each syndrome of associated autoimmune disorders requires specialized follow-up and treatment. Patients with APS-I often present in infancy with mucocutaneous candidiasis followed by Addison's disease and hypoparathyroidism. They often develop asplenism and require infectious prophylaxis, follow-up for multiple autoimmune disorders, and aggressive treatment for oral candida with associated oral cancers (see "Type 1 Diabetes: Cellular, Molecular & Clinical Immunology" at www.barbaradaviscenter.org). APS-I is caused by mutations in the autoimmune regulator (AIRE) gene and is an autosomal recessive disorder. It has recently been observed that 100% of patients with APS-1 are positive for anti-interferon-α antibodies compared with none of the normal control subjects or those with APS-II. These autoantibodies have been identified in children as young as 3 years of age with APS-I. Therefore, these autoantibodies may be a useful screen in patients in whom the diagnosis is being considered prior to sequencing the gene. The AIRE gene is large, with 14 exons. Multiple mutations have been identified as associated with the disorder. Sequencing may detect a mutation on only one chromosome, and it is likely that there are mutations in noncoding sequences. Therefore, in the face of clinical symptoms consistent with the diagnosis of APS-I without definitive mutations on both chromsomes, especially if anti-interferon autoantibodies are present, the patient should be considered to have APS-I and treated as such. APS-II is defined as the presence of two or more autoimmune processes, including type 1 diabetes, autoimmune thyroid disease, Addison's disease, hypogonadism, and/or celiac disease. It is characterized by polygenic inheritance, a female predisposition, and the development of disease in adulthood.

RISK OF TYPE 1A DIABETES

Type 1A diabetes occurs in 1 of 300 children. However, this is probably an underestimate of the total prevalence; adults with the autoimmune form of diabetes can now be diagnosed through AIAA assays. Table 2.3 shows the genetic risk of developing type 1A diabetes according to family history of diabetes. The highest risk for type 1A diabetes occurs in the identical twin of a patient with type 1 diabetes. With long-term follow-up, we have observed that ~50% of monozygotic twins who were initially discordant for diabetes progress to type 1A diabetes. In a combined series from the U.S. and Great Britain, almost half of initially discordant twins who developed diabetes became concordant for diabetes >5 years after the diagnosis in their twin-mate. The incidence of diabetes in the second twin is highest within 10 years of onset of diabetes in the first twin and declines steadily, but many monozygous twins develop diabetes decades after the first twin. The risk of diabetes for the second monozygous twin is influenced by the age at which the first twin developed diabetes (falling to <5% for index twins with onset after age 25 years). Even in Japan, a country with one of the lowest prevalences of type 1 diabetes, the risk for an identical twin is similar to that in the U.S.

Why offspring of a mother with type 1 diabetes have a lower risk of diabetes than offspring of a father with type 1 diabetes is unknown. Generally, the risk to a sibling of a patient with type 1A diabetes in childhood is ~1 in 20. Risk within a family is greatly influenced by HLA alleles of chromosome 6, particularly HLA-DR and -DQ alleles, with the dominant effect associated with DQ. DQ molecules consist of two chains, an α- and a β-chain, both of which are polymorphic in their amino acid sequence. DR molecules also consist of an α- and a β-chain, but only the β-chain gene is polymorphic. Each different polymorphic amino acid sequence is assigned a unique number. Thus, DR molecules can simply be described with one number for their β-chain gene (e.g., DRB1*0301 [DR3]), whereas both α- and β-chains must be specified for DQ molecules (e.g., DQA1*0501,DQB1*0201). The highest-risk genotype for type 1A diabetes consists of the common DR3 haplotype with the highest-risk DR4 haplotype (DQA1*0301,DQB1*0302 with DRB1*0401, 0402, or 0404 but not 0403).

In addition to being associated with risk for type 1A diabetes, HLA alleles are associated with protection from diabetes. In particular, DQA1*0102,DQB1*0602 provides dominant protection from type 1A diabetes in all populations studied to date. In most populations, this protective haplotype is present in ~20% of the general population and <1% of children with type 1A diabetes. The protection is not absolute, and, in particular, adults with type 1 diabetes have DQB1*0602 more often than children. DRB1*1401 and DQA1*0201,DQB1*0301 are also strongly protective.

Some HLA-DQ alleles are uncommon in the general U.S. population, but when present in families with type 1 diabetes, they may confer high diabetes risk. Such alleles include DQA1*0102,DQB1*0502 and DQA1*0401,DQB1*0402. Although most reviews do not list these molecules as high-risk alleles because only a small percentage of patients with type 1A diabetes express them, they confer a risk of diabetes. DQB1*0402 has aspartic acid at position 57 of its DQB chain (Asp57 positivity was reported to correlate with protection from diabetes). The gradation of risk for diabetes and the complexity (with so many alleles) suggests that genetic counseling on the basis of HLA alleles requires caution.

A large study in Denver is evaluating the presence at birth of DR and DQ alleles from cord blood in the general population. Of ~30,000 births, 2.4% of children express the highest-risk genotype (DR3/4 [DQB1*0302]). Such children may comprise ~40% of all children who develop type 1 diabetes and have an absolute risk of diabetes of ~6% (similar to having a father with type 1 diabetes). In contrast, for children with a first-degree relative with type 1A diabetes (parent or sibling), the risk of diabetes is >25% if the child has both DR3 and DR4 (DQB1*0302).

Groups of children at an even higher risk for the development of type 1 diabetes can be identified. Children who are identical by descent (i.e., they have inherited the exact same chromosomes) for both the DR3/4 (DQB1*0302) with their sibling with diabetes have a risk for diabetes-related autoimmunity of 80% and diabetes of 50% by age 10. This suggests that it is not just the DR3/4 (DQB1*0302) genotype alone that is important in determining diabetes risk but that there may be an additional gene or genes in linkage disequilibrium with DR3/4 (DQB1*0302) that contribute to the genetic risk for the disease. One such determinant is DP alleles. Children with multiple first-degree relatives with type 1 diabetes and high- or moderate-risk HLA genotypes have a similarly high diabetes risk. As previously mentioned, an identical twin whose twin-mate has type 1 diabetes has a very high risk (>50%) for the development of type 1 diabetes. Therefore, groups of patients with very high risk for type 1 diabetes can be identified on the basis of family history and genetic risk alone and may be ideal groups to target for diabetes prevention.

GENETIC, IMMUNOLOGICAL, AND METABOLIC TESTS

Genetic

The primary genetic test currently associated with defining risk for type 1A diabetes or aiding in its diagnosis is typing for DR and DQ alleles. The finding of DQA1*0102,DQB1*0602 in an individual thought to have type 1A diabetes should point to other causes of diabetes or autoimmune syndromes in which HLA alleles may have less influence. Approximately 10% of relatives of patients with type 1A diabetes express DQB1*0602 with its greatly reduced risk for type 1A diabetes. In addition, ~7% of cytoplasmic islet cell autoantibody (ICA)-positive relatives of patients with type 1A diabetes express DQB1*0602. Despite expression of cytoplasmic ICA, these relatives have a low risk of progression to type 1A diabetes, and most of these relatives express only a single biochemical AIAA. High risk for type 1A diabetes is usually associated with the expression of multiple biochemical autoantibodies. There are too few relatives with DQB1*0602 who express multiple biochemical autoantibodies to currently assess their risk of progression to diabetes.

Multiple additional genes associated with type 1 diabetes risk have been reported, but most with odds ratios <1.5 and limited ability to aid in prediction of diabetes for individuals, though defining potential important pathogenic pathways. A polymorphism at 5' end of the insulin gene contributes ~10% of the familial aggregation of type 1A diabetes. The diabetes protective polymorphism is associated with greater insulin messenger RNA in the thymus, potentially increasing tolerance to the key autoantigen insulin. Figure 2.1 shows odds ratios for diabetes for multiple genetic loci. Only HLA-DR/DQ and a polymorphism within the insulin gene have odds ratios >2.

Immunological

The best predictor of risk for type 1A diabetes is the expression of multiple islet autoantibodies (Table 2.4). This is a rapidly developing field. In the past 10 years, a series of specific islet autoantigens have been identified and sequenced. Reliable and convenient autoantibody assays for these autoantigens are now available. The standard autoantibody test for type 1A diabetes was the cytoplasmic ICA test, which used frozen sections of human pancreas. This test is difficult to standardize and measures some but not all of the autoantibodies that can be determined with biochemical autoantibody testing. The test still has specific research roles (especially in identification of additional unknown autoantigens). Generally, given a combination of testing for glutamic acid decarboxylase (GAD)-65, ICA512/IA-2, and insulin autoantibodies, testing for cytoplasmic ICA is of limited utility. More than 90% of individuals with typical autoimmune insulin-dependent diabetes express one or more of the three biochemical autoantibodies (each assay set with specificity >99th percentile).

Table 2.4 Major β-Cell Autoantigens Associated with Immune-Mediated Type 1 Diabetes

Autoantigen	Positive (%)	Comment
Insulin	49–92	>90% children <5 yr old, autoantibody positive
GAD	84	Low risk as single antibody
ICA512/IA-2	74	Highly specific for type 1
Phogrin/IA-2β	61	Usually a subset IA-2

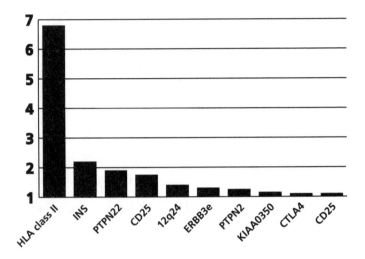

Figure 2.1 Odds ratios for type 1 diabetes for multiple genetic loci. Modified from Todd et al. (2007).

Among relatives at risk for type 1A diabetes, the highest risk is associated with expression of more than one of the biochemically defined autoantibodies. Figure 2.2 illustrates the risk of diabetes relative to autoantibody expression among a series of first-degree relatives of patients with type 1 diabetes. Adding the assay for cytoplasmic ICA to the determination of biochemical autoantibodies runs the risk that a single biochemical autoantibody (e.g., GAD65) may result in ICA positivity, suggesting that a relative may have two antibodies (ICA and GAD65) when he or she has only one. The form of ICA reacting only with GAD65 has been termed *restricted* or *selective* ICA and is associated with a lower risk of progression to diabetes than is nonrestricted ICA, which is usually associated with expression of multiple autoantibodies.

The autoantigen phogrin, or IA-2b, is related to ICA512/IA-2, and most (>95%) IA-2b–positive sera are detectable as ICA512/IA-2 positive. Several large studies indicate that the expression of multiple autoantibodies in the general population approximates the risk for type 1 diabetes.

Recently, the cation efflux transporter ZnT8 has been identified as an autoantigen in type 1 diabetes. Using a bioinformatics approach, investigators identified ZnT8 as a candidate autoantigen. Autoantibodies against ZnT8 have been identified in 60–80% of patients with new-onset type 1 diabetes compared with <2% of control subjects. Additionally, these autoantibodies were present in subjects with diabetes and negative GAD65, IA-2, and insulin autoantibodies.

Caveats of autoantibody testing include the following:

• Variation exists in the sensitivity and specificity of assays. Particularly wide variation is found between different assays for cytoplasmic ICAs. Most assays produce labeled autoantigens by transcribing and translating DNA of relevant clones in vitro. These assays are usually performed in a semiautomated 96-well format. Standard enzyme-linked immunosorbent assays (ELISAs), in which antigen is simply bound to plastic plates, usually perform poorly in terms of specificity and sensitivity, but more recent ELISA-like assays have been developed wherein autoantibodies react with both "labeled" fluid-phase autoantigens (e.g., GAD65) and antigens bound to plates.

- Insulin autoantibodies cannot be measured after insulin therapy. Within weeks, and certainly within a month, of the institution of insulin therapy, insulin antibodies are produced.
- Expression of insulin autoantibodies is inversely correlated with the age at onset of type 1A diabetes. Thus, this assay is particularly sensitive for children developing type 1A diabetes before age 12 years. However, with excellent insulin autoantibody assays, ~50% of adults developing diabetes also express such antibodies.
- Autoantibodies usually develop sequentially, and the first autoantibody often appears before 3 years of age. In some individuals, the first or subsequent autoantibodies can develop in late adulthood; hence, repetitive testing is necessary. When children are followed prospectively to diabetes, one autoantibody may be developing while another is disappearing,

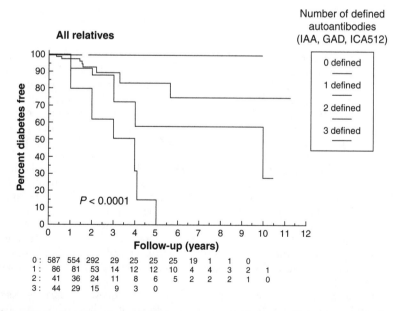

Figure 2.2 Progression of first-degree relatives to diabetes strongly depends on the number of biochemical autoantibodies expressed. IAA, islet autoantibody. From Verge et al. (1996).

and at diagnosis a small subset of children (<5%) have lost autoantibody expression.
- The prognostic significance of even multiple autoantibodies in the presence of the protective allele DQB1*0602 is unknown.
- Although most individuals stably express autoantibodies for years to decades before the development of diabetes, as many as 10% of young children may transiently express a single autoantibody.

Metabolic

Loss of first-phase insulin secretion during an intravenous glucose tolerance test (IVGTT) usually precedes the development of type 1A diabetes by several years. Fasting insulin and insulin levels 1 and 3 minutes after a glucose infusion can be measured, but in children developing type 1 diabetes, there are often impaired glucose tolerance and increases in A1C within the normal range preceding diabetes onset. Normal first-phase insulin secretion in a patient recovering from transient hyperglycemia is one of the best indications that the hyperglycemia will only be transient. Children aged <8 years old have lower first-phase secretion than adults, particularly on their first IVGTT. Given the variability of the test, at least two tests should be obtained to confirm an abnormality. Among multiple islet autoantibody–positive individuals, the level of insulin release inversely correlates with the approximate time to diabetes.

APPLICATIONS

Physicians caring for patients with type 1A diabetes should make patients and their relatives aware of the symptoms and signs of both type 1 diabetes and associated autoimmune disorders. We generally screen patients every 2 years for the disorders listed in Table 2.2.

Over the next 5 years, the diagnosis of autoimmune type 1 diabetes and other genetic diabetes syndromes will probably play a role in deciding therapy and assessing prognosis for these multiple diabetic disorders. An initial screening of new-onset patients for islet autoantibodies will help discern the subset of children who do not have type 1 diabetes as well as identify adults with diabetes who have the autoimmune form. With sensitive and specific radioassays for autoantibodies reacting with biochemically characterized autoantibodies, the presence of a single autoantibody would be consistent with autoimmune diabetes.

For children with mitochondrial mutations, associated neurological disorders should be sought (e.g., hearing impairment). With identification of MODY mutations, familial analysis and early diabetes diagnosis will be facilitated. Children with "mild" diabetes caused by glucokinase mutations may require no therapy or respond to oral agents.

Individuals with transient hyperglycemia, in whom the question concerns risk of progression to permanent diabetes, can be distinguished on the basis of expression of autoantibodies and whether first-phase insulin secretion on an IVGTT is normal.

An individual being considered as a living kidney donor for a relative with type 1A diabetes should be evaluated for expression of AIAAs and for metabolic function. When possible, relatives donating a kidney should lack high-risk characteristics.

Parents often request HLA typing to assess risk of autoimmune diabetes in siblings of a child with type 1A diabetes. If DQB1*0602 is present in a nondiabetic child, the parents can be reassured that the risk of type 1A diabetes approaches that of the general population (1 in 300). DQB1*0602 is present in ~10% of siblings of patients with type 1A diabetes. The benefit of such testing probably does not justify HLA typing outside of research studies.

With developments in in vitro fertilization and embryo transfer, the question has arisen whether DNA-based typing for diabetes risk of early-stage embryos should be considered. For example, would a family consider selecting embryos with DQB1*0602 or that lack DR3 and DR4? Although DQB1*0602 protects from autoimmune diabetes, it is a high-risk allele for multiple sclerosis.

Determination of biochemical autoantibodies can identify individuals at risk for type 1A diabetes among family members and the general population. A caveat is that expression of a single persistent autoantibody is often associated with a "low" risk (on the order of 20%) for progression to type 1A diabetes compared to multiple autoantibodies (>90%). Expression of no autoantibodies can be reassuring, but autoantibodies can appear later in life. The major benefit of identification of autoantibodies should be the prevention of severe disability or death at presentation in ketoacidosis. This is estimated to occur in ~1 in 200 children presenting with diabetes in the general population. The cons of such testing are potential anxiety and the potential for decreased insurability with "disease" detection. The best rationale for such screening is potential participation in a trial for the prevention of type 1A diabetes. First- and second-degree relatives of patients in the U.S. can be screened for expression of autoantibodies without charge as part of the program by calling 1-800-HALT-DM1.

BIBLIOGRAPHY

Barker JM, Gottlie PA, Eisenbarth GS: The immunoendocrinopathy syndromes. In *Williams Textbook of Endocrinology*. 11th ed. Kronenberg H, Melmed S, Polonsky KS, Larsen PR, Eds. Philadelphia, W.B. Saunders, 2008, p. 1747–1760

Cox NJ, Wapelhorst B, Morrison VA, Johnson L, Pinchuk L, Spielman RS, Todd JA, Concannon P: Seven regions of the genome show evidence of linkage to type 1 diabetes in a consensus analysis of 767 multiplex families. *Am J Hum Genet* 69:820–830, 2001

Eisenbarth GS (Ed.): *Type 1 Diabetes: Cellular, Molecular, and Clinical Immunology*. Available from http://www.barbaradaviscenter.org

Falorni A, Nikoshkov A, Laureti S, Grenback E, Hulting A, Casucci G, Santeusanio F, Brunetti P, Luthman H, Lernmark A: High diagnostic accuracy for idiopathic Addison's disease with a sensitive radiobinding assay for autoantibodies against recombinant human 21-hydroxylase. *J Clin Endocrinol Metab* 80:2752–2755, 1995

Hattersley AT, Ashcroft FM: Activating mutations in Kir6.2 and neonatal diabetes: new clinical syndromes, new scientific insights, and new therapy. *Diabetes* 54:2503–2513, 2005

Liu E, Li M, Emery L, Taki I, Barriga K, Tiberti C, Eisenbarth GS, Rewers MJ, Hoffenberg EJ: Natural history of antibodies to deamidated gliadin peptides and transglutaminase in early childhood celiac disease. *J Pediatr Gastroenterol Nutr* 45:293–300, 2007

Lyssenko V, Lupi R, Marchetti P, Del Guerra S, Orho-Melander M, Almgren P, Sjogren M, Ling C, Eriksson K-F, Lethagen A-L, Mancarella R, Berglund G, Tuomi T, Nilsson P, Del Prato S, Groop L: Mechanisms by which common variants in the TCF7L2 gene increase risk of type 2 diabetes. *J Clin Invest* 117:2155–2163, 2007

Meager A, Visvalingam K, Peterson P, Moll K, Murumagi A, Krohn K, Eskelin P, Perheentupa J, Husebye E, Kadota Y, Willcox N: Anti-interferon autoantibodies in autoimmune polyendocrinopathy syndrome type 1. *PloS Med* 3:e289, 2006

Pugliese A, Eisenbarth GS: Human type I diabetes mellitus: genetic susceptibility and resistance. In *Type I Diabetes: Molecular, Cellular, and Clinical Immunology.* Eisenbarth GS, Lafferty KJ, Eds. New York, Oxford University Press, 1996, p. 134–152

Rewers M, Bugawan TL, Norris JM, Blair A, Beaty B, Hoffman M, McDuffie RS Jr, Hamman RF, Kligensmith G, Eisenbarth GS, Erlich HA: Newborn screening for HLA markers associated with IDDM: Diabetes Autoimmunity Study in the Young (DAISY). *Diabetologia* 39:807–812, 1996

Saukkonen T, Savilahti E, Reijonen H, Ilonen J, Tuomilehto-Wolf E, Akerblom HK: Coeliac disease: frequent occurrence after clinical onset of insulin-dependent diabetes mellitus: Childhood Diabetes in Finland Study Group. *Diabet Med* 13:464–470, 1996

She J: Susceptibility to type I diabetes: HLA-DQ and DR revisited. *Immunol Today* 17:323–329, 1996

Todd JA, Walker NM, Cooper JD, Smyth DJ, Downes K, Plagnol V, Bailey R, Nejentsev S, Field SF, Payne F, Lowe CE, Szeszko JS, Hafler JP, Zeitels L, Yang JH, Vella A, Nutland S, Stevens HE, Schuilenburg H, Coleman G, Maisuria M, Meadows W, Smink LJ, Healy B, Burren OS, Lam AA, Ovington NR, Allen J, Adlem E, Leung HT, Wallace C, Howson JM, Guja C, Ionescu-Tîrgovişte C, Genetics of Type 1 Diabetes in Finland, Simmonds MJ, Heward JM, Gough SC, Wellcome Trust Case Control Consortium, Dunger DB, Wicker LS, Clayton DG: Robust associations of four new chromosome regions from genome-wide analyses of type 1 diabetes. *Nat Genet* 39:857–864, 2007

Verge CF, Gianani R, Kawasaki E, Yu L, Pietroapolo M, Jackson RA, Chase HP, Eisenbarth GS: Prediction of type I diabetes in first-degree relatives using a combination of insulin, GAD, and ICA512bdc/IA-2 autoantibodies. *Diabetes* 45:926–933, 1996

Wenzlau JM, Juhl K, Yu L, Moua O, Sarkar SA, Gottlieb P, Rewers M, Eisenbarth GS, Jensen J, Davidson HW, Hutton JC: The cation efflux transporter ZnT8 (Slc80A*) is a major autoantigen in human type 1 diabetes. *Proc Natl Acad Sci U S A* 104:17040-17045, 2007

Dr. Barker is an assistant professor of pediatrics at the Barbara Davis Center for Childhood Diabetes and The Children's Hospital, Denver, Colorado. Dr. Eisenbarth is the Executive Director of the Barbara Davis Center for Childhood Diabetes and a Professor at the University of Colorado Health Sciences Center, Denver, Colorado.

3. Gestational Diabetes Mellitus

Thomas A. Buchanan, MD

DEFINITION AND PREVALENCE

Gestational diabetes mellitus (GDM) is defined as glucose intolerance of any severity that has its onset or is first recognized during pregnancy. In essence, GDM occurs in women without known abnormalities of glucose whose circulating glucose concentrations are sufficiently high to impart some increase in perinatal risk to their infants. GDM also occurs in women who themselves are at increased risk for having or developing diabetes when they are not pregnant. The prevalence of GDM varies according to the diagnostic criteria used and the ethnicity of the patient population. When the criteria of the American Diabetes Association (see below) were applied to a Toronto cohort composed predominantly of white women, all of whom had 3-h oral glucose tolerance tests (OGTTs), the prevalence of GDM was 7%. Prevalence rates will likely be higher in ethnic and racial groups in the general population who have higher background rates of diabetes and impaired glucose tolerance.

SCREENING AND DIAGNOSIS

GDM almost never causes symptoms. Accordingly, the American Diabetes Association recommends screening all pregnant women to assess their risk for GDM and testing at-risk individuals' glucose tolerance. The process involves three steps:

1. Evaluate the patient for clinical characteristics that are associated with high, average, or low risk of glucose intolerance.
2. Among women with high or average clinical risk factors for GDM, perform a simple glucose challenge to distinguish women with little or no risk from women with some risk.
3. In the women with some risk, perform a more complicated glucose challenge test to determine whether the individual has GDM.

Specific aspects required for implementation of these three steps are summarized in Tables 3.1 and 3.2.

Table 3.1 Screening for GDM

Clinical Risk Assessment*		
Risk Category	**Clinical Characteristics**	**Recommended Screening**
High risk (any sufficient)	Marked obesity Diabetes in first-degree relatives Personal history of glucose intolerance Prior macrosomic infant Current glycosuria	Blood glucose screening at initial antepartum visit or as soon as possible thereafter; repeat at 24–28 wk if not already diagnosed with GDM by that time
Average risk	Fits neither low- nor high-risk profile	Blood glucose screening between 24 and 28 wk gestation
Low risk (all required)	Age <25 yr Low-risk ethnicity† No diabetes in first-degree relatives Normal prepregnancy weight and pregnancy weight gain No personal history of abnormal glucose levels No prior poor obstetrical outcomes	Blood glucose screening not required

Blood Glucose Screening‡		
Test§	50-g oral glucose challenge, measure serum or plasma glucose 1 h later	
Preparation	None (can be done any time of day)	
Interpretation	**Glucose cut point‖**	**Fraction of women with positive test¶**	**Sensitivity for GDM¶**
	≥140 mg/dl (≥7.8 mmol/l)	14–18%	~80%
	≥130 mg/dl (≥7.2 mmol/l)	20–25%	~90%

Adopted from the summary and recommendations of the 4th International Workshop-Conference on GDM (Metzger 1998) and American Diabetes Association (2009).
*Performed at initial antepartum visit.
†Ethnicities other than Hispanic, African, Native American, South or East Asian, Pacific Islander, or indigenous Australian, who have increased rates of GDM.
‡Women with very-high-risk clinical characteristics may proceed directly to measurement of fasting glucose or to a diagnostic OGTT (see Table 3.2).
§Performed in patients with high or average clinical risk characteristics.
‖Venous serum or plasma glucose measured by certified clinical laboratory.
¶May vary with ethnicity and with diagnostic OGTT used.

Table 3.2 Diagnosis of GDM

Overt Diabetes			
Serum or plasma glucose			
After overnight fast	≥126 mg/dl (≥7.0 mmol/l)		
Random*	≥200 mg/dl (≥11.1 mmol/l)		

GDM			
Procedure	Glucose cut points†		
100-g, 3-h OGTT‡	Time (h)	Glucose (mg/dl)	Glucose (mmol/l)
Fasting	95	5.3	
	1 h	180	10.0
	2 h	155	8.6
	3 h	140	7.8

Data are based on the recommendations of the 4th International Workshop-Conference on GDM (Metzger 1998).
*Venous serum or plasma glucose measured by certified clinical laboratory; two or more values that meet or exceed cut points are required for diagnosis.
†Outside of formal glucose challenge testing.
‡The glucose cut points for the 75-g, 2-h OGTT are identical to the fasting, 1-h, and 2-h values of the 100-g, 3-h OGTT, and two or more values are required to meet or exceed the cut points for diagnosis.

PATHOPHYSIOLOGY

The Mother

All forms of hyperglycemia result from an imbalance between tissue insulin requirements and the ability of pancreatic β-cells to meet those requirements. GDM is no exception. Physiological studies in several ethnic groups indicate ~50% lower β-cell compensation for insulin resistance in women with GDM compared with women who maintain normal glucose levels in pregnancy. Causes of the β-cell defect in GDM are as varied as the causes of β-cell defects underlying hyperglycemia in other settings. A minority of women have evidence for evolving type 1 diabetes (i.e., circulating antibodies to pancreatic islet cells or antigens). The frequency is highest in populations with the highest rates of type 1 diabetes but does not appear to be >20% in any population (and <5–10% in most). Causes of β-cell dysfunction vary among women without evidence for β-cell autoimmunity. Some have specific genetic problems affecting β-cells, such as genetic variants that also cause maturity-onset diabetes of the young (MODY). Most others have clinical (obesity) and physiological (chronic insulin resistance and poor β-cell compensation) characteristics that suggest evolving type 2 diabetes. At least two studies have shown that women with GDM and characteristics suggesting evolving type 2 diabetes do not have a fixed limitation in insulin secretion. Rather, they can increase or decrease their secretion in response to changes in insulin resistance. They do so, however, at a different glucose set point than normal women. More importantly, the set point changes over time as women with prior GDM lose β-cell function and develop diabetes. Recent evidence from Hispanic women at risk for type 2 diabetes indicates that declining β-cell function is caused or worsened by the high secretory demands placed on β-cells by chronic insulin resistance. Treatment of insulin resistance can preserve β-cell function and delay or prevent diabetes. The variability in pathophysiology means that clinicians should view GDM not as one disease, but as a montage of virtually all diseases that can cause hyperglycemia. Clinical management during pregnancy is generally aimed at improving the balance between insulin demand and supply by reducing the demands (e.g., nutrition and exercise) and/or increasing supply (e.g., exogenous insulin or glyburide). Ideally, management after pregnancy should be tailored to the specific disease process(es) causing hyperglycemia and subsequent diabetes in each patient. At the present time, those processes can only be assessed crudely by patients' clinical characteristics. Lean patients, especially those of European descent, should raise a suspicion of evolving type 1 diabetes. Testing for autoimmune markers of type 1 diabetes (e.g., antibodies to glutamic acid decarboxylase [GAD]) can confirm the suspicion. Patients with a strong family history of young-onset diabetes should suggest MODY. No specific interventions have been shown to delay or prevent diabetes in such patients. However, patients with evidence for autoimmune disease may deteriorate rapidly and warrant education and close follow-up to detect diabetes if it develops. Patients with MODY need genetic counseling. Moreover, some forms (e.g., MODY due to mutations in *HNF1α*) respond particularly well to insulin secretogogues. Obese patients or patients with other evidence for insulin resistance should suggest a risk of type 2 diabetes, which itself may prove to be a number of diseases when genetic etiologies are worked out. Treatment of insulin resistance after pregnancy appears to reduce the risk of type 2 diabetes in such patients (see below).

The Infant

Development in a diabetic environment can have effects on the human fetus that range from major birth defects and late-term death to mild increases in adiposity. In general, the more severe complications are associated with glycemia in the range of preexisting diabetes (Table 3.2), which is present in a minority of women whose hyperglycemia is first diagnosed during pregnancy. More often, hyperglycemia in GDM is mild and associated with an increased risk of fetal overgrowth and adiposity. The best evidence suggests that fetal overnutrition and hyperinsulinemia are mediators of the excessive growth. The risk of perinatal trauma increases with fetal size, especially at very high birth weights, and cesarean deliveries are often performed to reduce that risk. Unfortunately, there is now good evidence that the diagnosis of GDM per se raises cesarean delivery rates in the absence of increased fetal size. Two important concepts are often overlooked in the antepartum management of GDM. First, the risk of fetal overnutrition increases slowly and continuously across the range of maternal glucose levels. Second, different fetuses grow differently in response to the same glucose levels. Thus, there are no true thresholds of glucose that distinguish pregnancies at high risk from pregnancies at low risk for glucose-related perinatal complications. In fact, over the range of glucose levels most often encountered in women with GDM, only a minority of infants are at risk for complications related to maternal hyperglycemia.

In addition to perinatal complications, maternal GDM has been associated with unexpectedly high rates of obesity and abnormalities of glucose tolerance in children and adolescents. The relative contributions of genetics versus exposure to the intrauterine environment of GDM have not been worked out precisely, although it appears that both factors may play a role in the childhood problems.

ANTEPARTUM METABOLIC MANAGEMENT

General Approach

Given the highly variable relationship between fetal growth and related complications on the one hand and maternal glucose levels on the other, the general goal of management of GDM during pregnancy should be to achieve glucose levels that are appropriate to minimize the risk of perinatal complications in each individual pregnancy. This general goal can be achieved by either *1*) treating all women to a glucose level that, on average, results in good perinatal outcomes or *2*) tailoring interventions that modify maternal glucose to the growth pattern of the individual baby. The two approaches are not completely exclusive of one another. For example, glucose measurements can be used to define pregnancies with very high (i.e., in need of pharmacological intervention) or very low (appropriate for nutritional intervention alone) perinatal risks based on glucose alone. Fetal growth characteristics can then be used in the intermediate risk group to identify pregnancies with increased fetal risk that also need intervention, despite relatively mild hyperglycemia.

Nutrition Therapy

Diet is often stated to be the cornerstone of therapy for GDM. Nonetheless, there is a paucity of sound scientific evidence based on optimization of perinatal outcomes on which recommendations for dietary management can be based. A standard diet in the third trimester of pregnancy should provide 30–32 kcal/kg body weight. Modifications that lower glucose levels in the mother are *1*) restriction to ~25 kcal/kg body weight for overweight patients, *2*) restriction of carbohydrate to ~40% of calories, and *3*) a focus on complex rather than simple carbohydrates. Restriction of carbohydrates to ~40% of calories has been shown to improve perinatal outcomes as well. All three approaches can be combined to form the basis for general dietary recommendations. Medical nutrition therapy, in which individualized nutritional prescriptions are used to achieve clinical goals (e.g., glucose levels), is a sound approach to dietary management in GDM.

Monitoring Effectiveness of Therapy

The effectiveness of nutrition therapy and/or the need for additional interventions can be assessed in two ways: *1*) by measuring blood glucose concentrations in the mother and *2*) by measuring fetal size and growth patterns. Measurement of blood glucose concentrations can take two general forms: measurements performed in an office or clinic by certified laboratory methods (very accurate but cannot be done often) and self-measurement by the patient (not as accurate but can be done several times each day). If the general approach to management is based solely on maternal glucose levels, then all patients will need to perform glucose self-monitoring to assess whether they are achieving glycemic targets that are, on average, associated with a low risk of perinatal complications. The optimal timing and frequency of monitoring have not been determined. Some studies support a focus on postprandial monitoring, whereas others report good perinatal outcomes when the focus is on premeal monitoring. In reality, the timing of measurements and the glycemic goals together determine average glycemia, which is probably most important to the fetus. Goals recommended by the American Diabetes Association for pre- and postmeal glucose values in women managed according to glycemia alone appear in Table 3.3.

Management that takes into account fetal growth characteristics can be based on laboratory glucose measurements performed at 1- to 2-week intervals combined with assessment of fetal growth. Women who cannot maintain fasting glucose levels of >105 mg/dl after initiation of nutrition therapy are at a sufficient risk of fetal complications to warrant intensification of metabolic management, usually with insulin. Women with lower fasting glucose levels can continue nutritional management until ~30 weeks' gestation, at which time fetal ultrasound is performed to measure the abdominal circumference. Pregnancies in which the abdominal circumference is below the 70th percentile for gestational age are at low risk for excessive growth; the mothers can continue nutrition therapy. Pregnancies in which the fetal abdominal circumference is ≥70th percentile are the ones at risk for growth-related complications. These patients should have intensified management, again, usually with insulin. When insulin is started, patients should also begin glucose self-monitoring. Glycemic goals can be lowered below those recommended when management is based on maternal glycemia alone (Table 3.3) because there is little, if any, risk of inducing growth retardation by strict glucose control when the baby is already somewhat large.

Intensification of Treatment

Patients in whom maternal glycemia and/or fetal growth indicate a risk of excessive growth, despite nutritional treatment, should have their metabolic management intensified. The standard approach, and the one for which there is the best evidence of improving fetal outcomes, is addition of exogenous insulin. No one regimen has been proven optimally effective, and regimens should be tailored

Table 3.3 Glucose Targets for Antepartum Management of GDM

Approach	Self-Monitored Blood Glucose (mg/dl)*	Self-Monitored Plasma Glucose (mg/dl)*
Maternal glycemia alone†		
Fasting and before meals	≤95	≤105
1 h after meals	≤140	<155
2 h after meals	≤120	≤130
Fetal growth plus maternal glycemia‡		
Fasting and before meals	≤80	≤90
2 h after meals	≤110	≤120

*Refers to product information to determine which type of measurement a given meter makes.
†Adapted from the American Diabetes Association (2009).
‡For pregnancies identified as at-risk for excessive fetal growth on the basis of ultrasound measurement of abdominal circumference.

to meet glycemic goals (Table 3.3). Starting doses can be based on observed insulin requirements in pregnant women, which average 0.6–1.0 units/kg depending on the stage of gestation (i.e., requirements rise during pregnancy). Combinations of intermediate- or long-acting preparations with short- or rapid-acting preparations have been useful to reach glucose targets and improve fetal outcomes. Insulin requirements often fall dramatically at delivery; at the same time, glucose goals become less strict. Thus, insulin can be stopped at delivery to allow reassessment of maternal glucose levels.

Other approaches that have been used to intensify metabolic management include aerobic exercise and oral antidiabetic agents. Exercise (e.g., 45 min of exercise at ~50% of maximal aerobic capacity three times a week) has been shown to lower maternal glucose levels over 4–6 weeks. Effects on fetal outcomes are not well studied. Glyburide does not cross the human placenta in appreciable quantities. Treatment with doses of 2.5–20 mg/day has been reported to achieve glucose control and perinatal outcomes similar to insulin in one study of women whose glucose levels indicated a need for intensification of metabolic management. Metformin does cross the human placenta (Nanovskaya 2006), so direct fetal effects are possible. Initial reports of safety and efficacy came from small controlled trials in GDM or studies of pregnancy outcomes in women with polycystic ovarian syndrome who were treated with metformin during pregnancy. Maternal glucose levels were reduced by metformin, resulting in lower-than-expected frequency of GDM in women with polycystic ovarian syndrome who continued metformin during pregnancy (Glueck 2008) or in acceptable maternal glucose control and perinatal outcomes compared to insulin treatment (Glueck, Goldenberg, et al., 2004) in those with GDM. A single retrospective study suggested an increased frequency of preeclampsia in metformin-treated women (Glueck, Bornovali, et al., 2004, Thatcher and Jackson, 2006). A large randomized trial of metformin versus insulin as the initial approach to intensification revealed three main findings. First, metformin at a dose of 2,500 mg was associated with acceptable glycemic control in 54% of subjects, whereas 46% needed insulin in addition to metformin to achieve glycemic targets. Second, the two treatment approaches (insulin vs. metformin with insulin added if needed) yielded very similar perinatal outcomes, although spontaneous premature birth was slightly more common in the group assigned to metformin, whereas neonatal hypoglycemia (<30 mg/dl) was slightly less common compared with the group assigned to insulin as initial therapy. Third, more subjects in each treatment group stated that they would prefer metformin over insulin as initial therapy for GDM. Taken together, the available results suggest that metformin is a viable alternative to insulin as initial therapy when intensification is warranted. Long-term outcomes of infants exposed to metformin in utero remain to be determined (Rowan 2008).

OBSTETRIC MANAGEMENT

Assessment of Fetal Well-Being

The obstetric care provider is generally responsible for determining the mode and frequency of testing of fetal well-being. Several tests exist, and no single approach is superior. The most widely used approaches are as follows:

- *Fetal activity determinations (kick counts):* The patient notes each perceived fetal movement for a specific time interval each day or notes the amount of time that passes before a predetermined number of movements have occurred each day. A decline in the number of movements or an increase in the time it takes to attain the appropriate number of movements prompts the need for one of the tests described below. Fetal activity determinations have a high likelihood of false-positive results, but the test costs nothing and is convenient for the patient.
- *Nonstress test:* The fetal monitor is placed, and the patient notes fetal movements. The presence of accelerations of the fetal heart rate in conjunction with fetal movements denotes fetal well-being. Addition of ultrasound measurement of amniotic fluid volume enhances the sensitivity and specificity of the test for detection of fetal compromise.
- *Biophysical profile:* This test combines the nonstress test with ultrasound determination of fetal movement, tone, and breathing and of amniotic fluid volume. It is sensitive and specific but requires an ultrasound unit, an experienced operator, and a fetal monitor.

Hypertension in pregnancy is defined as a systolic blood pressure of >140 mmHg or a diastolic blood pressure of >90 mmHg on at least two occasions at least 6 h apart. Complications such as hypertension, inadequate diabetes control, or a previous perinatal loss dictate that testing begin sooner and/or be performed more frequently.

Timing and Mode of Delivery

GDM is not itself an indication for cesarean delivery before 38 completed weeks of gestation. Prolongation of pregnancy beyond 38 completed weeks has been associated with an increase in rates of large-for-gestational-age infants without a reduction in cesarean delivery rates. Thus, delivery during the 38th week is recommended unless other obstetrical considerations dictate otherwise. Most women can maintain serum or plasma glucose levels <120 mg/dl during labor and delivery without exogenous insulin. In those who cannot, continuous intravenous insulin may be used to lower glucose levels and reduce the risk of neonatal hypoglycemia.

MANAGEMENT AFTER PREGNANCY

The Mother

Nutritional management during breast-feeding should continue as prescribed during pregnancy. Any pharmacological treatments for diabetes can be stopped at delivery to allow reassessment of maternal glycemia in the hospital and, if the mother is not clearly diabetic at that time, at a follow-up visit 1–2 months after delivery. All women with GDM are at increased risk for diabetes, although the type may vary. No data are available on effective diabetes preventatives for women with evidence of autoimmune β-cell dysfunction (evolving type 1 diabetes). Because their course can be relatively rapid, follow-up should be relatively frequent (e.g., at 6-month intervals) for women with clinical characteristics that suggest type 1 diabetes and/or evidence of immunity directed against β-cells (e.g., anti-GAD antibodies). Most women have clinical features suggestive of a risk for type 2 diabetes (especially obesity). Current evidence suggests that interventions directed at reducing insulin resistance can delay or prevent diabetes. Regular exercise and weight loss, metformin, and thiazolidinedione drugs have all been effective in this regard. Women should be encouraged to exercise and, if they are overweight, to lose weight. They should be evaluated at least annually for diabetes, but probably more frequently. Rising glucose levels are indicative of progression toward diabetes and should indicate more aggressive efforts at treatment of insulin resistance to prevent diabetes. Because conception of another pregnancy in the presence of even mild diabetes can increase the risk of congenital malformations in the infant, patients should practice effective family planning to ensure that glycemia can be evaluated and optimized before any additional pregnancies. Low-dose combination oral contraceptives do not appear to increase the risk of diabetes after GDM. Two observation studies in Hispanic patients suggest that progestin-only contraception may increase the risk of diabetes (Kjos, Peters, Xiang, Thomas, et al., 1998; Xiang, et al., 2006)

The Child

No standard approach to evaluation and management of children of women with prior GDM has been established. Because these children may be at increased risk of obesity and diabetes at a relatively young age, they should have regular assessment of growth and development and be encouraged to pursue behaviors that minimize obesity. Children who are overweight should have regular assessment of glucose levels as well. The role of pharmacological treatment to prevent or delay diabetes in children has not been studied.

BIBLIOGRAPHY

American Diabetes Association: Diagnosis and classification of diabetes mellitus (Position Statement). *Diabetes Care* 32 (Suppl. 1):S62–S67, 2009

American Diabetes Association: Gestational diabetes mellitus (Position Statement). *Diabetes Care* 27 (Suppl. 1):S88–S90, 2004

Buchanan TA, Kjos SL, Schafer U, Peters RK, Xiang A, Byrne J, Berkowitz K, Montoro M: Utility of fetal measurements in the management of gestational diabetes mellitus. *Diabetes Care* 21 (Suppl. 2):B99–B106, 1998

Buchanan TA, Xiang AH, Peters RK, Kjos SL, Marroquin A, Goico J, Ochoa C, Tan S, Berkowitz K, Hodis HN, Azen SP: Preservation of pancreatic β-cell function and prevention of type 2 diabetes by pharmacological treatment of insulin resistance in high-risk Hispanic women. *Diabetes* 51:2796–2803, 2002

Expert Committee on the Diagnosis and Classification of Diabetes Mellitus: Report of the Expert Committee on the Diagnosis and Classification of Diabetes Mellitus. *Diabetes Care* 20:1183–1197, 1997

Glueck CJ, Pranikoff J, Aregawi D, Wang P: Prevention of gestational diabetes by metformin plus diet in patients with polycystic ovary syndrome. *Fertil Steril* 89:625–634, 2008

Glueck CJ, Goldenberg N, Pranikoff J, Loftspring M, Sieve L, Wang P: Height, weight, and motor-social development during the first 18 months of life in 126 infants born to 109 mothers with polycystic ovary syndrome who conceived on and continued metformin through pregnancy. *Hum Reprod* 19:1323-1330. 2004

Glueck CJ, Bornovali S, Pranikoff J, Goldenberg N, Dharashivkar S, Wang P: Metformin, pre-eclampsia, and pregnancy outcomes in women with polycystic ovary syndrome. *Diabet Med* 21:829–836, 2004

Jovanovic L, Pettitt DJ: Gestational diabetes mellitus. *JAMA* 286:2516–2518, 2001

Kjos SL, Peters RK, Xiang A, Schaefer U, Buchanan TA: Hormonal choices after gestational diabetes: subsequent pregnancy, contraception and hormone replacement. *Diabetes Care* 21 (Suppl. 2):B50–B57, 1998

Kjos SL, Peters RK, Xiang A, Thomas D, Schafer U, Buchanan TA: Oral contraception and the risk of type 2 diabetes in Latino women with prior gestational diabetes. *JAMA* 280:533-538, 1998

Metzger BE, Coustan DR, the Conference Organizing Committee: Summary and recommendations of the 4th International Workshop-Conference on Gestational Diabetes. *Diabetes Care* 21 (Suppl. 2):B161–B167, 1998

Nanovskaya TN, Nekhayeva IA, Patrikeeva SL, Hankins GD, Ahmed MS: Transfer of metformin across the dually perfused human placental lobule. *Am J Obstet Gynecol* 195:1081–1085, 2006

Rowan JA, Hague WM, Gao W, Battin MR, Moore MP, MiG Trial Investigators: Metformin versus insulin for the treatment of gestational diabetes. *N Engl J Med* 358:2003-2015, 2008

Thatcher SS, Jackson EM: Pregnancy outcome in infertile patients with polycystic ovary syndrome who were treated with metformin. *Fertil Steril* 85:1002–1009, 2006

Xiang AH, Kawakubo M, Kjos SL, Buchanan TA: Long-acting injectable progestin contraception and risk of type 2 diabetes in Latino women with prior gestational diabetes mellitus. *Diabetes Care* 29:613–617, 2006

Dr. Buchanan is Professor of Medicine, Obstetrics and Gynecology, and Physiology and Biophysics and Director of the General Clinical Research Center at the University of Southern California Keck School of Medicine, Los Angeles, California. He is also attending physician at the Los Angeles County–University of Southern California Medical Center.

4. Management of Pregnant Women with Diabetes

E. Albert Reece, MD, MBA, PhD, Carol Homko, RN, PhD, CDE, Lois Jovanovic, MD, and John L. Kitzmiller, MD, MS

PRECONCEPTIONAL METABOLIC CONTROL AND CONGENITAL MALFORMATIONS

The prevalence of congenital anomalies among children of women with pre-existing diabetes, both type 1 and type 2 diabetes, is 4–10 times higher than that among children of their nondiabetic counterparts. A1C determinations made soon after conception and by the end of the first trimester show that the frequency of malformations correlates with the degree of glycemic control rather than with the patient's White's classification (type of diabetes or presence of complications—Table 4.1).

Evidence suggests that the maternal metabolic milieu has a direct influence on embryogenesis during a critical and vulnerable developmental period. Tight control of blood glucose in the preconceptional period by intensive insulin treatment and the maintenance of normal glycemic control throughout this critical phase of organogenesis result in a reduced prevalence of major congenital malformations and early fetal loss. A1C levels should be as close to normal as possible without significant hypoglycemia before conception is attempted.

Women with diabetes who are contemplating pregnancy should be evaluated and, if indicated, treated for hypertension (≥130/80 mmHg in diabetes), dyslipidemia, thyroid disease, cardiovascular disease (CVD), depression, diabetic nephropathy, diabetic neuropathy, and diabetic retinopathy. Medications used by such women should be evaluated before conception, because drugs commonly used to treat diabetes and its complications may be contraindicated or not recommended in pregnancy, including statins, angiotensin-converting enzyme (ACE) inhibitors, angiotensin receptor blockers (ARBs), many antidepressants, and most noninsulin therapies.

MANAGEMENT OF UNCOMPLICATED PREGNANT WOMEN WITH TYPE 1 OR TYPE 2 DIABETES

From a management perspective, women with type 1 or type 2 diabetes can be classified into two groups, according to the presence or absence of diabetic vasculopathy. The first group includes White's classes B and C, and the second group consists of classes D, F, FR, and H. The fundamental differences in the management of the two groups are that patients in the second group have advanced disease, requiring more intense evaluation and surveillance, because advanced disease places the pregnancy at a greater risk for both maternal and fetal complications.

The third-trimester mean maternal blood glucose level correlates linearly with the perinatal mortality rate. Other complications associated with maternal hyperglycemia in the second and third trimesters include neonatal hypoglycemia, macrosomia, hyperbilirubinemia, hypocalcemia, erythrocytosis, and respiratory distress syndrome. Therefore, the major management goal of these pregnancies is to achieve and maintain euglycemia throughout pregnancy.

The recommended management approach for diabetic pregnancy and labor is outlined in Table 4.2 and includes the following:

- Blood glucose levels should be monitored at least four to seven times a day (e.g., before and after each meal and at bedtime) throughout the course of pregnancy.
- Blood glucose goals during pregnancy are 60–99 mg/dl (3.3–5.5 mmol/l) before meals and 100–129 mg/dl (5.5–7.2 mmol/l) after meals.
- An early ultrasound examination should be performed to date the pregnancy and to establish growth parameters against which future examinations can be compared.
- At 18–22 weeks, all patients with preexisting diabetes should receive a level 2 ultrasound and fetal echocardiogram to rule out malformations.
- Patients should be seen for clinical evaluation every 1–2 weeks (depending on degree of glucose control) until 34 weeks, after which they should be seen weekly.
- Nonstress tests and/or biophysical profiles should be done weekly beginning between 32 and 36 weeks' gestation.
- Fetal lung maturity studies should be undertaken for women in poor glucose control or with poor dating when elective delivery is planned before 39 weeks' gestation. Indicated urgent preterm deliveries for preeclampsia, hemorrhage, significantly nonreassuring fetal testing, etc., may be carried out without regard to fetal lung maturity evaluation.

Table 4.1 White's Classification

Class A1: gestational diabetes; diet controlled
Class A2: gestational diabetes; insulin controlled
Class B: preexisting diabetes; onset at age ≥20 years or with duration <10 years
Class C: preexisting diabetes; onset at age 10–19 years or duration 10–19 years
Class D: preexisting diabetes; onset before age 10 years or duration >20 years
Class F: preexisting diabetes; diabetic nephropathy
Class R: preexisting diabetes; proliferative retinopathy
Class RF: preexisting diabetes; retinopathy and nephropathy
Class H: preexisting diabetes; ischemic heart disease
Class T: preexisting diabetes; prior kidney transplant

Table 4.2 Management of Uncomplicated Pregnant Diabetic Patients

White's Classes B and C

- Self-monitoring of blood glucose (four to seven times daily)
- Biweekly visits until 34 wk, then weekly
- Ultrasound: level 2 at ~20 wk, then follow up every 4–6 wk
- A1C monthly
- Daily fetal movement counts
- Nonstress test at 32–34 wk, then weekly
- Ophthalmologic evaluation, follow up according to findings
- 24-h urine, initially and in each trimester, for protein and CrCl

White's Classes D–FR

- Above, plus electrocardiogram initially; uric acid, liver function test, fibrinogen, fibrin split product determinations; may repeat in each trimester

Delivery time

- Classes A and B: ≤42 wk gestation (if in good glycemic control)
- Classes C–FR: at term or pulmonary maturity

Labor

- Blood glucose to be maintained at ≤90 mg/dl (≤5.0 mmol/l)
- Intravenous normal saline solution to be started at a rate of 7 ml/h and insulin and/or glucose solutions to be administered based on hourly blood glucose checks

Medical Nutrition Therapy Recommendations

Pregnancy normally demands an additional intake of 300–400 kcal/day above basal requirements. No further additional calories are required for pregnant women with diabetes. Nutrition recommendations should be determined based on an individualized nutrition assessment. Monitoring blood glucose levels, appetite, and weight gain can be a guide to developing and evaluating an appropriate meal plan and to making adjustments to the meal plan. Weight-loss diets should not be prescribed. Three meals a day with two to three snacks are usually sufficient for patients with preexisting diabetes. Women should be taught to assess, control, and record carbohydrate intake for tight glycemic control and to minimize intake of saturated and trans-fats for long-term CVD risk reduction. A weight gain of 22–30 lb is considered acceptable, with 2–4 lb in the first trimester and 0.5–1 lb per week thereafter. Prevent excess weight gain to avoid short- and long-term complications. Obese women may not gain much weight, despite adequate food intake, and have normal fetal growth.

Exercise

The risk-to-benefit ratio of either occasional or regular exercise in pregnant women with type 1 or type 2 diabetes is unknown. Pregnancy generally is not a time for a woman who was previously sedentary to initiate strenuous activity. However, active women can continue to do similar activities during pregnancy. Almost all women should be encouraged to walk at least 30 minutes daily, which can be divided into three 10-minute periods. General guidelines for exercise during pregnancy are listed in Table 4.3. Exercise should not be prescribed for patients with uterine bleeding, antecedent hypertension, pregnancy-induced hypertension,

---

Table 4.3 Exercise Guidelines for Pregnant Women with Diabetes

- Gradually increase exercise intensity and duration
- Perform recommended exercises: upper-body exercises, swimming, walking
- Monitor blood glucose levels frequently

- Adjust insulin dose and food intake as indicated
- Be aware of the risks of late post-exertional hypoglycemia
- Palpate uterus for contractions
- Carry source of glucose and diabetes identification

---

macrovascular or microvascular disease, autonomic dysfunction, or lack of counterregulatory mechanisms. Medical input is necessary with the prescription of exercise to pregnant women with diabetes.

Insulin

A basal-bolus injection program should be designed for all pregnant diabetic women. When converting women with type 2 diabetes to insulin therapy, in general, two-thirds of the total dose for the day is given in the morning, in a 2-to-1 ratio of intermediate- to short-acting insulin (e.g., NPH to regular). The remaining third is given before dinner in a 1-to-1 ratio as short-acting insulin before dinner and NPH at bedtime. This regimen allows for smoother control of fasting blood glucose levels during overnight fasting. Often, patients need to be treated with rapid-acting insulin before each meal and with intermediate-acting insulin in the morning, midday, and at bedtime. Rapid-acting insulin analogs with peak insulin action 1–2 h after injection offer the potential for improved postprandial glucose control and are being increasingly used during gestation. Most studies have demonstrated improved metabolic control with less hypoglycemia and increased patient satisfaction when compared with regular insulin. No clinical trials have been reported using long-acting insulin analogs in pregnant women, and both are category C in pregnancy.

Insulin can also be continuously administered through the use of battery-operated pumps, which deliver insulin at a defined rate. Although insulin pumps most closely resemble the physiological insulin secretion of the pancreas, clinical studies have failed to show any significant advantages over intensified multiple daily injections in terms of fetal outcome, mean blood glucose, A1C, or mean amplitude of glycemic excursion. Insulin pump therapy is often chosen to minimize maternal hypoglycemia or to cover the increased insulin requirement at 4–8 A.M. in pregnant women with type 1 diabetes.

Hypoglycemia. Both chemical and clinical hypoglycemic episodes occur during the course of pregnancy and are believed to result, in part, from intensive insulin treatment (aimed at achieving good glycemic control), impaired glucose counter-regulation, and hypoglycemia unawareness. Prolonged hypoglycemia has been associated with teratogenic effects in rat offspring; however, there are no clinical data to confirm any potential teratogenic effect of hypoglycemia on human fetuses. The potential harm is maternal, and careful patient education is necessary to minimize the risks. Glucose targets may be raised for women with hypoglycemia unawareness until strict self-management has corrected the problem.

Ketosis. The presence of hyperketonemia denotes a state of cellular starvation due to hypoglycemia or to a relative lack of insulin with concomitant hyperglycemia. Ketoacidosis has been associated with a 30–60% fetal mortality rate. Ketonemia may have an adverse effect on neurological development in the fetus. Regular eating and intensified glucose control should prevent hyperketonemia.

MANAGEMENT OF PREGNANT WOMEN WITH DIABETES WITH VASCULOPATHY

Evidence of vascular complications places pregnant women with diabetes in a higher risk category for both maternal and fetal morbidity and mortality. The primary cause of maternal death among pregnant women with diabetes is no longer diabetic ketoacidosis but cardiorenal complications. Similarly, fetal mortality is significantly higher in diabetic patients with vasculopathy than in patients without vasculopathy. Although many organs can be affected by diabetic vascular complications, the kidneys, eyes, and heart are associated with the most significant clinical consequences.

Diabetic Nephropathy

Diabetic nephropathy (White's class F) is one of the most critical complications affecting the outcome of pregnancy and is the leading cause of death in diabetic patients aged <40 years. It is characterized by albuminuria (>300 mg/24-h collection), hypertension, reduced glomerular filtration rate (GFR), and end-stage renal disease. Its prevalence rises sharply after 10–15 years of diabetes. Because of the increase in GFR observed and the decreased tubular reabsorption of protein in pregnancy, the diagnosis of diabetic nephropathy in pregnancy is based on a value of ≥500 mg albumin/day during the first half of the pregnancy.

The physician caring for the pregnant woman with diabetic nephropathy should be interested in knowing whether pregnancy will alter the course of the renal damage and how the renal involvement will affect the pregnancy. The amount of proteinuria may increase during pregnancy (because of the combina-

Table 4.4 Perinatal Outcome of Class F Diabetic Patients Compared with Nonnephropathic Pregnant Diabetic Patients

■ No higher prevalence of spontaneous abortions	■ Preterm delivery labor: 25%
	■ Fetal distress: 30%
■ No higher prevalence of congenital malformations	■ Superimposed pregnancy-induced hypertension: 40–60%
■ Increased prevalence of intrauterine growth restriction: 15 vs. 2.2%	■ Respiratory distress syndrome: 23 vs. 8% of diabetic patients without kidney disease
■ Risk of stillbirth: higher than in diabetic patients without kidney disease	
	■ Neonatal jaundice: 36 vs. 20%
■ Risk of neonatal death: twice that of diabetic patients without kidney disease	■ 3% of babies have developmental problems in childhood; most do well

tion of factors mentioned above) and subside after delivery. However, the expected rise in creatinine clearance (CrCl) in pregnancy is only observed in one-third of patients. Whether tighter glycemic control allows for the normal expected rise in CrCl is unknown. The presence of hypertension is associated with heavier proteinuria, lower CrCl, mild azotemia, and poorer neonatal outcomes. The perinatal impact of diabetic nephropathy is outlined in Table 4.4.

The risks of preterm labor, stillbirth, neonatal death, and fetal distress are significantly increased among patients with diabetic nephropathy. However, with contemporary means of evaluation, glycemic control, and blood pressure control (110–129 mmHg systolic and 65–79 mmHg diastolic), perinatal survival in this group can exceed 90% if fetuses are delivered at or after 36 weeks with documentation of lung maturity. Experience with antihypertensive drugs in pregnant diabetic patients is limited. The drugs of choice include methyldopa, long-acting calcium channel blockers, selected β-blockers, and arteriolar vasodilators. ACE inhibitors and ARBs are contraindicated in any stage of pregnancy.

Assessment of kidney function, including a 24-h urine collection every trimester to determine CrCl and the rate of protein excretion, is recommended. Estimation of GFR with the Modification of Diet in Renal Disease (MDRD) equation based on serum creatinine, age, sex, and race is not accurate in pregnancy. The presence of kidney failure, defined as CrCl <30 ml/min, or creatinine >5 mg/dl (>442 mmol/l), constitutes a particular management problem for patients with diabetic nephropathy. If such patients are seen in a preconception clinic and are seriously contemplating becoming pregnant, they should be advised to consider kidney transplantation or dialysis before pregnancy. On the other hand, if kidney failure develops during pregnancy, peritoneal dialysis or hemodialysis may be used. Patients with uncontrollable hypertension should be advised against conception.

Retinopathy

Class R diabetes includes pregnant patients with diabetic retinopathy. Diabetic retinopathy is classified as mild, moderate, or severe nonproliferative retinopathy and as proliferative diabetic retinopathy (PDR). PDR is the most frequent cause of blindness among patients with type 1 diabetes, whereas macular edema is the primary cause for patients with type 2 diabetes.

Diabetic retinopathy can progress rapidly over short periods. Recent evidence suggests that there is an increased risk for both the development and progression of retinopathy during pregnancy, especially when blood glucose is rapidly normalized. Risk factors for progression include the status of retina at conception, degree of hyperglycemia, degree of hypertension, and duration of diabetes. Therefore, patients with diabetes should have a complete ophthalmologic evaluation at the beginning of pregnancy. Follow-up visits or treatments should be scheduled according to the findings. Although there is no contraindication for laser photocoagulation in pregnancy, not enough data are available regarding the safety of fluorescein use in pregnancy.

Coronary Artery Disease

White's class H diabetes is defined as the presence of coronary artery disease (CAD) in pregnant diabetic patients. CAD occurs more commonly at a younger age and with greater severity in diabetic patients than in nondiabetic patients.

Patients are defined as class H if they have a history of myocardial infarction (MI) or angina or if they develop these complications during pregnancy. Particular problems in the diagnosis of class H diabetes result from the inability of many pregnant patients to complete a standard stress-tolerance test. Additionally, neither radioisotopes nor angiography may be used safely to confirm the diagnosis. Therefore, clinicians must rely on signs and symptoms of advanced disease such as angina or MI to diagnose CAD in pregnancy. There are few data regarding the outcome of pregnancy in diabetic patients with CAD. Patients with angina seem to have had better prognoses than patients whose pregnancies were complicated by either a history of MI or the development of MI during pregnancy.

If CAD is diagnosed before pregnancy, patients should be advised against pregnancy. Patients may elect to undergo bypass surgery to improve their overall medical condition. When CAD is first diagnosed during pregnancy, however, management should depend on whether the patient presents with angina or MI.

Patients with angina can be treated with selective β-blockers. In addition, although the use of calcium channel blockers in pregnancy has not been tested, they may be an appropriate therapeutic choice. MI during pregnancy presents a particularly difficult management problem. The coexistence of pregnancy and MI is stressful; patients are at an increased risk of dying if they undergo surgery within 3–6 months after MI. This 3- to 6-month period is likely to overlap with the end of the pregnancy. Should the patient require a cesarean section for obstetric indications, the same risk applies. No recommendations can be made as to whether the termination or continuation of pregnancy is preferable.

BIBLIOGRAPHY

Abalos E, Duley L, Steyn D, Henderson-Smart DJ: Antihypertensive drug therapy for mild to moderate hypertension during pregnancy. *Cochrane Database System Rev* no. CD002252, 2007

Abalovich M, Amino N, Barbour LA, Cobin RH, De Groot LJ, Glinoer D, Mandel SJ, Stagnaro-Green A: Management of thyroid dysfunction during pregnancy and postpartum: an Endocrine Society Clinical Practice Guideline. *J Clin Endocrinol Metab* 92 (8 Suppl.):S1–S47, 2007

American Diabetes Association: *Medical Management of Pregnancy Complicated by Diabetes.* Alexandria, VA, American Diabetes Association, 2007

American Diabetes Association: Standards of medical care in diabetes—2009 (Position Statement). *Diabetes Care* 32 (Suppl. 1):S13–S61, 2009

American Diabetes Association: Nutrition recommendations and interventions for diabetes—2008 (Position Statement). *Diabetes Care* 31 (Suppl. 1):S61–S78, 2008

Carr DB, Koontz GL, Gardella C, Holing EV, Brateng DA, Brown ZA, Easterling TR: Diabetic nephropathy in pregnancy: suboptimal hypertensive control associated with preterm delivery. *Am J Hypertens* 19:513–519, 2006

Chew EY, Mills JL, Metzger BE, Remaley NA, Jovanovic-Peterson L, Knopp RH, Conley M, Rand L, Simpson JL, Holms LB, Aarons JH, The NICHD-DIEP:

Metabolic control and progression of retinopathy: the Diabetes in Early Pregnancy Study: National Institute of Child Health and Human Development. *Diabetes Care* 18:631–637, 1995

Diabetes Control and Complications Trial Group: Pregnancy outcomes in the Diabetes Control and Complications Trial. *Am J Obstet Gynecol* 174:1343–1353, 1996

Diabetes Control and Complications Trial Research Group: Effect of pregnancy on microvascular complications in the Diabetes Control and Complications Trial. *Diabetes Care* 23:1084–1091, 2000

Gordon M, Landon M, Samuels P, Hissrich S, Gabbe S: Perinatal outcome and long-term follow-up associated with modern management of diabetic nephropathy. *Obstet Gynecol* 87:401–409, 1996

Gordon MC, Landon MB, Boyle J, Stewart KS, Gabbe SG: Coronary artery disease in insulin-dependent diabetes mellitus of pregnancy (class H): a review of the literature. *Obstet Gynecol Surv* 51:437–444, 1996

Hare JW, White P: Pregnancy in diabetes complicated by vascular disease. *Diabetes* 26:953–955, 1977

Homko CJ, Khandelwal M: Glucose monitoring and insulin therapy during pregnancy. *Obstet Gynecol Clin N Am* 23:47–74, 1996

Homko CJ, Reece EA: Ambulatory management of the pregnant woman with diabetes. *Clin Obstet Gynecol* 41:584–596, 1998

Jovanovic L, Peterson CM: Insulin and glucose requirements during the first stage of labor in insulin-dependent diabetic women. *Am J Med* 75:607–612, 1983

Jovanovic L, Peterson CM, Reed GF, Metzger BE, Mills JL, Knopp RH, Aarons JH: Maternal postprandial glucose levels and infant birth weight: the Diabetes in Early Pregnancy study: the National Institute of Child Health and Human Development—Diabetes in Early Pregnancy Study. *Am J Obstet Gynecol* 164:103–111, 1991

Jovanovic L, Knopp RH, Kim H, Cefalu WT, Zhu X-D, Lee YJ, Simpson JL, Mills JL, Diabetes in Early Pregnancy Study Group: Elevated pregnancy losses at high and low extremes of maternal glucose in early normal and diabetic pregnancy: evidence for a protective adaptation in diabetes. *Diabetes Care* 28:1113–1117, 2005

Jovanovic L, Nakai Y: Successful pregnancy in women with type 1 diabetes: from preconception through postpartum care. *Endocrinol Metab Clin N Am* 35:79–97, 2006

Kitzmiller JL, Buchanan TA, Kjos S, Combs CA, Ratner RE: Preconception care of diabetes, congenital malformations, and spontaneous abortions (Technical Review). *Diabetes Care* 19:514–541, 1996

Kitzmiller JL, Block JM, Brown FM, Catalano PM, Conway DL, Coustan DR, Gunderson EP, Herman WH, Hoffman LD, Inturrisi M, Jovanovic LB, Kjos SI, Knopp RH, Montoro MN, Ogata ES, Paramsothy P, Reader DM, Rosenn

BM, Thomas AM, Kirkman MS: Managing preexisting diabetes for pregnancy: summary of evidence and consensus recommendations for care (Position Statement). *Diabetes Care* 31:1060–1079, 2008

Klein BEK, Moss SE, Klein R: Effect of pregnancy on progression of diabetic retinopathy. *Diabetes Care* 13:34–40, 1990

Leguizamon GF, Reece EA: Diabetic neuropathy and coronary heart disease. In *Diabetes in Women: Adolescence, Pregnancy, and Menopause*. Reece EA, Coustan DR, Gabbe SG, Eds. Philadelphia, PA, Lippincott Williams & Wilkins, 2004, p. 425–432

Manderson JG, Patterson CC, Hadden DR, Traub AI, Ennis C, McCance DR: Preprandial versus postprandial blood glucose monitoring in type 1 diabetic pregnancy: a randomized controlled clinical trial. *Am J Obst Gynecol* 189: 507–512, 2003

Nielsen LR, Muller C, Damm P, Mathiesen ER: Reduced prevalence of early preterm delivery in women with diabetes type 1 and microalbuminuria—possible effect of early antihypertensive treatment during pregnancy. *Diabet Med* 23:426–431, 2006

Nielsen LR, Pedersen-Bjergaard U, Thorsteinsson B, Johansen M, Damm P, Mathiesen ER: Hypoglycemia in pregnant women with type 1 diabetes: predictors and role of metabolic control. *Diabetes Care* 31:9–14, 2008

Reece EA, Coustan DR, Gabbe SG, Eds. *Diabetes in Women. Adolescence, Pregnancy, and Menopause*, Philadelphia, PA, Lippincott Williams & Wilkins, 2007

Smith MC, Moran P, Ward MK, Davison JM: Assessment of glomerular filtration rate during pregnancy using the MDRD formula. *BJOG* 115:109–112, 2008

Temple RC, Aldridge VJ, Murphy HR: Prepregnancy care and pregnancy outcomes in women with type 1 diabetes. *Diabetes Care* 29:1744–1749, 2006

Reece EA, Homko CJ, Wu YK: Multifactorial basis of the syndrome of diabetic embryopathy. *Teratology* 54:171–182, 1997

Reece EA, Leguizamon G, Homko C: Pregnancy performance and outcomes associated with diabetic nephropathy. *Am J Perinat* 15:413–421, 1998

White P: Diabetes mellitus in pregnancy. *Clin Perinatol* 1:331–347, 1974

Dr. Reece is Vice President and Dean of the University of Maryland College of Medicine, Baltimore, Maryland. Dr. Homko is a Nurse Manager at the General Clinical Research Center, a Research Assistant Professor in the Department of Medicine, and a Diabetes Nurse Specialist in the Department of Obstetrics, Gynecology, and Reproductive Sciences at Temple University School of Medicine, Philadelphia, Pennsylvania. Dr. Jovanovic is Director and Chief Scientific Officer, Sansum Diabetes Research Institute, Santa Barbara, California. Dr. Kitzmiller is consultant in Maternal-Fetal Medicine, Santa Clara Valley Medical Center, San Jose, California.

5. Antepartum and Intrapartum Obstetric Care

David A. Sacks, MD

The imposition of pregnancy upon preexisting diabetes, as is the case with type 1 or 2 diabetes, and the imposition of diabetes upon pregnancy, as is the case with gestational diabetes mellitus (GDM), pose unique challenges to the pregnant woman and to her caregivers. Some problems unique to pregnancy, such as spontaneous abortions, fetal malformations, stillbirths, and pregnancy-associated hypertensive disorders, may occur with greater frequency if the mother has diabetes. Many, if not most, of the complications of pregnancy in the diabetic woman are dependent, at least in part, upon the degree of maternal glycemic control. However, particularly in the woman who has type 1 diabetes, hypoglycemia and hypoglycemic unawareness are potential serious complications of treatment. This chapter will discuss the potential complications of pregnancy for the woman who has diabetes, the prevention and treatment of these complications, as well as some of the caveats regarding treatment during the antepartum and intrapartum periods.

PREPARING FOR PREGNANCY

The woman who has diabetes must be prepared for pregnancy from the time of discovery of her diabetes. The occurrence of two of the major complications of diabetes in pregnancy, namely spontaneous abortion and fetal anomalies, is related to maternal glycemic control during organogenesis. A number of studies have demonstrated a progressive positive relationship between measures of maternal glycemia in the first trimester and the incidence of spontaneous abortions and birth defects. In most studies, the maternal glycemic measure is A1C. It seems likely that there are threshold values above which the risk for each of these complications significantly increases. Because of ethnic and socioeconomic differences in populations studied, small sample sizes, and differences in glycohemoglobin assay methods, exactly what those thresholds are is unclear. One large study reported an incidence of major fetal anomalies of 3.7% if the first-trimester A1C was ≤9.3%. Although the incidence of major anomalies increased progressively with increasing A1C, a statistically significant increase over the lowest risk was not observed below an A1C of 12.1%. Data from the same center demonstrated an increased risk of spontaneous abortion above a first trimester A1C of 12%.

Because organogenesis begins about the time the woman first realizes that she is pregnant (5 weeks) and is completed 3 weeks later, and because the reduction of maternal glycemia to an optimal level for pregnancy frequently requires several weeks or months, it should be obvious that the time to establish maternal glycemic control for the woman who has type 1 or type 2 diabetes should be prior to conception. It therefore behooves the practitioner attending the reproductive-age diabetic woman or adolescent to inform his or her patient of the importance of preconception intensive control and to educate her about and to provide her with a reliable form of contraception. The latter should be used until glycemic control is achieved. Although some, if not most, pediatricians, internists, family practitioners, and endocrinologists may not feel comfortable or qualified to provide gynecologic evaluation and counseling, consultation from or referral to an obstetrician and/or a specialist in maternal-fetal medicine experienced in the care of pregnant women who have diabetes may serve not only to provide this necessary service, but to also introduce another member of the team involved in her maternity care.

Besides the provision of contraception and establishment of glycemic control, a program of preconception care provides an opportunity to educate the patient about the additional work that will be required of her during pregnancy because she has diabetes. She should learn of the need for more frequent visits, adherence to a detailed diet, self- and laboratory testing, and antepartum evaluation of her fetus. Care in anticipation of pregnancy also provides an opportunity to assess the patient's level of risk in relation to complications of diabetes that may affect her and her child. The initial history should include current diabetes management practices. The frequency of self-monitoring of glucose may have to be intensified or increased. A discussion of the alternatives of continuation of oral hypoglycemics versus changing to insulin should be initiated in women with type 2 diabetes. Medications that may be teratogenic should be replaced with others not known to be teratogenic for the same indication (e.g., replacement of other antihypertensives with α-methyldopa, labetalol, hydralazine, and calcium channel blockers). One class of drugs whose use during the preconception period is problematic is the angiotensin-converting enzyme (ACE) inhibitors. These drugs are not only effective antihypertensives, but also delay the progression of diabetic nephropathy (DN). Unfortunately, their use during the period of organogenesis and beyond has been associated with both structural and functional fetal defects. Weighing the fetal risk–to–maternal benefit ratio for continuation of these drugs to the time of first recognition of pregnancy is difficult. One potential resolution of this conundrum is to suspend the use of ACE inhibitors from the time of suspension of contraception to the time of delivery, carefully monitoring maternal blood pressure and renal function until pregnancy is established.

Once glycemic control has been optimized and the woman is ready to attempt to conceive, it is best to discontinue other potential teratogenic medications often used in the treatment of diabetes, such as statins and fibrates. Assessment of the woman's support system and the disruption of her everyday activities by the demands of her pregnancy (e.g., time out from school or work for snacks, insulin self-administration, and glucose self-monitoring) as well as available support from friends and family should be realistically assessed.

Physical examination should include evaluation of orthostatic changes in blood pressure, changes in pulse with exercise, and signs and symptoms of diabetic gastroparesis and autonomic neuropathy. Laboratory evaluation includes, but is not limited to, assessment of glycemic control (daily glucose reports as well as A1C) and assessment of renal function with urinalysis, culture, and 24-h urine protein and creatinine clearance. The latter two tests may prove to be particularly useful for women who have chronic hypertension in establishing the presence or absence of a gestational hypertensive disorder later in pregnancy because a rise in protein output and/or a decline in creatinine clearance may be the only signs of superimposition of preeclampsia on preexisting chronic hypertension. Particularly for the woman who has type 1 diabetes, thyroid function may also be assessed with thyroid-stimulating hormone and antithyroid antibodies. A dilated retinal examination by an ophthalmologist knowledgeable about retinal findings in the diabetic patient and an electrocardiogram for the woman at increased risk of cardiovascular complications (e.g., women with diabetes duration >10 years or who are hypertensive) seems prudent. Finally, as for all reproductive-aged women, daily intake of at least 400 µgm of folic acid (4 mg for the woman who has had a neonate with an open neural tube defect) should be recommended. A brief summary of these recommendations may be found in Table 5.1.

The benefits of preconception care programs have been demonstrated in a number of controlled and observational studies. Reductions in spontaneous abortions, major anomalies, preterm deliveries, and perinatal deaths have been reported. In at least one study of type 1 diabetic women, no increase in the frequency of severe maternal hypoglycemia was noted in the preconception care group.

Some issues pertaining to preconception care are currently unresolved. It is unclear what the frequency of visits and measures of glycemia should be during the period that conception is being attempted. Patient recruitment is more successful among women who are better educated, employed, and in a stable relation-

---

Table 5.1 Preconception Evaluation and Preparation for Pregnancy for the Diabetic Woman

Evaluation	Preparation
1. Dilated retinal examination	1. Provision of family-planning information and material until best glycemic control is achieved
2. Blood pressure, cardiovascular, and neurological examination	
3. Renal function tests (e.g., 24-h urine creatinine clearance and protein)	2. Consider changing from oral hypoglycemics to insulin
4. Thyroid-stimulating hormone	3. Stop ACE inhibitors, statins, and fibrates
5. A1C	
6. Electrocardiogram, if hypertension or cardiovascular complications are present	4. Start or continue folic acid 0.4–5 mg/day
	5. Control hypertension (see text for medications)
	6. Suggested glycemic goals (plasma glucose):
	a. Premeal, bedtime, and overnight: 60–99 mg/dl
	b. Peak postmeal: 100–129 mg/dl
	c. A1C < 6%

ship. Programs to attract women who are outside this demographic should be developed. The cost-effectiveness of preconception care in the long term has been demonstrated. In the U.S., where health care is not universally available and health insurance is privatized, many insurers do not include comprehensive preconception care as a covered benefit.

MINIMIZING RISKS FOR MOTHER AND BABY

Minimizing Fetal Risks

Fetal demise. Besides spontaneous abortions and congenital malformations, a persistent vexing complication of pregnancy for the woman who has diabetes is the increased frequency of fetal death. Compared with offspring of women who do not have diabetes, the infant of the pregestationally diabetic woman has 3–5 times increased risk of stillbirth. Although the etiology of this complication is unclear, animal and human data suggest a number of possible comorbid and/or causal factors. Approximately 20% of stillborn fetuses born to pregnant diabetic women have major congenital anomalies. While it is difficult to establish causality when the fetus has a major anomaly that is compatible with in utero survival, the fact remains that fetal anomalies are significantly more prevalent among stillbirths than among live births of diabetic women. Other findings associated with fetal demise in infants of diabetic women include small-for-gestational-age fetuses, placental abnormalities, placental abruption, chorioamnionitis, maternal hypertension, and maternal vascular disease.

A number of observations suggest a causal link between maternal hyperglycemia and fetal death. Diabetic ketoacidosis in humans carries with it a stillbirth rate in excess of 50%. Rat, sheep, and monkey studies in which both maternal hyperglycemia and minimal maternal hypoxia were induced found that this combination was associated with fetal lactic acidemia and fetal death. Similar degrees of maternal hypoxia among nonhyperglycemic animals produced significantly less fetal morbidity and mortality. These as well as some observations in humans suggest that maternal hyperglycemia likely leads to fetal hyperinsulinemia, which in turn stimulates an increase in fetal oxygen demand for aerobic glycolysis. In the presence of decreased fetal oxygen supply, such as may be found with placental vascular insufficiency, glycolysis may be switched to an anaerobic pathway, resulting in fetal accumulation of lactic acid and, ultimately, demise. The degree and duration of maternal hyperglycemia in pregnant diabetic women necessary to increase the risk of fetal death are unclear. However, given the plausible link between maternal hyperglycemia and this adverse outcome, it seems wise to recommend conventional maternal glycemic target values during pregnancy (Table 5.2).

Independent associations between maternal obesity, interpregnancy weight gain, and fetal demise have been reported in both diabetic and nondiabetic women. A BMI increase of 1–2 kg/m^2 from one pregnancy to the next has been correlated with an increased incidence of fetal demise in the second pregnancy.

Minimizing maternal risks

Diabetic retinopathy. Several studies have found that the rate of progression of diabetic retinopathy (DR) during pregnancy is greater than that of matched nonpregnant control subjects. Pregnant diabetic women with no retinopathy immediately prior to or during early pregnancy may develop benign to severe proliferative retinopathy as pregnancy advances. However, progression of disease is more commonly found in women whose background preproliferative and proliferative retinopathy antedates pregnancy. Other factors that have been associated with worsening diabetic retinal disease include long duration of diabetes, poor glycemic control before and during pregnancy, rapid normalization of maternal glucose concentrations, prepregnancy and pregnancy-associated hypertension, and coexisting DN. Much of the progression and development of DR during pregnancy appears to regress after delivery. Both cross-sectional and longitudinal studies comparing parous and nonparous women, respectively, found no long-term difference in prevalence of proliferative retinopathy or in progression of DR. These data suggest that pregnancy does not alter the long-term course of diabetic retinal disease. A confounding factor is that women who had severe proliferative DR did receive laser treatment during pregnancy.

Some hormonal and microcirculatory changes unique to pregnancy may help to explain the increased rate of development and progression of DR during gestation. An abrupt decrease in maternal glycemia has been associated, in vitro, with apoptosis of retinal capillary pericytes. The latter are the cells surrounding retinal capillaries in whose absence microaneurysms develop. Both placental and maternal angiogenic factors may contribute to retinal blood vessel proliferation. The concentrations of plasma progesterone are higher throughout gestation in women who have GDM compared with pregnant control subjects. Progesterone is associated with the development and release of intraocular vascular endothelial growth factor and the latter with development and progression of DR. Finally, one study reported a decrease in retinal venous diameter and blood flow in pregnant diabetic women compared with pregnant nondiabetic control subjects. This finding suggests the possibility that decreased retinal blood flow may increase retinal ischemia and hypoxemia in pregnant diabetic women and thus accelerate the pregnancy-related development and progression of DR.

From the foregoing, the ideal prevention of pregnancy-associated DR development and progression appears to be a gradual establishment of glycemic control

Table 5.2 Evaluation and Care During Pregnancy

Evaluation

1. Ultrasound
   a. At first visit for dating
   b. At 15–20 weeks for fetal anatomical survey
   c. Fetal echocardiogram
2. Genetic screening (first, second, and/or combined [sequential or contingent])

Treatment

1. Diet
2. Oral hypoglycemic or anti-hypoglycemic agent
3. Insulin
4. Fetal antepartum testing, beginning in third trimester
5. Testing for group B β-streptococcus at 35–37 weeks
6. Suggested glycemic goals (capillary blood glucose):
   a. Fasting: 60–90 mg/dl
   b. 1-h postprandial: <140 mg/dl
   c. 2-h postprandial: <120 mg/dl

Content of Table 5.1 also applies if patient first presents for pregnancy-related care after conception.

and treatment of proliferative DR prior to conception. Women who first appear for care during pregnancy should have a dilated retinal examination within close temporal proximity of the first prenatal visit. The desirable frequency and timing of subsequent dilated retinal examinations through the course of pregnancy is unclear. An arbitrary course of management might be to perform such an examination once or twice more during pregnancy for the woman who has no DR at her initial retinal examination. Women who have more advanced DR will likely need to have their retinas examined more often. Laser treatment of proliferative DR has been safely used during pregnancy.

Hypertensive disorders of pregnancy. Systemic hypertension antedating pregnancy is more common among diabetic women than among pregnant nondiabetic women. Chronic hypertension will be covered further in the discussion of DN in pregnancy. Gestational hypertensive disorders are seen more frequently in pregnancies complicated by both pregestational diabetes and GDM than in pregnancies unaccompanied by diabetes. Their classification is based on the presence of new-onset hypertension alone (gestational hypertension), new-onset hypertension plus proteinuria (preeclampsia), and seizures accompanying the latter (eclampsia), chronic hypertension, and superimposed preeclampsia. Insulin resistance is thought to be a common pathway for the development of gestational glucose intolerance and hypertension. In comparison with the nonpregnant state, increased insulin concentrations and increased insulin resistance are normal findings in all pregnancies. However, both in pregnancies complicated by GDM and in those complicated by pregnancy-associated hypertension, both serum insulin and insulin resistance are increased in comparison with pregnant women who do not have either of these two entities. Mechanisms that have been postulated to explain the association between insulin resistance and hypertension include activation of the sympathetic nervous system, sodium retention, and endothelial dysfunction. One proposed explanation for the augmented insulin resistance is an increase in inflammatory cytokines. Tumor necrosis factor (TNF)-α concentrations increase in both diabetes and preeclampsia. This cytokine disrupts the insulin signaling pathway, thus contributing to insulin resistance. It also induces plasminogen activator inhibitor-1. The latter is involved with deposition of fibrin in maternal and placental vessels, which in turn may lead to the endothelial dysfunction that characterizes preeclampsia. In addition, oxidative stress and antioxidant depletion are found more often with diabetes. Free oxygen radicals may cause endothelial thromboxane/prostacyclin imbalance, resulting in the vasoconstriction that characterizes preeclampsia.

Other factors that are independently associated with the development of hypertension in pregnancies complicated by diabetes include maternal overweight and obesity, preexisting hypertension, preeclampsia in a previous pregnancy, and DN. Maternal hyperglycemia of a degree less than that which defines GDM is also associated with hypertension in pregnancy. Among nondiabetic women who had a glucose tolerance test, the risk for developing hypertension in pregnancy was found to be independently associated with the 2-h result of the glucose tolerance test. Others have shown an independent correlation between GDM and preeclampsia. That control of maternal glycemia may decrease the incidence of preeclampsia was illustrated in a study of women who had GDM, in which the risk of preeclampsia increased proportionately to the severity of GDM in only poorly controlled women.

A number of measures have been used to attempt to prevent the development of gestational hypertension in women who have diabetes. Because aspirin inhibits thromboxane (a vasoconstrictor) more than it does prostacyclin (a vasodilator), it has been studied in pregnancies both complicated by and uncomplicated by diabetes to prevent preeclampsia. The results of most studies suggest that aspirin does not effectively prevent this disease. Similarly, the use of antioxidants (e.g., vitamins C and E) has not been found to be clinically useful in preventing preeclampsia. Because of the positive relationship between maternal glucose concentrations and the development of preeclampsia, normalization of maternal glucose throughout gestation appears to be of some value in preventing this disease.

The ultimate treatment of the gestational hypertensive disorders is delivery. Fortunately, most cases of preeclampsia occur at or near term. Unfortunately, some cases of severe preeclampsia also occur remote from term, when prematurity poses a substantial risk to the life of the neonate. In the event of severe disease occurring during the periviable period (e.g., 23–26 weeks), some evidence suggests that temporizing with antihypertensives and strict in-hospital clinical and laboratory observation may allow progression of pregnancy to the point of viability. Once the risk of neonatal demise due to prematurity is minimal (e.g., ≥26 weeks), severe preeclampsia may be managed by delivery. Because of the demonstrated benefit in preventing neonatal respiratory distress syndrome by giving the mother intramuscular steroids (betamethasone or dexamethasone) between 24 and 34 weeks, the administration of these drugs while the mother is under observation seems prudent. However, because hyperglycemia is a known side effect of steroids, careful observation of maternal glucose levels (e.g., every 1–2 h from the first injection to 24 h after the last) with intravenous administration of insulin as dictated by maternal glucose concentrations also seems wise.

Diabetic nephropathy. DN is a progressive disease that evolves over years, ultimately resulting in renal failure. It is the most common cause of end-stage renal disease (ESRD) in the U.S. and affects ~20–30% of patients who have type 1 and type 2 diabetes. DN also has been found in women with insulin-requiring GDM. As early as a few years after diagnosis of type 1 diabetes, and at the time of diagnosis with type 2 diabetes, scattered sclerosis of glomeruli may be found on renal biopsy. Kidney enlargement, glomerular hypertrophy, increased glomerular surface area, increased intraglomerular pressure, and hyperfiltration (glomerular filtration rate [GFR] >150 ml/min) ensue. At this stage, GFR may be returned to normal with good glycemic control. Microalbuminuria, defined as the excretion of 30–300 mg of albumen and/or 500 mg of protein per day, becomes manifest with the sclerosis of progressively more glomeruli, basement membrane thickening, and mesangial expansion. Hypertension may precede or follow the development of microalbuminuria in type 2 diabetes, whereas it lags the development of microalbuminuria in type 1 diabetes. Although microalbuminuria defines incipient nephropathy, macroalbuminuria (defined by the excretion of >300 mg of albumin per day) defines overt DN. Histologically, this stage is characterized by diffuse glomerulosclerosis, which is either generalized (in 75%) or nodular (the Kimmelsteil-Wilson lesion). The time to development of ESRD may be lengthened by good glycemic control and control of hypertension, especially with drugs that block the renin-angiotensin system.

The normal physiological changes in renal function that accompany pregnancy may cause confusion in the diagnosis of the renal manifestations of diabetes. Because of increased cardiac output, increased extracellular fluid, and decreased vascular resistance, GFR increases in normal pregnancy by 50% by early midtrimester. The mechanism of this hyperfiltration is, however, different from that found in diabetes; the latter is associated with increased intraglomerular pressure. Perhaps because of the increase in GFR and decrease in tubular reabsorption, proteinuria progressively increases throughout pregnancy, but to levels less than those defining overt DN. Thus, defining the presence or absence of DN in a woman whose kidney function was first evaluated during pregnancy must await repeat evaluation 2–3 months after delivery.

A number of studies have found that pregnancy is not causally related to the development of DN in women who do not have DN prior to pregnancy. However, some data do suggest that pregnancy in a woman who had moderate DN (e.g., those whose prepregnancy serum creatinine was 1.1–1.4 mg/dl and/or whose 24-h urine protein was >1,000 mg) may accelerate the development of ESRD. In contrast, the presence of any degree of DN may adversely affect both maternal and perinatal outcomes. Hypertension is a potential morbidity of great concern. Both chronic hypertension and gestational hypertensive disorders are seen more frequently in women who have diabetes. It is unclear whether lowering blood pressure in hypertensive pregnant women will avert the fetal consequences of this complication. The latter include fetal growth retardation, fetal demise, and prematurity (both spontaneous and iatrogenic due to severity of disease).

Whether control of maternal hypertension improves maternal and/or perinatal outcomes in all women who have DN was explored in a retrospective cohort study comparing 21 women whose mean arterial pressure (MAP) prior to 20 weeks' gestation was ≥100 mmHg with 22 women whose MAP was <100 mmHg. Although MAP and 24-h urine protein were not significantly different between groups by the third trimester and A1C was not different throughout pregnancy, the rate of prematurity in the higher early pregnancy MAP group was greater than that of the lower MAP group. These data suggest the possibility that control of blood pressure in women who have DN early in pregnancy may be of benefit in prolonging pregnancy. Drugs that are commonly used for the treatment of hypertension in pregnancy include α-methyldopa, labetalol, and others.

Pregnancies in patients undergoing hemo- and peritoneal dialysis have been reported. Anemia, electrolyte balance, acid-base balance, nutrition, and blood pressure control require intensive management in such patients. Pregnancies have also been reported in diabetic women who have had kidney transplants. The likelihood of a successful pregnancy is improved if no rejection was experienced for at least 1 year, graft function is stable, the dose of immunosuppressives is stable, and no infections that may endanger the fetus (e.g., cytomegalovirus) are present.

Diabetic Gastroenteropathy. Dysrhythmias of gastric pacemaker potential result in disordered gastric tone and contractility. The latter two findings are characteristic of both hyperemesis gravidarum and diabetic gastroparesis. Though rare, the latter complication is reported most often in pregnancy in women who have had type 1 diabetes for some years. Confusion in diagnosis may result from diabetic gastroparesis first manifesting during pregnancy. The difference is largely academic, because treatment for both entities in pregnancy, alone or in combination, is identical. Because of the risk of rapid onset of the serious complications of persistent vomiting in a woman who has overt diabetes (e.g., hypoglycemia, ketoacidosis, electrolyte imbalance, and malnutrition), it seems prudent to hospitalize the woman who has these symptoms. An attempt should be made to identify other causes of vomiting, such as a molar pregnancy, hyperthyroidism, and gastroesophageal reflux disease (GERD). Treatment consists of attempting to stop or decrease the vomiting. A variety of injectible and oral antiemetics, antihistamines, proton pump inhibitors, and antidepressants have been used for this purpose. If initial treatment fails, hydration and intravenous nutrition with a glucose/electrolyte solution might best be replaced with total parenteral nutrition for as long as severe nausea and vomiting persist. Throughout the course of treatment, meticulous attention must be paid to control of maternal glycemia. After stabilization, and assuming the availability of support for the patient, she may be discharged with instructions to her and her caregivers for continuation of total parenteral nutrition and medications at home.

TREATMENT OF DIABETES DURING PREGNANCY

Control of Maternal Glucose

Control of maternal glycemia is a guiding principle of the care of a pregnant woman with any type of diabetes. The rationale is that both maternal and fetal morbidity and mortality appear to increase incrementally with increases in maternal glucose concentrations. Likely the most frequently used yardstick for judging the success of management of maternal diabetes is the reduction in the rate of large newborns. It must be noted, however, that whether expressed as absolute birth weight or birth weight for gestational age, the majority of high-birth-weight babies are born to women who are glucose tolerant.

Despite meticulous control of maternal glycemia, some infants of diabetic mothers (IDMs) are >90th percentile in weight for gestational age. A number of potential explanations for this finding have been posited. One is that glucose may not be the sole or perhaps not even the major determinant of birth weight. Birth weight is positively and independently associated with maternal prepregnancy BMI as well as with maternal glucose concentrations. A second has to do with the observation that a distinguishing feature of both high- and average-birth-weight IDMs is that a greater proportion of their birth weight is fat weight. When easily applied instrumentation becomes available for the measurement of fat and lean tissue, the adequacy of glycemic control may be measured by the proportion of neonatal body composition that is fat, rather than birth weight alone. A third potential explanation is that other substrates besides glucose may be of importance in influencing fetal weight and body composition. Besides glucose, concentrations of triglycerides, free fatty acids, and free (especially branch-chained) amino acids are greater in the plasma of pregnant diabetic women than in that of their nondiabetic counterparts. Placental hormones and cytokines that alter maternal and fetal metabolism in pregnancy are present in different concentrations in pregnancies complicated by diabetes. For example, placental production of inflammatory cytokines, such as TNF-α, is associated with the increase in insulin resistance that characterizes normal pregnancy. However, in pregnancies complicated by GDM, the placental expression of genetic markers for inflammatory cytokines is greater than that in normal pregnancies.

For a variety of reasons, the appropriate target glucose values during pregnancy for women who have diabetes are unclear. Some have shown a stronger correlation between birth weight and maternal glucose early in pregnancy, whereas others have found maternal glucose to correlate best with third-trimester glucose. Whether birth weight correlates best with pre- or postmeal glucose and, if the latter is true, whether a stronger correlation exists with glucose measured 1 or 2 h postprandially is unresolved. In addition, studies using subcutaneously implanted glucose detectors that sample maternal glucose every 10 seconds and record averages of these readings every 5 min have reported that targeted glucose values for pregnant diabetic women substantially exceed normal values for nondiabetic women and that peak postmeal glucose values in nondiabetic women occur at times other than 1 and 2 h postprandially. Nevertheless, a number of studies have found a relatively low incidence of high-birth-weight babies when targeted glucose values identical with or similar to those found in Table 5.2 are utilized.

A word of caution should be expressed for pregnant women who have type 1 diabetes. Because of the greater lability of glycemic response to insulin in women who have type 1 diabetes, and because sudden hypoglycemia and hypoglycemic unawareness may result from attempting to reach the degree of control recommended in Table 5.2 during pregnancy in these women, higher glycemic targets, more frequent glucose checks, and the use of the insulin pump, either alone or in combination, may be beneficial, if not lifesaving, for these women. Studies comparing the results of applying higher or lower maternal glucose targets for all types of diabetes will hopefully help establish scientifically based maternal glycemic targets.

Medical Nutrition Therapy

Medical nutrition therapy (MNT) is often referred to as the cornerstone of therapy for diabetes in pregnancy. A goal of MNT is to provide adequate nutrients for fetal growth while maintaining appropriate maternal weight gain and glucose concentrations. Generally, the diet for the pregnant diabetic woman is similar to that prescribed for her pregnant nondiabetic counterpart. Weight gain is frequently used as a measure of adequacy of caloric supply, using guidelines based on maternal prepregnancy BMI, such as those in Table 5.3. One recommended formula is a diet consisting of 40–50% carbohydrates, 20% protein, and 20–40% (primarily unsaturated) fats, divided into three meals and three snacks. Carbohydrates (sugars, starch, and fiber) are best obtained from fruits, vegetables, whole grains, and low-fat milk. It must be noted that other diet contents (e.g., fats and starch-protein and starch-lipid combinations) may delay the absorption of carbohydrates and thus affect measures of maternal glycemia. It appears that the total amount of carbohydrates ingested, rather than type of carbohydrate, is the major determinant of maternal glycemic concentrations. Modest reduction in calories for obese women, substitution of unsaturated for saturated fats, and exercise during pregnancies complicated by diabetes have been shown to reduce maternal

Table 5.3   Institute of Medicine Guidelines for Weight Gain During Pregnancy

	Recommended Total Gain	
Category	kg	lb
Low (BMI <19.8 kg/m²)	12.5–18	28–40
Normal (BMI 19.8–26 kg/m²)	11.5–16	25–35
High (BMI 26.1–29 kg/m²)	7–11.5	15–25
Obese (BMI ≥29 kg/m²)	≥6.8	≥15

From Committee on the Impact of Pregnancy Weight on Maternal and Child Health, 2007.

glycemic and/or insulin responses to a meal. However, there is scant evidence that any of these measures affect important clinical outcomes (e.g., prevention of excessive birth weight).

A number of dietary supplements during pregnancies in diabetic women have been proposed. Although continued supplementation of folic acid throughout pregnancy is recommended by some, the greatest impact of folate in preventing neural tube defects is within the first 3 weeks after fertilization, when the neural tube is formed. Hyperglycemia via direct and indirect effects may also contribute to the development of birth defects. Hyperglycemia alters prostaglandin synthesis, producing free oxygen radicals. Activation of the Pax-3 gene necessary for neural tube closure is inhibited directly by hyperglycemia and indirectly by an excess of free oxygen species. Animal evidence suggests that supplementation with free oxygen radical scavengers, such as vitamins C and E, during organogenesis decreases the incidence of open neural tube defects. Whether dietary supplementation with antioxidants in the periconceptional period has a similar effect on preventing defects in humans remains speculative.

Artificial sweeteners have been in common use for several years. Currently, five nonnutritive sweeteners are approved by the Food and Drug Administration: saccharine, aspartame, neotame, sucralose, and acesulfame potassium. The FDA has designated these products as safe for use in pregnancy.

Restriction of dietary and/or carbohydrate calories for pregnant diabetic women in an effort to reduce maternal glycemia and its consequences has been explored. Compliance with caloric restriction has proven problematic for some. However, one study comparing isocaloric diets in which the study group's calories from carbohydrates were reduced and replaced by protein and fat found significant reductions in both postprandial glucose and in the incidence of large-for-gestational-age (LGA) neonates. A major concern in applying calorie-restricted diets to women who have diabetes is the threshold of restricted calories below which ketonemia and ketonuria increases. Older studies found a positive relationship between maternal ketonuria during pregnancy in diabetic women and impaired intellectual performance of their children. However, during normal pregnancy the physiological increase in and β-oxidation of free fatty acids results in the increased production of acetoacetate, 3-hydroxybutyrate, and acetone. Thus, during normal pregnancy the finding of (particularly fasting) ketonuria is not uncommon. In a more recent study of primarily diabetic women in which data were adjusted for socioeconomic status, ethnicity, and type of diabetes, children's intelligence scores at 2 years of age were found to be negatively associated with plasma β-hydroxybutyrate and with β-hydroxybutyrate and maternal free fatty acid concentrations when the children were tested between ages 3 and 5 years. At neither testing period was a relationship between maternal ketonuria and childhood intelligence found. Therefore, although restriction of total calories and exchange of carbohydrate calories for proteins and fats requires further exploration, childhood intelligence should likely be measured against maternal serum and not urine ketone concentrations.

Insulin and Insulin Analogs

Insulin is used for the treatment of pregnant women whose diabetes antedates pregnancy and for those gestationally diabetic women for whom MNT has not sufficiently lowered maternal glucose concentrations. After a glucose load, endogenous insulin is transported from the islet cells via the portal vein to the liver. Thus, the highest concentration of endogenous insulin first passes through the liver, suppressing the latter's production of glucose by gluconeogenesis. In contrast, insulin injected into the subcutaneous tissue does not reach the liver in as great a concentration as that naturally produced. Thus, the quantity of injected insulin required to adequately suppress hepatic gluconeogenesis and to drive glucose out of the blood and into insulin-dependent cells is greater than that produced physiologically. The progressive normal insulin resistance of pregnancy along with the β-cell insufficiency that characterizes type 2 diabetes and GDM contribute to the demand for progressively increasing doses of exogenous insulin as pregnancy advances to maintain desired maternal glucose concentrations.

Insulin lispro. The release of insulin occurs in two phases. The first, occurring in response to a glucose challenge, is a rapid release of a high concentration of insulin, lasting ~10 min and suppressing hepatic gluconeogenesis. The second, tapering phase, lasting 1–2 h, covers ingested carbohydrates. Between feedings, a basal level of insulin is maintained. In theory, the administration of an insulin (or a combination of insulins) that mimics the timing and release of physiologically produced insulin should produce ideal clinical results. Regular insulin has its onset in 30–60 min and peaks ~2–3 h after subcutaneous administration. In contrast, insulin lispro has its onset of action within 15 minutes of injection and has its peak action within 30–90 minutes. In some randomized controlled trials and cohort studies of pregnancies in women who have type 1 diabetes and GDM, postprandial glucose and A1C concentrations and both clinical and chemical hypoglycemia have been reported to be lower in women using lispro in comparison with those using regular insulin. However, no study to date has shown benefit with lispro in reducing the incidence of LGA babies.

One rationale for the use of all insulins is that unless antibody-bound, the drug does not pass the placenta. In the few reports that have addressed this issue, the frequency of insulin-specific and cross-reacting insulin antibodies are no different between lispro and regular insulin in pregnant diabetic women. One study found anti-insulin antibodies, but no lispro insulin, in the cord blood of fetuses of women using this analog.

Insulin aspart. Insulin aspart has pharmacokinetics and pharmacodynamics that are similar to those of lispro. In studies of nonpregnant individuals comparing these two analogs, the time to peak glucose concentrations, maximum postprandial glucose excursions, glucose disappearance rates, and endogenous glucose production were found to be not significantly different. In women who had GDM, the 1-h postprandial glucose concentration was significantly lower in women treated with lispro or aspart than in those treated with regular insulin. Comparing postmeal responses to regular insulin and aspart, maternal glucose levels were significantly lower 1, 2, and 3 h postprandially after the aspart than after regular insulin.

Because of small numbers of subjects, most studies of the use of insulin analogs during pregnancy lack the statistical power to evaluate differences in clinically meaningful endpoints. However, two reports from a randomized controlled study of >400 pregnant type 1 diabetic women comparing treatment with regular and insulin aspart have been published. The study was powered to show a 40% difference in major hypoglycemic episodes between groups. Although mean maternal postprandial glucose concentrations were lower for the aspart group at the end of the first and third trimesters, there was no significant difference in the overall rate of major maternal hypoglycemia. Birth weight for gestational age, though quantitatively less for the aspart group, was not statistically significantly less than that of the infants of women treated with regular insulin.

Insulin glulisine. Glulisine is one of the newer rapid-acting insulins. In nonpregnant patients who have type 1 or 2 diabetes, premeal glulisine was found to more effectively decrease 2-h postmeal glucose concentrations than did regular insulin. In nonpregnant patients who had type 2 diabetes, it was also found to better reduce 2-h postbreakfast and postdinner glucose concentrations as well as A1C than did regular insulin. The incidence of severe hypoglycemia in patients who have type 1 or 2 diabetes has been reported to be similar following injection of regular insulin or insulins lispro or glulisine. There are no published data on the use of glulisine during pregnancy.

Insulin glargine. By the addition of two arginine molecules at the COOH-terminal end of the β-chain and the substitution of glysine for asparagine at position 21 of the α-chain, the isoelectric point shifts from 5.4 to 6.7, making this insulin analog less soluble and more stable in subcutaneous tissue. The hypoglycemic effect begins 90 min after injection and lasts 22–24 h. Unlike other insulins, insulin glargine exhibits no peak in either insulin concentration or hypoglycemic activity. Only a few reports exist of its use during pregnancy. One study found no significant differences in mean maternal blood glucose and birth weights for women with either type 1 diabetes or GDM who were treated with glargine compared with matched control subjects treated with intermediate- and short-acting insulins. A few case reports of pregnancies in women who had type 1 diabetes found that major nocturnal hypoglycemia ceased by changing the treatment from an evening dose of NPH insulin to a daily dose of insulin glargine.

A major, albeit theoretical, concern for the use of glargine in pregnancy has to do with its binding to IGF-1 receptors. Both natural insulin and insulin analogs have minimal affinity for IGF-1 receptors. Natural insulin has 1,000-fold less affinity for IGF-1 receptors than does IGF-1. However, insulin glargine has a 6-fold greater binding affinity to IGF-1 receptors than does natural insulin. IGF-1 facilitates the implanting of the human embryo into the endometrium. Although not examined in animal models, a decrease in available IGF-1 may result in disturbances in implantation and perhaps disturbances in fetal organogenesis. Late in pregnancy, fetal growth is mediated in part by human placental growth hormone.

The effects of the latter are, in turn, mediated through IGF-1. Therefore, excessive binding of IFG-1 receptors may, in theory, disrupt fetal growth late in pregnancy. Finally, based on laboratory findings, concern has been expressed about glargine's potential mitogenicity. Osteosarcoma cells are rich in IGF-1 receptors. Insulin glargine, because of its relatively increased IGF-1 receptor affinity, was found in one study to have a 7-fold greater mitogenic potency for this cell line than did natural insulin. This finding, however, was not confirmed in other studies using other cell lines.

To summarize, drawing conclusions about the utility, risks, and benefits of insulin analogs during pregnancy is hampered by studies containing few subjects and the absence of evidence from well-designed controlled trials. Most reports of the use of insulins lispro and aspart in pregnancy have shown that they more closely imitate the first-phase response of natural insulin and that they are associated with lower postprandial maternal glucose concentrations when compared with regular insulin. To date, the use of these analogs has not been convincingly demonstrated to cause a decrease in clinically undesirable outcomes, such as maternal hypoglycemia and LGA neonates. The expense of these analogs relative to generic insulin gives pause to advocacy of their uniform application during pregnancy at this time. Until the clinical significance of increased IGF-1 receptor binding by insulin glargine is clarified, it may be prudent to confine its use during pregnancy to situations where it is clearly indicated, e.g., when severe nocturnal hypoglycemia cannot be effectively treated with other insulins.

Insulin detemir. Although its mechanism of prolonged action is different from that of glargine (preservation of its hexameric form by having a fatty acid side chain as well as albumen binding in subcutaneous tissue and blood), insulin detemir behaves similarly to glargine in its stability and duration of action. In nonpregnant patients, it has been shown to improve glycemic control and to reduce nocturnal hypoglycemia. There is no published human experience with detemir during pregnancy.

Continuous subcutaneous insulin infusion versus multiple daily injections. The availability of portable insulin pumps sparked interest in replacing intermittent doses of short-acting (usually regular) and intermediate-acting (usually NPH) insulin in pregnancy with continuously infused subcutaneously administered insulin. Whether there is maternal and/or fetal benefit in continuous subcutaneous insulin infusion (CSII) compared with conventional multiple daily injection (MDI) therapy has been investigated in a few small case-control and cohort studies. The majority of patients reported in these analyses had type 1 diabetes. Although some studies were confounded by such between-group differences as microvascular complications, duration of diabetes, utilization of preconception care, and maternal glycemia at the start of pregnancy, they found no differences between CSII and MDI in such outcomes as maternal glycemia, birth weight for gestational age, neonatal hypoglycemia, polycythemia, and hyperbilirubinemia.

A meta-analysis of two randomized controlled trials containing a total of 61 subjects found no differences between the CSII and MDI groups in second- and third-trimester 24-h mean maternal blood glucose concentrations, perinatal mortality, and neonatal hypoglycemia. Although there were no significant differences in gestational age at delivery, the neonates of mothers treated with CSII weighed significantly more than those in the MDI group. The authors of this meta-analysis concluded that the data were insufficient to draw conclusions for best practices.

An issue that has not been clearly addressed during pregnancy is the type of insulin to be used for CSII. A review of several open-label, randomized crossover trials performed on nonpregnant subjects who had type 1 diabetes concluded that CSII with either insulins lispro or aspart provided lower postprandial hyperglycemia, lower daily insulin requirements, and a similar or reduced frequency of hypoglycemic episodes than did CSII with regular insulin.

Glucose monitors. The development and adoption of memory-based devices for self-monitoring of capillary glucose has proven extremely useful during pregnancy, particularly in women using insulin or oral hypoglycemic agents. Most algorithms for adjustment of doses of these medications titrate against premeal and 1-, 1.5-, or 2-h postmeal capillary glucose values obtained by fingerstick. The utility of these readings relies on the ability and willingness of the patient to perform the tests as prescribed and especially to meticulously time her blood testing relative to her meals. In recent years, a subcutaneously implanted glucose-oxidase–embedded sensor that continuously records the mean of 30 readings of glucose values every 5 min (i.e., 288 data points per day) has been studied during pregnancy. Initial studies reported that the timing of peak postprandial glucose concentrations for diabetic women in the third trimester did not differ significantly between diet- and insulin-treated women who had GDM or women who had type 1 diabetes (means of 82, 85, and 93 min, respectively). Within each of the three groups, neither the time to peak glucose value nor the glucose value itself differed significantly between breakfast, lunch, and dinner.

More frequent detection of maternal hyperglycemia and hypoglycemia with continuous glucose monitoring than with intermittent monitoring has been reported for women with GDM and types 1 and 2 diabetes. A reduction in the occurrence of severe nocturnal hypoglycemia during pregnancy in a woman who had type 1 diabetes has been reported after initiation of a continuous glucose monitor programmed to alarm when subcutaneous glucose fell below 72 mg/dl. The development of closed-loop insulin delivery systems incorporating cross-talk between continuous glucose sensors and programmed insulin delivery devices is currently under investigation. Once perfected, these systems will likely have a significant positive impact on the glycemic control of pregnant women, particularly those who have type 1 diabetes.

Oral Hypoglycemic Agents

In recent years interest has been generated in the application of oral hypoglycemic agents to control maternal hyperglycemia during pregnancy. Classes of drugs studied include sulfonylureas, biguanides, thiazolidinediones, and α-glucosidase inhibitors. Because most of the literature pertaining to the use of oral hypoglycemic agents during pregnancy has focused on glyburide and metformin, these two drugs will be briefly discussed.

Glyburide. Sulfonylureas, the class of hypoglycemic drugs to which glyburide belongs, act by stimulating the β-cell to increase the release of insulin. Interaction between the drug and its receptors on the β-cell membrane initiates a series of intracellular biochemical changes resulting first in the immediate release of pre-formed insulin granules adjacent to the β-cell membrane, mimicking the first-phase response. Translocation of insulin granules from within the cell to the membrane results in a second phase–like release of insulin. In vitro studies of term placentas have found no to minimal transplacental transfer of glyburide. Glyburide was undetected in cord blood of infants of women who took the drug in one other study. Because of the long duration of action (peak 4 h; total 24 h postingestion) and because the action of the drug is independent of blood glucose concentrations, maternal hypoglycemia is a potential complication of glyburide. Timing of administration relative to meals is therefore critical. Most investigators have begun treatment with 2.5 mg glyburide before breakfast, adding another 2.5 mg before dinner, and then progressively adding incremental doses at either or both times, depending on maternal glycemic response. There are insufficient data on the administration of glyburide during the first trimester to comment on its potential as a teratogen. However, a retrospective analysis of women who took different sulfonylurea drugs during early pregnancy found no increased risk of teratogenesis. In randomized controlled trials, cohort studies, and case series of women who had GDM and who were treated with glyburide, the incidence of LGA neonates, maternal and/or neonatal hypoglycemia, and failure of the drug to achieve maternal glycemic goals varied. These differences may be explained by differences in diagnostic thresholds used to define GDM, maternal age, levels of maternal glycemia used to indicate use of the drug, when in gestation the drug was initiated, and targeted glucose values.

Continuation of glyburide by the breast-feeding mother was analyzed in a small patient sample of type 2 diabetic mothers and their neonates. Four hours after administration of 5 mg of glyburide, no drug was detected in either maternal serum or breast milk. No hypoglycemia was found in breast-fed neonates.

Metformin. Metformin is the only biguanide drug currently available in the U.K. and the U.S. The biguanides act by decreasing insulin resistance and are therefore classified as insulin sensitizers. Metformin's principal site of action is the liver, where it reduces excessive hepatic glucose production by decreasing gluconeogenesis and increasing glycogenesis. At the level of the skeletal muscle, it enhances glucose uptake and oxidation and increases muscle glycogen synthesis and storage. Its half-life is 2–5 h, and it is 90% eliminated by 12 h after ingestion. Unlike glyburide, its glucose-lowering effect does not cause hypgoglycemia, and it is therefore best described as an anti-hyperglycemic rather than hypoglycemic drug.

An in vitro study using third-trimester placentas found a rapid (<2 min) transit time from maternal to fetal circulations, with the concentration of metformin on the fetal side about half of that in the maternal circulation. No significant differences in drug transfer were found between placentas of women who did or did not have GDM. Another study found no differences in glucose concentrations on the fetal side of the placenta between those that were or were not perfused with metformin on the maternal side.

In a randomized controlled trial comparing metformin with insulin in women who had GDM, there were no significant between-group differences in a composite outcome including prematurity, birth trauma, neonatal hypoglycemia, and respiratory distress. However, to achieve this outcome, 46% of the group treated with metformin required supplementation with insulin. Because of some evidence of a reduction in spontaneous abortions when the drug is continued through first trimester in women who have polycystic ovary syndrome (PCOS), some case series have been published looking at the drug's effect in the first trimester. These uncontrolled data suggest no increase in teratogenicity incurred by the use of metformin. Other observational data from women who have PCOS suggest that administration of metformin from early pregnancy on may reduce the incidence of GDM. Confirmation of these observations awaits the execution of well-designed, adequately powered, randomized controlled trials.

There are a few reports of low concentrations of metformin in breast milk and no infant hypoglycemia in infants of lactating mothers taking metformin. One trial found no differences at ages 3 and 6 months in weight, height, and motor and social development between breast-fed infants of women taking metformin compared with formula-fed control subjects.

Antepartum Testing

As term approaches, most obstetricians will begin testing for fetal well-being. When in gestation such testing should begin and how often it should be repeated is a function of practice style and published protocols. Testing should not begin, however, before neonatal survival is possible. Likely the most commonly used tests include assessment of fetal heart rate (e.g., nonstress testing) and amniotic fluid volume assessment. When these tests are nonreassuring, they are usually promptly followed by further ultrasound assessment (e.g., biophysical profile, Doppler studies of flow through cord artery, middle cerebral artery, ductus venosus, maternal uterine artery, etc.). Reassuring tests are highly predictive of fetal well-being. Unfortunately a nonreassuring test or sequence of tests is not as reliable a predictor of the absence of fetal well-being. It must be noted, however, that no fetal testing protocol has been submitted to a prospective randomized controlled trial.

TREATMENT OF DIABETES DURING THIRD TRIMESTER, LABOR, AND DELIVERY

When to Deliver

There are two arguments for delivering prior to 40 weeks. One is that, given the increased risk of a large baby in a diabetic woman, intrapartum complications related to fetal macrosomia (e.g., shoulder dystocia, brachial plexus injury, humoral and clavicular fractures, intrapartum fetal death, maternal vaginal lacerations, and perineal damage) may be prevented with delivery prior to term. The counterarguments are that a large proportion of shoulder dystocias occur in diabetic women whose neonates weigh <4,000–4,500 g and that the majority of births to women whose babies have excessive growth are unaccompanied by shoulder dystocia.

The second argument for delivery prior to term is prevention of intrauterine fetal demise in pregnancies complicated by diabetes. Though rare, this complication is seen more often in women who have poor glycemic control.

Only one controlled trial in which insulin-requiring diabetic women were randomized to either induction of labor at 38 weeks or expectant management has been published. While those in the expectantly managed group delivered a week later and had significantly larger babies than those electively induced, there were no statistically significant differences in the incidence of cesarean delivery or shoulder dystocia between groups.

Analysis of amniotic fluid to predict fetal pulmonary maturity for deliveries prior to term was a standard practice for some years. Two major developments

Table 5.4 Preparation for and Management of Delivery

1. Consideration of amniocentesis if
   a. Poor glycemic control
   b. Poor confirmation of dates, or dates unknown
2. If steroids are administered, close observation and control of maternal glycemia for up to 24 h after the last dose are recommended
   a. Maternal glycemia checks every 1–2 h
   b. IV: D₅LR at 125 ml/h
   c. IV piggyback insulin with adjustments pending maternal glycemia checks
3. For elective delivery.
   a. On evening before delivery:
      – Usual intermittent-dose insulin and meal plan until midnight
      – Only water by mouth after midnight
      – If using intermittent insulin dosing,

   do not take any after midnight
      – If using CSII, do not program morning bolus
   b. On day of delivery.
      – Check blood glucose before starting IV
      – IV: D₅LR at 125 ml/h
      – Continuous IV piggyback insulin starting at 1.0 units/h, as needed
      – Check blood glucose hourly until within desired range, then every 2–4 h
      – Pending glucose results, adjust IV insulin infusion up or down from prior dose by 0.2 units/h
4. If patient presents in labor and has taken her insulin that day, manage as in 3b above, except check glucose hourly.

made these tests less necessary. One was the advent of accurate sonographic confirmation of gestational age when performed early in pregnancy. The second was a series of developments for the treatment of neonatal respiratory distress syndrome, reducing morbidity and mortality from that disease. Although unsupported by hard data, elective delivery at 38 weeks for the woman who has diabetes without prior amniotic fluid analysis seems reasonable if she has acceptable glycemic control and has good confirmation of dates.

Route of Delivery

The relative merits of elective cesarean delivery versus induction of labor for diabetic women versus awaiting spontaneous onset of labor have been debated for some time. Central to the debate is the observation from several studies that estimates of fetal weight, whether by ultrasound or obstetrician's or mother's clinical estimates, is highly inaccurate. Neither induction of labor nor cesarean is devoid of risk. No data are currently available to resolve this conundrum. However, the American College of Obstetricians and Gynecologists (ACOG) recommends consideration of cesarean delivery when the estimated weight of the fetus of a diabetic woman is >4,500 g. For women using multiple-dose insulin who are having an elective induction and those having an elective cesarean delivery, it is best to have neither food nor insulin after midnight of the night preceding delivery. For those using an insulin pump, the basal infusion rate should be continued overnight.

Intrapartum Glycemic Control

Neonatal glycemia is inversely related to maternal intrapartum glucose concentrations. One study of women who had pregestational diabetes found that the incidence of neonatal hypoglycemia was more reliably predicted by maternal hyperglycemia prior to the onset of labor, but that the severity of hypoglycemia was more accurately predicted by intrapartum maternal hyperglycemia. Whereas monitoring of maternal glucose during labor is likely unnecessary for women whose glucose is maintained during pregnancy by diet alone, all others who require either oral hypoglycemic agents or insulin may benefit from intrapartum glucose monitoring. ACOG recommends maintaining intrapartum glucose between 70 and 110 mg/dl. In labor, maintenance of maternal glycemia within these parameters may be maintained with piggyback intravenous infusion of insulin for all but the woman who uses an insulin pump and would like to continue its use during labor. The latter may have her dose adjusted as labor progresses.

CONCLUSIONS

Although the past few years have seen some advances in knowledge about and application of care for women who have diabetes, more work needs to be done. Better methods need be developed to educate reproductive-age women about the importance of preconception evaluation and control of their diabetes and to make such services as well as contraceptive information and materials universally available. Randomized controlled trials should be performed to better determine the relationship between measures of maternal glycemia during pregnancy and labor and clinically important outcomes. The development of insulin pumps allows the administration of this hormone to change with changing patterns of eating and activity. Continuous subcutaneous glucose monitors have provided new insights into diurnal fluctuations in maternal glucose values. Particularly for pregnant women who have type 1 diabetes, the development of effective communication between continuous pumps and glucose monitors may lead to more physiological control of diabetes during pregnancy, labor and delivery, and beyond.

REFERENCES

Ben-Haroush A, Yogev Y, Chen R, Rosenn B, Hod M, Langer O: The postprandial glucose profile in the diabetic pregnancy. *Am J Obstet Gynecol* 191:576–581, 2004

Carr DB, Koontz GL, Gardella C, et al.: Diabetic nephropathy in pregnancy: suboptimal hypertensive control associated with preterm delivery. *Am J Hypertens* 19:513–519, 2006

Catalano P, Thomas A, Huston-Presley L, Amini SB: Increased fetal adiposity: a very sensitive marker of abnormal in utero development. *Am J Obstet Gynecol* 189:1698–1704, 2003

Churchill JA, Berendes HW, Nemore J: Neuropsychological deficits in children of diabetic mothers. *Am J Obstet Gynecol* 105:257–268, 1969

Committee on the Impact of Pregnancy Weight on Maternal and Child Health, National Research Council Institute of Medicine: *Influence of Pregnancy Weight on Maternal and Child Health: Workshop Report.* Washington, DC, National Academies Press, 2007

Couch SC, Philipson EH, Bendel RB, Pujda LM, Milvae RA, Lammi-Keefe CJ: Elevated lipoprotein lipids and gestational hormones in women with diet-treated gestational diabetes mellitus compared to healthy pregnant controls. *J Diabetes Complications* 12:1–9, 1998

del Mar Colon M, Hibbard JU: Obstetric considerations in the management of pregnancy in kidney transplant recipients. *Adv Chronic Kidney Dis* 14:168–177, 2007

Farrer D, Tuffnell DJ, West J: Continuous subcutaneous insulin infusion versus multiple daily injections of insulin for pregnancy women with diabetes. *Cochrane Database System Rev* no. CD00541, 2007 [DOI: 10.1002/14651858. CD005542.pub2.]

Feig D, Briggs GG, Koren G: Oral antidiabetic agents in pregnancy and lactation: a paradigm shift? *Ann Pharmacother* 41:1174–1180, 2007

Fischer MJ: Chronic kidney disease and pregnancy: maternal and fetal outcomes. *Adv Chronic Kidney Dis* 14:132–145, 2007

Greene MF: Spontaneous abortions and major malformations in women with diabetes mellitus. *Semin Reprod Endocrinol* 17:127–136, 1999

Gunderson EP: Gestational diabetes and nutritional recommendations. *Curr Diab Rep* 4:377–386, 2004

Hawkins JS, Casey BM. Labor and delivery management for women with diabetes. *Obstet Gynecol Clin N Am* 34:323–334, 2007

Hod M, Damm P, Kaaja R, Visser GH, Dunne F, Demidova I, Hansen AS, Mersebach H, Insulin Aspart Pregnancy Study Group: Fetal and perinatal outcomes in type 1 diabetes pregnancy: a randomized study comparing insulin aspart with human insulin in 322 subjects. *Am J Obstet Gynecol* 198:e1–e7, 2008

Kitzmiller JL, Block JM, Brown FM, Catalano PM, Conway DL, Coustan DR, Gunderson EP, Herman WH, Hoffman LD, Inturrisi M, Jovanovic LB, Kjos SI, Knopp RH, Montoro MN, Ogata ES, Paramsothy P, Reader DM, Rosenn BM, Thomas AM, Kirkman MS: Managing preexisting diabetes for pregnancy: summary of evidence and consensus recommendations for care. *Diabetes Care* 31:1060–1079, 2008

Langer O, Conway DL, Berkus MD, Zenakis EMJ, Gonzales O: A comparison of glyburide and insulin in women with gestational diabetes mellitus. *N Engl J Med* 343:1134, 2000

Lapolla A, Dalfrà MG, Fedele D: Insulin therapy in pregnancy complicated by diabetes: are insulin analogs a new tool? *Diabetes Metab Res Rev* 21:241–252, 2005

Major CA, Henry MJ, deVeciana M, Morgan MA: The effects of carbohydrate restriction in patients with diet-controlled gestational diabetes. *Obstet Gynecol* 91:600–604, 1998

Metzger BE: Diet and medical therapy in the optimal management of gestational diabetes mellitus. *Nestle Nutr Workshop Ser Clin Perform Programme* 11:155–165, 2006

Modestin MA, Ananth CV, Smulian JC, Vintzileos AM: Birth weight and fetal death in the United States: the effect of maternal diabetes during pregnancy. *Am J Obstet Gynecol* 187:922–926, 2002

Naeye RL, Chez RA: Effects of maternal acetonuria and low pregnancy weight gain on children's psychomotor development. *Am J Obstet Gynecol* 139:189–193, 1981

Rizzo T, Metzger BE, Burns WJ, Burns K: Correlations between antepartum maternal metabolism and intelligence of offspring. *N Engl J Med* 325:911–916, 1991

Singh C, Jovanovic L: Insulin analogues in the treatment of diabetes in pregnancy. *Obstet Gynecol Clin North Am* 34:275–291, 2007

Solomon CG, Seely EW: Hypertension in pregnancy: a manifestation of the insulin resistance syndrome? *Hypertension* 37:232–239, 2001

Star J, Carpenter MW: The effect of pregnancy on the natural history of diabetic retinopathy and nephropathy. *Clin Perinatol* 23:897–916, 1998

Stehbens JE, Baker GL, Kitchell M: Outcome at ages 1, 3, and 5 years of children born to diabetic women. *Am J Obstet Gynecol* 127:408–413, 1977

Yogev Y, Ben-Haroush A, Chen R, Rosenn B, Hod M, Langer O: Diurnal glucose profile in obese and normal weight nondiabetic pregnant women. *Am J Obstet Gynecol* 191:949–953, 2004

Yogev Y, Xenakis EMJ, Langer O: The association between preeclampsia an the severity of gestational diabetes: the impact of glycemic control. *Am J Obstet Gynecol* 191:1655–1660, 2004

Dr. Sacks is an adjunct investigator of the Department of Research, Southern California Permanente Medical Group, Pasadena, California, and Clinical Professor of Obstetrics and Gynecology at the Keck School of Medicine, University of Southern California, Los Angeles, California.

6. Infants of Mothers with Diabetes

CRISTINA S. CANDIDO, MD, AND MARK A. SPERLING, MD

Preexisting diabetes complicates ~0.4–0.7% of all pregnancies. In 5–9% of all pregnant women, gestational diabetes (GDM) develops. As the prevalence of diabetes in pregnancy continues to increase, awareness of the importance of optimal diabetes control before and during conception must be promoted to achieve optimal outcomes for the mother and the newborn. Experience suggests that the best outcomes are more likely to occur in specialized units with dedicated teams of caregivers.

A diabetic intrauterine environment is rich in glucose, amino acids, and ketones. The relative concentrations of these nutrients vary depending on the metabolic control of the mother. A state of absolute inadequate maternal insulin production or relative inadequate insulin combined with deficient sensitivity to insulin's actions leads to hyperglycemia and sets the stage for "fuel-mediated teratogenesis." This leads to numerous possible fetal and neonatal complications. Rates of congenital malformations in infants born to diabetic mothers (IDM) with poorly controlled diabetes before conception are 4- to 10-fold higher compared to the general population. Stillbirths are five times more common, and perinatal mortality is four- to sevenfold higher. Offspring of diabetic mothers are also more likely to develop obesity and glucose intolerance later in life. There is irrefutable evidence that the risks of all complications (Table 6.1) are related to the degree of maternal metabolic control. Management begins from preconceptional planning until after delivery and beyond, when the offspring of a diabetic mother should continue to be followed closely for metabolic risks.

PATHOPHYSIOLOGY

The mechanisms involved in fetal and neonatal complications in diabetic pregnancies are not completely understood but are likely multifactorial. A proposed schema of pathophysiology of abnormalities in the infant of a diabetic mother is shown in Fig. 6.1. Inadequate insulin leads to maternal hyperglycemia; maternal glucose and other nutrients freely cross the placenta, but free insulin does not. In response to the constant increased provision of glucose, the fetal pancreas undergoes hyperplasia and hypertrophy and produces more insulin, which promotes increased growth and adiposity, leading to macrosomia. In turn, macrosomia

Table 6.1 Stigmata of the IDM and Possible Causes

PROBLEM	MECHANISM/CAUSE
Stillbirth	Placental insufficiency Hyperglycemia Hypoxia Congenital anomalies
Congenital malformations	Hyperglycemia Genetic linkage Insulin? Vascular accident?
Macrosomia	Hyperinsulinism
Hypoglycemia	Hyperinsulinism Decreased glucose and fat mobilization
Hyaline membrane disease (RDS Type 1)	Insulin antagonism of surfactant synthesis
Wet lung syndrome (RDS Type 2)	Cesarean section
Polycythemia	Fetal hypoxia Decreased oxygen delivery to fetus Increased erythropoiesis
RVT	Polycythemia Dehydration Birth asphyxia
Hyperbilirubinemia	Fetal hypoxia Increased erythropoietic mass Increased hemolysis Immature hepatic conjugation Oxytocin administration
Hypocalcemia	Prematurity Hypomagnesemia Decreased PTH secretion
Neonatal small left colon syndrome	Immature GI motility
Cardiomyopathy/cardiomegaly	Septal hypertrophy, transient Hyperglycemia-related oxidative stress

GI, gastrointestinal.

increases the risk for birth trauma and asphyxia. Increased insulin concentrations delay fetal lung maturity by decreasing surfactant production, contributing to respiratory distress. Fetal hyperinsulinemia can also lead to neonatal hypoglycemia precipitated by the cutting of the umbilical cord, which instantly curtails the source of glucose from the mother. This fall of blood glucose in the newborn is more profound if maternal hyperglycemia is exaggerated by excessive glucose infusion during labor.

Fetal asphyxia is thought to be a common pathway contributing to fetal compromise and death. Proposed pathophysiologic changes implicated in fetal asphyxia include *1*) changes in chorionic villi basement membrane, which decrease oxygen transfer; *2*) maternal diabetic vasculopathy and poor glycemic control, which lead to decreased uterine blood flow; and *3*) metabolic changes, particularly hyperinsulinemia, which increases fetal oxygen consumption and decreases arterial oxygen saturation levels. These changes also contribute to a state of chronic

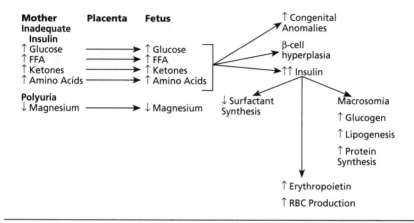

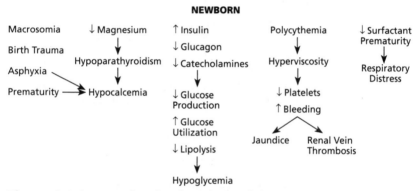

Figure 6.1 Proposed pathophysiology of abnormalities in an IDM. FFA, free fatty acid.

hypoxia in the fetus of a diabetic mother with poor metabolic control. Chronic fetal hypoxia is evidenced by studies of stillborn IDMs who demonstrate extramedullary hematopoiesis and elevated erythropoietin concentrations, leading to a state of hyperviscosity. Hyperviscosity may then predispose to hyperbilirubinemia and renal vein thrombosis (RVT), which occur more commonly in IDMs than in infants born to healthy mothers. Hyperviscosity also contributes to neonatal hypoglycemia via increased glucose consumption by red blood cells.

FETAL/NEONATAL COMPLICATIONS AND MANAGEMENT

Fetal Malformations

Maternal hyperglycemia during the first few weeks of pregnancy (period of organogenesis), as seen in poorly controlled preexisting diabetes, is strongly asso-

Table 6.2 Congenital Malformations in IDMs

Caudal regression syndrome
Situs inversus
Anencephaly
Spina bifida
Renal agenesis
Cystic kidney, ureter duplex
Cardiac anomalies (transposition of great vessels, VSD, ASD)
Anal/rectal atresia

ASD, atrial septal defect; VSD, ventricular septal defect.

Table 6.3 Management of the IDM

PROBLEM	MANAGEMENT
DAY 1	
Congenital malformations	Early detection Supportive measures Specific diagnostic modality and corrective treatment
Birth asphyxia	Supportive measures (including ventilatory support)
Birth trauma	Early detection ■ clinical examination ■ radiographic studies Supportive measures Orthopedic or neurosurgical referral, as appropriate
Macrosomia	Specific measures to avoid birth trauma
Cardiomyopathy	Confirmation by echocardiography Supportive measures Corrective surgery, if indicated
Hypoglycemia	Early feeding Intravenous glucose Rarely glucagon
RDS	Prevention ■ avoid prematurity ■ corticosteroids ■ surfactant therapy Supportive and ventilatory therapy
DAYS 2 AND 3	
Hypocalcemia	Calcium and magnesium supplementation
Hyperbilirubinemia	Hydration Phototherapy Exchange transfusion
Polycythemia	Hydration Partial exchange transfusion
RVT	Supportive measures Heparin Surgical management

ciated with spontaneous abortions and congenital malformations (Table 6.2). Caudal regression syndrome is almost exclusively seen in IDMs. Cardiac anomalies such as septal hypertrophy and subaortic stenosis are other examples of conditions seen in IDMs. The exact mechanisms involved in the development of these malformations are undefined but are likely mediated by hyperinsulinemia. Recent animal studies showed that hyperglycemia-related oxidative stress impedes cardiac neural crest cell migration, affecting cardiac outflow tract septation. Other than hyperglycemia, conditions implicated in other congenital problems include hypoglycemia, hyperinsulinemia, prostaglandin synthesis, and genetic factors.

There is evidence that the risk of congenital malformations increases as the degree of maternal metabolic control worsens. Attaining optimal diabetes control before planning a pregnancy is therefore recommended to prevent or decrease the risk of occurrence of these abnormalities. At delivery, a careful physical examination will identify the presence of congenital anomalies and facilitate proper management. Some clinical signs and symptoms may warrant further diagnostic modalities and appropriate referrals to relevant pediatric subspecialties (Table 6.3).

Stillbirth

Stillbirth is commonly defined as fetal death after 20 weeks of gestation. The 2003 National Center for Health Statistics report showed a fetal death rate of 6.23 per 1,000 births in the general population. This risk is increased by about fivefold in diabetic pregnancies. Studies identify uncontrolled hyperglycemia as accounting for ~50% of fetal deaths. Other causes include fetal malformations and aneuploidy, fetal infection, placental malformation or insufficiency, feto-maternal hemorrhage, maternal infection, and maternal vascular disease. In a number of cases, the reason for stillbirths cannot be defined.

Macrosomia

Fetal weight >4,000 g is considered to constitute macrosomia. Diabetes in pregnancy significantly increases the risk of fetal macrosomia, mostly due to fetal hyperinsulinemia as a response to maternal hyperglycemia, promoting growth by stimulating protein synthesis and lipogenesis. The risk of intrauterine death is increased two- to threefold with high birth weight, which contributes to prolonged labor, shoulder dystocia and plexus injury, cesarean delivery, fetal hypoxia, hypoglycemia, and risk of admission to the neonatal intensive care unit. Neonates who weigh >4,500 g are at heightened risk (9.2–24%) for shoulder dystocia even among mothers with normal glucose tolerance. The risk increases to 20–50% if the pregnancy is complicated by diabetes.

In its more severe form, poorly controlled maternal diabetes can lead to placental insufficiency, decreased uterine blood flow, and subsequent decrease in delivery of nutrients and oxygen supply to the fetus. This may lead to fetal intrauterine growth restriction (IUGR) or to a small-for-gestational-age neonate. IUGR in a fetus of a mother with a monogenic form of diabetes, particularly mutation in the glucokinase gene (MODY2), should raise the suspicion of gene transmission. In this case, the fetal glucose-sensing mechanism is impaired, decreasing fetal insulin-mediated growth.

Birth Asphyxia and Birth Injury

IDMs are at risk for birth asphyxia and birth injury. Contributing factors include macrosomia, decreased lung surfactant production, and fetal hypoxia. Expectant management should include preparation to administer standard respiratory support (e.g., oxygen, positive pressure ventilation, endotracheal intubation, if needed). Some premature neonates will require surfactant treatment.

Fetal macrosomia is a major contributing factor to birth injury, but attempts to accurately recognize fetal macrosomia have not been very effective. Despite the aid of ultrasonography, prediction remains imprecise, raising doubt on the value of inducing labor before 40 weeks of gestation in an attempt to avoid macrosomia. The route of delivery also is controversial. It is recommended by the American College of Obstetrics and Gynecology that cesarean section is indicated if the estimated fetal weight is ≥4,500 g. Cesarean section decreases the risk of shoulder dystocia and brachial plexus injury. With limited data on the best mode of delivery of an IDM, the decision should be based on the mother's past obstetrical history, estimated fetal weight, assessment of fetal lung maturity, and other clinical factors. Prolonged second stage of labor or arrest of fetal descent of macrosomic fetuses are other indications for cesarean delivery.

After delivery and stabilization, a careful neonatal physical examination should be done. Brachial plexus injury is suspected in the presence of asymmetry of a neonate's arm movements or Moro reflex. Clinical examination looking for crepitus over the clavicle or humerus, neurological examination, and radiological studies are helpful in identifying bone and nerve injuries. Traumatic deliveries may, at times, lead to brain injuries. If suspected, head ultrasonography or cranial computed tomography scan is warranted for diagnosis. Consultation with a pediatric neurologist and/or orthopedic surgeon is recommended when dealing with birth trauma and injuries.

Hypoglycemia

Ten to 25% of IDMs develop transient hypoglycemia in the first 4–6 h of life. Fetal hyperinsulinemia, as a response to maternal hyperglycemia and hyperaminoacidemia, contributes to hypoglycemia. Neonatal hypoglycemia has traditionally been defined as a blood glucose level <40 mg/dl. Some studies have questioned the physiologic basis of assigning a different normal cutoff value for newborns compared with older children and adults. Because data on long-term neurological outcomes of neonates with a history of hypoglycemia are limited, we recommend treating hypoglycemia with a goal of maintaining blood glucose ≥70 mg/dl. Hypoglycemia can present as poor feeding, apnea, lethargy, jitteriness, and seizure. Some cases are, however, asymptomatic. It is therefore mandatory to monitor all IDMs for hypoglycemia in the first 12–36 h of life. In some cases, early feeding with breast milk or formula suffices to maintain blood glucose. However, intravenous glucose infusion may be necessary. If necessary, intravenous glucose is given initially as a bolus of 2 ml/kg body wt of 10% dextrose followed by infusion at 5–15 mg • kg body wt^{-1} • min^{-1} to maintain blood glucose ≥70 mg/dl. The subsequent rate depends on the rate of glucose rise. Rarely, glucagon can be administered if intravenous access is not available. Side effects of glucagon include rebound hypoglycemia and vomiting.

Hypoglycemia secondary to maternal diabetes, per se, is usually transient and remitting, occurring in the first 3 days of life. Prolonged neonatal hypoglycemia can be seen in an IDM who also has a history of perinatal stress, such as prematurity or birth asphyxia. The underlying pathology is still hyperinsulinism. These cases are usually responsive to medical therapy with diazoxide at a dose of 5–15 mg • kg body wt^{-1} • day^{-1}.

Respiratory Distress Syndrome

IDMs are predisposed to developing respiratory distress syndrome (RDS) or hyaline membrane disease. Hyperglycemia and hyperinsulinemia are implicated in delaying fetal lung maturity by decreasing surfactant production. Prediction of fetal lung maturity is done through measurement of lecithin-to-sphingomyelin (L-to-S) ratio in the amniotic fluid. An L-to-S ratio of >2:1 indicates fetal lung maturity. This, however, is not always true in diabetic pregnancies. Secretion of fetal lung fluid may be affected in diabetic pregnancies, leading to increased removal of phospholipids from the alveolar lining, which falsely increases the L-to-S ratio. The presence of phosphatidylglycerol is a more reliable marker of fetal lung maturity. Its absence, however, does not equate to immaturity of the fetal lungs. Management of RDS includes surfactant therapy, judicious use of glucocorticoids to enhance lung maturation, arterial blood gas monitoring, and supportive measures.

Wet lung syndrome (also referred to as RDS2 or transient tachypnea of the newborn) is seen more commonly in IDMs. Cesarean delivery accounts for a big proportion of this syndrome. Some propose that an intrauterine diabetic state may cause alterations in secretion and absorption of fetal lung fluid that increases predisposition to wet lung syndrome.

Polycythemia

Delayed cord clamping or intrauterine hypoxia can contribute to polycythemia. Poor maternal metabolic control induces a state of chronic fetal hypoxia, which drives fetal erythropoiesis. The resulting polycythemia can increase the risk for hyperviscosity, hyperbilirubinemia, and RVT. Neonatal polycythemia is defined as a hematocrit (Hct) ≥65%. Some infants may be asymptomatic. Clinical signs include plethora, cyanosis, and, at times, pallor. Poor feeding, jitteriness, apnea, and lethargy may be seen. Hypoglycemia is commonly observed. Partial exchange transfusion is recommended if the Hct is >70% or if the neonate is symptomatic with Hct >65%. The goal is to bring Hct down to ~50–55%. Asymptomatic newborns with Hct between 65 and 70% can generally be managed with intravenous fluids and supportive treatment.

The formula to calculate the volume of blood to be exchanged is as follows:

$$\text{Volume of exchange} = \left(\frac{\text{Observed Hct} - \text{Desired Hct}}{\text{Observed Hct}}\right) \times \text{Blood volume}$$

$$\text{Blood volume} = 80 \text{ ml/kg} \times \text{body weight in kg}$$

Renal Vein Thrombosis

Polycythemia and hypercoagulability may lead to RVT. This entity is, however, rare in IDMs. If it occurs, prognosis is poor for the affected kidney. RVT is usually unilateral. There is evidence that it is more common on the left kidney. It is seen in the second or third day of life with variable presenting features. The classical triad of RVT, which may not always be seen at presentation, include presence of a palpable abdominal mass, macroscopic hematuria, and thrombocytopenia. Other signs and symptoms include vomiting, fever, shock, albuminuria, and leukocytosis. The diagnosis of RVT is confirmed via ultrasound. Recent management trends include use of low-molecular-weight heparin over unfractionated heparin. Most cases are, however, managed through supportive measures with fluid, electrolytes, and antibiotics. A small proportion of patients require surgical intervention. A multidisciplinary team approach is always recommended. Neonates who develop RVT should be followed for development of hypertension, renal insufficiency, atrophy, or functional loss.

Hyperbilirubinemia

Several factors may contribute to predisposition to hyperbilirubinemia in IDMs. These include prematurity or inadequate glucuronyl transferase activity, increased frequency of birth injuries leading to absorption of hematomas, increased hemolysis, and increased fetal erythropoiesis due to fetal hypoxia. Management includes hydration and/or phototherapy. Partial exchange transfusion is rarely necessary.

Hypocalcemia and Hypomagnesemia

Hypocalcemia, defined as serum calcium concentration of <7 mg/dl, is common in IDMs. Contributing factors include prematurity, birth asphyxia, and, more commonly, transient neonatal hypoparathyroidism. This hypoparathyroidism is attributed to maternal hypomagnesemia consequent to urinary magnesium losses in poorly controlled diabetes. Hypomagnesemia contributes to decreased parathyroid hormone (PTH) secretion and end organ resistance to PTH, likely through changes in calcium-sensitive, magnesium-dependent activity of adenylate cyclase.

Hypocalcemia is usually noted at day 2–3 of life. Management includes calcium and magnesium supplementation. Serum calcium should be maintained at ≥7 mg/dl. Intravenous calcium is sometimes indicated, particularly in the event of a hypocalcemic seizure. Care should be taken not to infuse calcium too rapidly to avoid bradycardia. Serum calcium, magnesium, and phosphorus should be monitored.

Metabolic Risks

Studies on epigenetic programming show that alterations in the intrauterine environment affect predisposition to pathologic conditions later in life. An intrauterine environment high in glucose with concomitant fetal hyperinsulinemia, as seen in a diabetic pregnancy, can cause lasting fetal changes that increase the risk for later obesity and development of type 2 diabetes. Studies show that children of diabetic mothers have higher prevalence of glucose intolerance, higher systolic and mean arterial blood pressures, higher concentrations of endothelial dysfunction markers, and higher total cholesterol–to–HDL cholesterol ratios compared with offspring of nondiabetic pregnancies, independent of BMI. These children should be identified and periodically monitored to prevent or recognize and manage metabolic abnormalities.

PREVENTIVE MEASURES

Preconceptional Counseling

Women with preexisting diabetes with childbearing potential should be counseled on the value of good metabolic control. Optimal diabetes control and lower A1C at conception decreases the risk for congenital anomalies in the fetus as well as the risk for preeclampsia. A diabetic woman contemplating pregnancy should be evaluated and treated appropriately for hypertension, cardiovascular disease, dyslipidemia, and other diabetic complications and comorbidities. A multidisciplinary patient-centered care team should be made available to the mother. Better maternal and fetal outcomes are achieved in centers where diabetologists, obstetricians, perinatologists, neonatologists, diabetes educators, and dietitians collaborate to provide care for the diabetic woman and her offspring. Services should focus on diet and lifestyle, smoking cessation, folic acid supplementation, assessment and management of complications of diabetes, setting of glycemic targets, and discussion of risks and management strategies.

Physicians should identify pregnant women who are at risk for GDM to facilitate screening between 24 and 28 weeks of gestation and start prompt and appropriate management. Risks for GDM include the following: prepregnancy weight >80 kg or BMI >28 kg/m², family history of type 2 diabetes in a first-degree relative, polycystic ovary syndrome, previous unexplained stillbirth, previous pregnancy with polyhydramnios, and a history of having a macrosomic infant.

Management during Pregnancy

The key management goal is maternal normoglycemia without significant hypoglycemia. Throughout the entire pregnancy, maternal glycemic goals include fasting glucose of 60–99 mg/dl, peak postprandial glucose of 100–129 mg/dl, mean daily glucose of <110 mg/dl, and A1C <6%. Frequent home blood glucose monitoring is advised. Insulin requirement should be frequently assessed because this generally increases as pregnancy advances. Pregnancy, in itself, is a relative state of insulin resistance due to increasing levels of human placental lactogen, growth factors, and certain cytokines.

Other important goals of therapy include provision of individualized medical nutrition therapy coupled with physical activity/exercise; continuation of monitoring and management of complications and comorbidities of diabetes, such as blood pressure monitoring, thyroid function testing, and assessment of renal function; and checking for proteinuria, retinopathy, gastroparesis, and neurological complications. Options for fetal monitoring include an 11- to 13-week nuchal translucency scan, detailed anomaly and fetal cardiac scans at 20 weeks, and regular growth scans at 28, 32, and 36 weeks to evaluate for macrosomia and polyhydramnios.

Care should be taken in the timing of delivery, considering both the risks of prematurity and respiratory distress in early delivery versus macrosomia and its associated complications, particularly birth injury, after 38 weeks of gestation. During delivery, maintenance of maternal normoglycemia is very important because more profound neonatal hypoglycemia is usually observed if the mother has higher serum glucose levels. It should also be noted that maternal insulin requirements generally decrease by half after delivery.

OUTCOMES

Improved awareness, better diabetes screening, and management increased the number of successful diabetic pregnancies. However, IDMs are still fraught with fetal and neonatal complications at much higher rates compared with those of nondiabetic pregnancies. Preconceptional counseling is an essential tool that is underutilized. The importance of tight maternal glycemic control cannot be over-emphasized. With better education, good metabolic control, and multidisciplinary management, perinatal outcomes of infants of diabetic mothers may approach those of the general population.

BIBLIOGRAPHY

Athukorala C, Crowther CA, Willson K, Australian Carbohydrate Intolerance Study in Pregnant Women (ACHOIS) Trial Group: Women with gestational diabetes mellitus in the ACHOIS trial: risk factors for shoulder dystocia. *Aust N Z J Obstet Gynaecol* 47:37–41, 2007

Bell R, Bailey K, Cresswell T, Hawthorne G, Critchley J, Lewis-Barned N, Northern Diabetic Pregnancy Survey Steering Group: Trends in prevalence and outcomes of pregnancy in women with pre-existing type I and type II diabetes. *BJOG* 115:445–452, 2008

Chatfield J: ACOG issues guidelines on fetal macrosomia: American College of Obstetricians and Gynecologists. *Am Fam Physician* 64:169–170, 2001

Dabelea D: The predisposition to obesity and diabetes in offspring of diabetic mothers. *Diabetes Care* 30 (Suppl. 2):S169–S174, 2007

Dudley D: Diabetic-associated stillbirth: incidence, pathophysiology, and prevention. *Clin Perinatol* 34:611–626, 2007

Graves CR: Antepartum fetal surveillance and timing of delivery in the pregnancy complicated by diabetes mellitus. *Clin Obstet Gynecol* 50:1007–1013, 2007

Henriksen T: The macrosomic fetus: a challenge in current obstetrics. *Acta Obstetricia et Gynecologica* 87:134–145, 2008

Kapoor N, Sankaran S, Hyer S, Shehata H: Diabetes in pregnancy: a review of current evidence. *Curr Opin Obstet Gynecol* 19:586–590, 2007

Kitzmiller JL, Block JM, Brown FM, Catalano PM, Conway DL, Coustan DR, Gunderson EP, Herman WH, Hoffman LD, Inturrisi M, Jovanovic LB, Kjos SI, Knopp RH, Montoro MN, Ogata ES, Paramsothy P, Reader DM, Rosenn

BM, Thomas AM, Kirkman MS: Managing preexisting diabetes for pregnancy: summary of evidence and consensus recommendations for care. *Diabetes Care* 31:1060–1079, 2008

Lau KK, Stoffman JM, Williams S, McCusker P, Brandao L, Patel S, Chan AK, Canadian Pediatric Thrombosis and Hemostasis Network: Neonatal renal vein thrombosis: review of the English-language literature between 1992 and 2006. *Pediatrics* 120:e1278–e1284, 2007

Nelson SM, Sattar N, Freeman DJ, Walker JD, Lindsay RS: Inflammation and endothelial activation is evident at birth in offspring of mothers with type 1 diabetes. *Diabetes* 56:2697–2704, 2007

Piazze JJ, Anceschi MM, Maranghi L, Brancato V, Marchiani E, Cosmi EV: Fetal lung maturity in pregnancies complicated by insulin-dependent and gestational diabetes: a matched cohort study. *Eur J Obstet Gynecol Reprod Biol* 83:145–150, 1999

Sperling MA, Menon RK: Infant of the diabetic mother. In *Current Therapy of Diabetes Mellitus*. DeFronzo RA, Ed. Philadelphia, PA, Mosby-Year Book, 1998, p. 237–241

Weintrob N, Karp M, Hod M: Short and long-range complications in offspring of diabetic mothers. *J Diabetes Complications* 10:294–301, 1996

Drs. Candido and Sperling are affiliated with the Department of Pediatric Endocrinology, Metabolism, and Diabetes Mellitus, Children's Hospital of Pittsburgh, University of Pittsburgh School of Medicine, Pittsburgh, Pennsylvania.

7. Diabetic Ketoacidosis in Children

Francine Kaufman, MD

Diabetic ketoacidosis (DKA) is a common occurrence in pediatric patients with type 1 diabetes. In North America and Europe, 15–70% of subjects with type 1 diabetes present with DKA, and in established patients, the risk for DKA is 1–10% per year. Worldwide, there is an inverse correlation between the background incidence of type 1 diabetes and the frequency of DKA. In addition, in pediatric subjects with type 2 diabetes, 33% have ketonuria, and 5–10% have ketoacidosis at diagnosis, with even higher rates described in African-American youth.

DKA is a major source of morbidity and mortality, with 1–2% of patients developing fatal or near-fatal cerebral edema, a complication of DKA and its treatment almost unique to children. As a result, there are aspects of the treatment of DKA that are different in children than in adults, particularly with regard to the rate and composition of initial fluids. The prevention of DKA should be the goal because, despite meticulous attention to its treatment, morbidity and mortality still occur. Hence, DKA accounts for two-thirds of overall childhood diabetes mortality.

DEFINITION

DKA is characterized by the following:

- hyperglycemia with blood glucose usually >300 mg/dl (>17 mmol/l)
- ketonemia with total ketones (β-hydroxybutyrate [β-OHB] and acetoacetate) in serum >3 mmol/l
- acidosis with blood pH <7.3 or serum bicarbonate <15 mEq/l
- hyperosmolar dehydration with serum osmolality >320 mmol/l

Pure lactic acidosis (blood lactate >7 mmol/l), salicylate ingestion, and nonketotic hyperglycemic coma should be distinguished from DKA. Occasionally, DKA can occur with near-normoglycemia. Vomiting and poor intake along with continued insulin therapy induce this condition. Hyperosmolar coma can occur in very young children, children with Down's syndrome or significant developmental delay, and adolescents with type 2 diabetes. Nonketotic hyperosmolar coma has been associated with mortality, particularly in obese adolescents and those with developmental delay at the onset of type 2 diabetes.

PATHOPHYSIOLOGY AND PRESENTATION

The metabolic derangements of DKA result from absolute or relative insulin deficiency amplified by an increased action of the counterregulatory hormones catecholamine, glucagon, cortisol, and growth hormone.

In new-onset patients, signs and symptoms of near-absolute insulin deficiency are often not recognized before the development of DKA. This is particularly true in young children aged <2 years because polyuria is often hard to appreciate prior to toilet training. Infants, children, and teens presenting to the emergency department with altered level of consciousness should have a fingerstick glucose obtained immediately to determine whether diabetes and DKA are present. Individuals presenting with signs and symptoms of the flu should be questioned about antecedent weight loss and polyuria. Failure to consider the diagnosis of diabetes leads to a delay in its diagnosis and a higher incidence of DKA at presentation. In established cases of diabetes, DKA is due to inappropriate sick-day management, intercurrent illness, physical and psychological stress, pump failure, and advertent or inadvertent skipping of insulin doses. Awareness that vomiting is almost universally associated with DKA mandates that, when emesis begins, blood glucose and urine or blood ketones should be tested immediately. If levels are compatible with DKA, immediate action must be taken and contact with the diabetes health care team established so that the safe reversal of early DKA can take place at home.

Normally, insulin is secreted with feeding, and the high-insulin state is associated with anabolism, whereas the fasting low-insulin state is associated with catabolism. Increased counterregulatory hormones compound and accelerate the catabolic state. Acting in concert, these hormones do the following:

- increase glucose production by glycogenolysis and gluconeogenesis (catecholamines, glucagon)
- impair glucose utilization by antagonizing the effects of insulin (catecholamines, cortisol, growth hormone)
- mobilize fatty acids by lipolysis (catecholamines, glucagon, growth hormone)
- induce ketogenesis with accumulation of the organic acids β-hydroxybutyrate (β-OHB) and acetoacetic acid (glucagon)

Excessive production and diminished use of these metabolites lead to hyperglycemia. Polyuria due to osmotic diuresis occurs when the renal threshold of ~180 mg/dl (~10 mmol/l) is exceeded. Osmotic diuresis is associated with electrolyte depletion. Vomiting occurs and dehydration rapidly progresses. Accumulating organic acids leads to metabolic acidosis with some lactic acidosis from poor perfusion and/or sepsis. Coma is the result of hyperosmolarity (>320 mmol/l) and not of acidosis.

CLINICAL MANIFESTATIONS

Clinical manifestations of ketoacidosis include the following:

- signs of dehydration: delayed capillary refill, postural changes of blood pressure and pulse, dry mucous membranes

Table 7.1 Treatment Approach for Patients with DKA

■ Initial approach: in the emergency department
  – Obtain and monitor vital signs, including blood pressure, on all patients.
  – Do a bedside glucose determination to determine glucose level, and then monitor at 30- to 60-min intervals.
  – Assess the degree of hydration and mental status.
  – Obtain a urine sample for glucose and acetone; continue to monitor every void.
  – Draw blood for electrolytes, blood urea nitrogen, venous pH, and complete blood cell count.
  – Start an intravenous line and give 10 ml/kg normal saline over 30–60 min.
  – Bolus bicarbonate therapy is contraindicated.
■ Begin therapy
  – Use 0.45–0.66% normal saline for maintenance (at a rate of 1.5 maintenance fluid requirements [1,500–2,000 ml/m^2]) plus replacement of dehydration over 36–48 h (>2 yr of age: 30 ml/kg for mild deficit, 60 ml/kg for moderate deficit, and 90 ml/kg for severe deficit; <2 yr of age: 50 ml/kg for mild deficit, 100 ml/kg for moderate deficit, and 150 ml/kg for severe deficit).
  – Begin an insulin drip of regular insulin at 0.1 units • kg^{-1} • h^{-1} within 2 h of fluid resuscitation (for younger children, the mildly ill, or within 6 h of subcutaneous dose, use 0.05–0.08 units • kg^{-1} • h^{-1}).
  – Add potassium chloride at 3–5 mEq • kg^{-1} • h^{-1} to intravenous fluids; potassium phosphate is not standard but may be used for half of the potassium dose.
  – Follow laboratory parameters, electrolytes, and pH every 1 h until pH is >7.2, then every 2–4 h, and then every 4–6 h.
  – Add dextrose to the intravenous fluids: 5% glucose when the blood glucose level is between 250 and 300 mg/dl and 10% glucose when the blood glucose level is between 180 and 200 mg/dl. Target the fall in blood glucose level to 80–100 mg • dl^{-1} • h^{-1}.
  – Consider obtaining a urine microscopy/culture, chest X-ray, blood culture, and throat culture.
  – Assess known patients for noncompliance, infection, and trauma.

- signs of acidosis: deep-sighing respirations (Kussmaul) in an attempt to blow off carbon dioxide, shortness of breath, chest pain due to accessory muscle exhaustion
- results of vomiting, dehydration, and hyperosmolality: abdominal pain mimicking pancreatitis or an acute surgical abdomen
- results of counterregulatory hormone release: elevated leukocyte count to 15,000–20,000/mm^3
- signs of hyperosmolality: progressive obtundation and loss of consciousness related to the degree of evolving hyperosmolality

CAVEATS

- Important calculations in DKA:
  o Anion gap = Na – (Cl + HCO$_3$): normal is 12 ± 2 mmol/l
    ▪ In DKA, the anion gap is typically 20–30 mmol/l; an anion gap >35 mmol/l suggests concomitant lactic acidosis

- o Serum sodium correction = add 1.6 mEq sodium for each 100 mg plasma glucose >100 mg/dl to the measured serum sodium value.

  - Corrected sodium = measured Na + $2\times\left(\dfrac{\text{glucose} - 100}{100}\right)$ mg/dl

  - Corrected sodium = measured Na + $2\times\left(\dfrac{\text{glucose} - 5.6}{5.6}\right)$ mmol/l

- o Effective osmolality calculated as mOsm = $2(\text{Na} + \text{K})$ mEq/l + $\dfrac{\text{glucose (mg/dl)}}{18}$

  - $2\times(\text{Na} + \text{K})$ + glucose (mmol/l): normal is 285 ± 5

- The degree of sodium loss may be overestimated because of the presence of hyperlipidemia and hyperglycemia. For each increase in glucose of 100 mg/dl (5.5 mmol/l), serum sodium may be decreased by ~2 mEq/l. An increase in corrected serum sodium is a goal of therapy.
- Serum potassium may be normal, but total-body potassium is commonly depleted. During acidosis, intracellular potassium moves to the extracellular compartment and may be lost in urine or vomitus. Hyperkalemia in DKA is therefore uncommon unless renal shutdown has occurred. In contrast, hypokalemia may develop rapidly after treatment is initiated because the provision of insulin in the presence of hyperglycemia and the correction of acidosis promote the return of potassium to the intracellular compartment. Hypokalemia may be life threatening in its predilection for cardiac arrhythmias; therefore, provision of potassium and monitoring of its plasma concentration is paramount in treating DKA.
- Ketone bodies may cause spurious elevation in creatinine values in some assays. Urine and blood ketone tests measure different metabolites: urine ketone tests measure acetoacetate, and blood ketone tests measure β-OHB. Because β-OHB is the predominant ketone body in DKA, urine measurement may give false-negative results. The concentration of β-OHB is 4- to 10-fold higher than that of acetoacetic acid at initial presentation. With correction of acidosis, the β-OHB is oxidized back to acetoacetate and is now measured. Hence, physicians should not be misled by the persistence of a strong ketone reaction as long as the patient manifests evidence of clinical and biochemical improvement in acidosis.
- Ketoacidosis takes longer to correct than hyperglycemia. Therefore, insulin therapy should not be discontinued if ketoacidosis has not cleared, even if glucose concentrations are approaching 300 mg/dl (17 mmol/l). Glucose should be provided in the intravenous solutions because the provision of substrate in the form of intravenous glucose and insulin will reverse ketogenesis.
- The provision of excessive chloride is almost inevitable and usually presents no problem, although it can lead to hyperchloremic acidosis in the recovery phase of ketoacidosis. The provision of some of the potassium deficit as potassium phosphate has certain theoretical and possible practical benefits. Potassium acetate has also been used. Acetate provides substrate to correct acidosis.

MANAGEMENT

Table 7.1 outlines the management approach to DKA, which includes correcting hyperglycemia, dehydration, and electrolyte disturbances using intravenous fluids, electrolytes, and insulin. Treatment protocols for adults advocate more rapid and aggressive reversal of DKA than what is recommended for children.

- The initial management is usually begun in the emergency department with isotonic saline. Recommendations vary from 10 to 20 ml/kg of isotonic saline during the first hour, followed by repeat boluses if the patient remains in hypovolemic shock.
- The patient should then be transferred to an appropriate inpatient unit, likely an intensive care unit, where the goal of treatment is to gradually correct the metabolic disturbances of the patient over the ensuing 36–48 h (Table 7.2).
- Within 2 h of presentation, intravenous insulin treatment at a dosage of 0.1 units/kg body wt/h should be begun. A lower dosage of 0.05–0.08 units • kg body wt^{-1} • h^{-1} should be considered for children <2 years of age, for those who have had prior insulin administration, and for those mildly ill. Hourly bedside blood glucose determinations help achieve the goal of lowering glucose by 50–100 mg • dl^{-1} • h^{-1}. As the glucose levels start to fall, 5 or 10% dextrose is added to the infusion to avoid rapidly lowering the glucose level and to help stabilize blood glucose concentrations between 150 and 200 mg/dl within the first 12–24 h. Maximal substrate (10% dextrose) and intravenous insulin will reverse ketogenesis, halt hepatic glucose production, and facilitate peripheral glucose uptake.
- After the initial fluid bolus(es), subsequent fluid management should be with a solution with tonicity ≥0.45 saline. This can be achieved with 0.9–0.75% saline, by a balanced salt solution such as Ringer's lactate, or with 0.45% saline with added potassium. IV rate should allow for correction of dehydration evenly over at least 48 h, without replacement of urinary losses. The IV infusion rate should be 1.5–2 times the usual daily requirements based on age, weight, or surface area (1,500 ml/m^2 per 24 h); use of effective osmolality may guide fluid and electrolyte replacement.
- Patients with DKA have total-body potassium depletion. This depletion can be corrected by infusing potassium chloride at 3 mEq • kg body wt^{-1} • day^{-1}, started after the patient is transferred. Potassium levels drop during the first 12–24 h concomitant with correction of acidosis and as potassium enters the cells. Potassium infusion often needs to be increased to maintain serum lev-

Table 7.2 Criteria for Admission to the Intensive Care Unit

■ pH <7.2	■ Prior administration of excess fluids with rapid dropping of glucose level
■ Age <2 yr	
■ Unconscious or other neurological symptoms	■ Low corrected serum sodium
	■ Administration of bolus bicarbonate
■ Blood glucose >800–1,000 mg/dl (>43–55 mmol/l)	

Management of Pediatric Patients (<20 years) with DKA* or HHS†

Complete initial evaluation‡. Start IV fluids: 10–20 ml/kg; 0.9% NaCl in the initial hour.

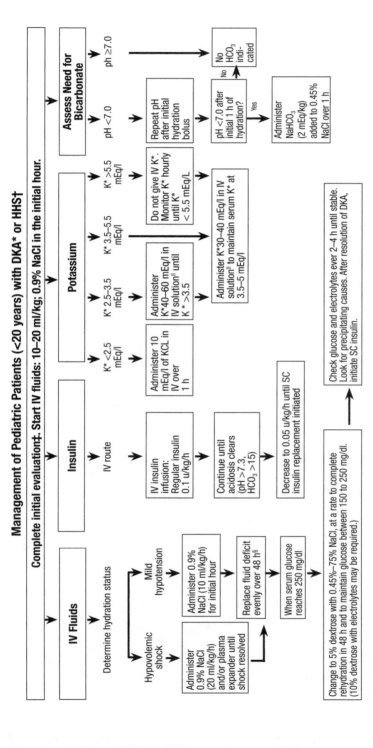

IV Fluids

Determine hydration status

Mild hypotension → Administer 0.9% NaCl (10 ml/kg/h) for initial hour

Hypovolemic shock → Administer 0.9% NaCl (20 ml/kg/h) and/or plasma expander until shock resolved

Replace fluid deficit evenly over 48 h§

When serum glucose reaches 250 mg/dl

Change to 5% dextrose with 0.45%–75% NaCl, at a rate to complete rehydration in 48 h and to maintain glucose between 150 to 250 mg/dl. (10% dextrose with electrolytes may be required.)

Insulin

IV route

IV insulin infusion: Regular insulin 0.1 u/kg/h

Continue until acidosis clears (pH >7.3, HCO₃ >15)

Decrease to 0.05 u/kg/h until SC insulin replacement initiated

Potassium

K* <2.5 mEq/l → Administer 10 mEq/l of KCL in IV over 1 h

K* 2.5–3.5 mEq/l → Administer K*40–60 mEq/l in IV solution‖ until K* >3.5

K* 3.5–5.5 mEq/l

K* >5.5 mEq/l → Do not give IV K*. Monitor K* hourly until K* < 5.5 mEq/L

Administer K*30–40 mEq/l in IV solution‖ to maintain serum K* at 3.5–5 mEq/l

Check glucose and electrolytes ever 2–4 h until stable. Look for precipitating causes. After resolution of DKA, initiate SC insulin.

Assess Need for Bicarbonate

pH <7.0

pH ≥7.0 → No HCO₃ indicated

Repeat pH after initial hydration bolus

pH <7.0 after initial 1 h of hydration? No → No HCO₃ indicated

Yes → Administer NaHCO₃ (2 mEq/kg) added to 0.45% NaCl over 1 h

From Kitabchi, 2001. Protocol for the management of pediatric patients (<20 years) with DKA or HHS. *DKA diagnostic criteria: blood glucose >250 mg/dl, venous pH <7.3, bicarbonate <15 mEq/l, and moderate ketonuria or ketonemia. †HHS diagnostic criteria: blood glucose >600 mg/dl, venous pH >7.3, bicarbonate >15 mEq/l, and altered mental status or severe dehydration. ‡After the initial history and physical examination, obtain blood glucose, venous blood gasses, electrolytes, blood urea nitrogen, creatinine, calcium, phosphorous, and urine analysis STAT. §Usually 1.5 times the 24-h maintenance requirements (~5 ml/kg/h) will accomplish a smooth rehydration; do not exceed two times the maintenance requirement. ‖The potassium in solution should be 1/3 KPO₄ and 2/3 KCl or K acetate.

Table 7.3 Signs, Symptoms, and Treatment of Cerebral Edema

Signs and symptoms

In children <10 yr old (especially children <5 yr old), anticipate possible clinical cerebral edema after 4–6 h of treatment. Remember that many children have some change in affect or increase in irritability. For example:

- Headache
- Change in consciousness level/response
- Unequal dilated pupils
- Delirium
- Incontinence
- Vomiting
- Bradycardia

Treatment

- Treat on clinical basis rather than waiting on imaging.
- Reduce intravenous infusion rate.
- Give mannitol 1 g/kg i.v. (or 10–20 g/m²). Repeat in 2–4 h.
- Consider intubation.

els >3.5 mEq/l. In severe hypokalemia, a cardiac monitor should be used to assess the development of U waves and arrhythmia. If the patient requires >4–5 mEq • kg body wt^{-1} • day^{-1}, half of the infusion can be given as potassium phosphate and/or acetate.

- The use of bolus bicarbonate in DKA is contraindicated. Hydration and insulin therapy alone will correct the acidosis; bolus bicarbonate places the patient at risk for paradoxical central nervous system acidosis, cardiac arrhythmias, and hyperosmolality. If used, it should be given at a rate of 1 mEq/kg over 2–4 h of $NaHCO_3$. Rechecking the pH level after the initial provision of a bolus of fluids may document a change in pH sufficient to make further treatment unnecessary.

- Close monitoring of the status of the patient must occur. Obtain hourly bedside blood glucose levels (laboratory values are required if blood glucose is >600 mg/dl). Record accurate input and output of fluid, along with urine glucose, ketones, and specific gravity, with each void. Observe electrolytes and acid-base status at 2-h intervals initially and then at 4- to 6-h intervals. Follow clinical progress and neurological status. Mannitol is available so that it can be rapidly administered at the first sign of neurological deterioration. Children with severe DKA (long duration of symptoms, compromised circulation, or depressed level of consciousness) or those who are at increased risk for cerebral edema (e.g., <5 years of age, severe acidosis, low PCO_2, high urea nitrogen) should be treated in an intensive care unit (pediatric, if available) or in a unit that has equivalent resources and supervision, such as a children's ward specializing in diabetes care.

COMPLICATIONS

Electrolyte Changes

Inappropriate levels of serum electrolytes, particularly hyperkalemia and hypokalemia, hypophosphatemia, and hypocalcemia from too-vigorous use of phosphate replacement, can be avoided by scrupulous monitoring and appropriate

Table 7.4 Method of Clinical Diagnosis for Cerebral Edema

Diagnostic criteria

Abnormal motor or verbal response to pain

Decorticate or decerebrate posture

Cranial nerve palsy (especially III, IV, and VI)

Abnormal neurogenic respiratory pattern (e.g., grunting, tachypnea, Cheyne-Stokes respiration, apneusis)

Major criteria

Altered mentation/fluctuating level of consciousness

Sustained heart rate deceleration (decrease >20 beats/min) not attributable to improved intravascular volume or sleep state

Age-inappropriate incontinence

Minor criteria

Vomiting

Headache

Lethargy or not easily arousable

Diastolic blood pressure >90 mmHg

Age <5 years

adjustment of the electrolyte composition. If acidosis is not resolved, check the composition of the insulin mixture to ensure that an error in dilution has not occurred. If no error is identified, and the acidosis is not resolved, despite appropriate fluids and insulin, consider the coexistence of severe sepsis causing lactic acidosis or another severe intercurrent illness.

Cerebral Edema

Cerebral edema is the gravest complication of DKA. It occurs in 1–2% of DKA episodes, and the rates of morbidity and mortality are high. The onset is usually within 6–12 h after the initiation of treatment, and the warning signs include headache, lethargy, incontinence, seizures, pupillary changes, decreasing heart rate, and increasing blood pressure (Table 7.3). Epidemiological studies have identified several potential risk factors at diagnosis or during treatment of DKA. These include:

- greater hypocapnia at presentation after adjusting for degree of acidosis
- increased serum urea nitrogen at presentation
- more severe acidosis at presentation
- bicarbonate treatment for correction of acidosis
- an attenuated rise in measured serum sodium concentrations during therapy
- greater volumes of fluid given in the first 4 h
- administration of insulin in the first hour of fluid treatment

The above criteria were mainly established from a retrospective multicenter study involving 61 children who developed symptomatic cerebral edema associated with DKA. These subjects were compared with 181 randomly selected children with DKA and 174 children with DKA, matched for age, new-onset versus known case, initial pH, and initial serum glucose concentration. Multivariate statistical methods showed that children with DKA-related cerebral edema had lower initial PCO_2 values and higher serum urea nitrogen concentrations than the control groups. A lesser rise in serum sodium concentration during treatment was seen in children with cerebral edema, although it is unclear whether this was due to therapy itself or to a physiological response to cerebral injury. The administration of bicarbonate bolus was also associated with the development of cerebral edema, suggesting that bicarbonate therapy, for the most part, is contraindicated in children with DKA.

A method of clinical diagnosis based on bedside evaluation of neurological state has been developed to diagnose cerebral edema (Table 7.4). One diagnostic criterion, two major criteria, or one major and two minor criteria have a sensitivity of 92% and a false-positive rate of only 4%.

The pathophysiological basis for the development of cerebral edema is incompletely understood. This complication can occur, despite meticulous attention to these or any other guidelines. Patients have developed cerebral edema before the institution of treatment. Individuals experienced in the treatment of DKA in children recognize that most children experience some mild transitory change in affect, state of alertness, or irritability during the course of treatment; however, only a few manifest clinical cerebral edema. Computed tomography (CT) of the head suggests that most patients with DKA have some evidence of raised intracranial pressure due to narrow ventricles during therapy, which then widen when the patient recovers. A study evaluating magnetic resonance imaging (MRI) in 41 children with DKA showed that the lateral ventricles were significantly smaller during DKA treatment in 22 subjects, and those children with ventricular narrowing were more likely to have mild mental status abnormalities and a lower initial PCO_2 level.

Patients at highest risk for cerebral edema are those aged <5 years, with new-onset diabetes. Clinical manifestations occur several hours after the institution of therapy and after clinical and biochemical indexes have suggested improvement. The symptoms and signs of raised intracranial pressure (e.g., headache, deterioration in conscious state, bradycardia, papilledema, development of fixed dilated pupils, and occasionally polyuria secondary to diabetes insipidus) should alert the physician to the existence of this potentially fatal complication. Once diagnosed, cerebral edema is treated by the administration of mannitol 0.25–1 g/kg IV over 20 min. This is repeated if there is no initial response in 30 min to 2 h. Hypertonic saline (3%), 5–10 ml/kg over 30 min, may be an alternative to mannitol, especially if there is no initial response to mannitol. Intubation may be required, but hyperventilation is not indicated. When instituted promptly (before coma), these measures can be lifesaving and may avoid neurological sequelae. In the case of severe cerebral edema, the use of high-dose dexamethasone therapy should be considered. After stabilization, a cranial CT or MRI scan should be obtained to rule out other possible intracerebral causes of neurological deterioration (~10% of cases), especially thrombosis or hemorrhage, which may benefit from additional therapy. Cerebral edema has been attributed to osmotic swelling. In a study of 14 children during DKA treatment and recovery, assessment of cerebral water distribution and cerebral perfusion showed that the process was predominately vasogenic rather than osmotic.

The most efficient way to decrease the incidence of cerebral edema, and other causes of morbidity and mortality associated with DKA, is by the prevention of DKA altogether. Worldwide studies have shown that DKA rates have been decreasing. This decrease in DKA is likely due to a number of factors, including increasingly effective patient/family education and support in established patients, enhanced public and professional awareness about the signs and symptoms of diabetes, and the need for early diagnosis in new-onset patients. In Parma, Italy, a public awareness campaign, conducted with physicians and schools, essentially eliminated DKA at diabetes onset in children. In the U.S., there is a suggestion that genetic screening combined with monitoring for signs of β-cell autoimmunity has decreased the severity of illness at diagnosis. Strategies should continue to be developed to eliminate DKA in pediatric patients.

BIBLIOGRAPHY

Barker JM, Goehrig SH, Barriga K, Hoffman M, Slover R, Eisenbarth GS, Norris JM, Klingensmith GJ, Rewers M: Clinical characteristics of children diagnosed with type 1 diabetes through intensive screening and follow-up. *Diabetes Care* 27:1399–1404, 2004

Dunger DB, Sperling MA, Acerini CL, Bohn DJ, Daneman D, Danne TP, Glaser NS, Hanas R, Hintz RL, Levitsky LL, Savage MO, Tasker RC, Wolfsdorf JI, European Society for Paediatric Endocrinology, Lawson Wilkins Pediatric Endocrine Society: European Society for Paediatric Endocrinology/Lawson Wilkins Pediatric Endocrine Society consensus statement on diabetic ketoacidosis in children and adolescents. *Pediatrics* 113:e133–e140, 2004

Finberg L: Why do patients with diabetic ketoacidosis have cerebral swelling, and why does treatment sometimes make it worse? *Arch Pediatr Adolesc Med* 150:785–786, 1996

Glaser N, Barnett P, McCaslin I, Nelson D, Trainor J, Louie J, Kaufman F, Quayle K, Roback M, Malley R, Kupperman N, Pediatric Emergency Medicine Collaborative Research Committee of the American Academy of Pediatrics: Risk factors for cerebral edema in children with ketoacidosis. *N Engl J Med* 344:264–269, 2001

Glaser NS, Wootton-Gorges SL, Buonocore MH, Marcin JP, Rewers A, Strain J, DiCarlo J, Neely EK, Barnes P, Kuppermann N: Frequency of sub-clinical cerebral edema in children with diabetic ketoacidosis. *Pediatr Diabetes* 7:75–80, 2006

Harris G, Fiordalisi I: Physiologic management of diabetic ketoacidemia: a 5-year prospective pediatric experience in 231 episodes. *Arch Pediatr Adolesc Med* 148:1046–1052, 1994

Hekkala A, Knip M, Veijola R: Ketoacidosis at diagnosis of type 1 diabetes in children in Northern Finland: temporal changes over 20 years. *Diabetes Care* 30:861–866, 2007

Kaufman FR, Halvorson M: The treatment and prevention of diabetic ketoacidosis in children and adolescents with type 1 diabetes mellitus. *Pediatr Ann* 28:576–582, 1999

Kitabchi AE, Umpierrez GE, Murphy MB, Barrett EJ, Kreisberg RA, Malone JI, Wall BM: Management of hyperglycemic crises in patients with diabetes. *Diabetes Care* 24:131–153, 2001

Mahoney C, Vlcek B, Del Aguila M: Risk factors for developing brain herniation during diabetic ketoacidosis. *Pediatr Neurol* 21:721–727, 1999

Marcin JP, Glaser N, Barnett P, McCaslin I, Nelson D, Trainor J, Louie J, Kaufman FR, Quayle K, Roback M, Malley R, Kuppermann N: Factors associated with adverse outcomes in children with diabetic ketoacidosis-related cerebral edema. *J Pediatr* 141:793–797, 2002

Muir A: Cerebral edema in diabetic ketoacidosis: a look beyond rehydration. *J Clin Endocrinol Metab* 85:509–513, 2000

Muir AB, Quisling RG, Yang MC, Rosenbloom AL: Cerebral edema in childhood diabetic ketoacidosis: natural history, radiographic findings, and early identification. *Diabetes Care* 27:1541–1546, 2004

Rewers A, Chase HP, Mackenzie T, Walravens P, Roback M, Rewers M, Hamman RF, Klingensmith G: Predictors of acute complications in children with type 1 diabetes. *JAMA* 287: 2511–2518, 2002

Rosenbloom AL, Hanas R: Diabetic ketoacidosis (DKA): treatment guidelines. *Clin Pediatr* 35:261–266, 1990

Sperling MA: Diabetic ketoacidosis. *Pediatr Clin North Am* 31:591–610, 1984

Vanelli M, Chiari G, Ghizzoni L, Costi G, Giacalone T, Chiarelli F: Effectiveness of a prevention program for diabetic ketoacidosis in children: an 8-year study in schools and private practices. *Diabetes Care* 22:7–9, 1999

Wootton-Gorges SL, Buonocore MH, Kuppermann N, Marcin JP, Barnes PD, Neely EK, DiCarlo J, McCarthy T, Glaser NS: Cerebral proton magnetic resonance spectroscopy in children with diabetic ketoacidosis. *Am J Neuroradiol* 28:895–899, 2007

Dr. Kaufman is Professor of Pediatrics and Communications at the Keck School of Medicine and the Annenberg School of Communications at the University of Southern California and is Head of the Center for Diabetes, Endocrinology and Metabolism at Childrens Hospital Los Angeles, Los Angeles, California.

8. Type 1 Diabetes in Children

WILLIAM V. TAMBORLANE, MD, KRISTIN A. SIKES, MSN, APRN, CDE, KARENA
SWAN, MD, AND STUART A. WEINZIMER, MD

The results of the Diabetes Control and Complications Trial (DCCT) and its follow-up, the Epidemiology of Diabetes Interventions and Complications (EDIC) Study, indicate that youth with type 1 diabetes should aim to achieve and maintain plasma glucose and A1C levels as close to normal as possible, as early in the course of the disease as possible, and with as few severe hypoglycemic events as possible. On the one hand, the adequacy of diabetes care during childhood may be the most important factor determining whether patients develop the late degenerative complications of diabetes. On the other hand, the rapid physiological and psychosocial changes that occur during childhood and adolescence make these patients among the most difficult to manage. A particular challenge in the care of children with type 1 diabetes is to make the treatment regimen fit as seamlessly as possible into the home and school environments, so that the primary childhood tasks of education, socialization, growth, and maturity continue unhindered by the extra responsibilities that diabetes care entails. Remarkably, a much greater proportion of young patients are able to meet these strict standards of care than was ever imagined possible just a few years ago. Moreover, an intensive approach to diabetes education and aggressive self-management by patients and families may actually reduce rather than increase the adverse psychosocial effects of this chronic illness.

INITIATION OF TREATMENT

We admit most of the children who are diagnosed with type 1 diabetes to the hospital for initiation of treatment. The diagnosis of diabetes in a child is a major shock and crisis for the family, who require time for adjustment and healing. The hospital provides a safe environment for this process to begin. In the absence of diabetic ketoacidosis, only 1.5–3 days of hospitalization are necessary to accomplish basic diabetes education and initiation of treatment. A comprehensive day-treatment program staffed by a multidisciplinary diabetes team can provide a suitable alternative to hospitalization in newly diagnosed patients.

INSULIN THERAPY

Plasma insulin profiles in nondiabetic individuals are characterized by basal levels upon which meal-related spikes in insulin concentrations are superimposed. Current intensive treatment regimens attempt to simulate this diurnal pattern of plasma insulin by using a basal-bolus approach to insulin replacement. However, in the absence of feedback control of insulin delivery, periods of excessive insulin that produce hypoglycemia and periods of inadequate insulin that permit hyperglycemia are impossible to avoid in youth with type 1 diabetes. The time-action characteristics of current insulin preparations are shown in Table 8.1.

Analog-Based Basal-Bolus Regimens

The most physiological approach to insulin replacement involves the continuous subcutaneous infusion of insulin (CSII) via an insulin pump. Originally introduced in the late 1970s, this approach to basal-bolus therapy only began to be used extensively in pediatrics over the past 7–8 years. The pumps are battery powered and about the size of a beeper/pager. Initially used with regular insulin, insulin pumps are now most often used with the rapid-acting insulin analogs, which are associated with improved meal coverage and less hypoglycemia. The newest "smart pumps" have advanced functions that include bolus dose calculators, the ability to record and summarize bolus and blood glucose histories, and the ability to receive sensor inputs from continuous glucose monitoring systems. The recommendations of the recent Pediatric Consensus Forum regarding the indications for pump therapy in children are summarized in Table 8.2.

With CSII, small amounts of rapid-acting insulin (down to 0.05- to 0.025-unit/h increments) are infused at a basal rate, and bolus doses are given at each meal or snack. The basal rate can be programmed to change every half hour, a function that is particularly helpful in regulating overnight blood glucose levels. Bolus doses are given before meals based on premeal plasma glucose level, car-

Table 8.1 Pharmacodynamic Properties of Common Insulin Formulations

Category	Onset (h)	Peak Action (h)	Duration (h)
Rapid-acting			
Insulin lispro, aspart, and glulisine	0.25–0.5	0.5–1.5	3–5
Short-acting			
Regular	0.5–1	2–3	3–6
Intermediate-acting			
NPH	2–4	4–10	10–24
Long-acting			
Insulin glargine	2–4	relatively flat	20–24
Insulin detemir	0.8–2 (dose dependent)	relatively flat	16–24

Table 8.2 Indications for CSII in Children and Adolescents with Type 1 Diabetes

CSII should be considered in patients with
1. Recurrent severe hypoglycemia
2. Wide fluctuations in blood glucose levels, regardless of A1C
3. Suboptimal diabetes control (i.e., A1C exceeds target range for age)
4. Microvascular complications and/or risk factors for macrovascular complications
5. Good metabolic control but insulin regimen that compromises lifestyle

CSII may also be beneficial in
1. Young children, especially infants and neonates
2. Adolescents with eating disorders
3. Children and adolescents with a pronounced dawn phenomenon
4. Children with needle phobia
5. Pregnant adolescents, ideally preconception
6. Ketosis-prone individuals
7. Competitive athletes

Recommendations of the Consensus Forum on the use of insulin pump therapy in the pediatric age-group (Phillip 2007).

bohydrate content of the meal, and anticipated exercise after the meal. Pump therapy also enhances flexibility in a child's diabetes regimen by allowing variable meal schedules and temporary increases or decreases in basal insulin rates. Due to their unpredictable eating and activity patterns, infants and toddlers are particularly well suited for insulin pump therapy. Although most patients can suspend the pump for up to 2 h without problems, families must be reminded that suspension or other causes of interruption of the insulin infusion for a prolonged period of time may lead to significant ketoacidosis and preventable hospitalization.

Basal-bolus therapy can also be accomplished with multiple daily insulin injections (MDI). In this method, once- or twice-daily injections of a long-acting insulin analog (glargine or detemir) provide basal insulin coverage, and meal-related insulin requirements are given by separate injections of a rapid-acting insulin analog, preferably given by insulin pens. Use of glargine-based MDI therapy in children has been associated with lower rates of nocturnal hypoglycemia as compared with MDI regimens using twice-a-day injections of NPH insulin, but the inability to "fine tune" basal insulin over the course of the day may be a problem. In addition, the flat time-action profiles of glargine and detemir put a premium on compliance with premeal bolus dosing. Indeed, the difficulty of administering four to five insulin injections daily accounted for the recent finding that adolescents randomized to glargine-based MDI therapy had higher A1C levels than those randomized to insulin pumps. Even the added convenience of insulin pumps fails to prevent some adolescents from omitting many of their prescribed premeal bolus doses. However, the bolus history function in newer pumps allows clinicians and parents to easily identify such problems with compliance.

With CSII and MDI, correction doses of rapid-acting insulin should be given when blood glucose values above the target range are discovered, according to a predetermined formula. For example, a younger child with premeal blood glucose values outside the goal range may be given an extra 0.5 units of rapid-acting insulin analog to reduce their blood glucose by 100 mg/dl in addition to the usual insulin dose at that mealtime, whereas an adolescent may use 2–3 units to "correct" the glucose by 100 mg/dl. Families should be advised to avoid "stacking" multiple correction doses too close together to avoid later hypoglycemia. The "insulin-on-board" feature of newer insulin pumps attempts to prevent stacking by accounting for boluses given within the last several hours and reducing the amount of subsequent boluses accordingly.

NPH-Based Conventional Treatment Regimens

The "split-mixed" regimen consisting of two daily doses of NPH and regular insulin that were mixed together in the same syringe was a standard approach to insulin replacement in pediatrics for many years. More recently, the regular insulin component was replaced by rapid-acting insulin analogs. Patients started on this approach generally receive two-thirds of the total daily dose before breakfast and one-third before dinner. Each injection starts with approximately two-thirds NPH and one-third rapid-acting analog. Individual components of the regimen are subsequently adjusted separately based on blood glucose testing results.

Although this conventional treatment regimen is almost always inadequate for patients with type 1 diabetes who have no residual endogenous insulin secretion, it may still play a role in the newly diagnosed patient who frequently goes through a "honeymoon" or partial remission period of their diabetes. During the honeymoon, insulin requirements rapidly decrease, and the doses of rapid-acting insulin may even be discontinued due to low prelunch and bedtime glucose levels. A major reason why the twice-daily injection regimen is effective during the honeymoon period is that endogenous insulin secretion provides much of the overnight basal insulin requirements as well as some of the meal bolus. Increased and more labile prebreakfast glucose levels often herald the loss of the relatively small amount of residual endogenous insulin secretion that is required for overnight glucose control, and the end of the honeymoon period.

When residual β-cell function wanes, problems with the two-injection regimen become apparent. One problem is that the peak of the predinner intermediate-acting insulin may coincide with the time of minimal insulin requirement (i.e., midnight to 4 A.M.). Subsequently, insulin levels fall off when basal requirements may be increasing (i.e., 4–8 A.M.), also known as the "dawn phenomenon." Increasing the predinner dose of intermediate-acting insulin to lower fasting glucose values often leads to hypoglycemia in the middle of the night without correcting hyperglycemia before breakfast. Another problem with the conventional two-injection regimen is high predinner glucose levels, despite normal or low prelunch and mid afternoon values. This is due, in part, to eating an afternoon snack when the effects of the prebreakfast dose of intermediate-acting insulin are waning.

One of the first true MDI regimens attempted to solve the problem of the dawn phenomenon by moving the predinner NPH to bedtime. A current alternative to this method that has been shown to be effective in children is to retain the prebreakfast mixture of NPH and rapid-acting insulin, cover dinner with rapid-acting analog, and use glargine or detemir (given before supper or bedtime) for overnight basal replacement. Indeed, some pediatric diabetes practices have come full circle, back to two shots a day by mixing the rapid- and long-acting insulins together in the same syringe at dinner, even though such mixing is not approved by the Food and Drug Administration.

SELF-MONITORING OF BLOOD GLUCOSE

The safety and success of any insulin regimen is dependent upon frequent self-monitoring of blood glucose (SMBG). Intensive diabetes control would have been impossible without the development of inexpensive, accurate, easy-to-use home glucose meters. Current models are fast (results in 5 s), accurate (within 5–8% of reference values), and require very small volumes of blood (0.1 ml). The smaller

Table 8.3 Plasma Blood Glucose and A1C Goals for Type 1 Diabetes by Age-Group

Values by age (years)	Plasma blood glucose goal range (mg/dl)		A1C	Rationale
	Before meals	Bedtime/ overnight		
Toddlers and preschoolers (0–6)	100–180	110–200	<8.5% (but >7.5%)	High risk and vulnerability to hypoglycemia
School age (6–12)	90–180	100–180	<8%	Risks of hypoglycemia and relatively low risk of complications prior to puberty
Adolescents and young adults (13–19)	90–130	90–150	<7.5%	•Risk of severe hypoglycemia •Developmental and psychological issues •A lower goal (<7.0%) is reasonable if it can be achieved without excessive hypoglycemia

Key concepts in setting glycemic goals:
- Goals should be individualized, and lower goals may be reasonable based on benefit-risk assessment.
- Blood glucose goals should be higher than those listed above in children with frequent hypoglycemia or hypoglycemia unawareness.
- Postprandial blood glucose values should be measured when there is a discrepancy between preprandial blood glucose values and A1C levels, and to help assess glycemia in those on basal/bolus regimens.

From American Diabetes Association, 2009.

blood volume requirement has allowed alternate site testing (i.e., forearm, thigh, or calf), which may minimize discomfort and improve adherence to self-monitoring regimens.

Children with type 1 diabetes should routinely test their blood glucose at least four times daily (premeal and prebedtime) and more frequently during intercurrent illnesses and to adjust insulin doses for exercise. It is very important for the family to record the results in either a written or electronic log and to review the data regularly to make self-adjustments of insulin doses between office visits. A target range is established (Table 8.3), but the targets may be altered based on the age of the child and the abilities of the family. Ideally, 80% of the blood glucose values should fall within the target range, but this is rarely the case in current clinical practice. Information gained from frequent testing is used to titrate insulin dosages according to need. Because daily insulin requirements continually increase in growing children, especially during puberty, and may acutely change with the start of a new sports season, it is important that the families be taught to look for trends that indicate a need to alter insulin doses. Virtually all of the meters are equipped with memory functions that record and store the date, time, and results of blood glucose tests. Although memory meters are extremely useful for checking compliance with and accurate reporting of glucose testing, all too often the patient and parents fail to retrieve and review these data for trend analysis.

Even when performed correctly, four (or even six) blood tests daily gives only a limited glimpse into the wide fluctuations in blood glucose that occur during a 24-h period in children with diabetes. Consequently, the introduction of real-time continuous glucose monitoring systems has the potential to be the most important advance in assessing diabetes control in the past 20 years. Recent studies from the Diabetes Research in Children Network (DirecNet) and the Juvenile Diabetes Research Foundation (JDRF) continuous glucose monitoring study groups demonstrated improvement in glycemic control, reduction in hypoglycemia, and high levels of patient and parent satisfaction when devices are worn continuously, although there remain obstacles to achieving full-time use in children, particularly adolescents. Because the error of current systems is considerably higher than that of conventional glucose meters, frequent SMBG is still required for making treatment decisions. Continuous monitoring may be particularly useful in reducing postprandial hyperglycemia, reducing hypoglycemia (particularly at night), and programming overnight basal rates in pump-treated patients. Ultimately, continuous glucose sensors may be employed as part of a closed-loop system, in which sensor data drive an insulin pump, thus creating an artificial β-cell.

Urine tests still have a role in management of diabetes. However, it is now restricted to measurements of urine ketone levels when the child is ill, nauseated, or vomiting. Home meters for blood β-hydroxybutyrate levels are also available.

Measurement of A1C provides the gold standard by which to judge the adequacy of the treatment regimen. Simple, point-of-service methods that can be performed in the office in a few minutes on small samples of blood offer the opportunity to make immediate changes in the insulin regimen while the patient is still being seen. Even more important, the results of this test when delivered during face-to-face encounters with the clinician serve as the quarterly "report cards" for the child and the parents. Teenagers may not be able to identify with the concept of working hard on their diabetes to be healthier many years in the future, but most are able to understand the value of good grades. Thus, the A1C level provides a tangible outcome for this age-group in particular. The goal of treatment is to achieve A1C levels as close to normal as possible. Based on DCCT results, our general goal of therapy is to try to keep all patients' A1C <7.5%. A1C levels are determined at least every 3 months.

DIET

Dietary guidance for children with type 1 diabetes requires careful instruction and frequent reinforcement. Involvement of a registered dietitian who is both experienced and comfortable working with children is strongly recommended. Generally, terms such as "diet" should be avoided in favor of "meal plan," both for the negative connotation associated with the former and for the simple fact that nutritional requirements for normal growth and development are the same in both diabetic and nondiabetic children. The increasing popularity of basal-bolus therapies has fundamentally changed the treatment paradigm. The traditional approach of adjusting the patient's lifestyle around fixed insulin doses and fixed amounts of carbohydrate intake with each meal has been replaced by a much more flexible approach that attempts to adjust the insulin regimen to the patient's food intake and lifestyle. The day-to-day variations in appetite in children and adolescents make the latter approach much more likely to be successful. It is important to note that in some patients and some families, the traditional approach maybe more successful because it fits their personalities and lifestyle better.

The currently favored model of nutritional therapy is carbohydrate counting, based on the conceptual model of matching carbohydrate "doses" to insulin doses. Because the total carbohydrate content rather than the type of carbohydrate has the greatest impact on blood glucose, the amount of carbohydrates ingested per meal or snack needs to be estimated as accurately as possible. Protein and fat intake, while important in the larger context of a healthy meal plan, are not counted to simplify the procedure. In the flexible approach to nutrition counseling, there is no set intake. Rather, the child or parents decide upon the meal content, the carbohydrates are counted, and an insulin dose is calculated, based on the insulin-to-carbohydrate ratio that is empirically determined by the diabetes practitioner. In younger children, a typical insulin-to-carbohydrate ratio is 1 unit per 20–30 g, whereas an older child may require 1 unit per 15 g, and an insulin-resistant adolescent 1 unit per 5–10 g. Actual insulin-to-carbohydrate ratios vary from child to child and even in the same child from meal to meal; breakfast often requires relatively more insulin than lunch or dinner. Carbohydrate counting can also be used in the traditional approach to dietary treatment to provide consistent amounts of carbohydrate per meal/snack.

Dietary recommendations should also take into account the long-term goal of prevention of macrovascular complications of diabetes. Consequently, heart-healthy diets low in cholesterol and saturated fats are encouraged. We face an epidemic of childhood obesity in developed countries, and one of the adverse consequences of intensive insulin treatment in the DCCT was a twofold increase in the risk of becoming overweight. Thus, any tendency for BMI Z-scores to excessively increase needs to be dealt with promptly. Continued access to a registered dietician can help to limit this unwanted side effect through regular reinforcement of appropriate portion control based on the age, sex, and activity level of children. Parents should also be counseled to monitor for an increase in episodes of mild hypoglycemia because not only are they disruptive to the activities of daily living, but treatment of multiple episodes can also significantly increase the daily caloric intake to well above recommended levels.

EXERCISE

Establishment and maintenance of an active lifestyle should be a goal for all children, but it is especially important for children with diabetes. Regular exercise is associated with improvements in insulin sensitivity, physical fitness, and self-esteem. Nevertheless, acute bouts of exercise in children with type 1 diabetes actually make regulation of blood glucose levels more difficult. Hypoglycemia is a common complication during exercise, and excessive snacking to prevent hypoglycemia can result in weight gain and hyperglycemia. These difficulties are compounded by the irregular pattern of physical activity that characterize most youth who are not participating in organized sports or regimented training programs, and by conventional methods of diabetes management that feature fixed basal insulin replacement doses.

The effects of exercise must be carefully considered in the context of the entire diabetes care plan. Children participating in school sports or other programs should be counseled to monitor blood glucose before, during, and after exercise because the hypoglycemic effects of exercise may be delayed for 7–11 h, markedly increasing the risk of nocturnal hypoglycemia. In pump patients, simply suspending the basal infusion rate can markedly reduce the risk of hypoglycemia during exercise, and similar benefits may accrue from reducing the overnight basal rates after very active days. Recent studies that have examined methods to manage glycemia during exercise illustrate that there is an almost infinite number of combinations of conditions that need to be considered. Because of this complexity, trial and error remains the principal method of managing glucose levels during and after exercise in children and adolescents with type 1 diabetes.

ROUTINE OUTPATIENT CARE

Children and adolescents with type 1 diabetes should be routinely referred to a diabetes center that uses a multidisciplinary team knowledgeable about and experienced in the management of young patients. This team should ideally consist of pediatric diabetologists, nurse clinicians, dietitians, and social workers or psychologists. During the first few weeks after diagnosis, patients and parents should maintain close contact with the treatment team. This is a critical period for the child and parent to learn the principles of adjusting insulin doses and overall diabetes self-management. The parent or older child should be in daily telephone contact with the clinician. Clinical well-being, SMBG results, and the effect of changes in diet and exercise should be reviewed. The patient's thoughts about changes in the insulin regimen should be sought before making recommendations. Usually within the first few weeks, the children (and parents) will feel more confident and should be able to begin to make their own insulin adjustments.

Regular office visits on a 3-month basis are recommended for established patients. The main purpose of these visits is to ensure that the patient is achieving the primary goals of treatment, namely, target A1C levels with as little hypoglycemia as possible. Glucose monitoring data are reviewed, and the treatment regimen is adjusted as needed. Familial, school, or other psychosocial problems are explored. In addition to serial measurements of height and weight, particular attention should be paid to monitoring of blood pressure and examinations of the thyroid and injection sites. Routine laboratory screening studies include measurement of lipids and microalbuminuria and thyroid function tests annually. Screening for celiac disease should also be obtained. The American Diabetes Association recommends annual dilated retinal examinations in patients who are aged >10 years and have had type 1 diabetes for ≥3 years. However, a recent study from our clinic population indicated that the yield from such examinations is very low in children and adolescents who have normal blood pressure, have A1C levels that meet current targets, and are without microalbuminuria.

HYPOGLYCEMIA

The nonphysiological nature of conventional insulin replacement, relatively large insulin doses required by adolescents, defective glucagon responses, irregularities in diet and exercise, and other problems contribute to the vulnerability of young patients to severe reductions in plasma glucose. Severe hypoglycemia is a more common problem in patients striving for strict glycemic control with intensive treatment regimens. In adolescents and adults in the DCCT, the risk of severe hypoglycemia was threefold higher in intensively treated patients than in conventionally treated patients. Severe hypoglycemic events are of particular concern in very young children with type 1 diabetes because of their potential adverse effects on brain development. The use of basal-bolus therapy with insulin analogs has reduced the frequency of severe hypoglycemia somewhat but has by no means eliminated this problem. Indeed, fear of hypoglycemia remains the most significant barrier to the pursuit and maintenance of tight glycemic control among young people with type 1 diabetes.

Treatment of a mild to moderate reaction consists of ≥15 g carbohydrate (e.g., orange juice, regular soda, or glucose tablets), but more may be needed for exercise-induced hypoglycemia. Children should carry glucose tablets to treat hypoglycemia efficiently and effectively. Friends should also be aware of how to treat low blood glucose levels. While in school, children should have ready access to glucose tablets and should not be required to walk alone to the nurse's office while hypoglycemic. Ideally, children with diabetes should have the ability to test and treat hypoglycemic events without having to leave the classroom. However, this currently is not allowed in some schools, and it should be reinforced with children and their caregivers that in the event of significant symptoms of hypoglycemia, a child should be treated right away, even if SMBG verification is not immediately available. Proper insulin and dietary adjustments should be made to prevent further hypoglycemia. Parents and school personnel must also be taught how to inject glucagon for treatment of more severe reactions.

SICK DAY GUIDELINES

Children with intercurrent illnesses such as infections or vomiting should be closely monitored for elevations in glucose and ketone levels. On sick days, blood glucose should be checked every 2–4 h, and urine (or blood) should be checked for ketones every 3–4 h. Supplemental doses of rapid-acting insulin (0.1–0.3 units/kg body wt) should be given every 2–4 h for elevations in glucose and ketones. If the patient uses an insulin pump and large or moderate ketones are present, we instruct the patient to change the infusion site, increase the correction bolus, and program a higher basal rate for 3–4 h. Adequate fluid intake is essential to prevent dehydration. Fluids such as Gatorade, flat soda, clear soups, popsicles, and gelatin water are recommended to provide some electrolyte and carbohydrate replacement. If vomiting is persistent and ketones remain large after several supplemental insulin doses, arrangements should be made for parenteral hydration. Recurrent episodes of ketonuria and vomiting are usually the result of missed insulin doses or overall poor metabolic control.

BIBLIOGRAPHY

Ahern JA, Boland EA, Doane R, Ahern JJ, Rose P, Vincent M, Tamborlane WV: Insulin pump therapy in pediatrics: a therapeutic alternative to safely lower HbA1c levels across all age groups. *Pediatr Diabetes* 3:10–15, 2002

American Diabetes Association: Standards of medical care in diabetes—2009. *Diabetes Care* 32 (Suppl. 1):S13–S61, 2009

Bangstad H-J, Danne T, Deeb LC, Jarosz-Chobot P, Urakami T, Hanas R, International Society for Pediatric and Adolescent Diabetes(ISPAD): Insulin treatment: ISPAD clinical practice consensus guidelines 2006-2007. *Pediatr Diabetes* 8:88–102, 2007 [Other ISPAD treatment guidelines can be found at www.ispad.org]

Diabetes Control and Complications Trial (DCCT)/Epidemiology of Diabetes Interventions and Complications (EDIC) Research Group: Beneficial effects of intensive therapy of diabetes during adolescence: outcomes after the conclusion of the Diabetes Control and Complications Trial (DCCT). *J Pediatr* 139:804–812, 2001

DirecNet Study Group: Positive impact of FreeStyle Navigator continuous glucose sensor use in children with type 1 diabetes. *J Pediatr* 151:388–393, 2007

JDRF CGM Study Group: Impact of continuous glucose monitoring in optimizing intensive treatment of type 1 diabetes in adults and children. *N Engl J Med* 359:1464–1476, 2008

Phillip M, Battelino T, Rodriguez H, Danne T, Kaufman F: Use of insulin pump therapy in the pediatric age-group: consensus statement from the European Society for Paediatric Endocrinology, the Lawson Wilkins Pediatric Endocrine Society, and the International Society for Pediatric and Adolescent Diabetes, endorsed by the American Diabetes Association and the European Association for the Study of Diabetes. *Diabetes Care* 30:1653–1662, 2007

Silverstein J, Klingensmith G, Copeland K, Plotnick L, Kaufman F, Deeb L, Grey M, Anderson BJ, Holzmeister LA, Clark N, American Diabetes Association: Care of children and adolescents with type 1 diabetes: a statement of the American Diabetes Association. *Diabetes Care* 28:186–212, 2005

Tamborlane WV, Bonfig W, Boland E: Recent advances in the treatment of youth with type 1 diabetes: better care through technology. *Diabet Med* 18:864–870, 2001

Weinzimer SA, Tamborlane WV: Diabetes mellitus in children and adolescents. In *Clinical Diabetes.* Fonseca V, Ed. Philadelphia, PA, Saunders Elsevier, 2006, p. 505–521

Drs. Tamborlane, Swan, and Weinzimer are members of the Pediatric Endocrinology Section of the Yale University School of Medicine, New Haven, Connecticut. Ms. Sikes is the Director of the Yale Children's Diabetes Clinic, New Haven, Connecticut.

9. Psychosocial and Family Issues in Children with Type 1 Diabetes

Barbara J. Anderson, PhD, Joseph I. Wolfsdorf, MD, and Alan M. Jacobson, MD

D aily treatment of children with diabetes affects and intrudes on everyday behavior in the family, alters family routines, and affects relationships among family members. How the family handles these intrusions determines the effectiveness with which childhood diabetes is managed. This chapter addresses these issues from a developmental perspective by examining the changing developmental tasks of different-aged children and their families.

CRISIS AT DIAGNOSIS

The diagnosis of diabetes in a child or adolescent hurls the parent from a secure and known reality into a frightening and foreign world. At diagnosis, they grieve the loss of their healthy child and cope with such normal distress reactions as shock, disbelief and denial, fear, anxiety, anger, and extreme blame or guilt. However, while grieving, parents are expected to acquire an understanding of the disease and behavioral skills to manage the illness at home and to assist the child in achieving acceptable blood glucose control.

Parents should receive the emotional support required to begin coping with the emotional distress and not be overwhelmed by unrealistic expectations from a well-meaning diabetes treatment team (Table 9.1). Parents must find a sense of balance after the diagnosis and should be encouraged to progress at their own pace, with emotional support offered by staff members or another parent.

Table 9.1 Recommendations for the Diabetes Treatment Team at Diagnosis

- Give the parent time to "grieve the diagnosis."
- Limit guidelines to basic skills.
- Keep to a minimum the number of medical staff providing information and treatment.
- Include both parents, in some fashion, in the diabetes education program.
- Encourage, in single-parent families, another adult (e.g., a grandparent or neighbor) to support the parent.

DIABETES AND CHILD DEVELOPMENT

Diabetes presents family members with the task of being sensitive to the balance between the child's need for a sense of autonomy and mastery of self-care activities and the need for ongoing family support and involvement. The struggle to balance independence and dependence in relationships between the child and family members presents a long-term challenge and raises different issues for families at different stages of child and adolescent development. Focusing on normal developmental tasks at each stage of the child's growth and development provides the most effective structure with which to address this concern.

INFANTS AND TODDLERS WITH DIABETES (0–3 YEARS OLD)

At this earliest stage of child development, the parent is the only appropriate patient with respect to diabetes management. Researchers have identified several problems facing parents of infants and toddlers with diabetes (Table 9.2).

Children diagnosed before age 5 years may be at risk for specific subtle cognitive deficits thought to be caused by recurrent severe hypoglycemic episodes, although recent evidence suggests that chronic hyperglycemia may also have an adverse effect on the developing brain. Hypoglycemia in very young children relates to difficulties in administering and adjusting the small insulin doses needed by most infants and toddlers as well as the preverbal child's inability to recognize and communicate symptoms of hypoglycemia.

At this stage of development, two important aspects of care are *1)* how treatment responsibilities are shared between parents and *2)* the prevention of severe hypoglycemic episodes. The primary developmental task during infancy is to achieve a stable, trusting relationship between infant and primary care provider.

The central task of the child from age 1 to 3 years is to establish an initial sense of mastery over the world. Toddlers do not have the cognitive skills to understand why cooperation with the intrusive, sometimes painful, procedures of the diabetes regimen is needed. Thus, injections or fingersticks for blood glucose monitoring may become battlegrounds when the toddler resists and will require significant emotional stamina by the parent.

PRESCHOOLERS AND EARLY-ELEMENTARY SCHOOLCHILDREN WITH DIABETES (4–7 YEARS OLD)

Nursery school, day care, or kindergarten may represent the first arena in which both parents and children face the social consequences of diabetes, including the need to educate others about the disease (Table 9.2). Thus, separation problems that often appear in children this age may be heightened in the child with diabetes.

Children who are 4–7 years old are beginning to use cause-effect thinking. Thus, the young child with diabetes may blame him- or herself for having the disease or see injections and restrictions as punishments. Youngsters with diabetes at this age may benefit from informal contact and group interactions with other children with diabetes.

Table 9.2 Challenges Facing Parents and/or Children with Diabetes

Parents of infants and toddlers (0–3 yr old)

- Monitoring diabetes control and avoiding hypoglycemia
- Establishing a meal schedule despite the child's normally irregular eating patterns
- Coping with the very young child's inability to understand the need for injections
- Managing the conflicts with older siblings that result from unequal sharing of parental attention

Preschoolers and early-elementary schoolchildren (4–7 yr old)

- Mastering separation from the family and adapting to the expectations of teachers
- Blaming self for having diabetes; regarding injections and restrictions as punishments
- Educating school personnel, coaches, and scout leaders about diabetes (parents)

Later-elementary schoolchildren (8–11 yr old)

- Engaging in a wide range of activities with peers
- Learning about the benefits of intensive diabetes management (child and parents)

- Becoming involved in diabetes self-care tasks (selecting snacks, selecting and cleaning injection sites, and identifying symptoms of low blood glucose) while sustaining parent involvement in major tasks

Early adolescence (12–15 yr old)

- Integrating physical changes into self-image and body image
- Acknowledging that the young teenager is on the threshold of becoming an adult (parents)
- Renegotiating parents' and young adolescents' roles in taking responsibility for diabetes management in the face of physiological changes caused by puberty, which complicate matters
- Fitting in with the peer group
- Maintaining good glycemic control while concerned about possible weight gain

Later adolescence (16–19 yr old)

- Making decisions regarding post–high school plans
- Living more independently of parents
- Strengthening relationships with fewer friends
- Assuming more independent responsibility for health and health care

At this stage of development, parents continue to be the primary recipients of diabetes education and the primary person to interact with the health care team. However, the child's increasing motor coordination and cognitive skills enable him or her to become a more involved partner in diabetes self-care tasks. Children can select appropriate snacks, select and clean injection sites, and begin to identify and report symptoms of low blood glucose. The goal is for elementary school–aged children to be positively drawn into their own care without premature and unrealistic expectations for independence while parental control and supervision continue.

OLDER-ELEMENTARY SCHOOLCHILDREN (8–11 YEARS OLD)

The preadolescent child forms close friendships with children of the same sex, strives to gain approval from this peer group, and seriously begins to evaluate him-

or herself by comparing abilities with those of peers. Children with diabetes, in the process of making these social comparisons, need to develop a strong positive self-image. In fact, preadolescent children with diabetes with adjustment problems may often be overlooked because they are not overtly rebellious and hostile, but rather are overdependent on family members and withdrawn from peers. Participation in activities with peers and positive self-image are key concepts at this age, and health care providers should emphasize to parents the importance of the child with diabetes participating in a wide range of activities with peers.

Parents should focus diabetes education on realistic blood glucose goals and safety guidelines for prevention of hypoglycemia. That is, parent and child should be ready to increase monitoring of blood glucose and plan ahead for additional snacks with extra activity.

It is important to continue emphasizing the long-term benefits of continued parent-child teamwork in diabetes care. Children this age can check blood glucose levels and give injections on occasion without supervision. Health care providers should begin to negotiate more directly with the child concerning issues and problems with diabetes rather than talking solely to the parents.

EARLY ADOLESCENCE (12–15 YEARS OLD)

At this stage of development, dramatic changes typically occur in five areas:

- Physical development
- Cognitive development
- Family dynamics
- School experiences
- Social networks

During all of these normal changes of early adolescence, the change in balance of responsibility for diabetes management tasks continues between the child and the family. It is common for families to change their expectations of the young adolescent and frequently "turn over" all responsibility for diabetes management. However, the physiological changes of puberty, which are associated with insulin resistance in both nondiabetic and diabetic adolescents, can complicate this transition. Reduced sensitivity to insulin is an important factor that contributes to the inability of many adolescents to achieve optimal glycemic control.

If the diabetes care regimen makes a teen stand out from the peer group, conflicts can arise. Some teenagers may stop their self-care and try to prove they are "normal." Others may use diabetes as an excuse to withdraw. Many who never before hid their diabetes may now refuse to talk about it with friends.

Young teenagers have an increasing cognitive ability to analyze themselves and the world around them and do not accept authority, but rather examine, criticize, and question. This growing ability leads many teenagers with diabetes to a new sensitivity about their disease (e.g., for the first time, they may vent their anger about having diabetes at parents). Parents and health care professionals frequently overestimate the teenager's conceptual understanding of diabetes. Parents also can overestimate the adolescent's ability to follow through with diabetes care tasks without immediate positive reinforcement and support, mistakenly assuming that long-term good health will provide motivation for adherence to the diabetes treatment plan.

Diabetes can further threaten the young teenager's self-confidence. Inexplicable fluctuating blood glucose levels that defy attempts at control contribute to younger teenagers feeling uneasy in their bodies. Insulin reactions, injections or pumps, and blood glucose monitoring can further undermine the child's ability to feel attractive or normal. Concerns about body image must be taken seriously by parents and health care providers. For example, a problem seen frequently in young adolescent girls who are distressed about weight gain is a dramatic increase in blood glucose levels. When adolescent girls are worried about their weight, and parents and the health care team focus exclusively on good control and A1C levels, many patients begin to secretly reduce their insulin dose and thereby purge calories and lose weight. This self-destructive behavior is a form of bulimia nervosa, and this diabetes-specific eating disorder may cause repeated hospitalizations for diabetic ketoacidosis in adolescent girls.

Because puberty causes such physiological challenges to controlling blood glucose and because of the psychological and social vulnerabilities of this age, parents should continue their involvement in and supervision of insulin administration and blood glucose checking throughout early adolescence. Negotiation of continued support and supervision is critical, even if the young adolescent initially rejects it. Similarly, parents should expect some participation from the youth, even if the youth is overly dependent on the parents and is content to have no active role in diabetes management. Negative family interactions surrounding diabetes management contribute to problems with adherence and metabolic control in adolescents with diabetes. The key is that both adolescents and parents must redefine their roles and renegotiate a balance of responsibility for diabetes that is acceptable to both parties.

Families should also be encouraged to change their pattern of relationships with diabetes health care providers. Young teenagers often have issues (e.g., concerns about sexuality) that they do not feel comfortable discussing in front of parents. Thus, health care providers should begin seeing parents and young teenagers individually and sequentially.

Both young adolescents and their parents may benefit from contact with other families coping with similar struggles. Diabetes summer camps and weekend retreats often provide an important forum for peer identification, and peer group educational and support programs may be helpful for both children and parents.

LATER ADOLESCENCE (16–19 YEARS OLD)

At this stage, physical growth and development is usually complete, and conflicts over diabetes self-care tend to decrease and stabilize. The central developmental tasks of the older adolescent are outlined in Table 9.2.

Some older teenagers with diabetes who feel overwhelmed with the pressures of high school and the need to plan for the future may ignore their self-care. When peer relationships are insecure or schoolwork seems beyond their abilities, some teenagers may use their diabetes to avoid conflicts at school. Some older teenagers with poor metabolic control reflect a chronic unmet need for more family support

Table 9.3 Families Benefiting from Additional Psychosocial Support

- All families at the time of diagnosis
- Single-parent families
- Families in which another member has a serious chronic physical illness (including diabetes) or mental illness (including a learning disability)
- Families with infants and toddlers with type 1 diabetes

for self-care tasks. Poor control in a teenager can be a reflection of chaos and dysfunction at home. In these instances, more (not less) parental involvement may be needed. Family counseling can help parents and teenagers negotiate roles with respect to sharing diabetes management responsibilities.

Conflicts over friendships are the primary cause of alienation between parents and teenagers. This is especially true when issues of alcohol and drugs, safety (driving), and sexual activity are raised. Older teenage girls (and their parents) should be educated about the importance of optimal metabolic control before conception and about the difficulties of managing a diabetic pregnancy.

During this stage of development, insulin requirements stabilize. Many older adolescent girls may continue to be concerned about weight gain caused by an inappropriate meal plan that provides significantly more calories than necessary after growth and physical development are complete. Patients should be evaluated for insulin manipulation whenever poor metabolic control remains unexplained in an adolescent girl concerned about her weight. More gradual separation from medical providers is not a sign of psychological problems or overdependence. Expectations are that the older adolescent can manage diabetes with less parental involvement; however, each family situation must be assessed individually.

REFERRAL TO A MENTAL HEALTH PROFESSIONAL

Several types of families should be considered high risk and may benefit from additional psychosocial support resources and more frequent appointments with

Table 9.4 Risk Factors Related to Individual Children

Children and their families should be referred for counseling if any one of the following is present:

- Failure to master the tasks of normal child or adolescent development
- Identification of the child/adolescent as a "problem" by the legal system or school (extended school absences, school failure)
- Serious depression, anxiety, learning disability, or other severe mental disorder
- Inability to show age-appropriate cooperation with the tasks of diabetes care
- More than one diabetes-related hospitalization for unexplained causes during a 1-yr period
- Weight loss and chronic hyperglycemia (elevated A1C), especially in adolescent girls

Table 9.5 Risk Factors Related to the Entire Family

Family therapy is recommended if any one of the following problems is present:
- Prolonged intense conflict between parent and child over division of responsibilities for diabetes care tasks
- Life crisis, such as divorce or death of a family member, that causes severe grief reactions within family
- Suspicion of child sexual/physical/emotional abuse or neglect, which should also be reported immediately to legal authorities

the health care team (Table 9.3). Similarly, several warning signals are used to identify a child (Table 9.4) or family (Table 9.5) for whom mental health intervention is required.

BIBLIOGRAPHY

Amiel SA, Sherwin RS, Simonson DC, Lauritano AA, Tamborlane WV: Impaired insulin action in puberty: a contributing factor to poor glycemic control in adolescents with diabetes. *N Engl J Med* 315:215–219, 1986

Anderson B, Coughlin C, Goldberg E, Laffel L: Comprehensive, family-focused outpatient care for very young children living with chronic disease: lessons from a program in pediatric diabetes. *Child Serv Soc Pol Res Pract* 4:235–250, 2001

Anderson BJ, Ho J, Brackett J, Finkelstein D, Laffel L: Parental involvement in diabetes management tasks: relationships to blood glucose monitoring adherence and metabolic control in young adolescents with insulin-dependent diabetes mellitus. *J Pediatr* 130:257–265, 1997.

Anderson BJ, Svoren B, Laffel L: Initiatives to promote effective self-care skills in young patients with diabetes. *Dis Manag Health Outcome* 15:101–108, 2007

Anderson BJ: Randomized controlled clinical trials of psychological interventions to improve glycemic control in pediatric and adult patients with T1DM. *Curr Diabetes Rep* 7:101–103, 2007

Jacobson AM: Psychological care of patients with insulin-dependent diabetes mellitus. *N Engl J Med* 334:1249–1253, 1996

Rydall AC, Rodin GM, Olmsted MP, Devenyi RG, Daneman D: Disordered eating behavior and microvascular complications in young women with insulin-dependent diabetes mellitus. *N Engl J Med* 336:1849–1854, 1997

Svoren BM, Volkening LK, Butler DA, Moreland EC, Anderson BJ, Laffel LMB: Temporal trends in the treatment of pediatric type 1 diabetes and impact on acute outcomes. *J Pediatr* 150:279–285, 2007

Wolfsdorf JI: Improving diabetes control in adolescents with type 1 diabetes. In *Practical Psychology for Diabetes Clinicians.* 2nd ed. Anderson B, Rubin R, Eds. Alexandria, VA, American Diabetes Association, 2002, p. 149–160

Dr. Anderson is Professor of Pediatrics at Baylor College of Medicine, Houston, Texas. Dr. Wolfsdorf is Professor of Pediatrics at Harvard Medical School, Boston, Massachusetts. Dr. Jacobson is Professor of Psychiatry at Harvard Medical School and Senior Vice President at the Joslin Diabetes Center, Boston, Massachusetts.

10. Obesity and Type 2 Diabetes in Children

CRISTINA CANDIDO, MD, FIDA BACHA, MD, TAMARA HANNON, MD,
INGRID LIBMAN, MD, PHD, AND SILVA ARSLANIAN, MD

INTRODUCTION

Both childhood obesity and type 2 diabetes are on an upward trajectory. Obesity, particularly abdominal adiposity, is strongly linked to insulin resistance in children. Insulin resistance is physiologically compensated by increased insulin secretion from the β-cell, resulting in the observed hyperinsulinemia in obese people. In individuals at genetic risk for type 2 diabetes, there is deficient compensation by a failing β-cell, leading to the clinical manifestation of type 2 diabetes. A myriad of genetic, environmental, social, and cultural factors contribute to the development of type 2 diabetes. To date, multiple genes have been identified associated with obesity and type 2 diabetes. Against this multigenic background, our present-day obesogenic environment, characterized with low levels of physical activity and overnutrition, promotes the development of type 2 diabetes. The gravity of the problem poses a challenge to health care professionals. Early screening of patients at risk is crucial for expedient diagnosis and treatment to prevent or delay diabetes-related comorbidities.

There has been a marked increase in the prevalence of childhood obesity in the U.S. for the past two decades. Results from the 2003–2004 National Health and Nutrition Examination Survey (NHANES) indicate that ~14% of 2- to 5-year-olds, 19% of 6- to 11-year-olds, and 17% of 12- to 19-year-olds are overweight, defined as having a sex-specific BMI for age ≥95th percentile. The overall prevalence in children and adolescents is estimated at ~17%. An additional 34% are at risk for overweight (defined as having a BMI for age of ≥85th but <95th percentile). The distribution of children and adolescents at risk for overweight by age-group is as follows: 26% of 2- to 5-year-olds, 37% of 6- to 11-year-olds, and 34% of 12- to 19-year-olds. Overall, the highest prevalence of overweight is seen among non-Hispanic blacks. For children and adolescents at risk for overweight, highest prevalence is noted among Mexican Americans.

Around two decades ago, type 2 diabetes accounted for <3% of cases of diabetes in adolescents. In the 1990s, several clinic-based studies reported an increase in the number of children with type 2 diabetes. Today, type 2 diabetes is reported to account for 8% to as high as 45% of pediatric diabetes clinic cases. A more recent multiethnic, population-based study, the SEARCH for Diabetes in Youth,

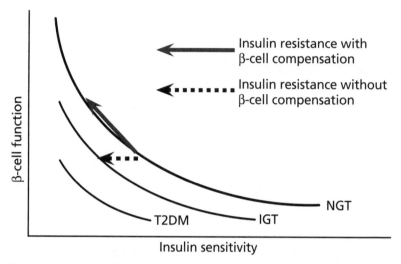

Figure 10.1   Hyperbolic relation between β-cell function and insulin sensitivity. NGT, normal glucose tolerance; T2DM, type 2 diabetes. Adapted with permission from Stumvoll (2005).

conducted from 2002 to 2003 among children and adolescents <20 years of age, noted an incidence of diabetes of 24.3 per 100,000 person-years. Overall, type 2 diabetes was relatively infrequent, but the highest rates (17.0–49.4/100,000 person-years) were documented among 15- to 19-year-olds in nonwhite populations. The highest rates were among American-Indian youth in the 10- to 14-year-old age-group (25.3/100,000) and the 15- to 19-year-old age-group (49.4/100,000), followed by African American, Asian/Pacific Islander, Hispanic, and then non-Hispanic youth. Moreover, type 2 diabetes rates were 60% higher in female than in male subjects. Based on the SEARCH data, the estimated annual number of newly diagnosed cases of type 2 diabetes in youth in the U.S. is ~3,700.

Pathophysiology of Youth Type 2 Diabetes

The regulation of blood glucose is maintained by a delicate balance between insulin secretion and insulin action or sensitivity, hepatic glucose production, and cellular glucose uptake. Fig. 10.1 shows the curvilinear relationship between β-cell function and insulin sensitivity. To maintain glucose tolerance, a decrease in insulin sensitivity is compensated by an increase in insulin secretion. Disruption of this normal hyperbolic relationship between insulin sensitivity and secretion may result in impaired glucose tolerance (IGT) and type 2 diabetes. Therefore, both insulin resistance (hepatic and peripheral) and insulin deficiency are the key components in the pathogenesis of type 2 diabetes. In obese youth with type 2 diabetes, peripheral insulin sensitivity is 50% lower and insulin secretion relative to insulin resistance is ~85% lower when compared with equally obese adolescents without diabetes. Even though the pathophysiology of type 2 diabetes in adults has long been debated, it is now accepted that the earliest abnormality is insulin resistance, and what eventuates diabetes is β-cell failure. In adults, studies suggest that the determinant of progression from normal glucose tolerance to IGT to type 2 diabetes is declining pancreatic β-cell function. In children, limited observations suggest the same. Based on this, our group proposed a pathophysiological sequence of type 2 diabetes consistent with findings in adults (Fig. 10.2).

RISK FACTORS FOR TYPE 2 DIABETES

Obesity

Obesity is the most important risk factor for the development of type 2 diabetes because the increasing prevalence of overweight in youth closely parallels the rise in the number of cases of type 2 diabetes. Measures of adiposity, including BMI, total body fat, and waist circumference, are strongly related to the degree of insulin resistance in children. Among these, however, waist circumference and excess abdominal fat, particularly visceral fat, confers a higher risk of insulin resistance. Moreover, there are limited data in pediatrics to suggest that ectopic fat deposition in the muscle may also be associated with insulin resistance. Although insulin resistance is a common feature of obesity, heterogeneity exists among obese individuals with regard to insulin sensitivity and risk for type 2 diabetes. Among obese adolescents pair-matched for age, pubertal stage, BMI, and total body fat, the ones with severe insulin resistance had higher visceral fat and waist-to-hip ratio and lower HDL than the ones with lesser degrees of insulin resistance. The former group was at greater risk for type 2 diabetes as manifested by impaired β-cell insulin secretion relative to insulin resistance.

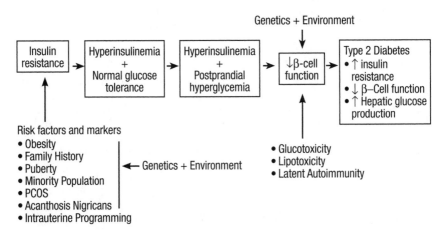

Figure 10.2 Proposed pathophysiology of youth-onset type 2 diabetes. Adapted with permission from Arslanian (2002).

Genetic Susceptibility

Most youths with type 2 diabetes report a strong family history of the disease in first- or second-degree relatives regardless of ethnic background, indicating a strong heritability of the disease. In our studies of healthy nondiabetic children, family history of type 2 diabetes was associated with lower insulin sensitivity and evidence of β-cell dysfunction when compared with peers without a family history of the disease. These findings were present as early as the first decade of life. An international linkage consortium, part of an extensive effort to identify susceptibility genes, has identified multiple genes associated with adult type 2 diabetes, some with known functions and others without. Data are not existent in pediatrics.

Ethnicity

Minority ethnic populations, including African Americans, Native Americans, Pima Indians, and Hispanics, represent the group with the highest incidence of pediatric type 2 diabetes. More than 5% of 15- to 19-year-old Pima Indians have type 2 diabetes related to a genetic predisposition to insulin resistance modified by lifestyle habits. Black and Hispanic children are also more insulin resistant and hyperinsulinemic than their white peers. In our studies, black normal-weight children have ~25% lower insulin sensitivity. Moreover, black obese adolescents, who typically have lower visceral fat than their white peers, do not have better insulin sensitivity than their white counterparts. In addition, black children have lower levels of the antidiabetogenic hormone adiponectin. These findings suggest an inherent insulin resistance in blacks that could stem from a combination of genetic and environmental factors.

Lifestyle

Highly technology-driven societies create an obesogenic environment, promoting low levels of physical activity and the consumption of easily available and abundant calorie-rich foods. This energy excess is stored as fat, leading to obesity. Lifestyle modification is a primary target for the prevention of obesity and type 2 diabetes.

Insulin Resistance Phenotype

Puberty, polycystic ovary syndrome (PCOS), metabolic syndrome, and exposure to gestational diabetes are all linked to insulin resistance. Childhood type 2 diabetes has its onset usually in the pubertal age-group. Insulin sensitivity is ~30% lower in pubertal adolescents compared with prepubertal children. The transient increase in growth hormone secretion during normal puberty appears to be the cause of the pubertal insulin resistance, and not sex steroids. It is likely that insulin resistance during adolescence may precipitate the imbalance between insulin action and secretion in a child with a predisposition to type 2 diabetes.

PCOS is considered a sex-specific form of the metabolic syndrome. It consists of oligo-/anovulation and signs of hyperandrogenism with hyperandrogenemia. Insulin resistance is an integral component of the syndrome and is present in overweight and normal-weight women with PCOS. Our research demonstrates that obese adolescents with PCOS have 50% lower in vivo insulin sensitivity compared with equally obese control girls of similar body composition and abdominal adiposity. Furthermore, the higher prevalence of IGT (~30%) and type 2 diabetes (~3.5%) in adolescents with PCOS appears to be due to impaired insulin secretion in IGT compared with normal glucose tolerance. The relative overrepresentation of female patients among youths with type 2 diabetes could be explained on this basis. Therefore, it is not unreasonable to screen these high-risk obese PCOS adolescents for the presence of IGT and/or type 2 diabetes, or to screen obese girls with type 2 diabetes for the possibility of PCOS.

Acanthosis nigricans is seen in 90% of children and adolescents with type 2 diabetes. Prevalence of acanthosis nigricans is 25-fold higher in blacks than in whites. Type 2 diabetes prevalence is six times higher in blacks who have acanthosis nigricans compared with blacks from the general population. Therefore, the presence of acanthosis nigricans on examination should raise suspicion for increased risk for type 2 diabetes.

Children of mothers with gestational diabetes have increased risk of developing obesity and IGT. This risk is 1.2% at <5 years of age and increases to 19.3% at 10.6 years of age, based on one prospective study. However, epidemiological studies revealed that adults with a history of intrauterine growth retardation (IUGR) are at higher risk for type 2 diabetes and cardiovascular disease. Clinical experience in youth with type 2 diabetes does not agree with the adult observations. Research is needed in pediatric type 2 diabetes to investigate the role of the intrauterine environment on youth type 2 diabetes.

Therefore, genetic as well as environmental factors appear to modulate the risk of type 2 diabetes in youth. Obesity and the presence of other risk factors should prompt appropriate screening in high-risk youths.

DIAGNOSIS

Criteria for diagnosis of diabetes are the same for children and adults and are based on fasting blood glucose, random blood glucose, and an oral glucose tolerance test (OGTT). Any one of these is diagnostic (Table 10.1). Each should, how-

Table 10.1 Criteria for Diagnosis of IFG, IGT, and Diabetes

Plasma glucose (PG)	Normal	IFG	IGT	Diabetes
Fasting PG	<100 mg/dl (5.6 mmol/l)	100–125 mg/dl (5.6–6.9 mmol/l)	N/A	≥ 126 mg/dl (7.0 mmol/l)
OGTT 2-hour PG	<140 mg/dl (7.8 mmol/l)	N/A	140–199 mg/dl (7.8–11.1 mmol/l)	≥ 200 mg/dl (11.1 mmol/l)
Random PG				≥ 200 mg/dl (11.1 mmol/l) + symptoms

2-hour PG, plasma glucose at 2 h after ingestion of glucose.

Adapted with permission from American Diabetes Association (2003).

ever, be confirmed on a subsequent day by any one of the three mentioned methods.

Metabolic stages between normal glucose homeostasis and diabetes constitute pre-diabetes, or IGT and impaired fasting glucose (IFG). IGT is defined as having a 2-h plasma glucose value of 140–199 mg/dl during an OGTT. The American Diabetes Association defines IFG as a fasting plasma glucose value of 100–125 mg/dl. The International Diabetes Federation (IDF) and the World Health Organization (WHO), however, use 110 mg/dl as the cutoff for IFG.

The clinical classification of the type of diabetes in an obese child is frequently difficult because many children present with an admixture of the clinical features of type 1 and type 2 diabetes. Different studies from the U.S. and Europe report that 30–75% of children and adolescents with clinically diagnosed type 2 diabetes have type 1 diabetes–associated autoantibodies, including glutamic acid decarboxylase-65, islet antigen 2, and insulin autoantibodies. The SEARCH data suggest that the presence of autoimmune markers in type 2 diabetes indicates a more aggressive diabetes disease process. Our preliminary data demonstrate that obese youth clinically diagnosed with type 2 diabetes who have positive autoantibodies have lower first- and second-phase insulin secretion compared with those with negative antibodies. The latter group, however, showed worse insulin resistance. Therefore, analysis of pancreatic autoantibodies may be necessary in some cases when the clinical picture is not clear because of an admixture. Proper diagnosis of diabetes type is important for assigning appropriate therapy.

Screening for Type 2 Diabetes in Youth

It is estimated that ~25% of adults with diabetes are undiagnosed. It is not known if this is similar in children. There is increasing evidence that some microvascular complications precede clinical diagnosis. Hence, early recognition and treatment may decrease the risk of complications. The ADA recommended guidelines for screening high-risk children are shown in Table 10.2. For children who do not fully meet the criteria, clinical judgment should be exercised. Furthermore, the ADA recommends using fasting plasma glucose as the screening test, whereas WHO recommends an OGTT as the screening tool. This is based on adult data showing that 30% of individuals with undiagnosed type 2 diabetes have nondiabetic fasting glucose. In our experience, we favor performing an OGTT if the risk for type 2 diabetes is deemed high.

Clinical Presentation of Type 2 Diabetes

The clinical presentation of youth with type 2 diabetes varies remarkably. Some youth are diagnosed incidentally during routine medical checkup when they are found to have glycosuria, and further workup reveals diabetes in the absence of symptoms. Others present with polyuria, polydipsia, or variable degrees of weight loss, with or without severe hyperglycemia. In extreme situations, patients will have hyperglycemic hyperosmolar nonketotic syndrome or present with severe ketoacidosis. The latter may or may not be precipitated by infection, stress, or other illness. The presence of diabetic ketoacidosis (DKA) in an obese child makes the distinction between pure type 2 diabetes or type 1 diabetes uncertain, necessitating measurement of pancreatic autoantibodies.

Table 10.2 Screening Guidelines for Type 2 Diabetes in Youth

Obesity defined as:
• BMI >85th percentile for age and sex, or
• Body weight for height >85th percentile, or
• Body weight >120% of ideal for height

Plus any two of the following risk factors:
• Family history of type 2 diabetes in first- and second-degree relatives
• Race/ethnicity (American Indian, African American, Hispanic, Asian/Pacific Islander)
• Signs/symptoms of insulin resistance (acanthosis nigricans, hypertension, dyslipidemia, PCOS)

When to screen: age 10 years or at onset of puberty, if puberty occurs at a younger age
Frequency of screening: every 2 years
Screening test recommended by ADA: fasting plasma glucose

Adapted with permission from American Diabetes Association (2000).

TREATMENT OF OBESITY

Management of obesity and type 2 diabetes should be through collaborative efforts among the patient, family, physician, behavioral specialist, nurse educator, dietitian, and school.

Clinical guidelines for identification and treatment of overweight in youth were recently published. Intensive family-based behavioral lifestyle modification is recommended for all children who are overweight. Type 2 diabetes prevention studies in adults clearly demonstrate the benefits of intensive lifestyle intervention on prevention of progression from IGT to type 2 diabetes. In children, similar studies are not yet available; however, there is some evidence to suggest that metabolic outcomes may be improved despite seemingly modest weight loss. The essential components in a family-based behavioral lifestyle intervention are cognitive behavior-based changes in nutritional habits and activity levels. Such an approach may prove effective in a research setting, but its translation to clinical practice remains to be determined. In a clinical setting, strategies that may be useful include *1)* quantification of relevant behaviors by trained personnel (e.g., behavioral psychologists, nutritionists, and exercise physiologists); *2)* emphasis on habits that can be modified, such as decreasing the consumption of sugar-sweetened beverages and fast food, decreasing sedentary habits, increasing physical activity, and controlling portion sizes; and *3)* reinforcement of positive change. The positive results of the adult prevention studies and the scarcity of pediatric data may indicate the need for farther-reaching societal change to promote healthy lifestyles in youth. Until there are evidence-based data upon which to make treatment recommendations, we suggest lifestyle modification be utilized as first-line therapy for obesity and IGT in youth.

Pharmacological Treatment of Obesity

Pharmacotherapy for pediatric obesity should be undertaken selectively and with caution under medical supervision and after adequate trial of lifestyle modification. The U.S. Food and Drug Administration (FDA)-approved medications include sibutramine and orlistat. Sibutramine is a nonselective inhibitor of neuronal uptake of serotonin and norepinephrine, which is FDA-approved for patients aged >16 years. Modest weight loss has been seen in some trials, but potential side effects, including tachycardia, hypertension, depression, and suicidal ideations, are a concern. Orlistat is a gastrointestinal lipase inhibitor, which is FDA-approved for adolescents aged >12 years. Potential side effects include fat-soluble vitamin deficiencies, diarrhea, flatulence, and rectal "leakage." Despite the availability of these pharmacological treatments, there is still a need for long-term data to assess their benefits and risks. Metformin is increasingly being used by some clinicians to induce weight loss without convincing robust long-term data in the literature about its effectiveness as a weight-loss drug. Metformin is FDA-approved for use in children with type 2 diabetes and not for the treatment of obesity alone. Metformin is an insulin sensitizer that in the adult Diabetes Prevention Program (DPP) reduced the rate of progression from pre-diabetes to type 2 diabetes, although much less effectively than lifestyle modification alone. Surgical approaches to obesity therapy, including adjustable gastric banding and Roux-en-Y gastric bypass, are available for adult obesity, but extreme caution must be exercised in the adolescent age-group in the absence of pediatric long-term data. These procedures should only be considered according to published recommendations.

Treatment of Type 2 Diabetes

For type 2 diabetes, the first goal of treatment is reversal of acute metabolic abnormalities and maintenance of glucose homeostasis. Other targets include prevention or elimination of symptoms of hyperglycemia, identification and treatment of comorbidities, attainment of ideal body weight, and improvement of insulin sensitivity. The prevention or delay of the development of complications comprises the ultimate goal. A proposed algorithm for the management of the child with type 2 diabetes is presented in Fig. 10.3. Once the patient is stabilized, the patient and family members should meet with a certified diabetes nurse educator to learn about diabetes, treatment options, and home blood glucose monitoring. In our center, we recommend that blood glucose be monitored fasting and before meals. In addition, the strength of psychosocial support, or lack thereof, is identified, and assistance is provided as needed. Lifestyle modification to achieve and maintain a healthy weight is stressed. This includes increased physical activity and nutritional modifications to encourage healthy food choices by the child with the support of the other household members. Pharmacological treatment is initiated with use of metformin. The treatment goal is fasting blood glucose <126 mg/dl and/or A1C <7%. When therapy is not adequate, use of insulin glargine or insulin detemir is added. Insulin therapy is intensified if goals are still not met in 3–6 months. Insulin use should be catered to the patient's needs and ability to comply.

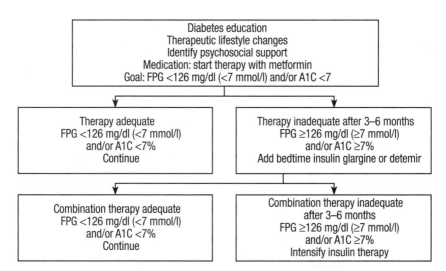

Figure 10.3 Proposed algorithm for the management of youth with type 2 diabetes. Adapted with permission from Hannon (2005).

Pharmacological Treatment of Type 2 Diabetes

Insulin should be used in patients who present with severe hyperglycemia (≥200 mg/dl or A1C >8.5%) or who are in ketosis/ketoacidosis. Insulin treatment will rapidly reverse the metabolic abnormalities. After recovery from the acute metabolic decompensation, metformin is added to the insulin regimen. Nonketotic patients with blood glucose between 126 and 200 mg/dl and A1C <8.5% can be treated with metformin coupled with lifestyle intervention. Metformin is the only oral medication approved by the FDA for use in children and adolescents with type 2 diabetes. Metformin is a biguanide that inhibits hepatic glucose production in the liver and increases insulin sensitivity in peripheral tissues. The initial dose is usually 500-1,000 mg/day and can be increased to a maximum of 1,000 mg twice a day in a period of 2–3 weeks. A 16-week, randomized, double-blind, placebo-controlled trial of metformin, 1,000 mg b.i.d., in newly diagnosed children (age 10–16 years) with type 2 diabetes showed a significant lowering of A1C in the metformin group. Side effects were minimal, with no lactic acidosis. Metformin should not be given to type 2 diabetic patients with acute ketosis (it can be given once the patient recovers from ketosis), with hepatic or renal impairment, with cardiopulmonary insufficiency, or who are undergoing evaluation with radiographic contrast materials because lactic acidosis may be precipitated.

There is no other FDA-approved oral medication for use in pediatric patients with type 2 diabetes. Sulfonylureas (i.e., glimepiride, glyburide, and glipizide) are insulin secretagogues routinely used in adults. A recent single-blind, 26-week study compared glimepiride and metformin in 263 obese youth with type 2 diabetes. Glimepiride was started at 1 mg once a day and increased to 8 mg once a day. Metformin was increased to a maximum of 1,000 mg twice a day. No significant difference in A1C reduction between the two groups was noted (glimepiride: change from baseline –0.85 ± 0.30%, metformin: –0.70 ± 0.30%). A difference in weight gain was noted, however (glimepiride: change from baseline +2.2 ± 0.6 kg, metformin: +0.7 ± 0.64 kg).

Currently, there is an ongoing National Institutes of Health–sponsored multi-site study called Treatment Options for Type 2 Diabetes in Adolescents and Youth (TODAY). This is a randomized, parallel-group clinical trial evaluating the effectiveness of metformin alone, metformin with rosiglitazone, and metformin combined with an intensive lifestyle intervention program in youth with type 2 diabetes. Results of this trial will shed much-needed light on the treatment of type 2 diabetes in youth.

ACUTE COMPLICATIONS

Patients with type 2 diabetes can present in DKA. Forty-two percent of black adolescents in a study in Cincinnati, Ohio, presented with ketonuria, wherein 25% met the criteria for DKA at presentation. A similar percentage was noted in Arkansas. A less common acute complication is hyperglycemic hyperosmolar coma. This is characterized by blood glucose >600 mg/dl and serum osmolality >330 mOsm/l, mild acidosis (bicarbonate >15 mmol/l), and mild ketonuria (<15 mg/dl). These complications can be life threatening. Management of such complications should only be carried out in tertiary medical centers with expertise in management of children with diabetes. The management includes fluid resuscitation, insulin therapy, electrolyte replacement and correction, neurological evaluation, and, in certain instances, airway and pressor support.

CHRONIC COMPLICATIONS AND OTHER COMORBIDITIES

Type 2 diabetic patients are routinely seen in clinic at least three to four times a year. Blood glucose monitoring is essential. Education provided by the physicians, diabetes educators, nurses, and dietitians remains important in subsequent follow-up clinic visits. Apart from giving emphasis on lifestyle intervention, glucose homeostasis, and social and behavior evaluation, physicians should be astute in screening for complications. Some studies in young adults suggest that progression of clinical complications may be more rapid if the onset of type 2 diabetes is at an earlier age. Some microvascular complications may even be present at the time of diagnosis.

Hypertension

Blood pressure should be checked and managed appropriately. Evaluation is based on height, sex, and age-specific (from 1 to 17 years of age) population-based blood pressure percentiles, as published by the National High Blood Pressure Education Group. A systolic or diastolic blood pressure between the 90th and 95th percentile is considered as prehypertension. A systolic or diastolic pressure ≥95th percentile is stage 1 hypertension. Stage 2 hypertension is classified when systolic or diastolic blood pressure is >95th percentile plus 5 mmHg. Once hypertension is identified, lifestyle intervention to achieve and maintain weight loss, dietary changes (including a low-salt diet), and increased physical activity is advised. ACE inhibitors are first-line therapy if lifestyle intervention is not successful in normalizing blood pressure. Angiotensin receptor blockers, calcium channel blockers, β-blockers, and diuretics have been used as other options or additional forms of therapy based on adult data and in the absence of pediatric data. Evaluation for target organ damage is recommended in those with established stage 1 and stage 2 hypertension. In patients with stage 2 hypertension, referral to specialists with expertise in pediatric hypertension should be considered.

Dyslipidemia

Once metabolic control is established, a fasting lipid profile should be obtained at diagnosis of type 2 diabetes. Recommended targets were proposed by the ADA as part of the treatment of type 2 diabetes in youth. Goals include LDL cholesterol <100 mg/dl, HDL cholesterol >35 mg/dl, and triglycerides <150 mg/dl. Initial treatment modalities include dietary changes, weight reduction, increasing physical activity, and glucose homeostasis. If hypercholesterolemia is not controlled in 6 months, HMG-CoA reductase inhibitors (statins) are first-line therapy. These are currently indicated in boys aged >10 years and in postmenarchal girls with familial hypercholesterolemia. Management, however, may vary at the physician's discretion upon weighing of other risk factors. The ADA-published guidelines in the management of dyslipidemia in youth with type 2 diabetes are shown in Table 10.3.

Table 10.3 Management of Dyslipidemia in Youth with Type 2 Diabetes

Goals		
LDL	<100 mg/dl	
HDL	>35 mg/dl	
TG	<150 mg/dl	
Treatment strategies		
LDL	100–129 mg/dl	Maximize nonpharmacological therapy
LDL	130–159 mg/dl	Consider pharmacological therapy based on other risk factors (blood pressure, family history, smoking)*
LDL	≥160 mg/dl	Start pharmacological treatment
Pharmacologic therapy		
LDL	≥160 mg/dl	Statins ± resins
TG	>1000 mg/dl	Fibric acid derivatives

*Continue ongoing management of other risk factors, including therapy for hypertension and smoking cessation. TG, triglyceride.

Adapted with permission from the American Diabetes Association (2003).

Vascular Complications

An annual eye exam is recommended to screen for diabetic retinopathy. This can be present at diagnosis of diabetes. Of the 1,065 patients with type 2 diabetes diagnosed before 30 years of age included in a large Japanese study, 9.3% had retinopathy before the first visit, 12.7% developed retinopathy before 35 years of age, and 24% of those were blind at ~32 years of age. Similar to retinopathy, nephropathy can predate diagnosis of type 2 diabetes. Urine is annually screened for microalbumin excretion. It is unclear as to when should the latter be started. This is left to the discretion of the physician until such time when research data are available.

Atherosclerotic cardiovascular disease is strongly linked to type 2 diabetes in adults. Aortic pulse wave velocity and carotid artery intima-media thickness are surrogate measures of cardiovascular events in adults. Data in children regarding these are limited. Our group demonstrated that obese adolescents with type 2 diabetes have higher aortic pulse wave velocity, indicative of increased arterial stiffness, compared with obese and normal-weight control subjects with no differences in intima-media thickness.

Other Comorbidities

Management of type 2 diabetes goes beyond treatment of metabolic abnormalities and hyperglycemia and prevention of complications. Health care professionals should be astute in recognizing possible comorbidities, such as psychiatric problems, especially in the form of depression. Once these patients are identified, appropriate referral should be made. Some health care providers advocate that screening for depression/behavioral problems by a psychiatrist or psychologist should be routine. Because type 2 diabetes is usually related to obesity, screening for signs of obstructive sleep apnea and appropriate management should be done.

CONCLUSION

Escalating obesity in childhood has clearly translated into an increased incidence of type 2 diabetes in youth. Obese individuals with genetic risk for type 2 diabetes are clearly at highest risk of progression to IGT and frank diabetes when their metabolic profile is overburdened by increased caloric intake and sedentary lifestyle, further exaggerating insulin resistance and enhancing β-cell failure. Pediatricians and family physicians should play an important role, not only in the recognition of obesity and other risk factors that predispose to diabetes, but also in educating the families and implementing lifestyle intervention early in childhood.

To date, lifestyle changes and pharmacological modalities have shown promising results in controlling type 2 diabetes in adults and in delaying or preventing its complications. The study of type 2 diabetes in youth is in its infancy, with great need for scientific information with regard to the natural history of β-cell failure, best therapeutic approaches for the clinical management of diabetes and its complications, and best approaches for its prevention. Ultimately, however, it will require major societal change, with governmental support to design strategies for the creation of healthier environments for the prevention of obesity and type 2 diabetes.

BIBLIOGRAPHY

American Diabetes Association: Management of dyslipidemia in children and adolescents with diabetes. *Diabetes Care* 26:2194–2197, 2003

American Diabetes Association: Type 2 diabetes in children and adolescents. *Diabetes Care* 23:381–389, 2000

Arslanian SA: Type 2 diabetes in children: clinical aspects and risk factors. *Horm Res* 57 (Suppl. 1):19–28, 2002

Bacha F, Saad R, Gungor N, Arslanian SA: Are obesity-related metabolic risk factors modulated by the degree of insulin resistance in adolescents? *Diabetes Care* 29:1599–1604, 2006

Balagopal P, George D, Patton N, Yarandi H, Roberts WL, Bayne E, Gidding S: Lifestyle-only intervention attenuates the inflammatory state associated with obesity: a randomized controlled study in adolescents. *J Pediatr* 146:342–348, 2005

Dietz WH: What constitutes successful weight management in adolescents? *Ann Intern Med* 145:145–146, 2006

Dunican KC, Desilets AR, Montalbano JK: Pharmacotherapeutic options for overweight adolescents. *Ann Pharmacother* 41:1445–1455, 2007

Ehrmann DA: Polycystic ovary syndrome. *N Engl J Med* 352:1223–1236, 2005

Expert Committee on the Diagnosis and Classification of Diabetes Mellitus: Report of the Expert Committee on the Diagnosis and Classification of Diabetes Mellitus. *Diabetes Care* 26 (Suppl. 1):S5–S20, 2003

Expert Committee on the Diagnosis and Classification of Diabetes Mellitus: Follow-up report on the diagnosis of diabetes mellitus. *Diabetes Care* 26:3160–3167, 2003

Frayling TM: Genome-wide association studies provide new insights into type 2 diabetes aetiology. *Nat Rev Genet* 8:657–662, 2007

Gungor N, Hannon T, Libman I, Bacha F, Arslanian S: Type 2 diabetes mellitus in youth: the complete picture to date. *Pediatr Clin North Am* 52:1579–1609, 2005

Hannon TS, Rao G, Arslanian SA: Childhood obesity and type 2 diabetes mellitus. *Pediatrics* 116:473–480, 2005

Inge TH, Krebs NF, Garcia VF, Skelton JA, Guice KS, Strauss RS, Albanese CT, Brandt ML, Hammer LD, Harmon CM, Kane TD, Klish WJ, Oldham KT, Rudolph CD, Helmrath MA, Donovan E, Daniels SR: Bariatric surgery for severely overweight adolescents: concerns and recommendations. *Pediatrics* 114:217–223, 2004

Lee S, Bacha F, Gungor N, Arslanian SA: Waist circumference is an independent predictor of insulin resistance in black and white youths. *J Pediatr* 148:188–194, 2006

Lee S, Gungor N, Bacha F, Arslanian S: Insulin resistance: link to the components of the metabolic syndrome and biomarkers of endothelial dysfunction in youth. *Diabetes Care* 30:2091–2097, 2007

Libman IM, Arslanian SA: Prevention and treatment of type 2 diabetes in youth. *Horm Res* 67:22–34, 2007

National Blood Pressure Education Program Working Group on High Blood Pressure in Children and Adolescents: The fourth report on the diagnosis, evalution, and threatment of high blood pressure in children and adolescents. *Pediatrics* 114:555–576, 2004

Ogden CL, Carroll MD, Curtin LR, McDowell MA, Tabak CJ, Flegal KM: Prevalence of overweight and obesity in the United States, 1999-2004. *JAMA* 295:1549–1555, 2006

Pinhas-Hamiel O, Zeitler P: Acute and chronic complications of type 2 diabetes mellitus in children and adolescents. *Lancet* 369:1823–1832, 2007

Ratner RE, Diabetes Prevention Program Research Group: An update on the Diabetes Prevention Program. *Endocr Pract* 12:20–24, 2006

Stumvoll M, Goldstein BJ, van Haeften TW: Type 2 diabetes: principles of pathogenesis and therapy. *Lancet* 365:1333–1346, 2005

Tfayli H, Bacha F, Gungor N, Arslanian S: Phenotypic type 2 diabetes in obese youth: insulin sensitivity and secretion i islet cell antibody-negative versus -positive patients. *Diabetes* 58:738–744, 2009

Warren-Ulanch J, Arslanian S: Insulin action and secretion in polycystic ovary syndrome. In *Polycystic Ovary Syndrome: Current Controversies from the Ovary to the Pancreas*. Dunaif A, Chang RJ, Franks S, Legro RS, Eds. Totowa, New Jersey, Humana Press, 2008, p. 159–184

Weiss R, Caprio S: The metabolic consequences of childhood obesity. *Best Pract Res Clin Endocrinol Metab* 19:405–419, 2005

Writing Group for the SEARCH for Diabetes in Youth Study Group, Dabelea D, Bell RA, D'Agostino RB Jr, Imperatore G, Johansen JM, Linder B, Liu LL, Loots B, Marcovina S, Mayer-Davis EJ, Pettitt DJ, Waitzfelder B: Incidence of diabetes in youth in the United States. *JAMA* 297:2761–2724, 2007

Drs. Candido, Bacha, Hannon, Libman, and Arslanian are from the Children's Hospital of Pittsburgh, Division of Weight Management & Wellness, Division of Pediatric Endocrinology, Metabolism and Diabetes Mellitus, University of Pittsburgh School of Medicine, Pittsburgh, Pennsylvania.

This work was supported by U.S. Public Health Service Grant nos. K24-HD-01357, RO1 HD 27503, and K12 DK063704, GCRC (M01-RR-00084), CTSA (UL1-RR-024153), the Pittsburgh Foundation, and the Thrasher Research Fund.

11. Psychosocial Aspects in Adults

Lawson R. Wulsin, MD, Alan M. Jacobson, MD,
and Mark F. Peyrot, PhD

ORIGIN OF PSYCHOSOCIAL COMPLICATIONS

Diabetes is associated with increased risk of psychiatric disorders. However, particular subgroups of the diabetic population are at risk for developing psychosocial complications. Women with type 1 diabetes seem to have a higher prevalence of eating disorders (e.g., anorexia nervosa, bulimia, and binge-eating disorder), and those with long-standing diabetes and major medical complications have a higher prevalence of symptoms of depression and anxiety. The estimated prevalence of major depression in patients with diabetes is ~20%, which is double the prevalence in individuals without chronic disease. Depression is associated with poorer glycemic control, and recovery from depression is associated with improvements in glycemic control. The mechanism for depression's contribution to hyperglycemia is not established but may include the well-documented alterations in the autonomic regulation of catecholamines and cortisol during a major depressive episode. Depression is also associated with an increased risk for diabetes complications and poor quality of life, so good management of diabetes includes the management of comorbid depression.

Stress

Stress is one of many factors that may interfere with glycemic control. Two pathways, one behavioral and one humoral, mediate the effect of stress on glucose levels. Stress may cause the person to change key behaviors that upset self-care habits, e.g., increased alcohol intake or decreased exercise. Alternatively, stress hormones (e.g., catecholamines and cortisol) directly alter glucose levels in response to stress.

Barriers to Self-Care

Psychological and social factors influence a patient's success in adhering to any prescribed self-care regimen (Table 11.1). Rubin and Peyrot (2001) have documented that patients often have beliefs about diabetes that are inconsistent with provider perspectives. Several medical problems can be reliable indicators of psychosocial barriers to adequate self-care (Table 11.2).

Table 11.1 Barriers to Self-Care

Patient attitudes and beliefs that affect self-care	Psychosocial factors affecting self-care
■ Anticipating an early cure ■ Believing that self-care regimen is too difficult ■ Believing that treatment is unlikely to improve or control health problems	■ Stressful events in a patient's life ■ Development of new complications ■ Availability and quality of social support for the patient ■ Psychiatric problems unrelated to the patient's diabetes ■ Health care provider's approach to medical care

Detection of Psychosocial Factors

The framework that favors early detection of complicating psychosocial factors is an effective working relationship with the patient and regular monitoring visits. Periodically, examine the patient's psychological functioning by asking open-ended questions (Table 11.3):

- Ask patients to describe any stressful events or situations.
- Determine whether patients have adequate social and family support.
- Ask about problems concerning mood, anxiety, and sense of well-being.
- Ask young women who might be at risk for eating disorders whether they have skipped insulin doses, dieted excessively, eaten in binges, or vomited.
- Engage the patient, and at times the family, in monitoring behaviors or events in addition to glucose levels.

Because depression is common and detrimental, all patients with diabetes should be screened for depression initially and at times of illness progression. The Beck Depression Inventory and the Patient Health Questionnaire (PHQ)-9 are useful screening and monitoring measures for depression.

Inquiries along these lines collect practical information that guide interventions and build the collaborative alliance. Over time, this alliance may lead to better glycemic control by helping the patient address such self-care barriers as low motivation, preconceived judgments about treatment, and fears about diabetes.

Table 11.2 Medical Problems Indicating Psychosocial Barriers to Diabetes Control

■ Recurrent hypoglycemia ■ Frequent episodes of ketoacidosis	■ Very high glycated hemoglobin levels ■ Brittle diabetes

Table 11.3 Open-Ended Questions for Patients with Self-Care Problems

Practitioners should ask for the patient's perception regarding the following:

- Importance of glycemic control
- Feasibility of adhering to a prescribed diet
- Importance of self-monitoring of blood glucose
- Susceptibility to developing complications
- Efficacy of treating complications
- Reasonableness of practitioner's recommendations and expectations

THERAPY

Table 11.4 summarizes the major principles of effective glycemic control when psychosocial factors impair that control. The first six steps are behavioral and focus on accomplishing a goal; the latter two steps recognize the importance of maintaining a strong long-term working relationship. Changing behavior to improve adherence is a complex task that requires assessment of readiness for change, tailoring interventions to the patient's stage of readiness, and motivating patients to take the appropriate next steps for behavior change. This process has been well described by Peyrot and Rubin (2007).

A systematic approach to glycemic control following these principles requires an initial investment of time and energy from the patient and clinician. The physician or diabetes educator should coordinate the effort, delegating responsibilities to the appropriate people and communicating the current plans to all involved. Once the plan has been developed, all team members can be helpful in carrying it out.

Diabetes self-help support groups are effective resources for patient education and for improving adherence to regimens.

Table 11.4 Guidelines for Improving Adherence to Diabetes Regimens

- Give specific instructions, written and oral, about who will do what, tailored to the patient's specific needs and situation.
- Train the patient and family in the skills necessary for the regimen and monitoring.
- Monitor self-care behaviors in several ways by several people.
- Increase the frequency of self-care behaviors with reminders.
- Reinforce or reward steps toward adherence to the regimen.
- Begin with small tasks and achievable goals; shape behaviors with successive revisions of the plan or contract as short-term goals are met.
- Meet the patient at the level of effort the patient is prepared to make.
- Avoid chastising patients when they fail to achieve a goal; instead, revise the goal or the approach.

From Wulsin and Jacobson (1988).

The treatment of comorbid depression is essential to good diabetes management, and it's cost-effective. According to a recent large study (Simon 2007), "For adults with diabetes, systematic depression treatment significantly increases time free of depression and appears to have significant economic benefits from the health plan perspective." For these reasons, the authors recommend that depression screening and systematic depression treatment become routine components of diabetes care. Cognitive behavioral therapy and selective serotonin reuptake inhibitors have been shown to be effective in resolving depressive episodes as well as in improving glycemic control. Exercise also can have the twin benefit of reducing depression and improving physical health.

REFERRAL TO A SPECIALIST

The practitioner will need to identify (for possible referral) mental health professionals who are knowledgeable about diabetes and who can serve as collaborators in treating the patient. The following people may need to be referred to a mental health specialist:

- patients who have had two or more episodes of severe hypoglycemia or diabetic ketoacidosis without obvious causes in 1 year
- patients who do not respond to your efforts to negotiate and implement a treatment plan
- patients with comorbid psychiatric disorders that complicate the management of diabetes

BIBLIOGRAPHY

Andersen B, Goebel-Fabbri A, Jacobson A: Behavioral research and psychological issues in diabetes: progress and prospects. In *Joslin's Diabetes Mellitus*. 14th ed. Kahn CR, Weir GC, King GL, Moses AC, Eds. Philadelphia, PA, Lippincott Williams & Wilkins, 2005

Anderson RJ, Freedland KE, Clouse RE, Lustman PJ: The prevalence of comorbid depression in adults with diabetes: a meta-analysis. *Diabetes Care* 24:1069–1078, 2001

Bradley C: Psychological aspects of diabetes. In *The Diabetes Annual*. Vol. 1. Alberti KGMM, Krall LP, Eds. New York, Elsevier, 1985, p. 374–388

Jacobson AM, Hauser S, Anderson B, Polonsky W: Psychosocial aspects of diabetes. In *Joslin's Diabetes Mellitus*. 13th ed. Kahn C, Weir G, Eds. Philadelphia, Lea & Febiger, 1994, p. 431–450

Kroenke K, Spitzer R, Williams JBW: The PHQ-9: validity of a brief depression severity measure. *J Gen Intern Med* 16:606–613, 2001

Lustman PJ, Clouse RE, Griffith LS, Carney RM, Freedland KE: Screening for depression in diabetes using the Beck Depression Inventory. *Psychosom Med* 59:559–560, 1997

Peyrot M, Rubin RR: Behavioral and psychosocial interventions in diabetes: a conceptual review. *Diabetes Care* 30:2433-2440, 2007

Rubin RR, Peyrot M: Psychological issues and treatments for people with diabetes. *J Clin Psychol* 57:457–478, 2001

Simon GE, Katon WJ, Lin EH, Rutter C, Manning WG, Von Korff M, Ciechanowski P, Ludman EJ, Young BA: Cost-effectiveness of systematic depression treatment among people with diabetes mellitus. *Arch Gen Psychiatry* 64:65–72, 2007

Wulsin LR, Jacobson AM: Management of stress and glycemic control in diabetes. *Intern Med Specialist* 9:100–116, 1988

Dr. Wulsin is a Professor of Psychiatry and Family Medicine at the University of Cincinnati, Cincinnati, Ohio. Dr. Jacobson is a Professor of Psychiatry at Harvard Medical School and Senior Vice President at the Joslin Diabetes Center, Boston, Massachusetts. Dr. Peyrot is a Professor of Sociology at Loyola College, Baltimore, Maryland.

12. Diabetic Ketoacidosis and Hyperosmolar Hyperglycemic Syndrome in Adults

Abbas E. Kitabchi, PhD, MD, and Aidar R. Gosmanov, MD, PhD, DMSc

Diabetic ketoacidosis (DKA) and hyperosmolar hyperglycemic syndrome (HHS) are two serious acute complications of type 1 and type 2 diabetes that require the immediate attention of health care professionals. The mortality rate for adult DKA, though improving, is <1% in experienced centers, whereas the mortality rate for HHS remains high, ~15%, depending on the age of the patient. The burden of both conditions on health care is indisputable. The cost of DKA admissions represent >$1 of every $4 spent on direct medical care for adults with type 1 diabetes and $1 of every $2 per episode in those patients experiencing multiple episodes. The average cost of DKA treatment is $17,559 per patient, which was ~$2.4 billion in 2006.

Patients with DKA present with hyperglycemia, ketonemia, and metabolic acidosis as a result of absolute or relative insulin deficiency. HHS is characterized by more severe hyperglycemia, absent to mild ketosis, and mental status changes (Table 12.1). A laboratory or clinical evaluation suggestive of DKA or HHS should prompt an immediate search for precipitating factors.

PRECIPITATING FACTORS

Omission of insulin and infection are the two most common precipitants of DKA and HHS. Noncompliance or inappropriate insulin therapy may account for up to 44% of DKA presentations; although infection is a top precipitant of HHS, occurring in up to 60% of cases, it is less frequently observed in DKA patients. Acute medical illnesses involving the cardiovascular system (e.g., myocardial infarction, stroke, and acute thrombosis) and gastrointestinal tract (e.g., bleeding and pancreatitis), diseases of the endocrine axis (e.g., acromegaly, Cushing's syndrome, and hyperthyroidism), and impaired thermoregulation or recent surgical procedures can contribute to the development of DKA and HHS by causing dehydration, an increase in insulin counterregulatory hormones, and worsening of peripheral insulin resistance. Administration of medications such as diuretics, β-blockers, corticosteroids, second-generation antipsychotics, and/or anticonvulsants may affect carbohydrate metabolism and volume status. Therefore, these factors could precipitate hyperglycemic crises. Patients who are elderly, bedridden, or nursing-home residents or who have mental disability are at significant risk for HHS because of altered thirst response, inability to seek help, and use of the above-mentioned medications. Psychological problems, eating disorders, insulin pump malfunction, and drug abuse can also be associated with DKA. It is now well recognized that new-onset type 2 diabetes can manifest with DKA. These patients are often obese, have undiagnosed hyperglycemia, and have impaired insulin secretion and insulin action. However, after treatment with insulin, β-cell function and insulin effects improve, so they are able to discontinue therapy. Similarly, HHS can be the initial presentation of diabetes in 30–40% of cases. A recent report suggests that cocaine abuse is an independent risk factor associated with DKA recurrence.

PATHOGENESIS

Reduced insulin concentration, increased insulin counterregulatory hormones (cortisol, glucagon, growth hormone, and catecholamines), and peripheral insulin resistance lead to hyperglycemia, dehydration, ketosis, and electrolyte imbalance, which underlie the pathophysiology of DKA and HHS. The fundamental difference between HHS and DKA is that small residual amounts of insulin in HHS can prevent significant ketosis and, therefore, acidosis.

Table 12.1 Diagnostic Criteria and Typical Total-Body Deficits of Water and Electrolytes in DKA and HHS

Diagnostic criteria and classification	DKA			HHS
	Mild	Moderate	Severe	
Plasma glucose (mg/dl)	>250 mg/dl	>250 mg/dl	>250 mg/dl	>600 mg/dl
Arterial pH	7.25–7.30	7.00 to <7.24	<7.00	>7.30
Serum bicarbonate (mEq/l)	15–18	10 to <15	<10	>15
Urine ketone*	Positive	Positive	Positive	Small
Serum ketone*	Positive	Positive	Positive	Small
Effective Serum Osmolality†	Variable	Variable	Variable	>320 mOsm/kg
Anion Gap‡	>10	>12	>12	<12
Mental Status	Alert	Alert/Drowsy	Stupor/Coma	Stupor/Coma
Typical deficits				
Total water (l)	6			9
Water (ml/kg body wt)	100			100–200
Na+ (mEq/kg)	7–10			5–13
Cl− (mEq/kg)	3–5			5–15
K+ (mEq/kg)	3–5			4–6
PO₄ (mmol/kg)	5–7			3–7
Mg++ (mEq/kg)	1–2			1–2
Ca++ (mEq/kg)	1–2			1–2

*Nitroprusside reaction method; †Calculation: effective serum osmolality: 2[measured Na+ (mEq/l)] + glucose (mg/dl)/18 = mOsm/kg; ‡Calculation: anion gap: [(Na+) − (Cl− + HCO₃−) mEq/l]

Fig. 12.1 depicts the evolution of both hyperglycemic syndromes. Hyperglycemia evolves through accelerated gluconeogenesis, glycogenolysis, and decreased glucose utilization. Due to increased lipolysis and decreased lipogenesis, abundant free fatty acids are converted to ketone bodies: acetoacetate, β-hydroxybutyrate (β-OHB), and acetone. It is noteworthy that measurement of β-OHB will most reliably indicate impending DKA. Hyperglycemia-induced osmotic diuresis, if not accompanied by sufficient oral fluid intake, leads to dehydration, hyperosmolarity, electrolyte loss, and subsequent decrease in glomerular filtration. With decline in renal function, glucosuria diminishes, and hyperglycemia/hyperosmolality worsens. With impaired insulin action and hyperosmolality, utilization of potassium by skeletal muscle is markedly diminished, leading to intracellular potassium depletion. In addition, potassium is lost via osmotic diuresis, causing profound total-body potassium deficiency. Therefore, patients in hyperglycemic crises can present with low, normal, or high serum potassium concentration. Nevertheless, a "normal" plasma potassium concentration indicates that potassium stores in the body are severely diminished, and the institution of insulin therapy and correction of hyperglycemia will lead to future hypokalemia.

Diagnostic criteria for DKA and HHS are presented in Table 12.1. In addition, clinicians should remember that a subset of patients with DKA can present with blood glucose <250 mg/dl. In HHS, the degree of hyperglycemia, serum osmolality, and mental status are important variables in assessing severity of the disease state. Notably, up to one-third of patients presenting with DKA may have elevated serum osmolality.

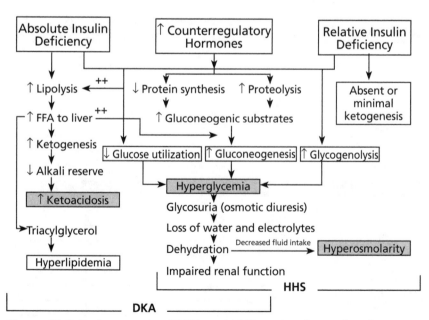

Figure 12.1 Pathogenesis of DKA and HHS. ++Accelerated pathway. FFA, free fatty acids.

DIAGNOSIS

Clinical Presentation

The process of HHS usually evolves over several days to weeks, whereas evolution of acute DKA tends to take hours to days. Clinically, polyuria, polydipsia, weight loss, vomiting, and abdominal pain usually are present in patients with DKA. Abdominal pain has been shown to be closely associated with acidosis and resolves with treatment. Physical examination findings, such as hypotension, tachycardia, poor skin turgor, and weakness support the clinical diagnosis of dehydration in both DKA and HHS. Mental status changes are a hallmark of HHS presentation but are infrequent in DKA. In HHS, obtundation correlates with the degree of osmolality and is unlikely to occur at effective osmolality values of <320 mOsm/kg. Other neurological changes, such as focal neurological deficits, aphasia, and seizures, may be associated with HHS as well; however, central nervous system changes without hyperosmolality should suggest other underlying etiologies besides hyperglycemia. Obtaining a history and performing an examination to diagnose precipitating causes are important. A search for signs or symptoms of infection, vascular events, or drug abuse should be initiated in the emergency room. Patients with hyperglycemic crises can be hypothermic because of peripheral vasodilation and decreased utilization of metabolic substrates.

Laboratory Findings

While evaluating clinical status and obtaining blood glucose by fingerstick, patients with suspected DKA or HHS should have measurements taken of plasma glucose, blood urea nitrogen, creatinine, electrolytes, osmolality, ketones, complete blood count with differential, urinalysis and urine ketones by dipstick, and arterial blood gases. Additional tests include an electrocardiogram, chest X-ray, and various tissues cultures, if indicated. Determination of A1C level will be indicative of degree of diabetes control for the last 2–3 months.

The presence or absence of acidosis/ketosis is the differentiating component between DKA and HHS (Table 12.1). Anion gap acidosis is calculated by subtracting the sum of chloride and bicarbonate from measured (not corrected) sodium concentration. The anion gap should be corrected by the degree of hypoalbuminemia (add 2.5 to the calculated anion gap for each 1-mg/dl decrease of albumin <4.5 mg/dl). An anion gap of >10–12 suggests anion gap acidosis, and usually a bicarbonate level of 18–20 mEq/l rules out metabolic acidosis. Arterial blood gases support the diagnosis. As was mentioned above, β-OHB is an early and abundant ketoacid and indicative of ketosis. Acetoacetate (determined by nitroprusside method) is measured by a majority of laboratories but may be negative in the blood in early DKA. Effective serum osmolality can be measured directly or derived from following formula:

$$2 \text{ [measured Na}^+ \text{ (mEq/l)]} + \text{glucose}/18.$$

Serum sodium concentration is markedly decreased because of intracellular water shift to the extracellular compartment in an attempt to equilibrate hyperosmolality; hence, high measured sodium indicates a significant degree of dehydration. Previous studies showed that the combined total deficit of potassium and sodium can be 500–700 mEq/l. Leukocytosis is often seen in hyperglycemic emergencies and is likely related to the stress response of ketonemia and hyperglycemia; however, a white blood cell count >25,000 should warrant a comprehensive search for infection. Amylase and lipase elevations are reported in DKA and are most often due to extrapancreatic sources; however, pancreatitis should be ruled out. Serum creatinine can be falsely elevated because of acetoacetate interference with the colorimetric creatinine assay. A urine drug screen is helpful to identify individuals at risk for DKA recurrence.

Differential Diagnosis

Other causes of ketoacidosis and anion gap metabolic acidosis should be considered in the differential diagnosis of DKA. Starvation and alcoholic ketoacidosis are not characterized by hyperglycemia >200 mg/dl and bicarbonate level <18 mEq/l. With hypotension and suspicion of sepsis, lactic acidosis should be suspected. Ingestion of methanol, isopropyl alcohol, and paraldehyde can also alter anion gap and/or osmolality and need to be investigated.

TREATMENT

The therapeutic goals of management are:

1. Restoration of volume status
2. Resolution of hyperglycemia and ketosis/acidosis
3. Correction of electrolyte abnormalities
4. Management of precipitating factors and prevention of complications

The majority of patients with DKA/HHS present to the emergency room. Therefore, therapy for resolution of hyperglycemic crises will be initiated by emergency physicians while a physical examination is performed, basic metabolic parameters obtained, and the diagnosis is made. There are several important steps to be followed in early stages of DKA/HHS management:

1. Collect blood for metabolic profile before initiation of intravenous fluids.
2. Infuse 1 liter of 0.9% sodium chloride in 1 h after drawing initial blood samples.
3. Potassium level should be >3.3 mEq/l before initiation of insulin therapy (supplement potassium intravenously, if needed).
4. Initiate insulin therapy only when steps 1–3 are executed.
5. Start 0.45% sodium chloride infusion when indicated (Fig. 12.2) along with insulin.

Protocols for the management of patients with DKA and HHS are presented in Figure 12.2. It must be also emphasized that successful treatment of DKA and HHS requires frequent monitoring of clinical and laboratory parameters to achieve resolution of hyperglycemic crises. Therefore, a flow sheet, such as the one illustrated in Fig. 12.3, should be maintained.

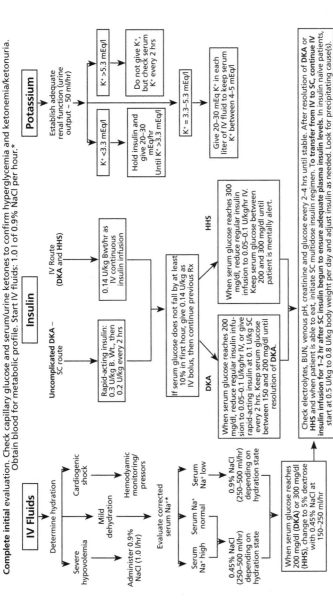

Figure 12.2 Protocol for management of adult patients with DKA or HHS. *DKA diagnostic criteria: serum glucose >250 mg/dl, arterial pH <7.3, serum bicarbonate <18 mEq/l, and moderate ketonuria or ketonemia. *HHS diagnostic criteria: serum glucose >600 mg/dl, arterial pH >7.3, serum bicarbonate >15 mEq/l, and minimal ketonuria and ketonemia. Normal laboratory values vary; check local lab normal ranges for all electrolytes. †After history and physical exam, obtain capillary glucose and serum or urine ketones (nitroprusside method). Begin 1 liter of 0.9% NaCl over 1 h after blood is drawn for arterial blood gases, complete blood count with differential, urinalysis, serum glucose, blood urea nitrogen (BUN), electrolytes, chemistry profile, and creatinine levels STAT. Obtain electrocardiogram, chest X-ray, and specimens for bacterial cultures, as needed. *Serum Na+ should be corrected for hyperglycemia (for each 100 mg/dl glucose >100 mg/dl, add 1.6 mEq to sodium value for corrected serum sodium value). IV, intravenous; SC, subcutaneous.

SUGGESTED
DKA/HHS FLOWSHEET

Height
Weight:
Initially
After 24hr:

DATE: HOUR:												
MENTAL STATUS*												
TEMPERATURE												
PULSE												
RESPIRATION/DEPTH**												
BLOOD PRESSURE												
SERUM GLUCOSE (MG/DL)												
SERUM KETONES												
URINE KETONES												
SERUM NA$^+$ (mEq/l)												
SERUM K$^+$ (mEq/l)												
SERUM Cl$^-$ (mEq/l)												
SERUM HCO$_3^-$ (mEq/l)												
SERUM BUN (mg/dl)												
EFFECTIVE OSMOLALITY 2 [measured Na (mEq/l)] + Glucose (mg/dl)/18												
ANION GAP												
pH VENOUS (V) ARTERIAL (A)												
p0$_2$												
pCO$_2$												
O$_2$ SAT												
UNITS in PAST HOUR												
ROUTE												
0.45% NaCl (ml) PAST HOUR												
0.9% NaCl (ml) PAST HOUR												
5% DEXTROSE (ml) PAST HOUR												
KCL (mEq) PAST HOUR												
PO$_4$ (mMOLES) PAST HOUR												
OTHER												
URINE (ml)												
OTHER												

Row group labels (left margin, bottom to top): ELECTROLYTES; ARTERIAL/VENOUS BLOOD GASES; INSULIN; INTAKE FLUID/METABOLITES; OUTPUT

*A-ALERT   D-DROWSY   S-STUPOROUS   C-COMATOSE
**D-DEEP   S-SHALLOW   N-NORMAL

Figure 12.3 Sample flow sheet for the monitoring of patients with DKA and/or HHS.

Fluid Therapy

Fluid loss averages ~6 l in DKA and ~9 l in HHS. The goal is to replace the volume loss within 24–36 h, with 50% of fluid resuscitation during the first 8–12 h. Current recommendations are to initiate restoration of volume loss with boluses of isotonic saline (0.9% NaCl) intravenously based on the patient's hemodynamic status. Thereafter, intravenous infusion of 0.45% NaCl solution, which is based on sodium serum level (corrected), will provide further reduction in plasma osmolality and help water move into the intracellular compartment. This intravascular and extravascular volume expansion will decrease hyperglycemia by stimulating osmotic diuresis, if renal function is not severely compromised, and enhance peripheral action of insulin (insulin effects on glucose transport are decreased by hyperglycemia and hyperosmolality). When glucose levels fall to <200 mg/dl in DKA and <300 mg/dl in HHS, intravenous fluids should be switched to dextrose-containing 0.45% NaCl solution to prevent hypoglycemia while insulin is infused.

Special considerations should be given to patients with congestive heart failure, chronic kidney disease, and end-stage renal disease. These patients tend to retain fluids; therefore, caution should be exercised during volume resuscitation in these patient groups. Urine output monitoring is an important step for patients with hyperglycemic crises.

Insulin Therapy

Intravenous infusion is a preferred route of insulin delivery in patients with DKA or HHS. Insulin infusion without initial volume resuscitation is not advised because it may only worsen dehydration. A recent prospective randomized study demonstrated that bolus or priming low dose insulin is not necessary if 0.14 units/kg body wt is infused per hour. This is equivalent to 10 units of insulin per hour in a 70-kg subject (Fig. 12.2). If plasma glucose does not fall by at least 10% in the first hour on the insulin infusion rate, the insulin dose should be doubled. Of clinical importance is the phenomenon of hyperglycemia-induced insulin resistance; hence, with reduction of glycemia, there can be a nonlinear decrease in insulin requirements. When plasma glucose reaches 200 mg/dl in DKA or 300 mg/dl in HHS, the insulin rate can be decreased by 50%.

Several prospective clinical trials indicate that a subcutaneous route of administration of rapid-acting insulin analogs in uncomplicated, mild forms of DKA can offer a cost-effective and, most importantly, noninferior mode of insulin delivery in the treatment of DKA (Fig. 12.2). Evaluation of hemodynamic status, degree of dehydration, acidosis, and possible signs of infection should always be conducted before selecting a subcutaneous route of insulin injection.

The length of intravenous insulin administration in DKA is determined by:

1. Resolution of hyperglycemia (plasma glucose <200 mg/dl)
2. Serum bicarbonate concentration >18 mEq/l
3. Venous blood pH >7.3
4. Anion gap <10

When ketonemia is used to assess for response to therapy, we advise measuring only β-OHB, the strongest and most prevalent ketoacid in DKA. Use of the nitroprusside method for monitoring ketonemia, which measures only acetoacetate and acetone in urine or blood, is not recommended. Venous pH is adequate to assess the degree of acidosis, as long as it is understood that it is 0.02–0.03 lower than that of arterial blood. If plasma glucose is <200 mg/dl but bicarbonate and pH are not normalized, insulin infusion must be continued and dextrose-containing intravenous fluids started. The latter approach will continue to suppress ketogenesis and prevent hypoglycemia.

In HHS, intravenous insulin is continued until:

1. Plasma glucose is 250–300 mg/dl
2. Plasma effective osmolality is <320 mOsm/l
3. Mental status is improved (reduction in osmolality usually closely correlates with level of alertness)

Serial measurements (every 2–4 h) of metabolic parameters are required to determine and then confirm resolution of hyperglycemic crisis (Fig. 12.2).

When the patient is able to tolerate oral intake and DKA/HHS is resolved, transition to subcutaneous insulin administration has to be initiated. Patients are given insulin or its analogs 1–2 h before termination of intravenous insulin to allow sufficient time for injected insulin to start to work. After resolution of hyperglycemic crises and when the patient can eat, we recommend injection of intermediate- or long-acting insulin to provide the basal insulin requirement and short- or rapid-acting insulin for prandial glycemic coverage. It is unfortunately common to see placement of a patient in transition from intravenous to subcutaneous insulin on sliding-scale insulin only. This strategy should be discouraged because it does not account for the short half-life of intravenous insulin and cannot provide the necessary insulin requirement in patients recovering from hyperglycemic crisis and β-cell failure. If patients used insulin prior to admission, the same dose can be restarted in the hospital. Insulin-naïve patients require insulin at total dose of 0.5–0.8 units/kg, divided into 30–50% basal insulin and the remainder as fast-acting insulin before each meal. Fingerstick glucose measurements before each meal and at night should be done after discontinuation of intravenous insulin to correct for possible fluctuations in insulin needs while in the hospital.

Potassium, Bicarbonate, and Phosphate Therapy

Insulin administration and correction of acidemia and hyperosmolality will drive potassium into cells and, if this situation is not monitored and treated, hypokalemia can result, potentially leading to arrhythmia and cardiac arrest. If the potassium level is <3.3 mEq/l at any point of therapy, insulin should be stopped and potassium replaced intravenously. If the potassium level is >5.3, replacement is not needed. Add 20–30 mEq of potassium to each liter of infusion fluids if the potassium level is between 3.3 and 5.3 mEq/l.

Bicarbonate use in DKA remains controversial. Based on existing evidence and expert opinion, it may be prudent to administer 50 mmol (1 ampule) of bicarbonate in 200 ml of water with 10 mEq of potassium chloride in 1 h in patients whose pH is 6.9–7.0 or plasma bicarbonate level <5 mEq/l. In adult patients with pH <6.9, we recommend doubling of the above bicarbonate dose. Venous pH should be monitored every 2 h when bicarbonate is administered.

Phosphate levels decrease during insulin therapy. Prospective randomized studies have failed to show any beneficial effect of phosphate on the clinical outcome in

DKA, and overzealous phosphate therapy may cause hypocalcemia. To avoid cardiac and skeletal muscle weakness and respiratory depression due to hypophosphatemia, careful phosphate replacement at a rate of 1.5 ml/h (4.5 mmol/h) of K_2PO_4 may sometimes be indicated in patients with cardiac dysfunction, anemia, or respiratory depression and in those with serum phosphate concentration <1.0 mg/dl. When needed, 20–30 mEq/l potassium phosophate can be added to replacement fluids. Studies are not available on the use of phosphate in the treatment of HHS.

COMPLICATIONS

Hypoglycemia and hypokalemia are the most frequent complications during the management of hyperglycemic crises with high-dose insulin. These are less frequent when low-dose insulin is used. They can be prevented by timely adjustment of insulin dose and frequent monitoring of potassium levels, with appropriate supplementation and judicious use of dextrose-containing infusion fluids.

Non–anion gap hyperchloremic acidosis occurs due to urinary loss of ketoanions, which are needed for bicarbonate regeneration, and preferential reabsorption of chloride in proximal renal tubules secondary to intensive administration of chloride-containing fluids and low plasma bicarbonate. The acidosis usually resolves and should not affect the treatment course.

Cerebral edema is rare in adult patients but could be a serious complication of DKA because it occurs in 1–2% of children presenting with DKA and has also been described in young adults with DKA and in patients with HHS. This condition is manifested by the appearance of headache, lethargy, papillary changes, or seizures. Mortality is high (up to 70%). Mechanisms underlying this condition could be cerebral edema, caused by rapid decline in plasma osmolality, and brain ischemia. Activation of Na^+/H^+ exchange or other ion transport mechanisms in neurons and toxic effects of ketonemia have been suggested to mediate water flux into cells and affect vascular integrity and permeability. Mannitol infusion and mechanical ventilation should be used to treat this condition. Prevention of cerebral edema may be achieved by avoiding overzealous hydration and by maintenance of the plasma glucose level at 150–200 mg/dl in DKA and 250–300 mg/dl in HHS until clinical and biochemical resolution of the hyperglycemic crisis.

Rhabdomyolysis is another possible complication. Hyperosmolality and hypoperfusion contribute to skeletal muscle damage. With recent evidence indicating that DKA is more common among cocaine abusers, a known cause of rhabdomyolysis, creatinephosphokinase level can be initially assessed in patients with DKA if clinically indicated.

Diabetes is characterized by a propensity to thrombosis. Hyperglycemic crises are associated with decreased blood flow and elevation of proinflammatory cytokines and may precipitate thromboembolism. Because the majority of patients present with some degree of renal failure, unfractionated heparin use is preferred for prevention of thromboembolism.

Particular attention should be paid to patients who have a history of severe chronic kidney disease, end-stage renal disease, or congestive heart failure. These individuals are at risk for volume overload. However, even in patients without known renal or cardiac problems, cardiogenic and noncardiogenic pulmonary edema can develop from excessive fluid replacement; as a result, hypoxemia can occur. Acute respiratory distress syndrome is a seldom but potentially fatal complication of DKA. Therefore, new pulmonary rales and increased A-a (alveolar-arterial) gradient should prompt the physician to initiate continuous pulse oxymetry monitoring and decrease fluid administration.

PREVENTION

Many cases of DKA and HHS can be prevented by better access to medical care, proper education, and effective communication with a health care provider during an intercurrent illness. This underscores the need for our health care delivery systems to address this problem. Sick-day management should be reviewed periodically with all patients. It should include specific information on *1*) when to contact the health care provider, *2*) blood glucose goals and the use of supplemental short- or rapid-acting insulin during illness, *3*) means to suppress fever and treat infection, and *4*) initiation of an easily digestible liquid diet containing carbohydrates and salt. Most importantly, the patient should be advised to never discontinue insulin and to seek professional advice early in the course of the illness. The patient/family member must be able to accurately measure and record blood glucose levels, the amount and type of insulin administered, temperature, and respiratory and pulse rates and be able to determine blood β-OHB or urine ketones (when blood glucose is >300 mg/dl). Adequate supervision and help from staff or family may prevent many admissions for HHS due to dehydration among elderly individuals who are unable to recognize or treat this evolving condition.

Many of these hospitalizations could be avoided by devoting adequate resources to apply the measures described above. Because of the significant cost of repeated admissions for DKA, resources need to be directed toward prevention by funding better access to care and educational programs tailored to individual needs, including cultural and personal health-care beliefs. In addition, resources should be directed toward the education of primary care providers and school personnel so that they can identify signs and symptoms of uncontrolled diabetes and so new-onset diabetes can be diagnosed earlier. Applying the above measures, hospitalization rates for DKA can be decreased by 69%. It has been also shown that this approach may decrease incidence of DKA at the onset of diabetes.

BIBLIOGRAPHY

Adrogue HJ, Lederer ED, Suki WN, Eknoyan G: Determinants of plasma potassium levels in diabetic ketoacidosis. *Medicine (Baltimore)* 65:163–172, 1986

Byrne HA, Tieszen KL, Hollis S, Dornan TL, New J: Evaluation of an electrochemical sensor for measuring blood ketones. *Diabetes Care* 23:500–503, 2000

Centers for Disease Control and Prevention: Diabetes data & trends [article online]. Available from http://www.cdc.gov/diabetes/statistics/complications_national.htm. Accessed March 2009

Charfen MA, Fernandez-Frackelton M: Diabetic ketoacidosis. *Emerg Med Clin North Am* 23:609–628, 2005

Della Manna T, Steinmetz L, Campos PR, Farhat SC, Schvartsman C, Kuperman H, Setian N, Damiani D: Subcutaneous use of a fast-acting insulin analog: an alternative treatment for pediatric patients with diabetic ketoacidosis. *Diabetes Care* 28:1856–1861, 2005

Fisher JN, Kitabchi AE: A randomized study of phosphate therapy in the treatment of diabetic ketoacidosis. *J Clin Endocrinol Metab* 57:177–180, 1983

Gaglia JL, Wyckoff J, Abrahamson MJ: Acute hyperglycemic crisis in the elderly. *Med Clin North Am* 88:1063–1084, 2004

Glaser N: New perspectives on the pathogenesis of cerebral edema complicating diabetic ketoacidosis in children. *Pediatr Endocrinol Rev* 3:379–386, 2006

Kitabchi AE, Ayyagari V, Guerra SM: The efficacy of low-dose versus conventional therapy of insulin for treatment of diabetic ketoacidosis. *Ann Intern Med* 84:633–638, 1976

Kitabchi AE, Wall BM: Diabetic ketoacidosis. *Med Clin North Am* 79:9–37, 1995

Kitabchi AE, Umpierrez GE, Murphy MB, Barrett EJ, Kreisberg RA, Malone JI, Wall BM: Management of hyperglycemic crises in patients with diabetes. *Diabetes Care* 24:131–153, 2001

Kitabchi AE: Ketosis-prone diabetes--a new subgroup of patients with atypical type 1 and type 2 diabetes? *J Clin Endocrinol Metab* 88:5087–5089, 2003

Kitabchi AE: Hyperglycemic crises: improving prevention and management. *Am Fam Physician* 71:1659–1660, 2005

Kitabchi AE, Nyenwe EA: Hyperglycemic crises in diabetes mellitus: diabetic ketoacidosis and hyperglycemic hyperosmolar state. *Endocrinol Metab Clin North Am* 35:725–751, 2006

Kitabchi AE, Umpierrez GE, Murphy MB, Kreisberg RA: Hyperglycemic crises in adult patients with diabetes: a consensus statement from the American Diabetes Association. *Diabetes Care* 29:2739–2748, 2006

Kitabchi AG, Murphy MB, Spencer J, Matteri R, Karas J: Is a priming dose of insulin necessary in a low-dose insulin protocol for the treatment of diabetic ketoacidosis? *Diabetes Care* 31:2081–2085, 2008

Lebovitz HE: Diabetic ketoacidosis. *Lancet* 345:767–772, 1995

Magee MF, Bhatt BA: Management of decompensated diabetes: diabetic ketoacidosis and hyperglycemic hyperosmolar syndrome. *Crit Care Clin* 17:75–106, 2001

Miller DW, Slovis CM: Hypophosphatemia in the emergency department therapeutics. *Amer J Emerg Med* 18:457–461, 2000

Morris LR, Murphy MB, Kitabchi AE: Bicarbonate therapy in severe diabetic ketoacidosis. *Ann Intern Med* 105:836–840, 1986

Nyenwe EA, Loganathan RS, Blum S, Ezuteh DO, Erani DM, Wan JY, Palace MR, Kitabchi AE: Active use of cocaine: an independent risk factor for recurrent diabetic ketoacidosis in a city hospital. *Endocr Pract* 13:22–29, 2007

Runyan JW Jr, Zwaag RV, Joyner MB, Miller ST: The Memphis diabetes continuing care program. *Diabetes Care* 3:382–386, 1980

Silver SM, Clark EC, Schroeder BM, Sterns RH: Pathogenesis of cerebral edema after treatment of diabetic ketoacidosis. *Kidney Int* 51:1237–1244, 1997

Stentz FB, Umpierrez GE, Cuervo R, Kitabchi AE: Proinflammatory cytokines, markers of cardiovascular risks, oxidative stress, and lipid peroxidation in patients with hyperglycemic crises. *Diabetes* 53:2079–2086, 2004

Umpierrez GE, Kelly JP, Navarrete JE, Casals MM, Kitabchi AE: Hyperglycemic crises in urban blacks. *Arch Intern Med* 157:669–675, 1997

Umpierrez G, Freire AX: Abdominal pain in patients with hyperglycemic crises. *J Crit Care* 17:63–67, 2002

Umpierrez GE, Cuervo R, Karabell A, Latif K, Freire AX, Kitabchi AE: Treatment of diabetic ketoacidosis with subcutaneous insulin aspart. *Diabetes Care* 27:1873–1878, 2004

Umpierrez GE, Latif K, Stoever J, Cuervo R, Park L, Freire AX, Kitabchi AE: Efficacy of subcutaneous insulin lispro versus continuous intravenous regular insulin for the treatment of patients with diabetic ketoacidosis. *Am J Med* 117:291–296, 2004

Umpierrez GE, Smiley D, Kitabchi AE: Narrative review: ketosis-prone type 2 diabetes mellitus. *Ann Intern Med* 144:350–357, 2006

Vanelli M, Chiari G, Ghizzoni L, Costi G, Giacalone T, Chiarelli F: Effectiveness of a prevention program for diabetic ketoacidosis in children: an 8-year study in schools and private practices. *Diabetes Care* 22:7–9, 1999

Wachtel TJ, Silliman RA, Lamberton P: Prognostic factors in the diabetic hyperosmolar state. *J Am Geriatr Soc* 35:737–741, 1987

Dr. Kitabchi is Professor of Medicine & Molecular Sciences and Director, Division of Endocrinology, Diabetes & Metabolism, Department of Medicine, University of Tennessee Health Science Center, Memphis, Tennessee. Dr. Gosmanov is Medical Resident at the Department of Medicine, University of Tennessee Health Science Center, Memphis, Tennessee.

13. Role of Diabetes Education in Patient Management

MARTHA M. FUNNELL, MS, RN, CDE, AND ROBERT M. ANDERSON, EdD

Recent advances in knowledge, therapies, and technology have greatly enhanced our ability to effectively care for patients with diabetes. Despite these advances, people with diabetes still experience less than optimal blood glucose levels as well as acute and long-term complications. Health care professionals are often frustrated by their patients' inability to make changes in their behavior, and people with diabetes sometimes feel that they are "just a blood sugar number" to their providers. Clearly, there is a gap between the promise and the reality of diabetes care. One of the keys to closing the gap is effective diabetes self-management.

DIABETES SELF-MANAGEMENT

Diabetes self-management refers to all of the activities in which patients engage to care for their illness; promote health; augment physical, social, and emotional resources; and prevent long- and short-term effects from diabetes. Education is the essential first step in becoming an effective self-manager. Traditional views of diabetes self-management education (DSME) were based on information transfer and compliance or adherence. Based on more recent evidence, DSME has evolved to recognize the right and responsibility of patients to make decisions and set self-selected goals that make sense within the context of their lives. The purpose of providing DSME is to help patients make informed decisions and evaluate the pros and cons of those choices.

Whereas patients need a comprehensive understanding of diabetes, its effect on their lives, and how to change behavior, it is unreasonable to think that a one-time educational intervention will be adequate to manage diabetes for a lifetime. Diabetes self-management support (DSMS) is the ongoing assistance patients need from health care professionals, the community, family and friends, and other relevant organizations to make informed self-management decisions and to make and sustain behavioral changes. It incorporates the provision of the needed intellectual, behavioral, emotional, psychosocial, and tangible resources to enable patients to manage their illness effectively. Strategies for providing DSMS include the following:

- Assess patient self-management knowledge, behaviors, confidence, and barriers.

- Incorporate effective behavior-change interventions and ongoing support from family, peers, and professionals.
- Incorporate strategies, including effective communication, to help patients cope with the distress that often results from the many demands of living with diabetes.
- Ensure collaborative care planning and problem solving with a team of health care professionals.

DSME AND SUPPORT

Recent reviews and meta-analyses have indicated that DSME is effective in improving metabolic and psychosocial outcomes, at least in the short term. More time with the educator increases the effect. In addition, DSME interventions that integrate the physiological, behavioral, and psychosocial aspects of diabetes are more effective than programs that focus strictly on knowledge. Table 13.1 summarizes findings related to DSME.

DSME is increasingly available through group programs that are often offered by hospitals or community-based organizations. Programs that achieve recognition from the American Diabetes Association (ADA) by meeting quality standards for process, structure, and outcomes are eligible to receive reimbursement from the Centers for Medicare & Medicaid Services. ADA recognition certifies that the program both meets quality standards and can be reimbursed for its services.

Essential content areas (Table 13.2) have been defined in the Standards for Diabetes Self-Management Education, which were developed by key diabetes organizations. These content areas were written in behavioral terms to maximize creativity on the part of the educator and to allow programs to match instruction and methodology to the culture, literacy, and other needs of their target populations. The information provided is based on an individual assessment of needs and learning style. Evaluation of the effectiveness of DSME is based on patient

Table 13.1 Recent Evidence for DSME

- DSME is effective for improving psychosocial and health outcomes.
- DSME is effective for patients with type 2 diabetes, especially in the short term.
- Traditional knowledge-based DSME is essential but not sufficient for sustained behavior change.
- No single strategy or programmatic focus shows any clear advantage, but interventions that incorporate behavioral and affective components are more effective.

- DSME has evolved from primarily didactic interventions into more theoretically-based empowerment models.
- Effective DSME is tailored to the patient's preferences and social and cultural situations. Group education is effective.
- DSME is most effective when coupled with appropriate care and reinforcement by all health care professionals.
- Behavioral goal-setting is an effective strategy to support self-management behavior.
- Ongoing support is critical to sustain progress made through DSME.

Table 13.2 National Standards for DSME Content Areas

- Describe the *diabetes disease process* and *treatment options*.
- Incorporate *nutritional* management into lifestyle.
- Incorporate *physical activity* into lifestyle.
- Use *medication(s)* safely and for maximum therapeutic effectiveness.
- *Monitor blood glucose* and other parameters, and interpret and use the results for self-management decision making.
- Prevent, detect, and treat *acute complications*.
- Prevent, detect, and treat *chronic complications*.
- Develop personal strategies to address *psychosocial issues and concerns*.
- Develop personal strategies to address *health and behavior change*.

achievement of self-selected behavior-change goals, metabolic measures, and other outcomes.

PROVISION OF DSME AND SUPPORT

Any health care professional who provides diabetes education is a diabetes educator. A certified diabetes educator (CDE) is a health care professional who has specialized knowledge and practical experience in diabetes education and has passed an examination developed by the National Certification Board for Diabetes Education. Board-certified–advanced diabetes managers (BC-ADM) are advanced-practice nurses, dietitians, or pharmacists who have passed an examination developed by the American Nurses Credentialing Center.

ROLE OF THE PROVIDER IN DSME AND DSMS

Based on the Chronic Care Model developed and tested by Wagner et al. (2001), successful management of a chronic illness requires actively involved patients working in partnership with a proactive practice team. Thus, effective diabetes care occurs at both the individual and system levels. Whereas it is unrealistic to expect providers to provide comprehensive DSME in the context of a busy practice, they do have an essential role to play in facilitating DSME and DSMS.

Starting at the time of diagnosis, providers need to provide key messages about diabetes and its treatment. Key messages include the following:

- All types of diabetes need to be taken seriously.
- Diabetes can be managed.
- Effective self-management is essential for positive outcomes.
- A collaborative partnership between the patient, the patient's family, and the health care team is essential for successful diabetes care.
- Effective chronic disease care requires active involvement on the part of the patient.

It is also useful to discuss the roles of the patient and the provider in diabetes care. Because chronic illness care differs from acute care, many patients will not have experienced working in partnership with their health care team. It is important to stress that the person with diabetes is the primary decision maker and is responsible for the daily care of diabetes. It takes the provider's knowledge about diabetes combined with the expertise of the patients about their own goals and priorities to create a truly workable care plan. A plan that is not working is not a negative reflection on either the patient or the provider but simply needs to be revised.

Providers also need to stress the importance of DSME for successful self-management and offer referral to ADA-recognized DSME programs and registered dietitians. Patients value physician opinions and recommendations. Providers need to let patients know that DSME is a wise investment in their future health and that it will provide the knowledge they need for making informed decisions as they care for themselves each day.

Providers can also acknowledge how difficult it is to live with diabetes, and provide reinforcement for the education that has been provided based on feedback from the patient and the DSME program. Although most practices cannot offer comprehensive DSME, practitioners can take advantage of teachable moments that present during any patient encounter. For example, pointing out at-risk areas during a foot examination or making the link between heart disease and diabetes when reviewing lab results are powerful educational moments. Spe-

Table 13.3 Effective Provider-Based Strategies for Self-Management Support

- Stress the seriousness of diabetes.
- Stress the importance of DSME.
- Stress the importance of the patient's role in self-management.
- Offer referral to an ADA-recognized DSME program and registered dietitian.
- Reinforce education provided in the DSME program.
- Begin each visit with an assessment of the patient's concerns, questions, and progress toward metabolic and behavioral goals.
- Assess and address patient-identified fears and concerns at the start of the visit.
- Assess patients' opinions about home blood glucose monitoring results and other laboratory and outcome measures.
- Review and revise the diabetes care plan as needed based on both the patients' and providers' assessment of its effectiveness.

- Provide ongoing information about the costs and benefits of therapeutic and behavioral options.
- Take advantage of teachable moments that occur during each visit.
- Establish a partnership with patients and their families to develop collaborative goals.
- Provide information about behavior change and problem-solving strategies.
- Assist patients to solve problems and overcome barriers to self-management.
- Support and facilitate patients in their role as self-management decision makers.
- Abandon traditional dysfunctional models of care (e.g., adherence and compliance).
- Close the loop at the end of the visit by asking parents to repeat back your instructions.
- End the visit by asking patients to identify one step they will take to care for their diabetes.

cific strategies that can be used with individual patients are listed in Table 13.3.

Physicians can not only ensure that individual patients receive DSME, but they can also design their practices to facilitate ongoing self-management support. Although DSME and DSMS work best when provided by a team of health care professionals, the team does not need to work in the same setting or in traditional roles. Better use of technology allows "virtual" teams to work and communicate effectively with each other and with patients. Table 13.4 lists strategies shown to be effective in facilitating DSME and ongoing DSMS in a variety of practice settings.

CONCLUSION

All types of diabetes are serious and can result in acute and long-term complications that diminish both the quality and length of patients' lives. Patients make multiple decisions each day that directly affect their outcomes, and they experience the consequences of their daily choices and self-care efforts. The key to closing the gap between the promise and reality of diabetes care is through the development of collaborative relationships and patient-centered practices that support patients' self-management efforts. Effective DSME recognizes the patient's role as a collaborator, decision maker, and expert on his or her own life and provides ongoing self-management support. DSME can help relieve the burden of diabetes care on practices by helping patients become informed, active participants in their own care. Staff members of an ADA-recognized DSME program can become a valuable resource for the health care provider, patients, and clinical staff. ADA-recognized DSME programs can be found at www.diabetes.org. Diabetes educators can be found in specific areas by visiting www.diabeteseducator.org.

Table 13.4 Effective Practice-Based Strategies for Self-Management Support

- Use continuous quality improvement to develop, implement, maintain, and enhance DSMS and improve practice.
- Link patient self-management support with provider support (e.g., systems changes, patient flow, and logistics).
- Supplement self-management education and support with information technology.
- Incorporate self-management support into practical interventions, coordinated by nurse case managers or other staff members.
- Create a team with other health care professionals in your system or area with additional experience or training in the clinical, educational, and behavioral or psychosocial aspects of diabetes care.
- Replace individual visits with group or cluster visits to provide efficient and effective self-management support.
- Assist patients to select one area of self-management on which to concentrate that can be reinforced by all team members.
- Create a patient-centered environment that incorporates self-management support from all practice personnel and is integrated into the flow of the visit.
- Use standard tools to assess concerns and establish the visit agenda (e.g., www.med.umich.edu/mdrtc/profs/index.htm).

BIBLIOGRAPHY

Anderson RM, Funnell MM: *The Art of Empowerment: Stories and Strategies for Diabetes Educators.* 2nd ed. Alexandria, VA, American Diabetes Association, 2005

Anderson RM, Patrias R: Getting out ahead: the Diabetes Concerns Assessment Form. *Clinical Diabetes* 25:141–143, 2007

Bodenheimer T, MacGregor K, Sharifi C: *Helping Patients Manage Their Chronic Conditions.* Oakland, CA, California Healthcare Foundation, 2005

Chodosh J, Morton SC, Mojica W, Maglione M, Suttorp MJ, Hilton L, Rhodes S, Shekelle P: Meta-analysis: chronic disease self-management programs for older adults. *Ann Intern Med* 143:427–438, 2005

Deakin T, McShane CE, Cade JE, Williams RD: Group-based education in self-management strategies improves outcomes in type 2 diabetes mellitus. *Cochrane Database System Rev* no. CD003417, 2005

Funnell MM, Tang TS, Anderson RM: From DSME to DSMS: developing empowerment-based self-management support. *Diabetes Spectrum* 20:221–226, 2007

Funnell MM, Brown TL, Childs BP, Haas LB, Hosey GM, Jensen B, Maryniuk M, Peyrot, M, Piette, JD, Reader D, Siminerio LM, Weinger K, Weiss MA: National standards for diabetes self-management education. *Diabetes Educ* 33:599–614, 2007

Glasgow RE, Funnell MM, Bonomi AE, Davis C, Beckham V, Wagner EH: Self-management aspects of the Improving Chronic Illness Care Breakthrough series: implementation with diabetes and heart failure teams. *Ann Behav Med* 24:80–87, 2002

Norris SL, Lau J, Smith SJ, Schmid CH, Engelgau MM: Self-management education for adults with type 2 diabetes: a meta-analysis on the effect on glycemic control. *Diabetes Care* 25:1159–1171, 2002

Polonsky WH, Earles J, Smith S, et al.: Integrating medical management with diabetes self-management training: a randomized control trial of the Diabetes Outpatient Intensive Treatment Program. *Diabetes Care* 26:3048–3053, 2003

Renders CM, Valk GD, Griffin SJ, Wagner EH, et al.: Interventions to improve the management of diabetes in primary care, outpatient, and community settings: a systematic review. *Diabetes Care* 24:1821–1833, 2001

Wagner EH, Glasgow RE, Davis C, Bonomi AE, Provost L, McCulloch D, et al.: Quality improvement in chronic illness care: a collaborative approach. *Jt Comm J Qual Improv* 27:63–80, 2001

Ms. Funnell is a research investigator and a diabetes educator and Dr. Anderson is an educational psychologist and professor of medical education in the Department of Medical Education at the University of Michigan Medical School, Ann Arbor, Michigan, and they are Co-Directors of the Behavioral, Clinical, and Health Systems Research Core at the Michigan Diabetes Research and Training Center, Division of Endocrinology and Metabolism, Department of Internal Medicine, University of Michigan, Ann Arbor, Michigan.

The authors were supported in part by grant nos. NIH5P60 DK20572 and 5 R18 DK070020 from the National Institute of Diabetes and Digestive and Kidney Diseases of the National Institutes of Health.

14. Monitoring in Diabetes

Satish K. Garg, MD, and Ramachandra G. Naik, MD

HISTORICAL PERSPECTIVE

It is interesting to note that the sweet taste of diabetic urine was recorded way back in the first century B.C.E. by Indian physicians, Sushruta and Charaka, in the Ayurveda, scripture of ancient Indian medicine. Much later, Paracelsus (1493–1541 C.E.) advocated the testing of urine for sugar, and later in 1674, Thomas Willis reemphasized the presence of "wonderfully sweet, like sugar or honey" urine in individuals suffering from diabetes. In the 18th century, Mathew Dobson (1776) documented that both urine and serum from a diabetic patient had a taste indistinguishable from sugar; this was later demonstrated to be glucose by the French chemist Chevreul (1815). Chemical tests for glucose then emerged, including polarimetry and the copper sulfate test, which was later modified in 1848 by Fehling (commonly referred to as Fehling's test). These innovative technologies then led to the pivotal physiological studies of Claude Bernard, von Mering, and Minkowski in the 19th century, and they recognized that pancreatectomy in dogs resulted in polyuria associated with the excretion of large quantities of sugar, i.e., diabetes. Micromethods for testing of glucose in blood became available in the early 20th century; knowledge about blood glucose in both normal and diabetic individuals soon followed. The first semiquantitative urine glucose test was devised in 1911 by Benedict (Benedict's test). Later in 1915, Benedict's method was introduced for the measurement of blood glucose.

More than five decades later, in 1962, self-sampling for blood glucose determination was introduced for the first time using a colorimetric technique of estimation of glucose in a dried blood sample applied to a small filter paper pad and assayed within a week of sampling. A rapid (1 min), enzyme test strip (Dextrostix, Ames), semiquantitative method for estimating capillary whole-blood glucose was described in 1964. Later, in 1970, an attempt was made to eliminate observer error when visually judging blood color changes to reflect glucose concentrations, and a portable, battery-operated, lightweight reflectance meter (Eyetone, Ames) used in conjunction with the Dextrostix was introduced and evaluated against the autoanalyzer method during oral glucose tolerance tests. In the late 1970s, it was demonstrated that rapid methods of self-monitoring of blood glucose (SMBG), predominantly in individuals with type 1 diabetes, were a means of improving diabetes control. These initial studies showed that the introduction of SMBG improved control in 83% of diabetic subjects, with almost two-thirds of them being able to maintain long-term blood glucose <180 mg/dl, and patients found adjusting their insulin dose and/or type of insulin to be much easier and more preferable than urine glucose testing. Less frequent episodes of hypoglycemia were also experienced using SMBG. Patients were able to use the technique accurately, and SMBG made these patients feel empowered and motivated in their self-care. Quickly, SMBG took on a central role in improving and maintaining glycemic control in diabetic patients. It helps minimize the long-term vascular risks associated with long-standing hyperglycemia. Today, we have >40 different U.S. Food and Drug Administration (FDA)-approved glucose meters available for day-to-day SMBG testing.

In conjunction with the capillary glucose measurements using rapid reagent test strips, the emergence of A1C assays in 1976 finally made it possible to address the questions of whether good glycemic control in humans prevents and/or delays the appearance and/or progression of the vascular complications related to diabetes.

BENEFITS OF MAINTAINING NORMOGLYCEMIA IN DIABETES AND THE ROLE OF GLUCOSE MONITORING IN ACHIEVING THIS GOAL

Large-scale clinical trials have shown that intensive insulin therapy, which is aimed at achieving glucose levels as close to the nondiabetic range as safely possible, decreases the incidence and progression of both micro- and macrovascular diabetes complications. Moreover, maintaining A1C at normal or near-normal levels reduces health care costs for adults with diabetes. The pivotal Diabetes Control and Complications Trial (DCCT) in individuals with type 1 diabetes convincingly demonstrated that improvement in glycemic control delayed the onset and progression of microvascular complications of diabetes, namely retinopathy, nephropathy, and neuropathy. Every 1% drop in A1C was associated with improved outcomes, and there was no threshold effect. Comparable results also emerged from another study in type 2 diabetes, the U.K. Prospective Diabetes Study (UKPDS), which demonstrated the benefit of improving blood glucose control and also blood pressure control in individuals with type 2 diabetes. It should be noted that although SMBG is a key factor in intensive therapy, it is intertwined with many other factors that may lower A1C.

Unfortunately, intensive insulin therapy is also associated with an increased risk of hypoglycemia. Subjects in the intensive insulin treatment arm of the DCCT, for example, experienced a 3.3-fold higher incidence of severe hypoglycemia than the control group. In the DCCT trial, the intensively treated group conducted SMBG at home more frequently (~4 times per day) in comparison with those in the conventional group, who monitored less frequently. Increased frequency of SMBG has been shown to significantly improve glucose control, as measured by A1C values. There are other compelling data that show a direct relationship between the frequency of SMBG and achieving better glucose control, as described by increased "within the target range" glucose values (70–150 mg/dl).

TESTS FOR GLYCEMIA IN DIABETES

Glycemic status monitoring, performed by both the patients and the health care providers, is the cornerstone of diabetes care today. Optimal monitoring of glycemic control involves blood glucose measurements by the patient at home (i.e., SMBG) and an assessment of long-term control by the physician, as measured by A1C. Both of these measurements are complementary; whereas A1C gives an average of glucose levels over the previous 2–3 months, SMBG guides the patients and providers on a day-to-day basis and helps in detecting hypoglycemia and hyperglycemia. Results of glucose monitoring are extremely useful in assessing the efficacy of therapy and in guiding adjustments in medical nutrition therapy, exercise, and medications in an attempt to achieve the best possible blood glucose control.

The American Diabetes Association (ADA) has formulated a position statement on the tests used most widely in monitoring the glycemic status of people with diabetes and addresses both patient and physician/laboratory-based testing. The current ADA recommendations are published in a technical review (Goldstein 2004).

SMBG

In a short span of a few years, SMBG has revolutionized diabetes management and has become the standard of care. In SMBG, a small drop of blood and an easily detectable enzymatic reaction allow measurement of capillary plasma glucose. A number of devices accurately measure glucose in blood obtained from the fingertip. SMBG has helped diabetic patients work to achieve and maintain specific glycemic targets.

SMBG is now well established in clinical practice, but its successful implementation relies on both education and motivation. Training in the technical aspect of blood glucose monitoring is essential to provide accurate and reliable results. Education allows the patient to understand and translate the readings into appropriate action when necessary. The frequency of testing needs to be tailored to the need and tolerance of the individual concerned. Other SMBG factors that also need to be considered include sustainability, convenience, execution, and cost.

Currently, the ADA recommends that all treatment programs in type 1 diabetes should encourage SMBG for routine daily monitoring. The frequency of SMBG measurements must be individualized and adapted to address the goals of diabetes care. Individuals with type 1 diabetes should routinely measure plasma glucose four to eight times per day to estimate and select mealtime boluses of short- or rapid-acting insulin and/or to modify long-acting basal insulin doses. This method of delivering insulin is commonly referred to as a multiple daily injection (MDI) regimen. The patients on MDI commonly use vials and syringes or insulin delivery devices such as pens. Some patients use continuous subcutaneous insulin infusion (CSII) pumps to deliver insulin. There are several insulin infusion pumps available in the market today.

Individuals with type 2 diabetes who are on oral medications should utilize SMBG as a means of assessing the efficacy of their medication and the impact of diet and monitoring for and preventing asymptomatic hypoglycemia. Most individuals with type 2 diabetes require less frequent monitoring, although the optimal frequency of SMBG has not been clearly defined. The literature on SMBG in type 2 diabetes suggests an improvement in glucose levels only for subjects in whom the data were used to make adjustments in therapeutic regimens. Because plasma glucose levels fluctuate less in these individuals, one to two SMBG measurements per day (or fewer) may be sufficient. Individuals with type 2 diabetes who are on insulin should utilize SMBG more frequently than those on oral agents.

When glucose control is less than optimal, having patients concentrate on premeal glucose levels is adequate. Once the premeal glucose levels reach the low 100s, it is recommended that patients switch to checking 1- to 2-h postprandial glucose levels because it amplifies the observed effect of diet on glycemic control and enables patients to see that moderate changes in meal plan, activity, and medications have a significant impact on glycemic control. Even after substantial appropriate changes in food intake, activity, or timing or dose of oral or injectable medication, blood glucose values often return to near-normal levels overnight or by the time of the next meal.

Existing data, however, indicate that only a minority of patients perform SMBG adequately. There are several barriers to the increasing use of SMBG, including cost of testing, inadequate understanding (by both health care providers and patients) of the health benefits and proper use of SMBG results, psychological and physical discomfort associated with fingerstick blood sampling by the patient, and inconvenience of testing in terms of time requirements, physical setting, and complexity of the technique. Given the importance of SMBG to diabetes care, government, third-party payers, and others should strive to make the procedure readily accessible and affordable for all patients who require it. Lack of feedback to guide in diabetes treatment is another important barrier for the use of SMBG.

Because the accuracy of SMBG is user dependent, it is important for health care providers to evaluate each patient's monitoring technique, both initially and at regular intervals thereafter. Use of calibration and control solutions on a regular basis by patients helps ensure accuracy of results. In addition, because laboratory methods measure plasma glucose, most blood glucose monitors approved for home use and some test strips now calibrate capillary whole-blood glucose readings to plasma values. Plasma glucose values are 10–15% higher than whole-blood glucose values.

Optimal use of SMBG requires proper interpretation of the data. Patients should be taught how to use the data to adjust medical nutrition therapy, exercise, or pharmacological therapy to achieve specific glycemic goals. Health professionals should, at regular intervals, evaluate the patient's ability to use SMBG data to guide treatment. A number of SMBG methods store test results and provide sophisticated analyses of blood glucose data when connected to a computer; it has been shown that these data management systems yield better glucose control. Recently, several websites, electronic tools, and insulin-guidance software have been made available to help patients make modifications in their treatment regimens. Thus, SMBG should be an important component of any health care benefits package.

With the availability of SMBG and A1C testing, routine laboratory blood glucose testing by health care providers should no longer be used to assess glycemic control except to supplement information obtained from other testing methods and to test the accuracy of SMBG. When adjusting oral glucose-lowering medication(s) in a patient not taking insulin, laboratory testing also may be appropriate. Comparisons between results from patient self-testing of blood glucose in the clinic and simultaneous laboratory testing are useful to assess the accuracy of patient results.

Alternative-Site Blood Glucose Testing

Currently, fingerstick capillary blood sampling is the traditional method used in SMBG. However, the pain associated with the fingerstick during sampling can often be limiting, and these challenges in fingerstick glucose measurements have led to the development of technologies to allow for sampling from sites other than the finger. At present, there are several meters that are FDA-approved for use on the forearm, upper arm, palm, abdomen, thigh, and calf.

Studies examining the efficacy of alternative-site blood glucose testing (AST) have shown that there is a strong positive correlation ($r > 0.95$) between fingertip and AST measurements; a majority of patients (70–90%) expressed that AST resulted in no pain or less pain than the conventional methods of testing. Despite the apparent advantages and accuracy, there are several limitations: it has been shown that the accuracy of AST is compromised when glucose levels are measured 1 h postprandially and immediately after exercise. The 1-h postprandial rise in blood glucose was blunted with AST as compared with conventional fingertip testing. Similarly, the drop in blood glucose expected with exercise exhibited a lag with AST, and glucose levels were higher when compared with fingertip testing. However, accuracy of AST was comparable with that of conventional SMBG at baseline, 90 min, and 2 h postprandial. Thus, AST appears to be most reliable in states of relatively stable glycemia and should be used with caution when the rate of change of blood glucose is rapid, exceeding >2 mg • dl^{-1} • min^{-1}; here, AST measurements tend to lag behind. Hence, the overall applicability in insulin-requiring subjects with diabetes is limited, given that these patients are at increased risk of rapidly fluctuating glycemia.

URINE GLUCOSE TESTING

With the availability of SMBG, urine glucose testing has become obsolete for most diabetic patients. It can still be useful among patients who cannot pay for SMBG, such as the homeless. Urine glucose testing by patients in the home setting consists of semiquantitative measurements based on a single voiding or, less often, by timed collections over 4–24 h. The rationale is that urinary glucose values reflect mean blood glucose during the period of urine collection. However, despite the relatively low cost and ease of specimen collection, the well-described limitations of urine glucose testing make SMBG the preferred method of monitoring glycemic status from day to day.

URINE/BLOOD KETONE TESTING

Ketone testing is an important part of monitoring in type 1 diabetic patients, in pregnant women with preexisting diabetes, and in women with gestational diabetes. The presence of ketones may indicate impending or even established ketoacidosis, a condition that requires immediate medical attention. Patients with type 1 diabetes should test for ketones when their plasma glucose is consistently >300 mg/dl; during a concurrent illness with symptoms such as nausea, vomiting, or abdominal pain; or during pregnancy. Ketones are normally present in urine, but concentrations are usually below the limit of detection with routine testing methods. However, positive ketone readings are found in normal individuals during fasting and in up to 30% of first morning urine specimens from pregnant women. Urine ketone tests using nitroprusside-containing reagents measure only acetoacetate and acetone and can give false-positive results in the presence of several sulfhydryl drugs, e.g., the antihypertensive drug captopril. False-negative readings have been reported when test strips have been exposed to air for an extended period of time or when urine specimens have been highly acidic, such as after large intakes of ascorbic acid. Ketone testing strips should be available in the office/clinic setting. It is important for health care professionals to remember that the currently available urine ketone tests are not reliable for diagnosing or monitoring treatment of ketoacidosis. Blood ketone testing methods that quantify β-hydroxybutyric acid, the predominant ketone body, are available and are preferred over urine ketone testing for diagnosing and monitoring ketoacidosis.

TESTING FOR GLYCATED PROTEINS: A1C MEASUREMENT

Although blood glucose testing and blood or urine ketone testing provide useful information for the day-to-day management of diabetes, these tests cannot provide the patient and health care professionals with a quantitative and reliable measure of glycemic control over an extended time period. Measurements of glycated proteins (primarily hemoglobin and serum proteins) can, with a single measurement, quantify average glycemia over weeks and months, thereby complementing day-to-day testing. *Glycated hemoglobin*, specifically A1C, is a term used to describe a series of stable minor hemoglobin components formed slowly and nonenzymatically from hemoglobin and glucose. When plasma glucose is consistently elevated, there is an increase in nonenzymatic glycation of hemoglobin; this alteration reflects the glycemic history over the previous 2 to 3 months because erythrocytes have an average lifespan of 120 days. The rate of formation of A1C is directly proportional to the ambient glucose concentration, and the A1C test has become the preferred standard for assessing glycemic control. As discussed earlier, this test has been shown to predict the risk for the development of many chronic complications in diabetes.

There were formerly numerous laboratory methods for measuring the various forms of glycated hemoglobin, and these had significant interassay variations. Optimal use of the A1C test for assessing glycemia required the standardization of A1C test assays. The National Glycohemoglobin Standardization Program (NGSP) (http://www.ngsp.org), sponsored in part by the ADA to standardize A1C test determinations to DCCT values, began in mid-1996. On an annual basis, manufacturers of A1C test assay methods are awarded a "certificate of traceability to the DCCT reference method" if their assay method passes rigorous testing criteria for precision and accuracy. The ADA recommends that laboratories use only A1C test assay methods that have passed certification testing. Currently, >95% of the laboratories in the U.S. are standardized to the NGSP standards. It is also desirable that all laboratories performing A1C testing participate in the College of American Pathologists proficiency testing survey for A1C testing started in mid-1996, which uses whole-blood specimens. Accordingly, after several years of work, the International Federation of Clinical Chemistry and Laboratory Medicine (IFCC) developed a new reference method that specifically measures glycated A1C values. The reference factor is only used to standardize the A1C assay and cannot be used by the clinical laboratory for measuring A1C values.

A1C testing should be performed routinely in all patients with diabetes, first to document the degree of glycemic control at initial assessment and then as part of continuing care. Because the A1C test reflects mean glycemia over the preceding 2–3 months, measurement approximately every 3 months is required to determine whether a patient's metabolic control has reached and been maintained within the target range. Thus, regular A1C testing permits detection of departures from the target range in a timely fashion. For any individual patient, the frequency of A1C testing should be dependent on the treatment regimen used and on the judgment of the clinician. It is recommended that A1C testing be done at least twice a year in patients who are meeting treatment goals (and who have stable glycemic control) and more frequently (i.e., quarterly) in patients whose therapy has changed, in those who are not meeting glycemic goals, and in those who are newly diagnosed with diabetes.

Proper interpretation of A1C test results requires that health care providers understand the relationship between test results and average blood glucose, kinet-

Table 14.1 Correlation between A1C level and mean plasma glucose levels (from DCCT and ADAG data)

A1C (%)	DCCT Mean plasma glucose		ADAG Mean plasma glucose	
	mg/dl	mmol/l	mg/dl	mmol/l
6	135	7.5	126	7.0
7	170	9.5	154	8.6
8	205	11.5	183	10.2
9	240	13.5	212	11.8
10	275	15.5	240	13.4
11	310	17.5	269	14.9
12	345	19.5	298	16.5

ics of the A1C test, and specific assay limitations. Depending on the assay methodology, hemoglobinopathies, anemias, and uremia may interfere with the A1C result. Table 14.1 shows the correlation between A1C levels and mean plasma glucose levels based on data from the DCCT and the A1C-Derived Average Glucose (ADAG) study. A1C test values in patients with diabetes are a continuum; they range from normal in a small percentage of patients whose average blood glucose levels are in or close to the normal range to markedly elevated values (e.g., >9.5%) in some patients, reflecting an extreme degree of hyperglycemia. The ADA recommends that the goal of therapy for most patients should be an A1C <7% and that physicians should reevaluate and, in most cases, significantly change the treatment regimen in patients with A1C test results consistently above this goal. Again, these specific A1C values apply only to assay methods that are certified as traceable to the DCCT reference method.

Estimated Average Glucose

More recent research has looked into reevaluating the biologic and clinical meaning of A1C; it has been suggested that there could be an accurate conversion algorithm that would result in an estimated average glucose (eAG); this may result in the laboratories eventually reporting A1C accompanied by its eAG. Results of the multicenter ADAG study, published in June 2008 (Action to Control Cardiovascular Risk in Diabetes [ACCORD] Study Group 2008), confirmed a close correlation of A1C with mean glucose in 507 subjects with type 1 diabetes ($n = 268$), type 2 diabetes ($n = 159$), and no diabetes ($n = 80$); analysis of the data in diabetic patients who completed the study demonstrated a sufficiently tight correlation between A1C and average glucose to provide a regression equation to translate A1C into an eAG. Final results of this study should allow more accurate reporting of the eAG and improve patients' understanding of this measure of glycemia. Table 14.1 compares the prior conversion from DCCT data to the conversion from the ADAG study. The differences in the DCCT-A1C comparison and the A1C-eAG results from the ADAG study are mainly attributed to the frequency of glucose measurements. The ADAG study used frequent glucose monitoring over 3 months in addition to continuous glucose monitoring monthly for 3 months, whereas, in contrast, DCCT data used only 1 day's seven-point profile for each comparison to A1C.

Role of A1C in Diagnosing Diabetes

There has been interest in the use of A1C values for screening and identification of impaired glucose tolerance and diabetes. However, there are significant problems with using A1C as a diagnostic tool, such as false-positive and false-negative results related to hemoglobinopathy and altered red cell survival and the imperfect correlation between A1C and 2-h plasma glucose, the traditional "gold standard" test. Previously, the ADA did not recommend its use for screening purposes. However, at the time of publication, an ADA, European Association for Study of Diabetes (EASD), and International Diabetes Federation (IDF) expert panel on the diagnosis of diabetes is considering cut points to diagnose diabetes with the now–globally standardized A1C test.

OTHER GLYCATED SERUM PROTEINS: SERUM FRUCTOSAMINE ASSAY

Because the turnover of human serum albumin is much shorter (half-life of 14–20 days) than that of hemoglobin, the degree of glycation of serum proteins (mostly albumin) provides an index of glycemia over a shorter period of time than does glycation of hemoglobin. Measurements of total glycated serum protein () and glycated serum albumin (GSA) correlate well with one another and with measurements of glycated hemoglobin (i.e., A1C). In situations where A1C cannot be measured or may not be useful (e.g., hemolytic anemias), the GSP assay may be of value in the assessment of the treatment regimen. Several methods have been described that quantify either total GSP or total GSA.

One of the most widely used is the fructosamine assay. The fructosamine assay (measuring glycated albumin) reflects the glycemic status over the prior 1–2 weeks. Values for GSP vary with changes in the synthesis or clearance of serum proteins that can occur with acute systemic illness or with liver or advanced renal disease. In addition, there is continuing debate as to whether fructosamine assays should be corrected for serum protein or serum albumin concentrations. Measurement of GSP (including fructosamine) has been used to document relatively short-term changes (e.g., 1–2 weeks) in glycemic status, such as in diabetic pregnancy or after major changes in therapy. However, further studies are needed to determine whether the test provides useful clinical information in these situations. Measurement of GSP, regardless of the specific assay method, should not be considered equivalent to the A1C test because it only indicates glycemic control over a short period of time. Therefore, GSP assays would have to be performed on a bimonthly basis to gather the same information as provided by the A1C test done three or four times a year. Unlike the A1C test, GSP has not yet been shown to be related to the risk of the development or progression of the chronic complications of diabetes. Current consensus statements do not favor the use of alternative assays of glycemic control because there are no studies to indicate whether such assays accurately predict the complications of diabetes.

ESTABLISHMENT OF BLOOD GLUCOSE TREATMENT TARGETS

The target for glycemic control (as reflected by A1C) must be individualized, and the goals of therapy should be developed in consultation with the patient after considering a number of medical, social, and lifestyle issues. Some important factors to consider include the patient's age, ability to understand and implement a complex treatment regimen, presence and severity of diabetes complications, ability to recognize hypoglycemic symptoms, presence of other medical conditions or treatments that might alter the response to therapy, occupation (e.g., possible consequences of experiencing hypoglycemia on the job), and level of support from family and friends.

The ADA has established suggested glycemic goals based on the premise that glycemic control predicts development of diabetes-related complications. For most patients, the target A1C should be <7.0%, but goals should be individualized, based on age, comorbidity, and history of hypoglycemia. Other consensus groups (such as the Veterans Administration) have suggested multiple A1C goals that take into account the patient's life expectancy at the time of diagnosis and the presence of microvascular complications. Such recommendations strive to balance the financial and personal costs of glycemic therapy with anticipated benefits (e.g., reduced health care costs, reduced morbidity). One limitation to this approach is that the onset of hyperglycemia in type 2 diabetes is difficult to ascertain and likely predates the diagnosis. In Table 14.2, guidelines from the ADA are presented. Other groups, such as the American Association of Clinical Endocrinologists (AACE) and the EASD, advocate A1C goals of <6.5%.

There are potential adverse events related to the pursuit of more aggressive targets. These include hypoglycemia, long-term exposure to poorly studied combinations of medications, cost, life disruption caused by greater attention and effort to achieve lower glycemic targets, and the potential that great efforts expended in achieving extremely stringent glycemic goals will result in less attention to other health risks.

The ADA target of fasting and premeal plasma glucose levels of 70–130 mg/dl was initially developed based on an estimate of the range of average glucose values that would be associated with a low risk of hypoglycemia and A1C <7%. It was modified based on recognition that to routinely achieve an A1C <7%, many patients would have moderate hypoglycemic events, with glucose levels in the 70- to 90-mg/dl range.

The ADA treatment target for peak postprandial glucose levels is set at <180 mg/dl, in part because those levels would be generally associated with an A1C of <7% and because nondiabetic individuals who have a large evening meal have been demonstrated to exhibit transient elevations of glucose to that level. There are no published studies in which even safety, much less outcome, is documented for targeting a particular level of postprandial glucose. However, it is clear that there are effective A1C-lowering agents that primarily target postprandial glucose levels and that monitoring postprandial glucose levels may be necessary to optimize dose adjustment of these agents. Furthermore, there are patients with diabetes who have average fasting glucose levels within targets but whose A1C is elevated. In these patients, monitoring and specifically treating postprandial elevations can provide improvements in A1C, perhaps with a lower risk of hypoglycemia and weight gain than further lowering fasting and premeal glucose levels.

A recent report of 20% increased mortality in the intensive-treatment arm (A1C <6%) of high-risk individuals with type 2 diabetes in the ACCORD study raises the question of the degree of intensity of glycemic control that is needed in such populations. There were 54 more deaths, or 3 per 1,000 participants, each

Table 14.2 Glycemic Targets

Parameter	Normal	ADA
Premeal plasma glucose (mg/d)	<100 (mean 90)	70–130
Postprandial plasma glucose (mg/dl)	<140	<180
A1C	4–6%	<7%

year (257 total deaths) in the intensively treated arm (A1C ~6.4%) versus 203 deaths in the less-intense, standard treatment arm (A1C ~7.4%). The intensively treated arm of the study was stopped 18 months early (February 2008) by the National Heart, Lung, and Blood Institute (NHLBI) of the National Institutes of Health due to safety concerns, and further analyses will provide insights into the cause-effect relationships of these circumstances. Subsequently, two other trials of intensive glucose control and cardiovascular disease, Action in Diabetes and Vascular Disease: Preterax and Diamicron MR Controlled Evaluation (ADVANCE) and Veterans Affairs Diabetes Trial (VADT), did not confirm an increase in mortality with intensive glycemic treatment. However, none of the three trials demonstrated a significant reduction in cardiovascular disease outcomes with intensive treatment compared with standard glucose treatment.

Patients for whom it may be appropriate to be more cautious about instituting intensive treatment regimens include children aged <13 years, people with hypoglycemia unawareness, elderly people, and patients with advanced complications such as end-stage renal disease or significant cardiovascular or cerebrovascular disease. Instituting aggressive insulin therapy in subjects with proliferative or severe nonproliferative retinopathy can lead to accelerated, but transient, progression of retinopathy. The target A1C should be achieved gradually over time in patients with eye disease, and treatment of the eye disease should be considered before instituting an aggressive insulin regimen. Patients who do not experience warning adrenergic symptoms of hypoglycemia (hypoglycemia unawareness) are at significantly greater risk for severe recurrent hypoglycemia, and this may prevent the safe institution of tight glucose control. Thus, individualization of the treatment to target A1C values is most important. The glycemic goals appearing in clinical guidelines should be expressed as IFCC units, derived NGSP units, and ADAC.

GLYCEMIC MONITORING AND TARGETS FOR PREGNANT WOMEN WITH DIABETES

In nonpregnant individuals, A1C reflects the mean blood glucose over the previous 8–12 weeks. This period is shorter in pregnancy because of the increased red blood cell production. It is recommended that the A1C be measured every 4–6 weeks during pregnancy. The goal is to achieve a value at or near the normal range (<6.1%) without inducing hypoglycemia. The rationale for choosing this target is that observational studies have shown that A1C values up to 1% above normal (5.0% is the nondiabetic mean) are associated with rates of congenital anomalies and miscarriage similar to the rates in the general population. However, it should be noted that the normal range of glucose concentration and A1C for pregnant women is lower than that for nonpregnant individuals because both average blood glucose concentration and A1C values fall by ~20% in nondiabetic pregnant women. This is the rationale for striving to achieve A1C levels at, or ideally below, the normal range in nonpregnant individuals. The frequency of SMBG should be increased during a pregnancy associated with diabetes, especially in the postprandial phase (1 and 2 h postmeal) to maintain target glucose values at those time points in the desired range. It is commonly believed that the fetal outcomes are directly proportional to postprandial blood glucose levels, especially the 1-h level.

It is also recommended that urinary ketones be measured when pregnant women with type 1 diabetes are ill or when any blood glucose value is >180 mg/dl. At these times, ketoacidosis may occur, a complication that is associated with high fetal mortality rate. Ketonemia may have adverse developmental effects as well. Women with moderate to severe ketonuria associated with hyperglycemia need to alert their physician immediately so that additional insulin can be prescribed promptly. Ideally, the woman should know exactly how much additional insulin is needed if her blood glucose elevation is associated with ketonuria.

Target blood glucose values proposed by the American College of Obstetricians and Gynecologists (ACOG) are fasting glucose concentrations ≤95 mg/dl, preprandial glucose concentrations ≤100 mg/dl, 1-h postprandial glucose concentrations ≤140 mg/dl, 2-h postprandial glucose concentrations ≤120 mg/dl, mean capillary glucose <100 mg/dl, and A1C ≤6%. The ADA recommends the following target: premeal, bedtime, and overnight glucose: 60–99 mg/dl; peak postprandial glucose 100–129 mg/dl; and A1C <6.0%.

INTERSTITIAL GLUCOSE MEASUREMENTS: USE OF CONTINUOUS GLUCOSE MONITORING IN DIABETES

The intermittent glucose monitoring by SMBG has now advanced toward continuous glucose monitoring (CGM) with built-in alarms for hypo- and hyperglycemia, and thus patients can respond to glucose trends and the rate of change of glucose. Interstitial detection of glucose may more closely relate to glucose readings at the organ level, where complications are likely to occur. Whereas SMBG measures blood glucose directly, most of the CGM devices monitor glucose in the interstitial space. CGM was first approved for retrospective analysis and now, with the approval of real-time glucose sensing, has advanced to the next step in diabetes management.

The first such real-time CGM product to be marketed was a transcutaneous device, the GlucoWatch Biographer. GlucoWatch use was limited due to adverse effects, including skin irritation, edema, and erythema at the site of reverse iontophoresis. Newer CGM devices are subcutaneously inserted (with a wired or wireless sensor) into the abdomen, arm, or leg and provide interstitial glucose readings every 1–5 min. CGM allows patients using MDI or insulin pumps to identify blood glucose trends and rates of glucose change. More recently, CGM has been shown to decrease A1C values while preventing the severity and time spent in hyperglycemic and hypoglycemic ranges. However, a meta-analysis of older CGM studies showed no significant decrease in A1C values in randomized controlled trials. More recently, glucose variability (GV) has been hypothesized to be an independent risk factor for microvascular and macrovascular complications. In part, mealtime hyperglycemia and overtreatment with insulin resulting in hypoglycemia can lead to greater GV, which in short-term studies has been documented to result in greater oxidative stress. Clearly, a large, long-term study needs to be conducted to prove that GV is an independent risk factor in the complications associated with diabetes.

The use of CGM in patients with type 1 diabetes provides them with the capability to prevent both hyper- and hypoglycemia, resulting in decreased GV, which may reduce the risk for short- and long-term diabetes complications.

Testing the Accuracy of CGM Devices

The accuracy of CGM has been evaluated in numerous clinical studies. Anecdotally, patient perceptions of the differences between CGM and SMBG readings can be a limiting factor to patient adherence with these devices, and proper patient education is critical and may help alleviate some of their concerns. The literature suggests that interindividual characteristics, such as age, sex, or insertion site have little effect on sensor performance.

The Clarke Error Grid has long been the gold standard for evaluating glucose monitoring meters for accuracy. Error Grid Analysis (EGA) divides the variance between test and reference blood glucose into zones. Zone A is the most accurate and represents ≤20% deviation of the test meter from standard or simultaneous blood glucose values <70 mg/dl for both machines. Zone B is >20% deviation, with no clinically significant adverse outcome from decisions made based on the value. Zones C through E represent wider disparities and erroneous readings that could result in potentially dangerous treatment decisions and are therefore unacceptable. A subsequent publication introduced a similar analysis for continuous glucose sensors, taking into account some characteristics of CGM, especially the time sequence of the data (lag time) to determine the accuracy of blood glucose readings (point EGA) and accuracy of evaluation of the rate of blood glucose change (rate EGA). The zones in both cases are similar to those in the SMBG EGA. The continuous glucose EGA was then derived by combination of both point and rate EGA in three clinically relevant blood glucose ranges (<70, 70–180, and >180 mg/dl) using the error grid matrix.

Another way to characterize glucose exposure using CGM data is by analyzing ambulatory glucose profiles (AGPs). All CGM profiles can be overlapped according to time of day and then used to calculate area under the median curve (AUC_{md}) using the trapezoidal method. This method better reflects overall glucose exposure in patients using CGM.

Use of CGM is also associated with a "lag time" (time for blood glucose to equilibrate with interstitial glucose concentrations) that is accentuated with a rapid rate of change of glucose. Therefore, as blood glucose quickly changes, either up or down, it may take longer for glucose concentrations in the blood and interstitial fluid to equilibrate. This often appears as an under- or overreading discrepancy in sensor readings. Calibrating during times of rapid blood glucose change may also result in inaccuracies in future sensor readings, even after blood glucose levels stabilize. Thus, it is recommended to calibrate during stable glucose levels. Generally, all CGM sensors are required to be calibrated initially and thereafter two to four times a day.

Currently, all of the FDA-approved CGM devices are considered to be adjunctive to SMBG to verify/confirm information that the CGM device provides, such as periods of hyper- and hypoglycemia. This means that patients need to understand when to perform confirmation SMBG (adjunctive claim), and insurance companies will have to continue to provide coverage of SMBG while they determine whether to provide individual coverage of the CGM. The use of

CGM may not expand until these products have a replacement claim (where cross-checking sensor glucose values with SMBG is not necessary) for SMBG and require no calibration. In addition, outcome studies need to show that glucose control can be improved long term and that hypoglycemia can be significantly reduced.

Clinical Efficacy of CGM Devices

Several studies have been published evaluating the impact of real-time CGM on A1C values in adults and children with type 1 diabetes and in adults with type 2 diabetes. The major clinical benefits of CGM include, as mentioned earlier, a decrease in the time spent in hypo- and hyperglycemia; improvement in the percentage of glucose readings in the euglycemic range (70–150 mg/dl), thus decreasing the GV; and an improvement in A1C during the period of sensor use. Short-term benefits may include early recognition of a rise in postprandial blood glucose and timing of injection of rapid-acting insulin analogs. In fact, many patients report that rapid-acting analog injection time may need to be 20–30 min prior to the meal, if euglycemia (1 and 2 h postprandial) is to be achieved. Intermittent SMBG data clearly indicated that at the higher end of A1C levels, fasting hyperglycemia makes a dominant contribution to the significant rise in A1C levels, more than postprandial blood glucose. For example, at an A1C of 10%, fasting hyperglycemia contributes 70% to the elevation of A1C. However, CGM data analysis indicates that increased postprandial blood glucose is equally responsible for increases in the A1C, even at higher levels.

Today, CGM is an important research tool in the monitoring required for the management of diabetes. There are limited human data on implantable sensors. A study in humans showed that in fairly well-controlled subjects with type 1 diabetes, the glucose excursions could be significantly reduced over a 6-month period, without any reduction in A1C values. To summarize, current data support the accuracy, safety, and clinical efficacy of incorporating CGM into the treatment of adults and children with type 1 diabetes.

Future Research on CGM

The Juvenile Diabetes Research Foundation Continuous Glucose Monitoring (JDRF CGM) Study Group has developed a randomized clinical trial to determine whether real-time CGM systems can improve glycemic control and quality of life in children and adults with type 1 diabetes. The initial 6-month data confirmed improvement of glucose control, with a reduction in A1C of 0.5% in adults (age >25 years) with type 1 diabetes. The study also reported improvement in the time spent in hypo- and hyperglycemia related to increased use of the sensor. The additiona data for the ongoing study at 1 year will be presented at the ADA meeting in 2009. Research in the area of CGM is also currently designed to improve the quality of existing products, including better sensor accuracies, longer use of sensors, creating different built-in algorithms for different rates of change of glucose, and attempts to develop noninvasive CGM devices. These endeavors make the spectrum of glucose monitoring likely to extend from the past methods of urine testing and blood glucose testing to the newer methods of interstitial glucose measurements. It is also imperative that we learn how to use the enormous amount of blood glucose data made available with CGM. For example, perhaps we can create (proactive) algorithms for adjusting insulin doses. Further research is also in progress to assess a closed-loop model incorporating insulin pump and CGM technology.

CONCLUSIONS

SMBG has completely replaced urine glucose measurements and has become an important tool in the day-to-day management of diabetes. SMBG should be done at least three times a day for insulin-requiring subjects with diabetes and less often in non–insulin-requiring patients. A1C should be measured between two and four times a year for assessing overall long-term glucose control. The role of measurements of glycated albumin and fructosamine remains controversial. The future of SMBG may evolve into interstitial glucose measurements (i.e., CGM), once the devices are more accurate and are made with better algorithms for guiding patients toward improved diabetes management. It is important to keep in mind the rising health care costs associated with diabetes. Thus, until CGM becomes easily accessible and long-term outcomes can be modified, these new technologies will continue to be important research tools but help few insulin-requiring diabetic patients. Attempts are in progress for "closing the loop" in insulin-requiring subjects. However, accuracy of CGM and better proactive guidance algorithms are needed before such a dream—the artificial or "bionic" pancreas—can be accomplished.

BIBLIOGRAPHY

Action to Control Cardiovascular Risk in Diabetes Study Group: Effects of intensive glucose lowering in type 2 diabetes. *N Engl J Med* 358:2545–2559, 2008

American College of Endocrinology: American College of Endocrinology consensus statement on the guidelines for glycemic control. *Endocr Pract* 8 (Suppl. 1):5–11, 2002

American Diabetes Association: Self-monitoring of blood glucose (Consensus Statement). *Diabetes Care* 17:81–86, 1994

American Diabetes Association: Standards of medical care in diabetes—2009. *Diabetes Care* 32 (Suppl. 1):S13–S61, 2009

American Diabetes Association: Consensus statement on the worldwide standardization of the hemoglobin A1C measurement: the American Diabetes Association, European Association for the Study of Diabetes, International Federation of Clinical Chemistry and Laboratory Medicine, and the International Diabetes Federation. *Diabetes Care* 30:2399–2400, 2007

Brewer KW, Owen S, Garg SK, Chase HP: Slicing the pie: correlating HbA—values with average blood glucose values in a pie chart form. *Diabetes Care* 21:209–212, 1998

Clarke WL, Cox D, Gonder-Frederick LA, Carter W, Pohl SL: Evaluating clinical accuracy of systems for self-monitoring of blood glucose. *Diabetes Care* 10:622–628, 1987

Diabetes Control and Complication Trial Research Group: The effect of intensive treatment of diabetes on the development and progression of long-term complications in insulin-dependent diabetes mellitus. *N Engl J Med* 329: 977–986, 1993

Garg SK: Glucose monitoring: an important tool for improving glucose control and reducing hypoglycemia. *Diabetes Technol Ther* 10 (Suppl. 1):S1–S4, 2008

Garg SK, Schwartz S, Edelman SV: Improved glucose excursions using an implantable real-time continuous glucose sensors in adults with type 1 diabetes. *Diabetes Care* 27:734–738, 2004

Garg S, Zisser H, Schwartz S, et al.: Improvement in glycemic excursions with a transcutaneous, real-time continuous glucose sensor: a randomized controlled trial. *Diabetes Care* 29:44–50, 2006

Garg SK, Kelly WC, Voelmle MK, Ritchie PJ, Gottlieb PA, McFann KK, Ellis SL: Improved glycaemic control with real life use of continuous glucose sensors in adult subjects with type 1 diabetes. *Diabetes Care* 30:3023–3025, 2007

Garg SK, Smith J, Beatson C, Lopez-Baca B, Voelmle M, Gottlieb PA: Comparison of accuracy and safety of the SEVEN and the Navigator continuous glucose monitoring systems. *Diabetes Technol Ther* 11:65–72, 2009

Garg SK, Voelmle MK, Gottlieb P: Feasibility of 10-day use of a continuous glucose-monitoring system in adults with type 1 diabetes. *Diabetes Care* 32:436–438, 2009

Goldstein DE, Little RR, Lorenz RA, Malone JI, Nathan D, Peterson CM, Sacks DB: Tests of glycemia in diabetes. *Diabetes Care* 27:1761–1773, 2004

JDRF CGM Study Group: JDRF randomized clinical trial to assess the efficacy of real-time continuous glucose monitoring in the management of type 1 diabetes: research design and methods. *Diabetes Technol Ther* 10:310–321, 2008

Juvenile Diabetes Research Foundation Continuous Glucose Monitoring Study Group, Tamborlane WV, Beck RW, Bode BW, Buckingham B, Chase HP, Clemons R, Fiallo-Scharer R, Fox LA, Gilliam LK, Hirsch IB, Huang ES, Kollman C, Kowalski AJ, Laffel L, Lawrence JM, Lee J, Mauras N, O'Grady M, Ruedy KJ, Tansey M, Tsalikian E, Weinzimer S, Wilson DM, Wolpert H, Wysocki T, Xing D: Continuous glucose monitoring and intensive treatment of type 1 diabetes. *N Engl J Med* 359:1464–1476, 2008

Little RR, Rohlfing CL, Wiedmeyer H-M, Myers GL, Sacks DB, Goldstein DE: The National Glycohemoglobin Standardization Program (NGSP): a five-year progress report. *Clin Chem* 47:1985–1992, 2001

Nathan DM, Kuenen J, Borg R, Zheng H, Schoenfeld D, Heine RJ, A1c-Derived Average Glucose Study Group: Translating the A1C assay into estimated average glucose values. *Diabetes Care* 31:1473–1478, 2008

Pickup J, Mattock M, Kerry S: Glycaemic control with continuous subcutaneous insulin infusion compared with intensive insulin injections in patients with type 1 diabetes: meta-analysis of randomised controlled trials. *BMJ* 324:705, 2002

Rohlfing CL, Wiedmeyer HM, Little RR, England JD, Tennill A, Goldstein DE: Defining the relationship between plasma glucose and HbA$_{1c}$: analysis of glucose profiles and HbA$_{1c}$ in the Diabetes Control and Complications Trial. *Diabetes Care* 25:275–278, 2002

Sacks DB, Bruns DE, Goldstein DE, Maclaren NK, McDonald JM, Parrott M: Guidelines and recommentations for laboratory analyses in the diagnosis and management of diabetes mellitus. *Diabetes Care* 25:750–786, 2002

UK Prospective Diabetes Study (UKPDS) Group: Intensive blood-glucose control with sulphonylureas or insulin compared with conventional treatment and risk of complications in patients with type 2 diabetes (UKPDS 33). *Lancet* 352:837–853, 1998

Dr. Garg is Professor of Medicine and Pediatrics and Director, Adult Program, at the Barbara Davis Center for Childhood Diabetes, University of Colorado Denver, Denver, Colorado. Dr. Naik is an Assistant Professor at the Barbara Davis Center for Childhood Diabetes, University of Colorado Denver, Denver, Colorado.

This work was funded in part by Grant 08 FLA 00250 from the State of Colorado Public Health and Environment; Grant P30 DK575616 from the Diabetes Endocrine Research Center, National Institutes of Health (NIH); Grant M01 RR00069 from the General Clinical Research Program, NIH; and Grants R01 HL61753, R01 HL079611, and R01 DK32493 from the Children's Diabetes Foundation (Denver, CO).

15. Rationale for Management of Hyperglycemia

Kathleen M. Dungan, MD

The principles involved in managing hyperglycemia in patients with diabetes are outlined in Table 15.1. Each patient should have an initial assessment to define the appropriate glycemic goal for his or her treatment program. Diabetes education in a structured program supervised by a qualified diabetes educator is essential for every patient with diabetes. Without adequate education, patients will not be able to self-monitor blood glucose, understand their disease, comply with their treatment program, or take appropriate action to minimize complications. Intervention is initiated with lifestyle modification and pharmacological agents. Changes in the therapeutic program are guided by the results of self-monitoring of blood glucose and A1C measurements.

Data from recent intervention studies in both type 1 and type 2 diabetic patients indicate that early initiation of intensive hyperglycemic management has profound long-term beneficial effects in reducing microvascular complications. The pathogenic effects of the level of hyperglycemia on the microvascular system persist for many years. This effect of the "memory" of the microvascular system for its history of glycemic control is noted in the remarkable delay between the time at which intensive glycemic control is achieved and the time at which the rate of development of microvascular complications begins to decrease. In the Diabetes Control and Complications Trial (DCCT), this delay was ~3–4 years, and in the U.K. Prospective Diabetes Study (UKPDS), it was ~9 years. The most definitive proof of this effect is being shown in the EDIC (Epidemiology of Diabetes Interventions and Complications) study, which is the long-term follow-up of individuals who had been in the DCCT. At the conclusion of the DCCT protocol, all of the patients were sent back to their primary care health facilities for continuing care. A substantial cohort of the individuals agreed to return to their DCCT

Table 15.1 Principles of Glycemic Control

- Initiate the treatment program when hyperglycemia is first diagnosed.
- Define the appropriate target goal.
- The glucose targets should be near normoglycemia, if possible.
- Diabetes education is essential.
- Monitor glycemic control.
- Initiate lifestyle modification.
- Use stepwise and combination pharmacological therapy.

research center yearly for continued monitoring for vascular complications. During the 7 years of follow-up, the mean A1C of the previously intensively treated group (mean A1C = 7.2%) increased and has averaged 8.0%. In contrast, the mean A1C of the control cohort (mean A1C = 9.0%) decreased and has averaged 8.0%. Despite the equal glycemic control over the last 4–5 years, the rate of development and progression of clinical retinopathy and nephropathy in the previously intensively treated cohort is less than one-third that of the previous control cohort. Similar findings were reported in the long-term follow-up of the UKPDS.

These results have prompted the current ADA recommendations for a target A1C of <7.0% for most individuals, with exceptions for more or less stringent goals in appropriate situations.

In contrast to microvascular complications, the benefits of intensive glycemic control for reducing macrovascular complications continues to be the subject of debate. The most compelling evidence stems once again from the EDIC results, which demonstrated a statistically significant 42% reduction in risk of any cardiovascular event and a 57% reduction in risk of nonfatal myocardial infarction, stroke, or death after a mean 17 years of follow-up. During the randomized portion of the UKPDS, only a nonsignificant 16% reduction in cardiovascular events ($P = 0.052$) was observed, despite an epidemiological analysis demonstrating a compelling continuous association of cardiovascular events with A1C. However, the 10-year follow-up of the UKPDS cohort revealed significant long-term reductions in myocardial infarction (15% with sulfonylurea or insulin as initial pharmacotherapy, 33% with metformin as initial pharmacotherapy) and in all-cause mortality (13 and 27%, respectively), suggesting that glycemic control early in the course of type 2 diabetes may have cardiovascular disease benefit.

Three large trials conducted in patients with type 2 diabetes and established cardiovascular disease or multiple risk factors did not demonstrate a significant benefit of more intensive glycemic therapy aimed at lowering A1C to ≤6.5% or <6%: Action in Diabetes and Vascular Disease—Preterax and Diamicron MR Controlled Evaluation (ADVANCE), the Veterans Affairs Diabetes Trial (VADT), and Action to Control Cardiovascular Risk in Diabetes (ACCORD). The intensive glycemic control arm of ACCORD was stopped early due to an increase in mortality in the more intensively treated arm. The reasons for the lack of results in these intensive glycemic control studies is uncertain but seem likely related to the specific strategies for intensive glucose lowering used in the populations studied as well as perhaps the duration of the trials. Furthermore, patients in these studies had more advanced diabetes and preexisting cardiovascular disease at baseline than in the DCCT or UKPDS. Subgroup analyses of these recent studies suggested that a window of opportunity exists, in which patients without macrovascular disease at baseline, shorter duration of diabetes, and/or better baseline glycemic control may obtain cardiovascular benefit from more intensive glycemic interventions.

The American Diabetes Association (ADA), American Heart Association, and American College of Cardiology have recently reviewed both older and the more recent studies and reaffirmed the current general glycemic targets of A1C <7% and the benefits of glycemic control for preventing microvascular complications, while emphasizing the importance of individualization of therapy. Lower targets could be considered in younger patients with a shorter duration of diabetes, longer expected life span, and no significant cardiovascular disease, provided that glycemic control could be achieved without substantial hypoglycemia or other adverse events. Conversely, less stringent A1C goals may be appropriate for patients with a history of severe hypoglycemia, limited life expectancy, advanced complications, and extensive comorbidities and for those with long-standing diabetes in whom A1C <7% is difficult to attain, despite diabetes self-management education, effective doses of multiple glucose-lowering agents (including insulin), and appropriate monitoring.

Hyperglycemia in patients with diabetes results from a combination of overproduction and underutilization of glucose. In establishing a rational approach to the management of hyperglycemia, it is important to understand the dominant influences in the patient for whom the strategy is being developed.

Patients who are absolutely insulin deficient (e.g., those with type 1 diabetes or surgical removal or destruction of the pancreas) must receive insulin replacement therapy as the main therapeutic agent. None of the available oral antidiabetic agents can effectively ameliorate hyperglycemia in the absence of endogenous insulin.

Patients in whom hyperglycemia results from an imbalance between insulin secretory function and peripheral insulin sensitivity, as occurs in type 2 diabetes, are excellent candidates for initiation of nonpharmacological therapies that reduce insulin secretory requirements (i.e., diet) or increase peripheral insulin effectiveness (i.e., exercise, weight loss). In addition, at least eight classes of pharmacological agents other than insulin are available for the treatment of type 2 diabetes. These agents may be classified according to their primary mechanisms of action:

1. Reduction in degree or rate of glucose absorption from the gut (α-glucosidase inhibitors, exenatide, glucagon-like peptide [GLP]-1 agonists, pramlintide, and possibly colesevelam)
2. Increase in peripheral glucose utilization (thiazolidinediones [TZDs])
3. Decrease in hepatic glucose production (metformin)
4. Insulin secretagogue (sulfonylureas, glinides, GLP-1 agonists, dipeptidyl peptidase [DPP]-IV inhibitors)
5. Inhibition of inappropriate glucagon secretion (GLP-1 agonists, DPP-IV inhibitors, pramlintide)
6. Reducing appetite or improving satiety (GLP-1 agonists, pramlintide)

Given the multitude of choices for the treatment of hyperglycemia, the ADA and the European Association for the Study of Diabetes (EASD) recently published a revised consensus statement for stepwise, goal-directed management. The need for such an algorithm is underscored by the observation of therapeutic inertia, in which patients remain on inadequate medication regimens with the promise of increasing lifestyle efforts or fail to efficiently and effectively receive adjustments in therapy in proportion to the degree of glycemic control. It is important that A1C levels are obtained every 3 months during treatment and that changes in therapy are promptly administered if patients are not meeting targets. In general, combination regimens should incorporate therapies with complementary mechanisms of action.

Recommendations for individual agents are based on factors such as glucose-lowering efficacy, long-term safety, side-effect profiles, ease of use, and cost. The

ADA/EASD consensus statement recognizes the high frequency of failure of diet and exercise alone and recommends the initiation of metformin in addition to lifestyle measures at the time of diagnosis. Metformin is inexpensive, efficacious, weight neutral, and has a long safety profile in patients for whom there are no contraindications (renal insufficiency) or unacceptable side effects (gastrointestinal complaints).

If A1C targets are not met within 3 months or if A1C later rises, the algorithm advocates the addition of one of two alternative "tier 1" second steps: insulin or sulfonylureas. Both are rapidly effective and relatively inexpensive but are associated with weight gain and hypoglycemia. The placement of insulin as an option early in the treatment algorithm represents a significant paradigm shift in treatment for hyperglycemia, in which insulin was formerly regarded as a therapy of last resort.

Pioglitazone and GLP-1 agonists are deemed to be less well-validated "tier 2" options in the ADA/EASD consensus algorithm for addition to metformin and lifestyle therapy. They are included in the algorithm because they both address fundamental pathophysiological features of type 2 diabetes without a risk of hypoglycemia. However, TZDs have a slow onset of action, cause weight gain, and in certain patients may increase the risk of heart failure and bone fracture. GLP-1 agonists are associated with moderate weight loss; however, there is insufficient clinical experience to be confident of long-term safety. Both TZD- and GLP-1–based therapies exhibit β-cell–protective properties that theoretically would improve the durability of the antihyperglycemic effect, although this is not well-validated in humans. It should be noted that the ADA/EASD consensus panel does not recommend the use of rosiglitazone, glyburide, or chlorpropamide due to lingering safety concerns and the availability of alternatives with fewer concerns (i.e., pioglitazone, glimepiride, glipizide, and gliclazide).

Alternatives to these preferred two tiers of drugs, including α-glucosidase inhibitors, glinides, pramlintide, DPP-4 inhibitors, and colesevelam, are certainly effective glucose-lowering therapies, but for various reasons, including side effects, cost, modest A1C reduction, or lack of long-term safety data, they were not included in the ADA/EASD consensus algorithm.

Insulin should be added at any time in the course of diabetes if patients are symptomatic or more severely hyperglycemic, defined as fasting plasma glucose levels >250 mg/dl, random glucose levels consistently >300 mg/dl, A1C >10%, or the presence of ketonuria. The insulin of choice is generally intermediate-acting or basal insulin at bedtime with subsequent methodical titration to achieve target fasting glucose. If fasting blood glucose is in the target range but a patient is not reaching A1C goals, the patient should monitor blood glucose at other times of day, and the addition of premeal insulin or a trial of premixed intermediate- and short-acting insulin is warranted.

The importance of glycemic control for preventing diabetes complications is evident, but it necessitates an individualized approach to maximize benefits and minimize risks. Therapy should be implemented using agents with complementary mechanisms of action. Adequacy of therapy should be evaluated with an A1C test every 3 months. Patients who are not meeting goals should have additional agents administered and promptly titrated to reach effective doses within 1–2 months. Insulin therapy should be encouraged at an early stage where indicated.

BIBLIOGRAPHY

Action to Control Cardiovascular Risk in Diabetes (ACCORD) Study Group: Effects of intensive glucose lowering in type 2 diabetes. *N Engl J Med* 358:2560–2572, 2008

ADVANCE Collaborative Group: Intensive blood glucose control and vascular outcomes in patients with type 2 diabetes. *N Engl J Med* 358:2560–2572, 2008

American Diabetes Association: Standards of medical care of diabetes—2009. *Diabetes Care* 32 (Suppl. 1):S13–S61, 2008

Bloomgarden ZT: Glycemic control in diabetes: a tale of three studies. *Diabetes Care* 31:1913–1919, 2008

Diabetes Control and Complications Trial Research Group: The effect of intensive treatment of diabetes on the development and progression of long-term complications in insulin-dependent diabetes mellitus. *N Engl J Med* 329:977–986, 1993

Duckworth W, Abraira C, Moritz T, Reda D, Emanuele N, Reaven PD, Zieve FJ, Marks J, Davis SN, Hayward R, Warren SR, Goldman S, McCarren M, Vitek ME, Henderson WG, Huang GD, VADT Investigators: Glucose control and vasular complications in veterans with type 2 diabetes. *N Engl J Med* 360:129–139, 2009

Holman RR, Paul SK, Bethel MA, Matthews DR, Neil HA: 10-year follow-up of intensive glucose control in type 2 diabetes. *N Engl J Med* 359:1577–1589, 2008

Lebovitz HE: Oral therapies for diabetic hyperglycemia. *Endocrinol Metab Clin North Am* 30:909–933, 2001

Lebovitz HE: Treating hyperglycemia in type 2 diabetes: new goals and strategies. *Cleve Clin J Med* 69:809–820, 2002

Nathan DM, Buse JB, Davidson MB, Ferrannini E, Holman RR, Sherwin R, Zinman B: Medical management of hyperglycemia in type 2 diabetes: a consensus algorithm for the initiation and adjustment of therapy: a consensus statement of the American Diabetes Association and the European Association for the Study of Diabetes. *Diabetes Care* 32:193–203, 2009

Nathan DM, Cleary PA, Backlund JY, Genuth SM, Lachin JM, Orchard TJ, Raskin P, Zinman B: Intensive diabetes treatment and cardiovascular disease in patients with type 1 diabetes. *N Engl J Med* 353:2643–2653, 2005

Skyler JS, Bergenstal R, Bonow RO, Buse J, Deedwania P, Gale EAM, Howard BV, Kirkman MS, Kosiborod M, Reaven P, Sherwin RS: intensive Glycemic Control and the Prevention of Cardiovascular Events: implications of the ACCORD, ADVANCE, and VA Diabetes Trials: a position statement of the American Diabetes Association and a scientific statement of the American College of Cardiology Foundation and the American Heart Association. *Diabetes Care* 32:187–192, 2009

Turner R, Cull C, Holman R: United Kingdom Prospective Diabetes Study 17: a 9-year update of a randomized controlled trial of the effect of improved metabolic control on complications in non-insulin-dependent diabetes mellitus. *Ann Intern Med* 124:136–145, 1996

UK Prospective Diabetes Study Group: Intensive blood-glucose control with sulphonylureas or insulin compared with conventional treatment and risk of complications in patients with type 2 diabetes (UKPDS 33). *Lancet* 352:837–853, 1998

UK Prospective Diabetes Study Group: Effect of intensive blood glucose control with metformin on complications in overweight patients with type 2 diabetes (UKPDS 34). *Lancet* 352:854–865, 1998

UKPDS Group: UK Prospective Diabetes Study 7: response of fasting plasma glucose to diet therapy in newly presenting type II diabetic patients. *Metabolism* 39:905–912, 1990

Writing Team for the Diabetes Control and Complications Trial/Epidemiology of Diabetes Interventions and Complications Research Group: Effect of intensive therapy on the microvascular complications of type 1 diabetes mellitus. *JAMA* 287:2563–2569, 2002

Yki-Jarvinen H, Kauppila M, Kujansuu E, Lahti J, Marjanen T, Niskanen L, Rajala S, Ryysy L, Salo S, Seppala P, et al.: Comparison of insulin regimens in patients with non-insulin-dependent diabetes mellitus. *N Engl J Med* 327:1426–1433, 1992

Dr. Dungan is Assistant Professor of Medicine at the Ohio State University, Columbus, Ohio.

16. Medical Nutrition Therapy

ANNE DALY, MS, RD, CDE, AND MARGARET A. POWERS, PHD, RD, CDE

Medical nutrition therapy (MNT) is an essential component of comprehensive diabetes care and management. Within 6–12 weeks of initiating MNT, A1C levels often decrease 1–2%. Additionally, MNT is effective in lowering blood pressure and improving lipid profiles. With such a clinically significant treatment tool available, why do so many health care professionals not encourage its full use? Perhaps it is because they are unaware of the effectiveness of MNT. Perhaps some think it is too hard to follow a "diet." Perhaps a referral process for MNT has not been established. Perhaps health care professionals or their patients do not believe that MNT can be reimbursed. This chapter will address these issues so that patients can receive the full benefit of MNT.

OVERVIEW OF MNT

The ultimate goal of diabetes nutrition therapy is for people with diabetes to be comfortable and confident in making daily food choices that contribute to improved metabolic status. This goal is achieved through the development of a personalized food plan that incorporates an individual's favorite foods and typical eating patterns. Additionally, counseling and coaching about behavioral strategies particular to the individual support the achievement of short- and long-term goals related to the food plan.

Table 16.1 lists the goals of MNT. Because 75% of deaths in individuals with diabetes are attributed to cardiovascular disease, it is critical that the focus of care be expanded beyond glycemic control. That is why the first goal encompasses the ABCs of diabetes care—managing A1C, blood pressure, and cholesterol. Nutrition therapy is the first-line therapy for managing elevations in each of these areas and heightens the effectiveness of medication when it is necessary. Table 16.2 highlights the effectiveness of MNT in lowering blood glucose, cholesterol, and blood pressure.

Diabetes medications support the food plan and should be prescribed to correspond with eating times and food patterns. The medication should not force an individual to eat at inappropriate or unusual times. The fact that the medication needs of individuals with type 2 diabetes become more complex as their diabetes progresses is typical and should be expected. Combinations of oral agents and/or noninsulin injectable medications are eventually needed, with 40–60% of patients requiring insulin. Continuous reliance on MNT alone, or MNT and one diabetes

Table 16.1 Goals of MNT

1. Attain and maintain optimal metabolic outcomes.
   ■ Blood glucose goals in a normal range to reduce risk for diabetes complications
   ■ Blood pressure levels in a normal range to reduce risk for vascular disease
   ■ Lipid levels in a normal range to reduce risk for macrovascular disease
	2. Prevent, delay, or treat nutrition-related complications: obesity, dyslipidemia, cardiovascular disease, hypertension, and nephropathy.
	3. Improve health through healthy food choices and physical activity.
	4. Address individual nutrition needs.

agent, to achieve glycemic control may not be sufficient to achieve desired glycemic control. As medication therapy advances, MNT needs to be continuously evaluated and may also need to advance.

Tables 16.3 and 16.4 outline MNT principles for type 1 and type 2 diabetes. Table 16.5 summarizes new nutrition paradigms based on the 2008 nutrition recommendations.

DIABETES PREVENTION

Key clinical research, including the Diabetes Prevention Program (DPP), concludes that the incidence of type 2 diabetes can be decreased by 58% in at-risk individuals. The success of such programs depends on the implementation of lifestyle-structured intervention programs (Table 16.6). These programs emphasize reduced fat and energy intake, regular physical activity, and frequent participant contact. The intervention is well defined and available via the Internet at www.diabetes.niddk.nih.gov/

Table 16.2 MNT Effectiveness in Diabetic Patients

Glycemic control

■ ~1% decrease in A1C in newly diagnosed type 1 diabetic patients (10–12% decrease)
■ ~2% decrease in A1C in newly diagnosed type 2 diabetic patients (22% decrease)
■ ~1% decrease in A1C with an average 4-yr duration of type 2 diabetes (12% decrease)
■ 50–100 mg/dl decrease in fasting plasma glucose
■ Outcomes will be known by 6 wk to 3 mo

Lipids (7–10% saturated fat, 200–300 mg cholesterol intake)

■ 10–13% decrease in total cholesterol (24–32 mg/dl)
■ 12–16% decrease in LDL cholesterol (18–25 mg/dl)
■ 8% decrease in triglycerides (15–17 mg/dl)
■ Without exercise, HDL cholesterol decreases by 7%; with exercise, no decrease

Hypertension (2,400 mg sodium)

■ 5 mmHg decrease in systolic blood pressure and 2 mmHg decrease in diastolic blood pressure in hypertensive patients

Table 16.3 Principles of Nutrition Therapy for Type 1 Diabetes

■ Integrate insulin with individual eating and lifestyle. ■ Conventional therapy: synchronize food with insulin, eat at consistent times, and teach types of foods and portion sizes. ■ Intensive therapy: adjust insulin to fit food intake, physical activity, and lifestyle factors.	■ Use self-monitored blood glucose results to adjust meal plan and insulin doses. ■ Monitor potential weight gain with intensive therapy. ■ Monitor blood glucose, A1C, lipids, blood pressure, and microalbuminuria.

dm/pubs/preventionprogram. Primary care providers can partner with dietitians to provide their patients similar care in order to prevent or delay the onset of type 2 diabetes. Dietitians were involved in the many facets of the study and were integral to designing and achieving the significant reduction in new cases of diabetes. Through intensive lifestyle intervention, DPP participants achieved a:

- mean weight loss of 7% after 1 year and maintained a 5% weight loss at 3 years, and
- mean level of physical activity of 208 min/week at 1 year and 189 min/week at 3 years.

These results have the potential to reduce the onset of diabetes or treat other medical conditions, such as hypertension and elevated cholesterol levels, making the impact of lifestyle intervention greater on health outcomes.

Individuals at risk for type 2 diabetes include those described in Chapter 19. Special attention can be given to people who are overweight and women who have had gestational diabetes. Children pose difficult challenges that involve public health and school policy issues. Diabetes care providers may need to become involved in these issues to ensure access to appropriate food and activity throughout the day.

INITIATING THERAPY

Nutrition therapy must be goal directed and individualized according to a person's usual food intake and lifestyle. It is not appropriate to prescribe a precise caloric intake or a precise distribution of food. It takes a series of visits to develop and

Table 16.4 Principles of Nutrition Therapy for Type 2 Diabetes

■ Focus on glucose, blood pressure, and lipid goals. ■ Modify fat intake. ■ Improve food choices. ■ Space intake of carbohydrate foods throughout day. ■ Increase physical activity.	■ If obese, modify calories for moderate weight loss. ■ Monitor blood glucose, A1C, blood pressure, and lipids. ■ Add and advance diabetes medication therapy, as needed.

Table 16.5 The Old Versus the New Nutrition Paradigm

Outdated Nutrition Advice	Updated Nutrition Advice
MNT was a calculated ADA diet (calories and percentage of macronutrients).	There no longer is an ADA diet that applies to all individuals with diabetes. An ADA diet can only be defined as an individualized food/meal plan based on assessment, therapy goals, and use of approaches that meet the patient's needs. Diet sheets or a one-time "diet instruction" rarely is sufficient to change eating habits. For people to make lifestyle changes that result in positive clinical outcomes, both education and counseling, especially in the areas of nutrition and physical activity, and support over time are required.
Weight loss was encouraged.	Weight loss is typically a helpful but not essential treatment for improving blood glucose. Weight loss may be a barrier for individuals who have tried multiple times to lose weight unsuccessfully. It is often possible to improve glucose control by changing food habits without weight loss. For those who are already at or below an appropriate weight, weight loss is not a treatment goal.
Standard treatment included 1–2 visits.	Frequent contact with individualized goal setting and implementation plans recommended.
Ideal body weight was used as the goal, and this goal often required a weight loss of 40–50 lb (18–23 kg).	Weight loss of 5–10% of current weight is proven effective to reduce health risk. Long-term follow-up is used to improve or maintain eating behaviors and increase physical activity.
Sugars and sweets were forbidden because they were believed to be more rapidly digested and absorbed and to cause blood glucose levels to go higher than starches.	Evidence from many clinical studies has demonstrated that sugars do not increase glycemia more than isocaloric amounts of starch. Therefore, the total amount of carbohydrate eaten is more important than the source of the carbohydrate.
Protein was recommended because it was believed to slow the absorption of carbohydrates and to prevent hypoglycemia.	Ingested protein does not slow the absorption of carbohydrate, and neither does adding protein prevent late-onset hypoglycemia or assist in the treatment of hypoglycemia.
Chromium and vitamin E were often recommended to improve blood glucose or lipid levels.	If individuals are not deficient in a micronutrient, supplements are unlikely to be beneficial. It is difficult to determine who is and who is not deficient in chromium. Supplementation with vitamin E has not been shown to be beneficial in the intervention trials.
"When diet and exercise fail," add medications: at this point, there was no need to pay attention to lifestyle.	Type 2 diabetes is a progressive disease, and MNT should always be part of the diabetes care plan. β-Cells fail, not diet and exercise.

Table 16.6 Components of a Structured Lifestyle-Change Program

- Calorie intake deficit achieved through calorie counting and/or fat gram counting, with strict attention to portion control
- Increased physical activity
- Individual goal setting

- Specific plan making
- Individual and/or group sessions
- Standardized curriculum
- Follow-up contact during weight-maintenance phase

refine the food plan, and more visits may be required for the patient to learn how to maintain the plan in a variety of situations and to incorporate a variety of food choices (see Table 16.7 for time frames for nutrition intervention). Modifying eating patterns is not a simple procedure, yet reasonable, achievable goals can be set and successfully met with the guidance of a skilled counselor. When initiating or adjusting MNT, increased frequency of blood glucose monitoring may be necessary to guide changes in food intake, activity, and medications, if prescribed. More frequent blood glucose monitoring is needed to determine whether changes to the food plan are necessary or whether adjusting another therapy is more appropriate.

The five primary nutrition messages that apply to most people with diabetes are as follows:

1. Eat similar amounts of carbohydrate throughout the day each day (e.g., eat similar amounts at breakfast from day to day) and distribute the carbohydrate fairly evenly throughout the day.
2. Practice portion control by measuring foods to become more aware of how much is eaten and to be able to eat similar amounts of carbohydrate.
3. Decrease fat by reducing frequency and portion sizes of high-fat foods, choosing foods prepared with less fat, and using less fat as spreads and sauces.
4. Add a total of 30 min of physical activity each day.
5. Be at a healthy weight or, if overweight and interested in losing weight, lose ~10 lb and observe how blood glucose, blood pressure, and/or cholesterol improves.

Table 16.7 Time Frames for Nutrition Intervention

Initial workup/assessment (can be part of group DSMT)	**Follow-up for therapy evaluation, adjustment, and education**
■ 1–2 h, one to two appointments	■ As needed
Self-management education (can be part of group DSMT)	■ With lifestyle and life-cycle changes ■ Minimum follow-up for children every 3–6 mo; for adults, every 6–12 mo
■ Biweekly or monthly sessions for 2–4 mo, 30–60 min each ■ Daily/weekly phone calls to discuss self-monitored blood glucose records, as needed	■ Intensive therapy requires 4–6 visits a year plus phone contact

DSMT, diabetes self-management training.

There are many details to understand to make these behavioral changes. Simply stating them to a patient will not promote adherence. The education process described below will help patients achieve these goals.

OBESITY TREATMENT

The U.S. has experienced epidemics of both obesity and diabetes in the last decade. Approximately 36% of people diagnosed with diabetes have a BMI ≥30 kg/m², which classifies them as obese. Risk for developing diabetes increases from a BMI as low as 22 kg/m². The relative risk for diabetes increases by ~25% for each additional unit of BMI >22 kg/m². Obesity increases insulin resistance and may aggravate hyperlipidemia and hypertension. Aggressive intervention is warranted to treat obesity in patients diagnosed with diabetes as well as individuals with pre-diabetes, or those with one or more risk factors for developing diabetes. Long-term weight maintenance poses a major challenge. Structured, intensive lifestyle-change programs (Table 16.6), similar to those used in the DPP and Look AHEAD (Action for Health in Diabetes) trials, produce more successful weight loss and weight maintenance than conventional treatment consisting of one initial visit to the registered dietitian (RD), followed by two follow-up visits. Look AHEAD is a large National Institutes of Health–sponsored clinical trial currently underway that is designed to determine the effects long-term weight loss has on cardiovascular disease outcomes.

Recent nutrition recommendations encourage setting goals for a reasonable body weight, defined as a weight that the patient confirms as being achievable and sustainable. Baseline calorie needs depend on height, weight, the need for weight loss or gain, and usual activity/exercise patterns.

Diabetes in obese, inactive children has become a major concern and takes special skill in treating so as to not create eating disorders or a negative attitude toward health care. Encouraging physical activity and a well-balanced food plan that maintains weight is often a goal. Counseling support may be necessary to supplement a variety of interventions. When working with children, it is helpful to remember that the family is a valuable addition to the support team.

Nonpharmacological Treatment of Obesity

Assessing patient readiness is an important first step to successful weight management. Readiness means that a patient is interested in weight reduction, understands that weight management is a lifelong commitment, and is willing to do what is appropriate and necessary to support success. Selection of weight-reduction treatment options can be based on health risk (Table 16.8).

Pharmacological Treatment of Obesity

Pharmacological agents for obesity can be a useful adjunct to, but not a substitute for, the necessary changes in food intake and physical activity. The effectiveness of any pharmacological intervention depends on its use with appropriate nutrition intervention, increased physical activity, and lifestyle change. Pharmacological intervention is recommended for use only in patients with a

Table 16.8 Selected Weight-Reduction Treatment Options Based on Health Risk

Health Risk	Based Solely on BMI (kg/m²)	Adjusted for Comorbid Conditions and/or Risk Factors	Treatment Options Available
Minimal	<25	—	Healthful eating
			Increased physical activity
Low	25 to <27	<25	All the above plus moderate calorie deficit
Moderate	27 to <30	25 to <27	All the above plus low-calorie diet
High	30 to <35	27 to <30	All the above plus pharmacotherapy
Very high	35 to <40	30 to <35	All the above plus very-low-calorie diet
Extremely high	≥40	≥35	All the above plus surgical intervention

BMI ≥27 kg/m² in the presence of a comorbid condition and ≥30 kg/m² when no comorbid condition is present.

NUTRITION CARE PROCESS

The nutrition care process includes a continuous four-step process:

1. **Nutrition Assessment:** The assessment process includes obtaining, verifying, and interpreting data that is needed to identify and understand nutrition needs. Five categories of data are reviewed: *1*) food/nutrition history; *2*) biochemical data, medical tests, and procedures; *3*) anthropometric measurements; *4*) physical examination findings; and *5*) patient history.

2. **Nutrition Diagnosis:** The purpose is to describe the presence of, risk of, or potential for developing a nutritional situation that can be addressed by nutrition therapy. Diagnoses include a diagnostic label, etiology, and signs and symptoms. Diagnoses are organized into three categories: *1*) clinical, *2*) intake related, or *3*) behavioral-environmental.

3. **Nutrition Intervention:** Interventions are specific actions to remedy the nutrition diagnosis and includes the planning phase as well as the intervention. The focus is on *1*) food and/or nutrient intake and *2*) nutrition education, nutrition counseling, and coordination of care. There is no gold standard single strategy or method of nutrition intervention because various methods have been tested and demonstrated to facilitate attainment of nutrition goals. During initial phases of education (soon after diabetes diagnosis), simplified resources are recommended. Subsequently, more

Table 16.9 Nutrition Intervention Options

Level of Care		
Initial	Continuing	Intensive
Basic nutrition guidelines	Carbohydrate counting	Carbohydrate counting using insulin-to-carbohydrate ratios
Healthy food choices		
Food-guide pyramid	Exchange lists: basic	Exchange lists: advanced
First step in diabetes meal planning	Calorie counting	Structured lifestyle-change program
	Lifestyle changes	Medically supervised very-low-calorie diets
Carbohydrate counting: basic	Fat counting	

complex approaches may be appropriate. Commonly used nutrition interventions are listed in Table 16.9. Use of various nutrition interventions provides greater flexibility and choices to the person with diabetes and is especially useful for those who have been discouraged or frustrated by previous nutrition instruction methods. The different nutrition interventions have distinctive and varying characteristics of structure and complexity. The choice of a food plan depends on both the dietitian's experience with different strategies and which approach best meets the individual needs of the patient.

4. **Nutrition Monitoring and Evaluation:** The purpose of this step is to determine the amount of progress made and whether goals are met. It is a continuous process of observing metabolic outcomes and patient perceptions of how things are going as well as designing additional education and support services to meet instructional and lifestyle needs.

Follow-up educational sessions with the dietitian focus on various topics, such as food composition, food labeling, shopping, recipe adaptations, and eating in restaurants. Dietitians guide patients in using food records in conjunction with blood glucose records to observe patterns in blood glucose control. A problem-solving approach is used to analyze individual blood glucose responses to food, activity, and medications. Patients are then able to make adjustments in food intake and/or insulin dosage to maintain target blood glucose levels. Algorithms for food, medication, and activity can be developed to help manage diabetes on a daily basis. Small careful steps over weeks or months help move the patient toward nutrition goals. Follow-up sessions by the dietitian can be accomplished via clinic visits and telephone conversations to facilitate problem solving. Family members and significant others should be involved in the nutrition education process and are encouraged to follow the same healthy lifestyle recommendations as the person with diabetes.

Contact with a dietitian is recommended at least annually (Table 16.7) to monitor metabolic parameters and assess the appropriateness and effectiveness of the nutrition therapy. When patients experience lifestyle changes, such as schedule changes, marriage, divorce, change of job or home, or pregnancy, nutrition therapy should be reviewed. If nutrition therapy goals are not met, changes can be made in the overall diabetes care and management plan. See Table 16.10 for the top seven reasons to refer a patient to a dietitian.

WHO SHOULD PROVIDE MNT?

The complexity of nutrition issues requires a coordinated team effort, including the person with diabetes. To achieve nutrition goals, the American Diabetes Association (ADA) recommends that an RD, who is knowledgeable and skilled in implementing current principles and recommendations for diabetes, play the leading role in providing nutrition care. However, it is important that all team members, including physicians and nurses, be knowledgeable about MNT and support its implementation.

ACCESS TO MNT

Although referrals for diabetes self-management education (DSME) are increasing, the sad fact remains that only ~30–40% of individuals with diabetes have had structured education. Of those individuals, a smaller percentage has seen an RD for MNT. Studies of referral patterns indicate that the lack of referral by physicians and other health care professionals remains a major barrier. Lack of awareness of the availability of improved reimbursement may be a factor. Table 16.11 provides information about how to access dietitians and diabetes education.

REIMBURSEMENT FOR DIABETES MNT AND DSME

Over the last decade, reimbursement/coverage for diabetes MNT and DSME have improved greatly. More health plans than ever before are covering MNT and DSME due to the significant impact they have on health outcomes. Providers should encourage people with diabetes to learn about their benefits and to be proactive in obtaining coverage for MNT and DSME. For more information, Table 16.12 lists information resources about DSME and MNT.

Table 16.10 Top Five Reasons to Refer to a Dietitian

Refer a patient to a dietitian when a patient:

- is new to diabetes and doesn't know what to eat
- has had diabetes awhile but needs to get back on track
- wants help in deciding how to eat their favorite foods
- has a schedule that makes it difficult to eat well
- wants to feel better and improve their diabetes control
- would like to improve food choices and/or lose weight

Table 16.11 Accessing Dietitians and Diabetes Education

- Find the ADA's Recognized Education Programs in your area (see Table 16.12).
- Locate a diabetes educator who is a dietitian by calling the American Association of Diabetes Educators (AADE) at 1-800-TEAMUP4 (800-832-6874) or go to AADE's website www.diabeteseducator.org and go to "Find a Diabetes Educator" in the "General Public" section.
- Find a dietitian by calling The American Dietetic Association at 800-366-1655 or go to their website www.eatright.org.
- Ask colleagues about dietitians and diabetes education programs in your area.

State Legislation

Forty-six states and the District of Columbia have passed laws that require health insurance companies and managed care plans to cover DSME, which includes MNT. These laws have also typically required coverage of diabetes supplies, such as blood glucose meters and testing strips. Unfortunately, however, these state laws cover only ~30% of people with diabetes because they do not cover Medicaid or Medicare recipients or individuals employed by large businesses with federally regulated insurance. In some states, efforts to roll back these benefits have been attempted; the ADA aggressively opposes these roll-back initiatives.

Medicare

Medicare covers DSME for people with diabetes who meet specific eligibility criteria and when it is provided by programs that have been reviewed and recognized by the ADA Education Recognition Program or by the Indian Health Service. These programs must follow the National Standards for Diabetes Self-Management Education programs. There are 10 h of outpatient training available initially during the first 12 months of submitting for this service, and up to 2 h annually thereafter, with provider referral. Medicare requires that the DSME be provided in groups unless the provider has identified a specific barrier to group education.

Table 16.12 Information Resources about DSMT and MNT Reimbursement

State laws	www.diabetes.org/advocacy
	www.diabeteseducator.org
List of recognized diabetes programs in each state	ADA Recognition Programs: call 1-800-DIABETES (800-342-2383)
	www.professional.diabetes.org
Medicare coverage for MNT and DSMT	www.diabetes.org
	www.aadenet.org
	www.eatright.org

In addition, Medicare coverage for MNT for Part B beneficiaries with type 1, type 2, and gestational diabetes and renal disease (exclusive of beneficiaries on dialysis and 6 months after renal transplant) went into effect January 2002. The beneficiary must be referred by the treating provider, and the service must be provided by a qualified nutrition professional (i.e., an RD) who has obtained a Unique Physician/Practitioner Identification Number (UPIN) from Medicare. The nutrition professional can then be directly reimbursed for MNT and DSME or can assign reimbursement to his or her place of employment. The beneficiary is entitled to 3 h within a 12-month period for initial MNT and 2 h in the following years. Eligible beneficiaries are allowed to use both the MNT and DSME benefit. The only restriction is that the services cannot be provided on the same day.

WHAT TO EXPECT

MNT is effective in lowering A1C, blood pressure, and lipid levels when used without medications, and it improves the effectiveness of medication when needed (Table 16.2). MNT is the initial treatment of these metabolic conditions, although at some point in their progression, medications often are needed to support MNT. Continued support and reinforcement of behavioral goals needed to be successful are necessary and can usually be reimbursed as part of established changes in federal and state laws governing health care. Establishing a referral network to dietitians has become easier as these reimbursement changes occur. Patients will ultimately benefit as they achieve their goals and decrease the risk of developing complications from diabetes, hypertension, or cardiovascular disease. This result is achieved through the implementation of individualized food plans that take into consideration the patient's lifestyle and metabolic needs.

BIBLIOGRAPHY

American Diabetes Association: Nutrition recommendations and interventions for diabetes (Position Statement). *Diabetes Care* 31 (Suppl. 1):S61–S78, 2008

American Diabetes Association and National Institute of Diabetes, Digestive and Kidney Diseases: The prevention or delay of type 2 diabetes (Position Statement). *Diabetes Care* 27 (Suppl. 1):S47–S54, 2004

Chobanian AV, Bakris GL, Black HR, et al.: The seventh report of the Joint National Committee on Prevention, Detection, Evaluation, and Treatment of High Blood Pressure. *JAMA* 289:2560–2572, 2003

Cutler JA, Follmann D, Allender PS: Randomized trials of sodium restriction: an overview. *Am J Clin Nutr* 54 (Suppl. 1):643S–651S, 1997

Franz MJ, Monk A, Barry A, McClain K, Weaver T, Cooper N, Upham P, Gergenstal R, Mazze R: Effectiveness of medical nutrition therapy by dietitians in the management of non-insulin-dependent diabetes mellitus: a randomized, controlled clinical trial. *J Am Diet Assoc* 95:1009–1017, 1995

Franz M, Warshaw H, Pastors JG, Daly A, Arnold M: The evolution of diabetes medical nutrition therapy. *Postgrad Med J* 79:30–35, 2003

Franz M, Boucher J, Green-Pastors J, Powers MA: Evidence-based nutrition practice guidelines for diabetes and scope and standards of practice. *J Am Diet Assoc* 108 (4 Suppl. 1):S52–S8, 2008

Kulkarni K, Castle G, Gregory R, Holmes A, Leontos C, Powers M, Snetselaar L, Splett P, Wylie-Rosett J: Nutrition practice guidelines for type 1 diabetes mellitus positively affect dietitian practices and patient outcomes. *J Am Diet Assoc* 98:62–70, 1998

Monk A, Barry B, McClain K, Weaver T, Cooper N, Franz M: Practice guidelines for medical nutrition therapy provided by dietitians for persons with non-insulin-dependent diabetes mellitus. *J Am Diet Assoc* 95:999–1006, 1995

National Institutes of Health (NIH) National Heart, Lung & Blood Institute (NHLBI): Clinical guidelines on the identification, evaluation and treatment of overweight and obesity in adults: the evidence report. *Obes Res* 6 (Suppl. 2):51S–209S, 1998

Pastors JG, Warshaw H, Daly A, Franz M, Kulkarni K: Evidence for effectiveness of medical nutrition therapy in diabetes management. *Diabetes Care* 25:608–613, 2002

Powers M: *American Dietetic Association Guide to Eating Right When You Have Diabetes.* Hoboken, NJ, John Wiley and Sons, 2003

Rickheim P, Weaver TW, Flader JL, Kendall DM: Assessment of group versus individual diabetes education. *Diabetes Care* 25:269–274, 2002

Rosett JW, Delahanty L: An integral role of the dietitian: implications of the Diabetes Prevention Program. *J Am Diet Assoc* 102:1065–1068, 2002

Sacks FM, Swetkey LP, Vollmer WM, Appel LJ, Bray GA, Harsha D, Obarzanek E, Conlin PR, Miller ER 3rd, Simons-Morton DG, Karanja N, Lin PH, DASH-Sodium Collaborative Research Group: Effects on blood pressure of reduced dietary sodium and the Dietary Approaches to Stop Hypertension (DASH) diet. *N Engl J Med* 344:3–10, 2001

U.K. Prospective Diabetes Study: Response of fasting plasma glucose to diet therapy in newly presenting type II patients with diabetes. *Metabolism* 39:905–912, 1990

Yu-Poth S, Zhao G, Etherton T, Naglak M, Jonnalagadda S, Kris-Etherton PM: Effects of the National Cholesterol Education Program's step I and step II dietary intervention programs on cardiovascular disease risk factors: a meta-analysis. *Am J Clin Nutr* 60:632–646, 1999

Ms. Daly is Director of Nutrition and Diabetes Education at the Springfield Diabetes and Endocrine Center, Springfield, Illinois. Ms. Powers is a Research Scientist at the International Diabetes Center at Park Nicollet, Minneapolis, Minnesota.

17. Pharmacological Treatment of Obesity

Donna H. Ryan, MD, and George A. Bray, MD

Obesity has become a major focus of modern medicine, driven by the U.S. epidemic of overweight and obesity. The 1999–2000 National Health and Nutrition Examination Survey (NHANES) pegs obesity rates (BMI ≥30 kg/m²) at 30.5% of the U.S. population. The concern, of course, is the morbidities that accompany obesity. In particular, attention has recently focused on the metabolic syndrome—the constellation of lipid, vascular, and metabolic abnormalities associated largely with insulin resistance. A reanalysis of NHANES data shows that the metabolic syndrome affects 24% of the U.S. population. The 2001 National Cholesterol Education Program Adult Treatment Panel III (ATP III) guidelines target the metabolic syndrome as a focus for cardiovascular risk reduction. This shift from lipid management to "therapeutic lifestyle change" as a way to control metabolic syndrome stems from the knowledge that type 2 diabetes is a cardiovascular risk equivalent. By the time type 2 diabetes is diagnosed, cardiovascular disease is already entrenched, a concept bolstered by evidence that individuals with type 2 diabetes have the same risk for subsequent cardiovascular events as individuals without diabetes who have had a first cardiovascular event.

At the same time that there is alarm over the links between obesity and diabetes and cardiovascular risk, there is an appreciation by our public health officials that even modest weight reduction can produce substantial health benefits. The U.S. Diabetes Prevention Program and the Finnish Diabetes Prevention Study both demonstrated significant reduction in risk for diabetes in individuals with impaired glucose tolerance who lost as little as 5–7% of baseline weight.

Physicians must develop effective office-based approaches to obesity management. Medicating for obesity is a tool unique to physicians, and if we are to stem the tide of obesity-related morbidities, physicians must be knowledgeable about the use of medications in at-risk patients. This chapter is a guide to current practices in evaluating and medicating for obesity management.

REALITIES OF TREATMENT

First, obesity is a chronic, relapsing, neurochemical disease that has many causes. Environmental, biological, and psychological factors all play a role in the current prevalence of obesity, which exceeds 30% of the U.S. population. In most patients presenting with obesity, a clear etiologic diagnosis is usually not possible. Because of its chronic nature and relative unknown cause, cure of obesity is rare, but palliation is a realistic clinical goal. Weight loss occurs with most treatments, and, except for surgery or very-low-calorie diets, it is usually slow (0.5–1.0 kg/week). Recidivism, or regain of body weight, is common after a weight loss program is terminated. In contrast to the relatively slow rate of weight loss, weight regain may be rapid. A regain in weight after termination of drug treatment is often ascribed to a failure of the drugs or other treatment. A more appropriate interpretation is that medications do not work if not taken. This is true of medications for the treatment of obesity, just as it is for medications used to treat hypertension, diabetes, heart disease, or asthma.

EVALUATION OF THE OBESE PATIENT

Classification and Risk Assessment of Obesity

The first step in assessing the obese patient is to consider potential causes of the condition. Table 17.1 outlines an etiologic classification of obesity. Whereas secondary causes of obesity are rare, endocrine and hypothalamic syndromes, such as hypothyroidism, Cushing's syndrome, Prader-Willi syndrome, and hypothalamic injury, must be considered. Although diet and a sedentary lifestyle are always contributory, physicians must remember that the amount of energy imbalance required to result in significant weight gain does not usually indicate sloth or gluttony. With a net excess energy intake of only 100 kcal/day, >10 lb will be gained in a year and 100 lb in 10 years. Whereas there are strong genetic influences on weight and body habitus, the cause of the obesity epidemic of the last 30 years is an environmental, rather than a genetic, shift.

Table 17.2 lists drugs that may be associated with weight gain. Many common medications promote weight gain, and physicians must be cognizant of the additional health risks imposed by such weight gain and seek alternative therapy for susceptible individuals. Another problem is the excessive gain and weight retention that can follow pregnancy or that is associated with menopause. Not all women are susceptible, but at least a subset report the onset of obesity with these life events.

Operationally, BMI is a useful way of communicating the degree of overweight. Table 17.3 shows BMI values for various heights and weights. Whereas BMI may be elevated in bodybuilders without a concomitant increase in body fat, a high BMI generally reflects an increased percentage of total body fat. BMI may overestimate health risks from obesity in African American women and underestimate them in Asian and Indian individuals. The most reliable way to measure total body fat is with dual-energy X-ray absorptiometry, where body fat >25% for

Table 17.1 Etiologic Classification of Obesity

■ Hypothalamic ■ Endocrine	■ Dietary ■ Sedentary lifestyle	■ Genetic ■ Drug-induced	■ Idiopathic

Table 17.2 Drugs Associated with Weight Gain

Psychiatric/neurological	Others
■ Antipsychotics: olanzapine, clozapine, risperidone	■ Hormonal contraceptives
■ Antidepressants: tricyclic antidepressants, some selective serotonin-reuptake inhibitors	■ Corticosteroids
	■ Progestational agents
■ Lithium	■ Antihistamines
■ Antiepileptics: valproate, gabapentin, carbamazepine	■ β-Blockers, α-blockers

Diabetes treatment

■ Insulin
■ Sulfonylureas
■ Thiazolidinediones

men and >33% for women can define obesity. On a practical level, clinical judgment usually suffices in interpreting BMI in relation to health risk. In particular, consideration of waist circumference, in addition to BMI, can aid in risk assessment and diagnosis of the metabolic syndrome.

Intra-abdominal fat increases with age and carries the highest risk for developing cardiovascular and other disease consequences. Visceral fat distribution can be estimated by several techniques. The ratio of the circumference of the waist to the circumference of the hips has been widely used in epidemiological studies, but this is no better than the waist circumference alone. Men with a waist circumference >40 inches (102 cm) and women with a waist circumference >35 inches (88 cm) are in the high-risk category. The top tertile in abdominal fat distribution nearly doubles the risk of mortality and morbidity from heart disease, diabetes, and hypertension. This extra risk is observed in men and women and rises sharply for the top 10th percentile of abdominal fat distribution. When the difference in fat distribution is corrected, the excess mortality observed between men and women is largely, if not completely, eliminated. The risk associated with excess central accumulation of fat probably reflects the increase in visceral fat. Abnormal glucose tolerance, hypertension, hypertriglyceridemia, and low HDL cholesterol are more closely associated with the amount of visceral fat than with total body fat. The sagittal diameter has been proposed as a way to estimate visceral fat, but currently the only reliable way to determine visceral fat is with a computed tomography or magnetic resonance imaging scan. The availability of newer, less expensive methods will be an important clinical advance.

METABOLIC SYNDROME

The National Cholesterol Education Program ATP III indicates the metabolic syndrome as a secondary target (in addition to lipid levels) for cardiovascular disease prevention. Table 17.4 lists the ATP III criteria for the metabolic syndrome. The levels chosen are less stringent than those generally used by physicians for categorizing disease states; for example, the blood pressure cut point is 130/85 mmHg, which is less than the 140/90 mmHg cut point usually indicating

Table 17.3 BMI Using Either Pounds and Inches or Kilograms and Centimeters

BMI (kg/m²)

Inches	19	20	21	22	23	24	25	26	27	28	29	30	31	32	33	34	35	36	37	38	39	40	Centimeters
58	*91*	*95*	*100*	*105*	*110*	*115*	*119*	*124*	*129*	*134*	*138*	*143*	*148*	*153*	*158*	*162*	*167*	*172*	*177*	*181*	*186*	*191*	147
	41	**43**	**45**	**48**	**50**	**52**	**54**	**56**	**58**	**61**	**63**	**65**	**67**	**69**	**71**	**73**	**76**	**78**	**80**	**82**	**84**	**86**	
59	*94*	*99*	*104*	*109*	*114*	*119*	*124*	*128*	*133*	*138*	*143*	*148*	*153*	*158*	*163*	*168*	*173*	*178*	*183*	*188*	*193*	*198*	150
	43	**45**	**47**	**50**	**52**	**54**	**56**	**59**	**61**	**63**	**65**	**68**	**70**	**72**	**74**	**77**	**79**	**81**	**83**	**86**	**88**	**90**	
60	*97*	*102*	*107*	*112*	*118*	*123*	*128*	*133*	*138*	*143*	*148*	*153*	*158*	*164*	*169*	*174*	*179*	*184*	*189*	*194*	*199*	*204*	152
	44	**46**	**49**	**51**	**53**	**55**	**58**	**60**	**62**	**65**	**67**	**69**	**72**	**74**	**76**	**79**	**81**	**83**	**85**	**88**	**90**	**92**	
61	*100*	*106*	*111*	*116*	*121*	*127*	*132*	*137*	*143*	*148*	*153*	*158*	*164*	*169*	*174*	*180*	*185*	*190*	*195*	*201*	*206*	*211*	155
	46	**48**	**50**	**53**	**55**	**58**	**60**	**62**	**65**	**67**	**70**	**72**	**74**	**77**	**79**	**82**	**84**	**86**	**89**	**91**	**94**	**96**	
62	*104*	*109*	*115*	*120*	*125*	*131*	*136*	*142*	*147*	*153*	*158*	*164*	*169*	*175*	*180*	*186*	*191*	*196*	*202*	*207*	*213*	*218*	158
	47	**50**	**52**	**55**	**57**	**60**	**62**	**65**	**67**	**70**	**72**	**75**	**77**	**80**	**82**	**85**	**87**	**90**	**92**	**95**	**97**	**100**	
63	*107*	*113*	*118*	*124*	*130*	*135*	*141*	*146*	*152*	*158*	*163*	*169*	*175*	*180*	*186*	*192*	*197*	*203*	*208*	*214*	*220*	*225*	160
	49	**51**	**54**	**56**	**59**	**61**	**64**	**67**	**69**	**72**	**74**	**77**	**79**	**82**	**84**	**87**	**90**	**92**	**95**	**97**	**100**	**102**	
64	*110*	*116*	*122*	*128*	*134*	*140*	*145*	*151*	*157*	*163*	*169*	*174*	*180*	*186*	*192*	*198*	*203*	*209*	*215*	*221*	*227*	*233*	162
	50	**52**	**55**	**58**	**60**	**63**	**66**	**68**	**71**	**73**	**76**	**79**	**81**	**84**	**87**	**89**	**92**	**94**	**97**	**100**	**102**	**105**	
65	*114*	*120*	*126*	*132*	*138*	*144*	*150*	*156*	*162*	*168*	*174*	*180*	*186*	*192*	*198*	*204*	*210*	*216*	*222*	*228*	*234*	*240*	165
	52	**54**	**57**	**60**	**63**	**65**	**68**	**71**	**74**	**76**	**79**	**82**	**84**	**87**	**90**	**93**	**95**	**98**	**101**	**103**	**106**	**109**	
66	*117*	*124*	*130*	*136*	*142*	*148*	*155*	*161*	*167*	*173*	*179*	*185*	*192*	*198*	*204*	*210*	*216*	*223*	*229*	*235*	*241*	*247*	168
	54	**56**	**59**	**62**	**65**	**68**	**71**	**73**	**76**	**79**	**82**	**85**	**87**	**90**	**93**	**96**	**99**	**102**	**104**	**107**	**110**	**113**	
67	*121*	*127*	*134*	*140*	*147*	*153*	*159*	*166*	*172*	*178*	*185*	*191*	*198*	*204*	*210*	*217*	*223*	*229*	*236*	*242*	*248*	*255*	170
	55	**58**	**61**	**64**	**66**	**69**	**72**	**75**	**78**	**81**	**84**	**87**	**90**	**92**	**95**	**98**	**101**	**104**	**107**	**110**	**113**	**116**	
68	*125*	*131*	*138*	*144*	*151*	*158*	*164*	*171*	*177*	*184*	*190*	*197*	*203*	*210*	*217*	*223*	*230*	*236*	*243*	*249*	*256*	*263*	173
	57	**60**	**63**	**66**	**69**	**72**	**75**	**78**	**81**	**84**	**87**	**90**	**93**	**96**	**99**	**102**	**105**	**108**	**111**	**114**	**117**	**120**	

(continued)

BMI (kg/m²)

Inches	19	20	21	22	23	24	25	26	27	28	29	30	31	32	33	34	35	36	37	38	39	40	Centimeters
69	*128*	*135*	*142*	*149*	*155*	*162*	*169*	*176*	*182*	*189*	*196*	*203*	*209*	*216*	*223*	*230*	*237*	*243*	*250*	*257*	*264*	*270*	
	58	**61**	**64**	**67**	**70**	**74**	**77**	**80**	**83**	**86**	**89**	**92**	**95**	**98**	**101**	**104**	**107**	**110**	**113**	**116**	**119**	**123**	175
70	*132*	*139*	*146*	*153*	*160*	*167*	*174*	*181*	*188*	*195*	*202*	*209*	*216*	*223*	*230*	*236*	*243*	*250*	*257*	*264*	*271*	*278*	
	60	**63**	**67**	**70**	**73**	**76**	**79**	**82**	**86**	**89**	**92**	**95**	**98**	**101**	**105**	**108**	**111**	**114**	**117**	**120**	**124**	**127**	178
71	*136*	*143*	*150*	*157*	*165*	*172*	*179*	*186*	*193*	*200*	*207*	*215*	*222*	*229*	*236*	*243*	*250*	*258*	*265*	*272*	*279*	*286*	
	62	**65**	**68**	**71**	**75**	**78**	**81**	**84**	**87**	**91**	**94**	**97**	**100**	**104**	**107**	**110**	**113**	**117**	**120**	**123**	**126**	**130**	180
72	*140*	*147*	*155*	*162*	*169*	*177*	*184*	*191*	*199*	*206*	*213*	*221*	*228*	*235*	*243*	*250*	*258*	*265*	*272*	*280*	*287*	*294*	
	64	**67**	**70**	**74**	**77**	**80**	**84**	**87**	**90**	**94**	**97**	**100**	**104**	**107**	**111**	**114**	**117**	**121**	**124**	**127**	**131**	**134**	183
73	*144*	*151*	*159*	*166*	*174*	*182*	*189*	*197*	*204*	*212*	*219*	*227*	*234*	*242*	*250*	*257*	*265*	*272*	*280*	*287*	*295*	*303*	
	65	**68**	**72**	**75**	**79**	**82**	**86**	**89**	**92**	**96**	**99**	**103**	**106**	**110**	**113**	**116**	**120**	**123**	**127**	**130**	**133**	**137**	185
74	*148*	*155*	*163*	*171*	*179*	*187*	*194*	*202*	*210*	*218*	*225*	*233*	*241*	*249*	*256*	*264*	*272*	*280*	*288*	*295*	*303*	*311*	
	67	**71**	**74**	**78**	**81**	**85**	**88**	**92**	**95**	**99**	**102**	**106**	**110**	**113**	**117**	**120**	**124**	**127**	**131**	**134**	**138**	**141**	188
75	*152*	*160*	*168*	*176*	*184*	*192*	*200*	*208*	*216*	*224*	*232*	*240*	*247*	*255*	*263*	*271*	*279*	*287*	*295*	*303*	*311*	*319*	
	69	**72**	**76**	**79**	**83**	**87**	**90**	**94**	**97**	**101**	**105**	**108**	**112**	**116**	**119**	**123**	**126**	**130**	**134**	**137**	**141**	**144**	190
76	*156*	*164*	*172*	*180*	*189*	*197*	*205*	*213*	*221*	*230*	*238*	*246*	*254*	*262*	*271*	*279*	*287*	*295*	*303*	*312*	*320*	*328*	
	71	**74**	**78**	**82**	**86**	**89**	**93**	**97**	**101**	**104**	**108**	**112**	**115**	**119**	**123**	**127**	**130**	**134**	**138**	**142**	**145**	**149**	193
BMI	19	20	21	22	23	24	25	26	27	28	29	30	31	32	33	34	35	36	37	38	39	40	BMI

BMI is shown as **bold underlined** numbers at the top and bottom.
To determine your BMI, select your height in either inches or centimeters and move across the row until you find your weight in pounds or inches. Your BMI can be read at the top or bottom.
Italic numbers are pounds and inches; **bold numbers are kilograms and centimeters.**
Copyright 1999 George A. Bray

Table 17.4 Revised ATP III Metabolic Syndrome Criteria

Presence of three or more of the following risk factors:

Risk Factor	Defining Level
Abdominal obesity (waist circumference)	
Men	>40 inches (102 cm)
Women	>35 inches (88 cm)
Fasting glucose	≥100 mg/dl
Triglycerides	≥150 mg/dl
HDL cholesterol	
Men	<40 mg/dl
Women	<50 mg/dl
Blood pressure	≥130/≥85 mmHg

hypertension. The aim of using these criteria is to identify individuals with insulin resistance and the accompanying dyslipidemia (small, dense LDL particles; low levels of HDL cholesterol; and elevated triglycerides), vascular dysfunction (elevations in blood pressure), and increased risk for development of type 2 diabetes. Metabolic syndrome is best managed by weight reduction, as evidenced by the results of the U.S. Diabetes Prevention Program and Finnish Diabetes Prevention Study. We believe that the presence of the metabolic syndrome is an indication for pharmacological interventions to aid weight loss because the health risks of the disorder justify that approach. We also provide a scheme to adjust risk using some of these risk factors, which we shall discuss later (Table 17.5).

EVALUATING RISK TO GUIDE TREATMENT

Because all treatments for obesity entail some risk, it is important to decide whether drug treatment is appropriate for the risks involved. This requires an assessment of the risk associated with total fat and fat distribution, as well as an assessment of metabolic status and complicating factors. In general, clinical judgment can be used to "adjust" BMI to assess risk. We propose here a scheme that relies on fat distribution assessed by waist circumference and evaluating other risk factors. Our scheme helps physicians codify the judgment decisions (adapted from Bray [2007]).

Body weights associated with a BMI of 19–25 kg/m^2 are good weights for most people. Body weights associated with BMI >30 kg/m^2 are almost invariably associated with increasing health risk. Risk assessment for a BMI between 25 and 30 kg/m^2 should include accounting for visceral fat and other comorbid factors that are affected by body weight, such as diabetes, hypertension, and dyslipidemia.

Table 17.5 illustrates our schema for the adjustment that can be made to reflect the increased risk imparted by the presence of comorbid risk factors, such as lipid levels, fasting glucose, blood pressure, sleep apnea, and osteoarthritis, and for degrees of weight gain since age 18 years. Once relative risk is evaluated,

Table 17.5 BMI Adjustments for Metabolic Variables and Other Risk Factors

	Adjustment Scores			BMI Adjustment Score
	0	+1	+3	
Weight gain since age 18 (kg)	<5	5–15	>15	_____
Fasting glucose (mg/dl)	<110	≤110–125	≥125	_____
Triglycerides (mg/dl)	<150	≥150	≥200	_____
HDL cholesterol (mg/dl)				
Men	≥40	<40	<35	_____
Women	≥50	<50	<60	_____
Blood pressure (mmHg)	<130/<85	≥130/≥85	>140/≥90	_____
Sleep apnea	Absent		Present	_____
Osteoarthritis	Absent	Present		_____
Adjustment to BMI for central fat (Table 17.4)				_____
Calculated BMI				_____
Adjusted BMI				_____

the appropriateness of various treatments can be determined from Fig. 17.1. For adjusted BMI ≥30 kg/m², pharmocotherapy is indicated. By adjusting the BMI for risk factors, one can identify patients who will benefit most from weight loss and in whom the risks associated with medications are justified.

INITIATING PHARMACOLOGICAL THERAPY

Practice guidelines, such as those of the National Institutes of Health, National Heart, Lung, and Blood Institute (1998), recommend a trial of behavioral approaches before medications are initiated. We endorse this approach. In practice, however, most obese patients who are candidates for medications have had prior weight loss attempts without lasting success, and physicians need only document this history.

Before initiating drug therapy, a counseling session with patients is important. Because the amount of weight reduction is correlated with the degree of behavior change, assessing readiness to change is an important first step. The medications will, through biological measures, reinforce the intention to restrict food intake and modify eating behavior. However, patients can override their biological signals. If patients are to maximize the amount of weight lost during the active weight-loss phase, they must be ready to change entrenched behavior patterns. Patients must also have a realistic weight-loss goal. It is unrealistic for very obese patients to expect to achieve the ideal BMI of 25 kg/m². However, loss of 5–10% initial body weight can translate into significant health benefits. A focus on a

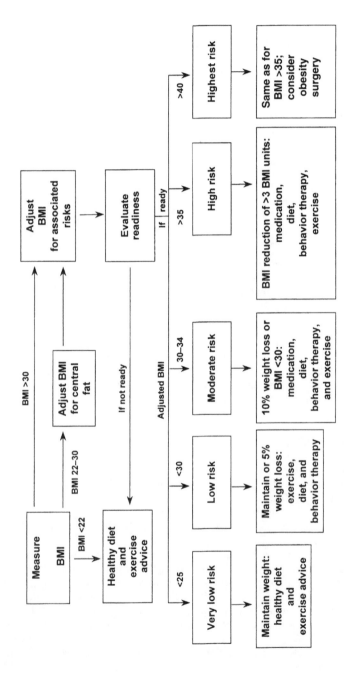

Figure 17.1 Algorithm for adjusting BMI for other comorbid risk factors and obtaining an overall assessment of risk, goal for weight loss, and rank order for potential treatments.

realistic weight loss goal of 10% and on health, rather than cosmetic benefits, is essential for the very obese. Once reached, the patient can then establish a new weight loss goal. One theory to the success of lifestyle change is setting small achievable goals to prevent failure.

A frank discussion of side effects must be preliminary to a patient's consent to undergo treatment. Sibutramine can cause blood pressure elevation, and patients must be prepared to return for monitoring. Orlistat causes fat malabsorption and anal leakage by blocking up to 30% of fat digestion, and occasional steatorrheal diarrhea must be anticipated. Another facet of the counseling interview is to describe the weight gain that is certain to occur if medications are stopped and there has not been permanent lifestyle adaptation to maintain weight loss.

MEDICATION AS ADJUNCTIVE TREATMENT

Medications for the treatment of obesity are considered adjuncts to the overall treatment plan. The other components of a standard treatment protocol include:

- Use of meal replacements (e.g., shakes, nutrition bars, and frozen entrees) as means of portion and calorie control. These are important adjuncts in the active weight loss and weight loss maintenance phases.
- Counseling on how to reduce fat and calorie intake
- An exercise program that will increase activity (by walking or other suitable means)
- The use of techniques for behavior modification that can help the patient monitor food intake, increase physical activity, and develop constructive cognitive strategies for dealing with the everyday demands to eat

STRATEGIES FOR RELAPSE PREVENTION AFTER WEIGHT LOSS

Physicians should develop a list of local resources for weight loss and lifestyle adaptation. Health clubs, hospital- or clinic-based programs, commercial programs (e.g., Weight Watchers, Jenny Craig, and Nutri/System), and support organizations (e.g., Overeaters Anonymous and TOPS Club, Inc.) can all play a role.

If the patient is an appropriate candidate, treatment options are discussed and medications are initiated with the behavioral program. Failure to lose >4 lb after 4–8 weeks of treatment is considered "treatment failure." Nonresponsive patients should not continue on medication. Evidence from clinical trials demonstrates that weight loss plateaus after ≤6 months. When patients discontinue the treatment, as they often do, they regain weight unless lifestyle changes have become a permanent part of daily life. Enrollees in our weight loss programs must commit to 1 year of treatment and then are given the option of either continued medication or an intensive lifestyle program that incorporates exercise (burning >2,000 kcal/week) and behavior modification techniques. We encourage them to resume medication whenever weight regain exceeds 5% and provide "refresher courses" of more intensive therapy.

The physician plays an important role in monitoring progress by providing positive reinforcement for success and devising constructive strategies for problem areas. Once weight has plateaued, the physician must shift emphasis to the lifelong goal of weight maintenance.

DRUGS APPROVED BY THE U.S. FOOD AND DRUG ADMINISTRATION FOR CLINICAL USE IN THE TREATMENT OF OBESITY

Drugs on the Market

There are only two drugs approved by the U.S. Food and Drug Administration (FDA) for long-term obesity management: orlistat (Xenical) and sibutramine (Meridia or Reductil). Phentermine is still widely prescribed but has approval only for short-term obesity management (usually interpreted to mean use up to 12 weeks). Phentermine is no longer patent protected and is thus inexpensive. There are other noradrenergic drugs still available, although they are rarely used. Table 17.6 shows all drugs with an obesity indication currently listed in the *Physician's Desk Reference*.

Sibutramine. Sibutramine, marketed as Meridia in the U.S., entered the market in March 1998. It is a β-phenethylamine with a cyclobutyl group on the side chain. Sibutramine inhibits the reuptake of serotonin, norepinephrine, and, to a lesser extent, dopamine. Sibutramine produces weight loss by a dual mechanism of action. It promotes satiety and increases energy expenditure, blocking the reduction in metabolic rate that accompanies weight loss. One key to successful use of sibutramine is to prescribe an appropriate dietary approach. Because sibutramine promotes satiety (it does not produce anorexia), it works best in a program that enforces regular portion-controlled meals. One regimen for the active weight loss period is to use two meal replacements (breakfast and lunch) and a sensible dinner (~600–700 kcal or two frozen entrees) in addition to sibutramine.

There are three key factors to sibutramine's efficacy. First, weight loss is dose related. The usual starting dose is 10 mg, but the drug may be increased to 15 mg (or decreased to 5 mg if there are side effects). An advantage is sibutramine's once-a-day dosing. Second, the amount of initial weight loss is related to the intensity of the behavioral intervention. Highly structured, portion-controlled schemes produce the most weight loss. Third, sibutramine is very effective during weight loss maintenance. Placebo-controlled studies demonstrate successful weight loss maintenance with sibutramine for up to 2 years.

In general, clinical trials inform us that about three-quarters of patients treated with 15 mg/day sibutramine will achieve >5% weight loss, and 80% of those will maintain that loss for 2 years. About 5% of patients will not tolerate the drug because of adverse effects on blood pressure and pulse. Some patients (~20%) are nonresponders.

Sibutramine, like other sympathomimetic agents, produces a small increase in mean heart rate and mean blood pressure observed in clinical trials. However, the blood pressure response is variable. A subset (~5% of patients) appear to be sensi-

Table 17.6 Drugs Approved by the FDA for Treatment of Obesity

Drug	Trade Names	Dosage	DEA Schedule
Pancreatic Lipase Inhibitor Approved for Long-Term Use			
Orlistat	Xenical	120 mg t.i.d. before meals	—
	alli	60 mg t.i.d. before meals	
Norepinephrine-Serotonin Reuptake Inhibitor Approved for Long-Term Use			
Sibutramine	Meridia (U.S.) Reductil (outside U.S.)	5–15 mg/day	IV
Noradrenergic Drugs Approved for Short-Term Use			
Diethylpropion	Tenuate Tenuate Dospan	25 mg t.i.d. 75 mg q. AM	IV
Phentermine	Adipex Ionamin Slow Release	15–37.5 mg/day 15–30 mg/day	IV
Benzphetamine	Didrex	25–50 mg t.i.d.	III
Phendimetrazine	Bontril Prelu-2	17.5–70 mg t.i.d. 105 mg q.d.	III

tive to the blood pressure effects and cannot tolerate sibutramine. Some patients may need to discontinue sibutramine because of blood pressure elevations to a hypertensive range. Other side effects, including dry mouth, insomnia, and asthenia, are similar to those of other noradrenergic drugs. Sibutramine is not associated with valvular heart disease, primary pulmonary hypertension, or substance abuse.

Sibutramine should be used with caution in patients with cardiovascular disease and in individuals taking selective serotonin reuptake inhibitors. It should not be used within 2 weeks of taking monoamine oxidase inhibitors and should not be used with other noradrenergic agents.

Orlistat. Orlistat is marketed as Xenical and as alli (over the counter). Fat digestion can be inhibited by blocking the enzymatic action of pancreatic lipase. In experimental studies, orlistat (tetrahydrolipstatin) has been shown to be a potent inhibitor of lipase activity that decreases intestinal triglyceride hydrolysis in a dose-dependent manner. In clinical trials, it also has a dose-dependent effect on fat absorption and weight loss. After a high-fat meal, steatorrheal diarrhea is expected, but in practice gastrointestinal events are mild to moderate, resolve spontaneously, and are usually limited to one or two episodes per patient. Deficiency of fat-soluble vitamins can occur, and vitamin supplementation should be used. In general, patients tolerate the drug very well, especially if it is combined with advance patient education.

Orlistat works best when given with a diet that has ~30% fat content, so patient counseling is important. If a high-fat meal or snack is consumed, gastrointestinal distress can result. For a very-low-fat meal, orlistat is not going to produce a caloric deficit, and patients on a low-fat diet will not lose weight on orlistat.

Orlistat is effective in producing and sustaining weight loss. It is given at a dose of 120 mg before meals three times daily. Data from clinical trials support that ~70% of patients will achieve >5% weight loss, and at 2 years, 70% of them will have maintained that loss. There are clinical trials documenting orlistat use for up to 4 years.

One advantage to orlistat's use is its beneficial effect on LDL cholesterol. Because orlistat blocks fat absorption, the LDL reduction is about twice that seen with weight loss alone.

Phentermine, diethylpropion, phendimetrazine, and benzphetamine. Phentermine and diethylpropion are classified by the U.S. Drug Enforcement Agency (DEA) as schedule IV drugs, and phendimetrazine and benzphetamine are classified as schedule III drugs. This regulatory classification indicates the government's belief that these drugs have the potential for abuse, although this potential appears to be very low. These drugs are only approved for a "few weeks" of use, which is usually interpreted as up to 12 weeks. Weight loss with phentermine and diethylpropion persists for the duration of treatment, suggesting that tolerance to these drugs does not develop. If tolerance developed, the drugs would lose their effectiveness, or increased amounts of drugs would be required for patients to maintain weight loss. Of the agents in this group, phentermine is prescribed most frequently in the U.S., probably because it is no longer protected by patents and is therefore inexpensive. Phentermine is not available in Europe. A review in the *New England Journal of Medicine* (Yanovski and Yanovski, 2002) recommends obtaining written informed consent if phentermine is prescribed for longer than 12 weeks, because there are not sufficient published reports on the long-term use of phentermine.

The only published studies of these medications involve small numbers of patients treated for a short duration. Because of the lack of long-term studies and the lack of sufficient safety data, we do not recommend the use of these agents routinely. There is one 36-week study using phentermine that shows that intermittent (1 month on, 1 month off) use of phentermine is just as effective in producing weight loss as continuous therapy. This approach is occasionally useful.

The side effect profile for sympathomimetic drugs is similar. They produce insomnia, dry mouth, asthenia, and constipation. Sympathomimetic drugs can also increase blood pressure.

OFF-LABEL PRESCRIBING

Weight loss has been reported with bupropion (an approved antidepressant and aid to smoking cessation), venlafaxine (an antidepressant with structural similarity to sibutramine), and topiramate (an anticonvulsant). We discourage off-label prescribing for obesity. However, because many antidepressants produce weight gain, bupropion or venlafaxine are good choices for the depressed obese patient. Clinical trials of topiramate as an anti-obesity agent are underway. Because of the central nervous system effects (cognitive slowing) and other serious side effects (renal stones and acute blindness), physicians should not prescribe this medication for obesity management until adequate safety has been assessed.

SPECIAL ISSUES IN DIABETES

In regard to patients with diabetes, diabetes management improves with weight reduction, and hypoglycemia becomes a possibility for those patients on insulin or oral hypoglycemic medications. Some patients may develop increased hunger due to hypoglycemia, and weight loss may slow or stop. Physicians must remember to monitor glucose carefully and reduce or stop diabetes medications as weight loss occurs. In our clinics, we halve or discontinue insulin and sulfonylureas at the start of the weight loss program.

BIBLIOGRAPHY

Bray GA: *The Metabolic Syndrome and Obesity.* Totowa, NJ, Humana Press, 2007

Bray GA, Greenway FL: Pharmacological treatment of the overweight patient (Review). *Pharmacol Rev* 59:151–184, 2007

National Institutes of Health, National Heart, Lung, and Blood Institute: Clinical guidelines on the identification, evaluation, and treatment of overweight and obesity in adults: the evidence report. *Obes Res* 6 (Suppl. 2):51S–210S, 1998

Yanovski SZ, Yanovski JA: Drug obesity. *N Engl J Med* 346:591–602, 2002

Dr. Ryan is Associate Executive Director for Clinical Research and Dr. Bray is Chief of the Division of Obesity and Metabolic Diseases at the Pennington Biomedical Research Center, Baton Rouge, Louisiana.

18. Exercise

Edward S. Horton, MD

Regular physical exercise has long been considered to be a cornerstone in the management of people with diabetes. However, the goals of an exercise program, as well as the specific risks and benefits, will vary from one patient to another and are often quite different for people with type 1 or type 2 diabetes. For example, a young person with type 1 diabetes may wish to participate in recreational or competitive sports and participate in vigorous or prolonged exercise as part of their normal lifestyle, whereas an overweight, middle-aged person with type 2 diabetes may undertake a program of regular physical exercise as part of his or her treatment program to improve glycemic control, lose or maintain body weight, and improve blood pressure, lipids, and other cardiovascular risk factors.

For the management of exercise in type 1 diabetes, it is important to understand the hormonal regulation of metabolic fuels at rest, during exercise of varying intensities and durations, and during the postexercise recovery period. For example, in patients with type 1 diabetes who are insulin deficient, exercise may cause a further rise in blood glucose and the rapid development of ketosis, and even in well-controlled patients, vigorous exercise may result in sustained hyperglycemia. However, if insulin levels are excessive, hypoglycemia may occur during or after exercise. Because of these problems with regulation of blood glucose and ketones during or after exercise, many patients with type 1 diabetes find it difficult to participate in sports or other recreational activities or to manage exercise as part of their daily lives. This result has led to the opinion that exercise should not be recommended for all patients with type 1 diabetes, but that efforts should be focused on making it possible for those who want to exercise to be able to do so as safely as possible. The availability of self-monitoring of blood glucose (SMBG) and the increased use of multiple-dose insulin regimens or insulin pumps have led to the development of individualized strategies for the management of exercise in type 1 diabetic patients, making it possible for them to safely participate in a wide range of physical activities and thus to have a normal or near-normal lifestyle.

In patients with type 2 diabetes, regular activity is an important component of treatment and should be prescribed along with appropriate diet and oral antidiabetic agents or insulin as part of a comprehensive treatment program. Recent prospective studies have also demonstrated the beneficial effects of lifestyle modification programs focusing on a healthy diet, weight reduction, and increased physical activity to prevent or delay progression from impaired glucose metabolism (pre-diabetes) to overt type 2 diabetes and to reduce risk factors for cardio-

Table 18.1 Benefits of Exercise for Patients with Diabetes

- Lower blood glucose concentrations during and after exercise
- Lower basal and postprandial insulin concentrations
- Improved insulin sensitivity
- Lower A1C levels
- Improved lipid profile
  - Decreased triglycerides
  - Slightly decreased LDL cholesterol
  - Increased HDL2 cholesterol

- Improvement in mild to moderate hypertension
- Increased energy expenditure
  - Adjunct to diet for weight reduction
  - Increased fat loss
  - Preservation of lean body mass
- Cardiovascular conditioning
- Increased strength and flexibility
- Improved sense of well-being and quality of life

vascular disease (CVD). Designing an appropriate exercise program for type 2 diabetes requires a careful assessment of the expected benefits and associated risks of exercise in individual patients and the development of an exercise program with appropriate monitoring to avoid injuries and other complications.

BENEFITS

The benefits of exercise for patients with diabetes are listed in Table 18.1. Moderate-intensity, sustained exercise in patients with either type 1 or type 2 diabetes may be used to help regulate glucose on a day-to-day basis and may be the mechanism by which regular physical exercise assists in achieving improved long-term metabolic control. Physical training results in lower fasting and postprandial insulin concentrations and increased insulin sensitivity. In patients with type 1 diabetes, increased insulin sensitivity results in lowered insulin requirements. In patients with type 2 diabetes, the improvement in insulin sensitivity resulting from regular physical exercise may be of major importance in improving long-term glycemic control. Several studies have demonstrated that both aerobic and strength training programs improve insulin sensitivity and glycemic control as measured by improvement in A1C.

Another benefit of regular exercise is a reduction in cardiovascular risk factors through improvement of the lipid profile, reduction in both systolic and diastolic blood pressure, decreased biomarkers of subclinical inflammation, and improved endothelial function. Although several population studies have demonstrated an inverse correlation between the amount of habitual physical exercise and cardiovascular events, prospective randomized controlled trials of lifestyle intervention have not yet been completed, so it has not yet been determined whether the improvement in cardiovascular risk factors will result in reduced cardiovascular events over time.

In addition to improvement in cardiovascular risk factors, physical exercise may be an effective adjunct to diet for weight reduction and weight maintenance. Physical exercise programs alone are usually associated with little or no weight loss and must be combined with a calorie-restricted diet to achieve significant weight loss. However, numerous studies have demonstrated that regular physical

Table 18.2 Risks of Exercise for Patients with Diabetes

■ Hypoglycemia, if treated with insulin or oral agents
– Exercise-induced hypoglycemia
– Late-onset postexercise hypoglycemia
■ Hyperglycemia after very strenuous exercise
■ Hyperglycemia and ketosis in insulin-deficient patients
■ Precipitation or exacerbation of CVD
– Angina pectoris
– Myocardial infarction
– Arrhythmias

■ Worsening of long-term complications of diabetes
– Proliferative retinopathy
  □ Vitreous hemorrhage
  □ Retinal detachment
– Nephropathy
  □ Increased proteinuria
– Peripheral neuropathy
  □ Soft tissue and joint injuries
– Autonomic neuropathy
  □ Decreased cardiovascular response to exercise
  □ Decreased maximum aerobic capacity
  □ Impaired response to dehydration
  □ Postural hypotension

exercise is an important part of the lifestyle modification program and is particularly important for achieving weight maintenance after weight loss goals have been achieved.

Finally, regular exercise improves cardiovascular fitness and physical working capacity and also improves the sense of well-being and quality of life.

RISKS

There are several risks associated with exercise for patients with diabetes (Table 18.2). In patients with type 1 diabetes, either hyperglycemia or hypoglycemia can occur during exercise depending on its intensity and duration as well as on the amount and timing of insulin injections. In addition, last-onset postexercise hypoglycemia can occur 6–15 h after completion of the exercise and may persist for up to 24 h after prolonged, strenuous exercise. In contrast to hypoglycemia, high-intensity exercise may result in a rapid increase in blood glucose that can persist for several hours after exercise is discontinued. Even moderate-intensity exercise may result in hyperglycemia and in the rapid development of ketosis or ketoacidosis in patients with type 1 diabetes who are insulin deficient.

Careful screening for underlying cardiac disease is important for all patients with diabetes before starting a vigorous exercise program that involves an exercise intensity that is unusual for the patient and is greater than that achieved by brisk walking or its equivalent. In addition, degenerative joint disease is more common in obese individuals and may be exacerbated by weight-bearing exercises.

Several complications of diabetes may be aggravated by exercise, and all patients should be screened before they start an exercise program. The most important of these is proliferative retinopathy, in which exercise may result in retinal or vitreous hemorrhage.

Exercises that increase blood pressure, e.g., heavy lifting or exercise associated with Valsalva-like maneuvers, should be avoided by patients with proliferative retinopathy requiring laser therapy until cleared by an opthalmologist, usually 3–6 months following laser photocoagulation. Physical exercise is also associated with increased proteinuria in patients with diabetic nephropathy, probably because of changes in renal hemodynamics. It has not been shown, however, that exercise leads to more rapid progression of renal disease, and the use of angiotensin-converting enzyme (ACE) inhibitors does appear to decrease the amount of exercise-induced albuminuria.

Patients with peripheral neuropathy have an increased risk of soft tissue and joint injuries, and, if autonomic neuropathy is present, the capacity for high-intensity exercise is impaired because of a decreased maximum heart rate and aerobic capacity. In addition, patients with autonomic neuropathy may have impaired responses to dehydration and develop postural hypotension after exercise. With proper selection of the type, intensity, and duration of exercise, most of these complications can be avoided.

GUIDELINES FOR EXERCISE

Screening

Before starting an exercise program, all patients should have a complete history and physical examination, with particular attention paid to identifying any long-term complications of diabetes. The role of exercise stress testing before beginning an exercise program is controversial. For young, generally healthy people with type 1 or type 2 diabetes, an exercise stress test is not needed prior to starting an exercise program. However, in older individuals, particularly those who have increased CVD risk factors, a stress test will be useful to help identify silent ischemic heart disease and may identify patients who have an exaggerated hypertensive response to exercise and/or may develop postexercise orthostatic hypotension. The American College of Sports Medicine (ACSM) recommends that people with type 2 diabetes aged ≥35 years have a stress test conducted prior to participating in physical activity that exceeds that which is associated with the activities of daily living. A careful ophthalmologic examination to identify proliferative retinopathy; renal function tests, including screening for microalbuminuria; and a neurological examination to determine peripheral and/or autonomic neuropathy should be performed. If abnormalities are found, exercises should be selected that will not pose significant risks for worsening complications or result in injuries. In general, active young patients with diabetes of brief duration and no evidence of long-term complications do not require formal exercise prescriptions, although they need specific recommendations regarding strategies for managing exercise and avoiding injuries.

Selection of Type of Exercise

If there are no contraindications, the types of exercise a patient performs can be a matter of personal preference. In general, moderate-intensity aerobic exercises that can be sustained for ≥30 minutes are preferred, although there is now also good evidence that intermittent high-intensity and resistance exercises can be managed successfully and will also result in improved insulin sensitivity and improved glycemic control. Most exercise programs for people with diabetes now include a combination of aerobic exercises and strength-building exercises to achieve the maximum benefits from a physical training program.

Frequency and Structure of Exercise Sessions

It is generally recommended that most people participate in moderate intensity for ≥30 min most days of the week. However, exercise at least three times a week has been shown to result in significant improvement in cardiovascular fitness, improved glycemic control, and reduction in cardiovascular risk factors in people with type 2 diabetes. The effect of a single bout of aerobic exercise on insulin sensitivity lasts 24–72 h, depending on the duration and intensity of the exercise. Consequently, it is recommended that the time between exercise sessions should not be >2 consecutive days. The carryover effect of resistance exercise training may be somewhat longer because of the associated increase in muscle mass. A commonly recommended program would be to alternate days of predominantly aerobic exercise with days of strength training with a goal of achieving ≥30 min of exercise on 5 or 6 days each week.

The importance of including a 5- to 10-min warmup of low-intensity aerobic exercise and stretching to prevent musculoskeletal injuries has been traditionally emphasized, but recent studies have failed to show that this is necessary. The higher-intensity portion of the exercise session should last 20–45 min and then gradually be increased up to 60 min if possible, depending on the level of physical conditioning. The general rule is to start slowly and build up gradually as cardiovascular condition and strength training improve. Aerobic exercises should be of moderate intensity, i.e., 40–60% of maximum aerobic capacity or 50–70% of maximum heart rate for at least a total of 150 min/week. Alternatively, more vigorous aerobic exercise at levels >60% of maximum aerobic capacity or 70% of maximum heart rate can be done for ≥90 minutes per week. Increased amounts of time doing moderate or vigorous aerobic exercise will result in greater cardiovascular conditioning and greater CVD risk reduction compared with shorter durations of activity. In general, exercise intensity should be limited so that systolic blood pressure doesn't exceed 180 mmHg. The intensity of exercise can also be estimated from the heart rate response (i.e., the resting pulse rate determined before arising in the morning and the maximum heart rate determined during exercise). Fifty percent of a subject's maximal effort can be estimated by the formula 0.5 (maximum heart rate – resting heart rate) plus resting heart rate. When the true maximum heart rate is unknown, it can be estimated by the formula 220 – patient's age in years. However, this is less accurate than a direct determination of the maximum heart rate under controlled conditions and may significantly overestimate the maximum heart rate in patients with autonomic neuropathy. An alternative approach is to use the Borg scale of relative perceived exertion, which provides a numerical scale for estimating the patient's own sense of the level of exertion during aerobic exercise. Once the heart rate response to exercise is determined for an individual patient, exercise intensity can be conveniently monitored by teaching the patient to measure his or her own pulse periodically during exercise and recording the results.

For resistance training the ACSM recommends a minimum of 8–10 exercises involving the major muscle groups, with a minimum of one set of 10–15 repetitions resulting in near fatigue. Alternatively, fewer repetitions (8–10) of the heaviest weight that can be lifted eight to ten times to near fatigue can also be used. A general plan would be to start with a single set of 10–15 repetitions two to three times weekly at moderate intensity and then gradually increase to two sets and finally to three sets of repetitions of high-intensity exercise, while gradually increasing the amount of resistance as strength improves.

By undertaking a program of aerobic exercise equivalent to brisk walking ≥3 days/week and resistance training ≥2 days/week, one can expect improved glucose, blood pressure, and dyslipidemia control as well as better maintenance of weight loss if the program is combined with reduced caloric intake.

Monitoring and Compliance

For patients who have not participated regularly in exercise in the past or who have significant complications of diabetes or other impediments to exercise, supervised exercise programs may be beneficial. Often cardiac rehabilitation programs will be of assistance in supervising exercise programs for people with diabetes, particularly if the patients are at high risk for CVD. There is an increasing number of diabetes treatment centers that offer supervised exercise programs for patients with either type 1 or type 2 diabetes. Many patients, however, do not need formal supervision once an initial assessment has been completed and an appropriate exercise plan has been established.

Several things can be done to improve the patient's motivation and participation on a regular basis. These include choosing activities the patient enjoys, providing a variety in types and settings for exercise, performing exercise at convenient times and locations, encouraging participation in group activities, involving the patient's family and associates for reinforcement, and measuring progress to provide positive feedback. Most important is to start slowly, build up gradually, and not set excessive or unrealistic goals.

Patients should be instructed to avoid injuries or other complications while participating in physical exercise. Feet should be inspected daily and always after exercise for cuts, blisters, and infections. Exercise should be avoided in extreme hot or cold environments and during periods of poor metabolic control. Special guidelines for patients taking insulin are described below.

MANAGEMENT OF EXERCISE IN PATIENTS WITH TYPE 1 DIABETES

Whereas changes in blood glucose are small in nondiabetic individuals during exercise, several factors may complicate glucose regulation during and after exercise in people with type 1 diabetes. Plasma insulin concentrations do not decrease normally during exercise, thus upsetting the balance between peripheral glucose utilization and hepatic glucose production. With insulin treatment, plasma insulin concentrations stay the same or may even increase if exercise is undertaken within 1 h of an insulin injection. Enhanced insulin absorption during exercise is most likely to occur when the insulin injection is given immediately before or within a few minutes of the onset of exercise, particularly when using rapid-onset, short-acting insulin preparations. The longer the interval between injection and

Table 18.3 Pre-exercise Checklist for Patients with Type 1 Diabetes

1. Consider the exercise plan.
   - What is the duration and intensity of the planned exercise?
   - Is the exercise habitual or unusual?
   - How does the exercise relate to the level of physical conditioning?
   - What is the estimated calorie expenditure?
2. Consider the insulin regimen.
   - What is the usual insulin dosage schedule? Should it be decreased?
   - What is the interval between injection of insulin and the onset of exercise?
   - Should the site of injection be changed to avoid exercising areas?
3. Consider the plan for food intake.
   - What is the interval between the last meal and the onset of exercise?
   - Should a pre-exercise snack be eaten?
   - Should carbohydrate feedings be taken during exercise?
   - Will extra food be required after exercise?
4. Check blood glucose.
   - If <100 mg/dl (<5.5 mmol/l), eat a pre-exercise snack.
   - If 100–250 mg/dl (5.5–14 mmol/l), it should be all right to exercise.
   - If >250 mg/dl (>14 mmol/l), check urine ketones.
5. Check urine ketones (if glucose is >250 mg/dl [>14 mmol/l]).
   - If negative, it is all right to exercise.
   - If positive, take insulin; do not exercise until ketones are negative.

onset of exercise, the less significant this effect will be, and the less important it is to choose the site of injection to avoid an exercising area.

The sustained insulin levels during exercise increase peripheral glucose uptake and stimulate glucose oxidation by the exercising muscles. In addition, insulin inhibits hepatic glucose production. The hepatic glucose production rate cannot match the rate of peripheral glucose utilization, and blood glucose concentration falls. During mild to moderate exercise of short duration, this may be a beneficial effect of exercise, but during more prolonged exercise, hypoglycemia may result. If exercise is very intense, sympathetic nervous stimulation of hepatic glucose production may result in a rapid and sustained rise in blood glucose concentra-

Table 18.4   Strategies for Avoiding Hypoglycemia and Hyperglycemia with Exercise

1. Eat a meal 1–3 h before exercise.
2. Take supplemental carbohydrate feedings at least every 30 min during exercise if exercise is vigorous and of long duration.
3. Increase food intake for up to 24 h after exercise, depending on intensity and duration of exercise.
4. Take insulin at least 1 h before exercise. If <1 h before exercise, inject in a nonexercising area.
5. Decrease insulin dose before exercise.
6. Alter daily insulin schedule.
7. Monitor blood glucose before, during, and after exercise.
8. Delay exercise if blood glucose is >250 mg/dl (>14 mmol/l) and ketones are present.
9. Learn individual glucose responses to different types of exercise.
10. Continuous glucose monitoring (CGM) may be a useful tool.

tions. If there is also insulin deficiency, hepatic ketone production is stimulated, and ketosis or ketoacidosis may occur.

A checklist of factors to consider before the onset of exercise is provided in Table 18.3. Obviously, it is not possible to predict all situations, because exercise is often spontaneous or intermittent and varies greatly in intensity and duration.

By considering the exercise plan and making adjustments in insulin dosage and food intake, patients with type 1 diabetes can avoid severe hypoglycemia or hyperglycemia. If exercise is of moderate intensity and long duration, blood glucose levels will fall, whereas vigorous exercise of short duration will often cause blood glucose to rise. Attention should be paid to the amount, timing, and site of insulin administration. Food intake before, during, and after exercise should be considered. It is also important to measure blood glucose before starting exercise and, if necessary, during and after exercise. With this information, the strategies outlined in Table 18.4 can be used to avoid either hypoglycemia or hyperglycemia.

Usually, a snack containing 20–25 g carbohydrate every 30 min is sufficient to provide enough glucose to maintain normal blood levels during prolonged exercise. Carbohydrate requirements will depend on factors such as the intensity and duration of exercise, the level of physical conditioning, the antecedent diet, and the circulating insulin levels.

If the exercise is planned, the insulin dosage schedule may be altered to decrease the likelihood of hypoglycemia. Individuals who take a single dose of intermediate-acting insulin may decrease the dose by 30–35% on the morning before exercise or may change to a split-dose regimen, taking 65% of the usual dose in the morning and 35% before the evening meal. Those who are taking a combination of intermediate- and short-acting insulin may decrease the short-acting insulin by 50% or omit it altogether before exercise; they also may decrease the intermediate-acting insulin before exercise and take supplemental doses of short-acting insulin later if needed. Many patients now are treated with once-daily long-acting insulin glargine or detemir with multiple daily doses of rapid-onset, short-acting insulin (i.e., aspart, lispro, glulisine). In these patients, the short-acting insulin dose before exercise may be decreased by 30–50%, and postexercise doses may be adjusted based on glucose monitoring and experience with postexercise hypoglycemia. If insulin infusion devices are used, the basal infusion rate may be decreased during exercise and premeal boluses decreased or omitted.

EXERCISE PROGRAMS FOR TREATING TYPE 2 DIABETES

In people with type 2 diabetes, exercise programs may improve insulin sensitivity and lower average blood glucose concentrations. The increased energy expenditure associated with exercise, when combined with calorie restriction, may improve weight reduction. Thus, regular exercise is an important component of treating patients with type 2 diabetes.

However, type 2 diabetic patients are usually older, are frequently obese, and may have significant long-term complications, making the initiation of exercise programs difficult. In this group of patients, exercises that enhance motivation and participation and have a low risk of injury should be selected. Increasing daily activities such as walking, climbing stairs, and other familiar activities is an excellent start.

Unlike patients with type 1 diabetes, problems in glucose regulation do not occur, with the exception of occasional problems with hypoglycemia in patients taking insulin or insulin secretogogues. In patients treated with diet alone, supplemental feedings before, during, or after exercise are generally unnecessary.

In patients being treated with low-calorie diets, physical exercise is generally well tolerated and does not pose any additional risks if the diet is adequately supplemented with vitamins and minerals and adequate hydration is maintained. In patients treated with very-low-calorie diets (600–800 kcal/day), the diet should contain ≥35% of calories as carbohydrate to maintain normal muscle glycogen stores, which are needed to maintain high-intensity exercise. On the other hand, very-low-calorie diets severely restricted in carbohydrate are compatible with moderate-intensity exercise after an adaptation period of ≥2 weeks. It is important to note that increasing activity while on a very-low-calorie diet in someone on a hypoglycemic agent will increase the risk of hypoglycemia.

An exercise program for obese patients with type 2 diabetes should start slowly, build up gradually, and include exercises that are familiar to the patient and least likely to cause injuries or worsening of long-term diabetes complications.

BIBLIOGRAPHY

Ruderman N, Devlin JT, Kriska A (Eds.): *American Diabetes Association Handbook of Exercise in Diabetes*. Alexandria, VA, American Diabetes Association, 2001

Steppel JH, Horton ES: Exercise in patients with diabetes mellitus. In *Joslin's Diabetes Mellitis*. 14th ed. Kahn CR, Weir GC, King GL, Jacobson AM, Moses AC, Smith RJ, Eds. Philadelphia, PA, Lippincott Williams and Wilkins, 2005, p. 649–657

Sigal RJ, Wasserman DH, Kenny GP, Castaneda-Sceppa C: Physical activity/exercise and type 2 diabetes (Technical Review). *Diabetes Care* 27:2518–2539, 2004

Dr. Horton is Professor of Medicine at Harvard Medical School, Joslin Diabetes Center, Boston, Massachusetts.

19. The Prevention of Type 2 Diabetes

Vanita R. Aroda, MD, and Robert E. Ratner, MD

Diabetes is an escalating worldwide epidemic. Predictions made in the 1990s on the prevalence rates for diabetes in the 21st century have disconcertingly proven to be underestimates. In 1997, Amos et al. (1997) estimated that the prevalence of diabetes worldwide would increase from 124 million in 1997 to 221 million by the year 2010. Startlingly, the prevalence of diabetes in the world reached 171 million by the year 2000 (Wild 2004) and has already prematurely surpassed its prediction with an estimated 246 million people with diabetes in 2006 (IDF 2008). Assuming a constant level of obesity, >366 million individuals will have diabetes by the year 2030 (Wild 2004). With the epidemics of obesity and diabetes rising in parallel, this too will likely be an underestimate.

Diabetes carries with it a marked increase in premature mortality and morbidity. Data from the Framingham Study indicate that men and women aged ≥50 years with diabetes live an average 7.5 years and 8.2 years less than men and women without diabetes, respectively (Franco 2007). Similarly, Narayan et al. (2003) estimated that if an individual is diagnosed with diabetes at age 40 years, a man would lose 11.6 life-years and 18.6 quality-adjusted life-years (QALYs), and a woman would lose 14.3 life-years and 22.0 QALYs. Diabetes is also a source of significant comorbidity, posing a major risk for cardiovascular disease (CVD) and accounting for a majority of new cases of blindness, renal failure, and nontraumatic lower-limb amputations (CDC 2007).

The increasing prevalence of diabetes and its associated complications are bound to increase associated costs. In the U.S., for example, the total estimated cost of diabetes in 2007 was $174 billion, already an adjusted $21 billion higher than in 2002 (ADA 2008). Not only do diabetes-associated costs directly impact individuals and families afflicted with the disease, but they also impact health care resources and national productivity.

With the increasing prevalence of diabetes and its associated morbidity, mortality, and cost, the need to prevent diabetes is becoming increasingly clear. The last two decades have provided us with abundant evidence for the prevention of diabetes, and we are continuing to learn about the long-term effects of prevention. In this chapter, we provide background on the natural history of pre-diabetes, the goals and evidence for prevention of diabetes, and an update on published guidelines for the prevention of diabetes.

DEFINING PRE-DIABETES ALONG THE CONTINUUM OF DISEASE

An influential factor in considering the benefit of preventing diabetes is the long natural history of normoglycemia and intermediate hyperglycemia preceding the overt hyperglycemia of type 2 diabetes. Data from the U.K. Prospective Diabetes Study (UKPDS) suggest that β-cell function progressively declines an average of 12 years before the diagnosis of type 2 diabetes. By the time of diagnosis of type 2 diabetes, ~50% of β-cell function is already lost and continues to decline (UKPDS 1995).

The key factors promoting the progression from intermediate hyperglycemia to diabetes include insulin resistance in combination with progressive pancreatic β-cell dysfunction, compounded by environmental risk factors such as obesity on a background of genetic predisposition (Weyer 1999). As shown in the Insulin Resistance Atherosclerosis Study, normoglycemia is maintained primarily through a compensatory increase in insulin secretion to overcome insulin resistance. However, the failure to increase insulin secretion followed by a decrease in insulin secretion results in the development of hyperglycemia and, eventually, diabetes (Festa 2006).

This long period of intermediate hyperglycemia preceding the clinical entity of type 2 diabetes is termed pre-diabetes. Pre-diabetes consists of both impaired fasting glucose (IFG) and impaired glucose tolerance (IGT). IFG refers to a fasting plasma glucose (FPG) ≥100 mg/dl (5.6 mmol/l) but <126 mg/dl (7.0 mmol/l) according to the American Diabetes Association (ADA), whereas the World Health Organization (WHO) defines IFG at an FPG ≥110 mg/dl (6.1 mmol/l) but <126 mg/dl (7.0 mmol/l). Both the ADA and WHO define IGT as an abnormal 2-h response to a 75-g oral glucose tolerance test (OGTT) of ≥140 mg/dl (7.8 mmol/l) and <200 mg/dl (11.1 mmol/l) (ADA 2009a, WHO/IDF 2006).

These categories of classifying normoglycemia, pre-diabetes, and diabetes stem from both assessments of disease risk and population distributions of plasma glucose (WHO/IDF 2006). Specifically, fasting plasma glucose (FPG) and 2-h postprandial glucose cut points, above which the incidence of retinopathy significantly increases, were used to help define the current diagnostic criteria for diabetes. However, it is becoming increasingly clear that there is increased risk of complications even at levels below this categorical cutoff point, suggesting a continuous rather than a categorical relationship between glucose and disease risk. A cross-sectional study in the Diabetes Prevention Program (DPP), for example, showed that 7.9% of subjects with IGT had findings consistent with diabetic retinopathy, whereas 12.6% of subjects with diabetes had evidence of diabetic retinopathy early after the conversion to diabetes (DPP 2007). Similarly, there is a growing recognition of a possible relation between IGT and neuropathy. The neuropathy seen in IGT is clinically similar to early diabetic neuropathy, preferentially affecting the small nerve fibers (Smith 2008). Data from the Framingham Heart Study also suggest a relationship between pre-diabetes (IFG and/or IGT) and the subsequent development of chronic kidney disease. Baseline glomerular filtration rate was found to increase across the spectrum of hyperglycemia, a finding typical of hyperfiltration seen in the early stages of diabetes. Baseline IFG or IGT also conferred an increased risk of developing chronic kidney disease after a mean 7 years, which appeared to be related to associated cardiovascular risk factors (Fox 2005).

There is also evidence to support a continuous relationship between glucose and risk of macrovascular disease and mortality at levels well below the diagnostic cutoff for diabetes. Both the DECODE study and Paris Prospective study showed J-shaped relationships between mortality and FPG (DECODE 2003, Balkau 1999). The lowest mortality rates in the Paris Prospective study centered on FPG of 99 mg/dl (5.5 mmol/l), and in the DECODE study they corresponded with FPG 81–110 mg/dl (4.50–6.09 mmol/l) (DECODE 2003, Balkau 1999). Furthermore, the DECODE study observed a linear relationship between cardiovascular mortality and 2-h postprandial glucose without an obvious threshold (DECODE 2003). The Baltimore Longitudinal Study of Aging also reported an almost linear increase in coronary artery disease and all-cause mortality above FPG levels of 110–120 mg/dl (6.1–6.7 mmol/l) and 2-h postprandial glucose >140 mg/dl (7.8 mmol/l) (Sorkin 2005). A meta-analysis of prospective studies further supports a linear relationship between 2-h postprandial glucose levels and CVD risk and a possible threshold of risk for FPG at a level of ~100 mg/dl (5.6 mmol/l) (Levitan 2004).

Additional evidence supporting the continuous association of risk at glucose levels comes from the HAPO (Hyperglycemia and Adverse Pregnancy Outcomes) study. Data from 75-g oral glucose tolerance tests (OGTTs) obtained from >23,000 pregnant women between weeks 24 and 32 of gestation suggested a strong continuous association between maternal glucose levels (FPG, 1-h glucose, and 2-h glucose) below those diagnostic of diabetes and adverse pregnancy outcomes, including increased birth weight and increased cord-blood serum C-peptide levels. Again, there was no obvious threshold of glucose above which risk sharply increased (HAPO 2008).

In summary, observations from the UKPDS suggest that the pathophysiological processes leading to progressive hyperglycemia begin long before the actual diagnosis of diabetes. Furthermore, there is evidence of an increased risk of both macrovascular and microvascular disease during this long intermediate stage of hyperglycemia. The traditional terms "normoglycemia," "pre-diabetes," and "diabetes" represent arbitrary delineations attempting to separate risks, but clearly, the risk of developing diabetes and many of its complications are linear, without an unambiguous threshold. Indeed, in the WHO/International Diabetes Federation (IDF)'s report on the "definition and diagnosis of diabetes and intermediate hyperglycemia," consideration is given to "replacing this category of intermediate hyperglycemia by an overall risk assessment for diabetes, CVD, or both, which includes a measure of glucose as a continuous variable" (WHO/IDF 2006). This approach incorporating glucose in an overall risk assessment provides the framework for establishing goals in the prevention of diabetes.

PREVENTION OF DIABETES: WHAT ARE THE GOALS?

In evaluating the evidence to prevent diabetes, it is important to consider the goals. As discussed in detail in the 2007 ADA consensus statement on IFG and IGT, the goals depend on how we define the natural history of pre-diabetes (Nathan 2007). On the one hand, it is clear that progression along the continuum of hyperglycemia is associated with a marked increase in mortality, CVD, and microvascular disease. Thus, one of the primary goals should be the maintenance of glycemia or at least the prevention of glycemic deterioration. However, is it enough to just maintain normoglycemia by treating the hyperglycemia earlier in the course of disease or should we be focusing on therapies that not only maintain normoglycemia but also biologically delay the pathophysiological processes leading to diabetes? Viewing the prevention of diabetes in this way, a pivotal measure of prevention would be the ability to halt the progressive decline in insulin secretion and/or improve insulin resistance to maintain glycemic stability. Last, if we consider the big picture of prevention, the goal in preventing diabetes extends beyond the prevention of hyperglycemia. The ultimate goal in the prevention of diabetes is the prevention of the increased morbidity and mortality associated with the disease. It is important to consider these three separate but related goals in understanding the evidence surrounding the prevention of diabetes.

Evidence for Prevention of Diabetes

There is now overwhelming evidence that diabetes can indeed be prevented. In evaluating the available evidence, it is important to ask how the evidence supports the aforementioned goals. Does the intervention reduce the likelihood of developing hyperglycemia consistent with diabetes? Are the effects of the intervention sustainable beyond the intervention? In other words, is the intervention delaying the biological progression of disease, or merely treating hyperglycemia early? Lastly, does the intervention have an impact on long-term outcomes?

Goal #1 in Prevention of Diabetes: Prevention of Glycemic Deterioration

Individuals with pre-diabetes are at high risk of developing type 2 diabetes. The average annual risk of developing diabetes in the general population is ~0.7% per year (NDSS 2008). Whereas this risk is ~5–10% per year in individuals with IFG or IGT, it is even higher in individuals with combined IFG and IGT (Gerstein 2007). In the DPP, for example, 11% of subjects annually with elevated fasting glucose (≥95 mg/dl [≥5.3 mmol/l]) and IGT progressed to diabetes in the standard treatment arm (Knowler 2002). It is estimated that up to 70% of individuals with pre-diabetes will eventually develop type 2 diabetes without intervention (Nathan 2007).

Numerous lifestyle and pharmacotherapy intervention studies have proven the benefit in reducing the likelihood of progression from IGT to diabetes. We highlight here a select number of these intervention studies (Table 19.1).

Lifestyle Changes for the Prevention of Diabetes. The earliest study evaluating lifestyle changes to prevent the progression from IGT to diabetes was the Chinese Da Qing study. Over 500 subjects with IGT were randomized to a control group or to diet-only intervention, exercise-only intervention, or diet-plus-exercise intervention and followed for 6 years. Compared with the control group, diet-only intervention reduced the risk of developing diabetes by 31%, exercise-only intervention by 46%, and diet-plus-exercise intervention by 42% (Pan 1997).

The Finnish Diabetes Prevention Study also randomized >500 high-risk subjects (mean age 55 years, mean BMI 31 kg/m^2) with IGT to either a control or intensive lifestyle-intervention group and followed them annually (with OGTTs) for a mean of 3.2 years. Intervention goals included weight reduction of >5%, reduction in total fat and saturated fat intake, increase in fiber consumption, and

Table 19.1 Summary of Select Diabetes Prevention Trials

Study	*n*	Mean Duration of Follow-up (Years)	Intervention	Relative Risk Reduction in Diabetes Compared with Placebo (%)
Da Qing Study (Pan 1997)	577	6	Diet	31
			Exercise	46
			Diet + Exercise	42
Finnish Diabetes Prevention Study (Tuomilehto 2001)	522	3.2	Diet and Activity	58
Kosaka et al. (2005)	458	4	Diet and Activity	67.4
DPP (Knowler 2002)	3,234	2.8	Diet and Activity	58
			Metformin	31
IDPP-1 (Ramachandran 2006)	531	3	Lifestyle	28.5
			Metformin	26.4
			Lifestyle + Metformin	28.2
STOP-NIDDM (Chiasson 2002)	1,429	3	Acarbose	25
XENDOS (Torgerson 2004)	3,305	4	Orlistat	37.3
DPP (Knowler 2005)	1,167	0.9	Troglitazone	75
TRIPOD (Buchanan 2002)	236	2.5	Troglitazone	55
DREAM (DREAM 2006)	5,269	3	Rosiglitazone	60
ACT NOW (DeFronzo 2008)	602	2.6	Pioglitazone	81

moderate exercise for ≥30 min daily. Instruction was individualized, with seven sessions with a nutritionist during the first year of the study and supervision of circuit-type resistance training. Diabetes was reduced by 58% in the lifestyle-intervention group, with a clear association between achieving the outlined goals and ability to prevent progression to diabetes (Tuomilehto 2001).

Adding to the universal benefit of lifestyle intervention, a recent study of Japanese male subjects with IGT resulted in a 67.4% reduction in type 2 diabetes over 4 years. The aims in this study focused on a BMI goal of ≤22 kg/m² in the intensive lifestyle group compared with <24 kg/m² in the standard group. Subjects in the intensive lifestyle group lost a mean 2.18 kg compared with 0.39 kg in the control group (Kosaka 2005).

The largest diabetes prevention study to date is the DPP, which randomized >3,000 participants aged ≥25 years with elevated fasting glucose (≥95 mg/dl) and IGT to placebo, 850 mg metformin twice daily, or intensive lifestyle intervention. Goals of the lifestyle modification program included 7% body weight loss and moderate physical activity of ≥150 min/week. Conducted in 27 centers in the U.S., the study enrolled a population that was ethnically diverse, with nearly one-half of the population representing racial or ethnic minorities. Compared with standard lifestyle advice, intensive lifestyle intervention showed categorical benefit, with a 58% reduction in the progression from IGT to type 2 diabetes over 3 years (Knowler 2002). Extrapolating from the DPP, intensive lifestyle interven-tion would be expected to delay the onset of diabetes by 11.1 years (Herman 2005). Lifestyle intervention appeared to benefit both sexes and all ethnic sub-groups and was particularly advantageous in older individuals (aged ≥60 years) and in those with a lower baseline BMI (22 to <30 kg/m²) (Knowler 2002).

Metformin for the Prevention of Diabetes. In the DPP, metformin at 850 mg twice daily decreased the risk of progressing from IGT to diabetes by 31%. Com-pared with lifestyle intervention, metformin appeared to be more effective in younger individuals and in individuals with a higher baseline BMI. To illustrate, there was only a mean 3% reduction in incidence of diabetes with metformin in individuals with BMI 22 to <30 kg/m² compared with a mean 53% reduction in individuals with BMI >35 kg/m². Likewise, there was only a mean 11% reduction in diabetes incidence in individuals aged ≥60 years with metformin, but a mean 44% reduction in individuals aged 25–44 years. Metformin was well tolerated, with the exception of an increase in gastrointestinal side effects (e.g., diarrhea, flatulence, nausea, and vomiting) compared with placebo. These side effects lim-ited the tolerability of the treatment, with only 84% able to tolerate the full dose of metformin at 850 mg twice daily (Knowler 2002). Extrapolations from the DPP estimate that over a lifetime, compared with standard treatment, treatment with metformin would delay the onset of diabetes by 3.4 years (Herman 2005).

The Indian Diabetes Prevention Programme (IDPP-1) uniquely evaluated the effects of the combination of metformin with intensive lifestyle changes on diabe-tes prevention. Over 500 subjects with IGT (mean age 45.9 years, mean BMI 25.8 kg/m²) were randomized to control, lifestyle modification, metformin, or a combi-nation of metformin with lifestyle modification. The IDPP-1 cohort had a remark-ably high progression rate to diabetes of 55% over 3 years. Compared with the control group, lifestyle modification reduced the incidence of diabetes by 28.5%, and metformin reduced the incidence by 26.4%. The combination of lifestyle changes with metformin reduced the incidence by 28.2%, indicating no additive benefit than either intervention alone. However, the tolerated dose of metformin in the IDDP-1 was only 250 mg twice daily, compared with 850 mg twice daily in the DPP, which may have influenced outcomes (Ramachandran 2006).

Gastrointestinal Agents in the Prevention of Diabetes. The STOP-NIDDM (Study to Prevent Non–Insulin-Dependent Diabetes Mellitus) trial evaluated the effects of acarbose, an α-glucosidase inhibitor, compared with placebo in >1,400 individuals with IGT. Compared with placebo, acarbose at doses of 100 mg three times daily was associated with a 25% reduction in the progression from IGT to diabetes over 3 years. Flatulence and diarrhea were the most common side effects (Chiasson 2002). The XENDOS (XENical in the Prevention of Diabetes in Obese Subjects) study also showed a reduction in the incidence of type 2 diabetes over 4 years with the gastric lipase inhibitor orlistat. This study had a high attrition rate, and the baseline group was a heterogeneous population of subjects with normo-glycemia and IGT (Torgerson 2004).

Thiazolidinediones in the Prevention of Diabetes. The two available thiazoli-dinediones, rosiglitazone and pioglitazone, have also demonstrated effects on dia-betes prevention. In the DREAM (Diabetes Reduction Assessment with Ramipril and Rosiglitazone Medication) trial, rosiglitazone reduced the composite outcome of diabetes or death by 60% over 3 years. There was an increased risk of congestive heart failure in subjects treated with rosiglitazone (0.5%) compared with placebo (0.1%), but no effects on cardiovascular outcomes (DREAM 2006).

Results from ACT NOW (ACTos NOW for the Prevention of Diabetes) were recently reported at the ADA's 68th Scientific Sessions. Compared with placebo, pioglitazone reduced the conversion from IGT to type 2 diabetes by 81% over a mean 2.6 years. De Fronzo et al. (2008) reported a 1.5% rate of progression to diabetes per year in subjects treated with pioglitazone compared with 6.8% per year with placebo. This was despite a 3.9-kg weight gain in subjects treated with pioglitazone compared with 0.8 kg in subjects treated with placebo (DeFronzo 2008).

In summary, multiple prospective studies have demonstrated that intensive lifestyle changes and/or pharmacotherapy can effectively prevent the progression to diabetes. Depending on the therapy and the population, the risk of progressing to diabetes can be reduced by 25–81% (Table 19.1). Intensive lifestyle changes are accepted as safe and universally beneficial, but require significant time and commitment by the patient and the health care system. Pharmacotherapy also has a proven benefit, but the lack of long-term data necessitates a detailed discussion of risks, benefits, and goals of therapy.

Goal #2 in the Prevention of Diabetes: Sustainable Prevention of Diabetes

There are two ways for an intervention to have benefit beyond the active intervention period. In the case of lifestyle changes, it is possible for individuals to acquire the habits necessary to continue intensive lifestyle intervention beyond the active intervention period of a clinical trial setting. Alternatively, the intervention may deter the progression to diabetes by helping to preserve pancreatic β-cell function, which would represent a biological delay of the disease rather than early treatment of hyperglycemia.

Sustainability of Intensive Lifestyle Intervention. Long-term follow-up from both the Da Qing study and the Finnish Diabetes Prevention Study indicate that lifestyle intervention benefits the population well beyond the cessation of the intervention (Li 2008, Lindström 2006). After the initial 6-year intervention, subjects in the Da Qing study were followed for an additional 14 years. Of the subjects in the control group, 93% developed diabetes during this time frame, pointing to the high likelihood of progression without intervention. Even without ongoing intervention, subjects who were part of the initial lifestyle intervention groups sustained a significant 43% lower incidence of development of diabetes over the entire 20-year period (Li 2008).

In the Finnish Diabetes Prevention Study, follow-up 3 years after the intervention period demonstrated ongoing reduction in the risk of developing diabetes in the active intervention group. Compared with control subjects, the intervention group also sustained a 43% reduction in relative risk of developing diabetes during the total follow-up period. The greatest risk reduction was seen in individuals who maintained the lifestyle goals of weight loss, reduced fat intake, increased fiber intake, and increased physical activity (Lindström 2006).

Another lifestyle study in Japan, the JOETSU study, highlights the sustainability of a brief intensive lifestyle intervention. Over 400 subjects with IGT were randomized to a 2-day short-term hospitalization combined with diabetes and education support every 3 months, diabetes and education support every 3 months without hospitalization, or to a control group. The 2-day hospitalization covered a nine-lesson curriculum, covering diet, exercise, and behavior modification, whereas the structure of the follow-up support sessions was similar in the two intervention groups. Over a mean 3.1 years, subjects in the short-term hospitalization with support had a 42% reduction in diabetes incidence compared with a 27% reduction in the diabetes and education support group. All else being equal, the brief 2-day intensive lifestyle modification curriculum conferred sustainable benefit for a mean 3.1 years (Kawahara 2008).

Sustainable Benefit from Pharmacotherapy. Whether pharmacotherapy delays diabetes or treats the progressive hyperglycemia early in these intervention studies is addressed by evaluating the incidence of diabetes following a washout period. In the DPP, OGTTs were repeated following a 1- to 2-week washout period of metformin. Metformin demonstrated a persistent reduction in diabetes by 25%, supportive of the delay of the onset of diabetes rather than the early treatment of diabetes (DPP 2003). A longer washout period would have offered more insight as to whether metformin therapy reset the clock of diabetes.

In contrast, acarbose did not sustain a reduction in diabetes incidence following a 3-month washout period in the STOP-NIDDM trial, suggesting that perhaps acarbose was treating hyperglycemia early in its progression to diabetes (Chiasson 2002). Consistent with the washout findings, a mechanistic study evaluating the effect of acarbose on insulin secretion and insulin sensitivity by hyperglycemic clamp, and its effect on OGTT demonstrated no effect of acarbose on insulin secretion and insulin sensitivity, but improvements in 2-h postprandial glucose. Thus, acarbose appears to maintain glycemic control by treating postprandial glucose levels, rather than improving β-cell function per se (Nijpels 2008).

Data from Buchanan et al. (2002) provide mechanistic insight on how thiazolidinediones may biologically reset the clock of diabetes by preserving pancreatic function. In the TRIPOD (Troglitazone in Prevention of Diabetes) and PIPOD (Pioglitazone in Prevention of Diabetes) studies, Buchanan et al. (2002) studied Hispanic women with a history of gestational diabetes (Xiang 2006). In the initial TRIPOD study, troglitazone reduced the annual incidence of diabetes by >50%, an effect that persisted after an extended washout period. Protection from diabetes was associated with improvements in whole-body insulin sensitivity and marked preservation of insulin output from β-cells observed in the intravenous glucose tolerance tests. In contrast to the placebo group, the troglitazone group maintained stable β-cell compensation, suggesting a biological delay of the processes leading to diabetes (Buchanan 2002). Once troglitazone was removed from the market, these women were then studied in the PIPOD study. Here, too, Buchanan et al. found that pioglitazone stabilized β-cell function. Those subjects who were treated with placebo in TRIPOD had a stabilization of β-cell function with pioglitazone, and subjects previously treated with troglitazone in TRIPOD maintained stable β-cell function with pioglitazone. These effects also persisted following an extended 8-month washout period, supporting the biological delay of disease (Xiang 2006).

Despite such findings with troglitazone and pioglitazone in the TRIPOD and PIPOD studies in women with a history of gestational diabetes, rosiglitazone did not sustain a reduction in diabetes incidence following a washout period in the DREAM trial (Holman 2006). Results from the washout period of ACT NOW are underway. Although there were improvements in insulin sensitivity and β-cell function, suggesting a preservation of β-cell function, clinical end points will provide the definitive answer (DeFronzo 2008).

In summary, 20-year data from the Da Qing study and 7-year data from the Finnish Diabetes Prevention Study support the sustainable benefit of intensive lifestyle modification to prevent diabetes. The current DPP Outcomes Study will help address whether these benefits are similarly sustainable in an ethnically diverse population. Data are more variable with pharmacotherapy, with the possibility of a persistent benefit with metformin therapy and conflicting data with the thiazolidinediones. Ongoing outcome studies will provide answers to better guide the practitioner on the necessary length of time of intervention to impart long-standing benefit.

Goal #3 in the Prevention of Diabetes: Prevention of Long-Term Morbidity and Mortality

This is perhaps the most important goal, but also the area for which we have the least data. The Da Qing Study represents the longest lifestyle intervention follow-up to date and did not show any significant mortality or cardiovascular benefit. However, the incidence of first-time CVD events and mortality were relatively low (2.3–2.5 and 1.4–1.7 per 100 person-years per year, respectively), and this study was not statistically powered to evaluate whether the prevention of diabetes translated to decreased mortality and decreased cardiovascular events (Li 2008).

In the DPP, lifestyle intervention conferred benefits beyond the prevention of diabetes. Lifestyle intervention improved hypertension and dyslipidemia and reduced cardiovascular risk factors such as C-reactive protein and fibrinogen, suggesting potential cardiovascular benefit (Ratner 2005, Haffner 2005). Furthermore, computer modeling from the DPP predicts that over a lifetime, intensive lifestyle intervention would increase life expectancy by 0.5 years and reduce the incidence of blindness by 39%, end-stage renal disease by 38%, amputation by 35%, stroke by 9%, and coronary heart disease by 8% (Herman 2005). The current DPP Outcomes Study should provide long-term data and clinical outcomes on mortality and cardiovascular impact.

The only pharmacotherapy intervention associated with reduction in CVD was acarbose in the STOP-NIDDM trial. Even though the reduction in diabetes incidence did not persist following the 3-month washout phase, acarbose treatment was associated with a 49% relative risk reduction in CVD (Chiasson 2003). Supporting this benefit was a reduction in hypertension and a reduction in progression of carotid intima-media thickness in the acarbose-treated participants (Chiasson 2003, Hanefeld 2004). Similarly, although rosiglitazone did not maintain its reduction in diabetes incidence following a washout period, rosiglitazone treatment also reduced the risk of renal disease (DREAM 2008). Thus, considering the long-term goals of reducing macrovascular and microvascular disease, perhaps the maintenance of normoglycemia early in the course of diabetes is just as important as preventing the progression to diabetes itself.

COST-EFFECTIVENESS OF DIABETES PREVENTION

Herman et al. (2005) examined the cost-effectiveness of interventions in the DPP and found lifestyle intervention to be relatively cost-effective. They estimated the cost per QALY gained from a societal perspective to be $8,800. Eddy et al. (2005) predicted higher cost-effectiveness ratios, predicting the cost per QALY of the lifestyle intervention compared to doing nothing to be ~$62,600 from a societal perspective. However, the estimates used by Eddy et al. were based on assumptions of a slower, linear rate of progression to diabetes and assumed a limited glycemic exposure, resulting in fewer estimated complications (Herman 2006).

Metformin therapy is also thought to be cost-effective. In the DPP, the estimated cost per QALY gained for metformin intervention was ~$31,300, but this would be substantially lower (at $1,755) if the cost of generic metformin was used instead of the branded product (Herman 2005). Two models outside of the DPP have evaluated estimated costs for metformin therapy in diabetes prevention and have found it to be relatively cost-saving (Norris 2008).

PUBLISHED GUIDELINES FOR THE DIAGNOSIS, TREATMENT, AND MONITORING OF PRE-DIABETES

The increasing prevalence of diabetes, the associated costs and complications, and the overwhelming evidence in favor of prevention of diabetes has resulted in the formulation of official guidelines to aid the practitioner in the management of pre-diabetes (Table 18.2). The Indian Health Services (IHS) (2006) published guidelines on the care of adults with pre-diabetes and/or the metabolic syndrome in clinical settings in 2006. The ADA, Australian Diabetes Society/Australian Diabetes Educators Association, and IDF published consensus/position statements in 2007 (Nathan 2007, Twigg 2007, Alberti 2007), and in 2008 the American Association of Clinical Endocrinologists (AACE) followed suit (AACE 2008). All of these published statements are similar in recognizing the need to prevent diabetes, but they have subtle differences in the approach. The authors have similarly published a practical, case-based approach to weigh the available options for screening, diagnosis, treatment, and monitoring of pre-diabetes (Aroda 2008).

Screening/Diagnosis of Pre-Diabetes

Traditional risk factors that prompt screening for pre-diabetes/diabetes include overweight/obesity, age, family history of type 2 diabetes, hypertension, low HDL cholesterol, elevated triglycerides, metabolic syndrome, history of gestational diabetes or polycystic ovary syndrome, history of vascular disease, physical inactivity, or belonging to a high-risk ethnic group (Nathan 2007, ADA 2009b). More recently, the U.S. Preventive Services Task Force (2008) specifically recommended screening for type 2 diabetes in asymptomatic adults with sustained blood pressure, treated or untreated, >135/80 mmHg and did not find sufficient evidence to screen asymptomatic adults with a blood pressure ≤135/80 mmHg.

There is not a clear consensus on the optimal screening interval. The ADA recommends testing for pre-diabetes and diabetes at age 45 years, earlier if one is overweight and has at least one risk factor for diabetes. If initial testing is normal,

Table 19.2 Key Features of Select Published Recommendations on Diabetes Prevention

	Who Should Be Screened?	Screening Method	Recommended Treatment(s) for Prevention	Follow-Up
IHS Guidelines for Care of Adults with Pre-diabetes and/or the Metabolic Syndrome in Clinical Settings (IHS 2006)	Annual testing of individuals at risk for developing diabetes	1) FPG 2) Optional 2-h OGTT if resources permit	• Lifestyle changes for everyone • Consideration of metformin on an individualized basis	Monitor glucose values every 6 months.
ADA Consensus Statement (Nathan 2007)	Individuals with risk factors for diabetes	1) FPG 2) 2-h OGTT, particularly if metformin therapy is considered	• Lifestyle modification for IFG or IGT • Lifestyle modification and/or metformin: IFG and IGT and at least one of the following: age <60 years, BMI ≥35 kg/m^2, family history of diabetes in first-degree relative, elevated triglycerides, reduced HDL cholesterol, hypertension, A1C >6.0%	Lifestyle intervention: annual follow-up Metformin treatment: semiannual A1C
IDF Consensus (Alberti 2007)	Opportunistic screening by health care personnel; use brief questionnaires to identify people at higher risk of type 2 diabetes	1) FPG 2) OGTT if FPG is ≥110–125 mg/dl (6.1–6.9 mmol/l)	• Lifestyle intervention for everyone • Consideration of pharmacotherapy if desired weight loss and/or improved glucose tolerance goals is not achieved	Not specified
Australian Diabetes Society and Australian Diabetes Educators Association Position Statement (Twigg 2007)	No specified screening for diabetes prevention; incidental detection of pre-diabetes while screening for diabetes	Not specified	Intensive lifestyle intervention for a minimum of 6 months before consideration of pharmacotherapy	OGTT, initially performed annually, then individualized retesting every 1–3 years
American College of Endocrinology Task Force on Pre-Diabetes (American College of Endocrinology 2008)	Individuals at increased risk for developing type 2 diabetes	Discusses methods of diagnosis (FPG, OGTT)	• Intensive lifestyle modification • Consider additional pharmacotherapy in individuals at high risk	• Annual OGTT and urine microalbumin • FPG, A1C, lipids: at least semiannually

repeat testing is recommended every 3 years, but it may be done earlier depending on initial results and risk status (ADA 2009b). With the high prevalence of diabetes in the Native American population, the IHS recommends screening all American Indian or Native Alaskan adults aged ≥18 years with at least one other risk factor for diabetes on an annual basis. If no risk factors are present, the IHS recommends screening every 3 years beginning at age 35 years (IHS 2006).

Potential screening tests include FPG, 2-h postprandial glucose, or A1C. Most agree that FPG should be performed in screening for pre-diabetes. Recommendations for an OGTT in the initial management of a patient with pre-diabetes are variable and take into consideration costs, available resources, and impact on management. The IHS recommends OGTT if resources permit (IHS 2006). The ADA advocates performance of an OGTT to identify individuals with IGT, particularly if metformin therapy is under consideration for the prevention of diabetes (Nathan 2007). Similarly, the IDF recommends screening with a FPG followed by an OGTT if FPG is elevated (≥110–125 mg/dl [6.1–6.9 mmol/l]) (Alberti 2007).

If FPG is elevated, it is important to consider an OGTT for several reasons. First, fasting glucose alone can miss the detection of ~30% of cases of type 2 diabetes (WHO/IDF 2006, ADA 2009b). In some reports, this is even higher. In the DPP, in which FPG was performed semiannually and OGTT was performed annually, 87% of new cases of diabetes were detected based on elevated 2-h glucose, as opposed to only 34%, detected based on initial elevation of FPG (DPP 2006). In the Rancho Bernardo cohort, 70% of women and 48% of men aged 50–89 years had new diabetes diagnosed on the basis of an elevated 2-h postprandial glucose alone (Barrett-Connor 1998). In addition, as discussed earlier, risk of progression to diabetes is approximately twofold higher if an individual is diagnosed with both IFG and IGT compared with a diagnosis of isolated IFG or IGT alone (Gerstein 2007). Furthermore, cardiovascular risk is greater in individuals diagnosed with IGT or diabetes based on their 2-h postprandial glucose (DECODE 2003, Tominaga 1999).

There is also growing interest in the inclusion of A1C in the evaluation and screening of diabetes. A1C reflects chronic glycemic changes over time. Furthermore, at lower levels (e.g., A1C <7.3%), A1C largely reflects the postprandial contribution to hyperglycemia, which is an early feature in the progression to diabetes (Monnier 2003). In addition, A1C is a good risk predictor for both macrovascular and microvascular complications (Stratton 2000, Khaw 2001, Myint 2007, Selvin 2005, Klein 1984, Magliano 2008). However, it is important to note that A1C is not sensitive enough to be used alone in the screening of pre-diabetes/diabetes. Further, A1C is not standardized across various populations, as found in the DPP, in which A1C levels were consistently higher across ethnic minorities compared with Caucasians after adjustment for factors affecting glycemia (Herman 2007).

In light of the data supporting A1C in risk assessment for diabetes and long-term complications, a recent panel recommendation by Saudek et al. (2008) advocates the adjunctive use of A1C in the screening for diabetes. An A1C ≥6.5–6.9% should prompt further evaluation with FPG or OGTT to evaluate for diabetes, and an A1C ≥7% should increase suspicion of the possibility of diabetes, requiring confirmation with an FPG, OGTT, or repeat A1C ≥7% (Saudek 2008).

In summary, screening for pre-diabetes/diabetes should occur in individuals at risk of developing diabetes. FPG is considered the initial test of choice in screening for pre-diabetes and diabetes, but consideration should be given to an adjunctive OGTT and A1C to provide complete information on hyperglycemia.

Treatment Recommendations for the Prevention of Diabetes

The published guidelines all accept intensive lifestyle interventions as a cornerstone of therapy to prevent diabetes. However, there are differences in the consideration of pharmacotherapy for the prevention of diabetes. The Australian position statement recommends initial intensive lifestyle therapy for a minimum of 6 months prior to the consideration of pharmacotherapy (Twigg 2007). The IHS guidelines consider metformin on an individual basis (IHS 2006). The ADA consensus statement considers the use of metformin in individuals with IFG and IGT with an additional risk factor for progressing to diabetes (e.g., family history of diabetes in a first-degree relative, elevated triglycerides, reduced HDL cholesterol, hypertension, or A1C ≥6.0%) or in individuals similar to those in the DPP who had a greater benefit from metformin therapy compared with lifestyle (i.e., age <60 years and BMI ≥35 kg/m^2) (Nathan 2007). The AACE guidelines consider the use of pharmacotherapy in individuals at high risk of progressing to diabetes, such as individuals with combined IFG and IGT, worsening glycemia, polycystic ovary syndrome, history of gestational diabetes, CVD, or nonalcoholic fatty liver disease. In addition to glycemic goals, the AACE guidelines recommend strict nonglycemic targets for patients with pre-diabetes, advocating similar goals for lipids, blood pressure, and antiplatelet therapy as is followed for patients with diabetes (American College of Endocrinology 2008). The IDF considers the addition of pharmacotherapy in individuals who have not achieved desired weight loss and/or improved glucose tolerance goals (Alberti 2007).

It is worthwhile to evaluate practices in the DPP as well as published guidelines in diabetes to help address the issue of when to escalate therapy in the treatment of pre-diabetes/diabetes. In the DPP, therapy was advanced in individuals who had FPG ≥140 mg/dl (Knowler 2002). In individuals who had FPG ≥140 mg/dl on two occasions, therapy was advanced and included pharmacotherapy to achieve preprandial capillary glucose measurements of 80–120 mg/dl and to maintain A1C levels at <7% (DPP 2001). Likewise, the European Association for the Study of Diabetes (EASD)/ADA guidelines for the clinical management of diabetes support advancement of therapy if A1C is ≥7% in order to minimize long-term complications (Nathan 2006). Thus, one practical approach would be to advance therapy if FPG increases to ≥140 mg/dl (7.8 mmol/l), as was done in the DPP, or if A1C increases to ≥7.0% in order to minimize long-term complications (Knowler 2002, Aroda 2008, Nathan 2006).

Monitoring the Prevention of Diabetes

The Australian position statement acknowledges that the interval for retesting is arbitrary, with a suggestion to retest with an OGTT at 12 months with subsequent follow-up intervals based on individualized risks and results of testing (Twigg 2007). The AACE guidelines recommend an annual OGTT for all patients with pre-diabetes (American College of Endocrinology 2008). The IHS recommends monitoring of glucose values every 6 months, and the ADA consensus statement recommends annual follow-up for patients being treated with lifestyle intervention and semiannual A1C in patients with IFG and IGT treated with metformin (Nathan 2007, IHS 2006).

The OGTT offers valuable information in timing the exact conversion from pre-diabetes to diabetes, but one must consider whether the information obtained from the 2-h postprandial glucose will alter management. For example, if a patient's FPG remains stable at 118 mg/dl and A1C is stable at 6.5%, but the 2-h glucose has progressed from 180 to 210 mg/dl in 1 year, would management change? The glycemic management would probably not change. If, however, the A1C also increased to ≥7.0%, indicating deterioration of chronic glycemic control, progression of disease, and increased long-term risk of complications, one would definitely consider an escalation of current therapy. Furthermore, the OGTT is less reproducible and has greater intraindividual variation. An abnormal OGTT would therefore require a repeat confirmation within a reasonable time frame, as demonstrated in the DPP, where only 47% of suspected cases of diabetes identified by OGTT were confirmed with repeat OGTT (DPP 2006).

Thus, in consideration of the published guidelines, the costs of the OGTT, the need to repeat an abnormal OGTT, and the practical consideration of whether an OGTT would change clinical management, an approach to the management of pre-diabetes is as follows: *1)* if FPG is elevated, complete the glycemic evaluation with an OGTT to exclude diabetes and to evaluate for isolated IFG or combined IFG/IGT, in addition to A1C for baseline risk assessment, and *2)* monitor glycemic status with interval (e.g., semiannual) FPG and A1C tests to evaluate for glycemic deterioration. An OGTT may be considered on an individual basis if it will change glycemic or nonglycemic management in the course of disease.

In summary, diabetes represents a significant personal and societal burden and is increasing in epidemic proportions worldwide. The clinical diagnosis of diabetes is preceded by many years of an intermediary stage termed pre-diabetes. Both pre-diabetes and diabetes are on the same spectrum of disease and the glucose represented by these categories reflects a continuum of risk for macrovascular and microvascular sequelae. In many regards, treating pre-diabetes and treating diabetes are no different. The goals for both are the same, including the maintenance of glycemic control to prevent morbidity and mortality. There are now many effective methods, including intensive lifestyle intervention and various modes of pharmacotherapy, that can deter the progression from pre-diabetes to diabetes. Research and clinical efforts in diabetes prevention will continue to revolve around the sustainability of the intervention(s) and of the benefits themselves, as well as the practical implementation of the evidence into practice and society.

BIBLIOGRAPHY

Alberti KG, Zimmet P, Shaw J: International Diabetes Federation: a consensus on type 2 diabetes prevention. *Diabet Med* 24:451–463, 2007

American College of Endocrinology Task Force on Pre-Diabetes: American College of Endocrinology consensus statement on the diagnosis and management of pre-diabetes in the continuum of hyperglycemia: when do the risks of diabetes begin? Available from http://www.aace.com/meetings/consensus/hyperglycemia/hyperglycemia.pdf, 2008. Accessed 24 August 2008

American Diabetes Association: Economic costs of diabetes in the U.S. in 2007. Diabetes Care 31:596–615, 2008

American Diabetes Association: Diagnosis and classification of diabetes mellitus. Diabetes Care 32 (Suppl. 1):S62–S67, 2009a

American Diabetes Association: Standards of medical care in diabetes –2009. Diabetes Care 32 (Suppl. 1):S13-S61, 2009b

Amos AF, McCarty DJ, Zimmet P: The rising global burden of diabetes and its complications: estimates and projections to the year 2010. *Diabet Med* 14 (Suppl. 5):S1–S85, 1997

Aroda VR, Ratner R: Approach to the patient with prediabetes. *J Clin Endocrinol Metab* 93:3259–3265, 2008

Balkau B, Bertrais S, Ducimetiere P, Eschwege E: Is there a glycemic threshold for mortality risk? *Diabetes Care* 22:696–699, 1999

Barrett-Connor E, Ferrara A: Isolated postchallenge hyperglycemia and the risk of fatal cardiovascular disease in older women and men: the Rancho Bernardo Study. *Diabetes Care* 21:1236–1239, 1998

Buchanan TA, Xiang AH, Peters RK, Kjos SL, Marroquin A, Goico J, Ochoa C, Tan S, Berkowitz K, Hodis HN, Azen SP: Preservation of pancreatic β-cell function and prevention of type 2 diabetes by pharmacological treatment of insulin resistance in high-risk Hispanic women. *Diabetes* 51:2796–2803, 2002

Centers for Disease Control and Prevention: National diabetes fact sheet 2007. Available from: http://www.cdc.gov/diabetes/pubs/pdf/ndfs_2007.pdf, 2007. Accessed 25 August 2008

Chiasson JL, Josse RG, Gomis R, Hanefeld M, Karasik A, Laakso M, STOP-NIDDM Trail Research Group: Acarbose for prevention of type 2 diabetes mellitus: the STOP-NIDDM randomised trial. *Lancet* 359:2072–2077, 2002

Chiasson JL, Josse RG, Gomis R, Hanefeld M, Karasik A, Laakso M, STOP-NIDDM Trial Research Group: Acarbose treatment and the risk of cardiovascular disease and hypertension in patients with impaired glucose tolerance: the STOP-NIDDM trial. *JAMA* 290:486–494, 2003

DECODE Study Group, European Diabetes Epidemiology Group: Is the current definition for diabetes relevant to mortality risk from all causes and cardiovascular and noncardiovascular diseases? *Diabetes Care* 26:688–696, 2003

DeFronzo R, Banerji MA, Bray G, Buchanan T, Clement S, Henry R, Kitabchi A, Mudaliar S, Musi N, Ratner R, Reaven P, Schwenke D, Stenz F, Tripathy D: ACTos NOW for the Prevention of Diabetes (ACT NOW) Study. Paper presented at the American Diabetes Association 68th Scientific Sessions, June 2008, at Moscone Convention Center, San Francisco, California

Diabetes Prevention Program: Protocol for the Diabetes Prevention Program version 4.4—May 18, 2001. Available from http://www.bsc.gwu.edu/dpp/3armprot.htmlvdoc, 2001. Accessed 15 September 2008.

Diabetes Prevention Program Research Group: Effects of withdrawal from metformin on the development of diabetes in the diabetes prevention program. *Diabetes Care* 26:977–980, 2003

Diabetes Prevention Program: Repeat glucose testing to confirm glucose tolerance status: implications for diagnosing diabetes in high risk adults (Abstract). *Diabetes* 55 (Suppl. 1):894P, 2006

Diabetes Prevention Program Research Group: The prevalence of retinopathy in impaired glucose tolerance and recent-onset diabetes in the Diabetes Prevention Program. *Diabet Med* 24:137–144, 2007

DREAM (Diabetes REduction Assessment with ramipril and rosiglitazone Medication) Trial Investigators, Gerstein HC, Yusuf S, Bosch J, Pogue J, Sheridan P, Dinccag N, Hanefeld M, Hoogwerf B, Laakso M, Mohan V, Shaw J, Zinman B, Holman RR: Effect of rosiglitazone on the frequency of diabetes in patients with impaired glucose tolerance or impaired fasting glucose: a randomised controlled trial. *Lancet* 368:1096–1105, 2006

DREAM Trial Investigators, Dagenais GR, Gerstein HC, Holman R, Budaj A, Escalante A, Hedner T, Keltai M, Lonn E, McFarlane S, McQueen M, Teo K, Sheridan P, Bosch J, Pogue J, Yusuf S: Effects of ramipril and rosiglitazone on cardiovascular and renal outcomes in people with impaired glucose tolerance or impaired fasting glucose: results of the Diabetes REduction Assessment with ramipril and rosiglitazone Medication (DREAM) trial. *Diabetes Care* 31:1007–1014, 2008

Eddy DM, Schlessinger L, Kahn R: Clinical outcomes and cost-effectiveness of strategies for managing people at high risk for diabetes. *Ann Intern Med* 143:251–264, 2005

Festa A, Williams K, D'Agostino R Jr, Wagenknecht LE, Haffner SM: The natural course of β-cell function in nondiabetic and diabetic individuals: the Insulin Resistance Atherosclerosis Study. *Diabetes* 55:1114–1120, 2006

Fox CS, Larson MG, Leip EP, Meigs JB, Wilson PW, Levy D: Glycemic status and development of kidney disease: the Framingham Heart Study. *Diabetes Care* 28:2436–2440, 2005

Franco OH, Steyerberg EW, Hu FB, Mackenbach J, Nusselder W: Associations of diabetes mellitus with total life expectancy and life expectancy with and without cardiovascular disease. *Arch Intern Med* 167:1145–1151, 2007

Gerstein HC, Santaguida P, Raina P, Morrison KM, Balion C, Hunt D, Yazdi H, Booker L: Annual incidence and relative risk of diabetes in people with various categories of dysglycemia: a systematic overview and meta-analysis of prospective studies. *Diabetes Res Clin Pract* 78:305–312, 2007

Haffner S, Temprosa M, Crandall J, Fowler S, Goldberg R, Horton E, Marcovina S, Mather K, Orchard T, Ratner R, Barrett-Connor E, Diabetes Prevention Program Research Group: Intensive lifestyle intervention or metformin on inflammation and coagulation in participants with impaired glucose tolerance. *Diabetes* 54:1566–1572, 2005

Hanefeld M, Chiasson JL, Koehler C, Henkel E, Schaper F, Temelkova-Kurktschiev T: Acarbose slows progression of intima-media thickness of the carotid arteries in subjects with impaired glucose tolerance. *Stroke* 35:1073–1078, 2004

HAPO Study Cooperative Research Group, Metzger BE, Lowe LP, Dyer AR, Trimble ER, Chaovarindr U, Coustan DR, Hadden DR, McCance DR, Hod M, McIntyre HD, Oats JJ, Persson B, Rogers MS, Sacks DA: Hyperglycemia and adverse pregnancy outcomes. *N Engl J Med* 358:1991–2002, 2008

Herman WH, Hoerger TJ, Brandle M, Hicks K, Sorensen S, Zhang P, Hamman RF, Ackermann RT, Engelgau MM, Ratner RE, Diabetes Prevention Program Research Group: The cost-effectiveness of lifestyle modification or metformin in preventing type 2 diabetes in adults with impaired glucose tolerance. *Ann Intern Med* 142:323–332, 2005

Herman WH, Hoerger TJ, Hicks K, Brandle M, Sorensen SW, Zhang P, Engelgau MM, Hamman RF, Marrero DG, Ackermann RT, Ratner RE: Managing people at high risk for diabetes. *Ann Intern Med* 144:66–67, 2006

Herman WH, Ma Y, Uwaifo G, Haffner S, Kahn SE, Horton ES, Lachin JM, Montez MG, Brenneman T, Barrett-Connor E, Diabetes Prevention Program Research Group: Differences in A1C by race and ethnicity among patients with impaired glucose tolerance in the Diabetes Prevention Program. *Diabetes Care* 30:2453–2457, 2007

Holman RR: DREAM washout period results. Late-breaking trial presented at the 19th World Diabetes Congress, 3–7 December 2006, at Cape Town, South Africa

International Diabetes Federation: Diabetes atlas 2006. Available from http://www.eatlas.idf.org/media, 2006. Accessed 25 Aug 2008

Indian Health Services: 2006 IHS guidelines for care of adults with prediabetes and/or the metabolic syndrome in clinical settings. Available from http://www.ihs.gov/MedicalPrograms/Diabetes/resources/r_index.asp, 2006. Accessed 27 August 2008

Kawahara T, Takahashi K, Inazu T, Arao T, Kawahara C, Tabata T, Moriyama H, Okada Y, Morita E, Tanaka Y: Reduced progression to type 2 diabetes from impaired glucose tolerance after a 2-day in-hospital diabetes educational program (the JOETSU diabetes prevention trial). *Diabetes Care* 31:1949–1954, 2008

Khaw KT, Wareham N, Luben R, Bingham S, Oakes S, Welch A, Day N: Glycated haemoglobin, diabetes, and mortality in men in Norfolk cohort of

European prospective investigation of cancer and nutrition (EPIC-Norfolk). *BMJ* 322:15–18, 2001

Klein R, Klein BE, Moss SE, David MD, DeMets DL: The Wisconsin epidemiologic study of diabetic retinopathy: III: prevalence and risk of diabetic retinopathy when age at diagnosis is 30 or more years. *Arch Opthalmol* 102:527–532, 1984

Knowler WC, Barrett-Connor E, Fowler SE, Hamman RF, Lachin JM, Walker EA, Nathan DM, Diabetes Prevention Program Research Group: Reduction in the incidence of type 2 diabetes with lifestyle intervention or metformin. *N Engl J Med* 346:393–403, 2002

Knowler WC, Hamman RF, Edelstein SL, Barrett-Connor E, Ehrmann DA, Walker EA, Fowler SE, Nathan DM, Kahn SE, Diabetes Prevention Program Research Group: Prevention of type 2 diabetes with troglitazone in the Diabetes Prevention Program. *Diabetes* 54:1150–1156, 2005

Kosaka K, Noda M, Kuzuya T: Prevention of type 2 diabetes by lifestyle intervention: a Japanese trial in IGT males. *Diabetes Res Clin Pract* 67:152–162, 2005

Levitan EB, Song Y, Ford ES, Liu S: Is nondiabetic hyperglycemia a risk factor for cardiovascular disease? A meta-analysis of prospective studies. *Arch Intern Med* 164:2147–2155, 2004

Li G, Zhang P, Wang J, Gregg EW, Yang W, Gong Q, Li H, Li H, Jiang Y, An Y, Shuai Y, Zhang B, Zhang J, Thompson TJ, Gerzoff RB, Roglic G, Hu Y, Bennett PH: The long-term effect of lifestyle interventions to prevent diabetes in the China Da Qing Diabetes Prevention Study: a 20-year follow-up study. *Lancet* 371:1783–1789, 2008

Lindström J, Ilanne-Parikka P, Peltonen M, Aunola S, Eriksson JG, Hemiö K, Hämäläinen H, Härkönen P, Keinänen-Kiukaanniemi S, Laakso M, Louheranta A, Mannelin M, Paturi M, Sundvall J, Valle TT, Uusitupa M, Tuomilehto J, Finnish Diabetes Prevention Study Group: Sustained reduction in the incidence of type 2 diabetes by lifestyle intervention: follow-up of the Finnish Diabetes Prevention Study. *Lancet* 368:1673–1679, 2006

Magliano D, Barr ELM, Zimmet PZ, Cameron AJ, Dunstan DW, Colagiuri S, Jolley D, Owen N, Phillips P, Tapp RJ, Welborn TA, Shaw JE: Glucose indices, health behaviors, and incidence of diabetes in Australia: the Australian Diabetes, Obesity and Lifestyle Study. *Diabetes Care* 31:267–272, 2008

Monnier L, Lapinski H, Colette C: Contributions of fasting and postprandial plasma glucose increments to the overall diurnal hyperglycemia of type 2 diabetic patients: variations with increasing levels of HbA_{1c}. *Diabetes Care* 26:881–885, 2003

Myint PK, Sinha S, Wareham NJ, Bingham SA, Luben RN, Welch AA, Khaw KT: Glycated hemoglobin and risk of stroke in people without known diabetes in the European Prospective Investigation into Cancer (EPIC)-Norfolk prospective population study: a threshold relationship? *Stroke* 38:271–275, 2007

Narayan KM, Boyle JP, Thompson TJ, Sorensen SW, Williamson DF: Lifetime risk for diabetes mellitus in the United States. *JAMA* 290:1884–1890, 2003

Nathan DM, Buse JB, Davidson MB, Heine RJ, Holman RR, Sherwin R, Zinman B: Management of hyperglycemia in type 2 diabetes: a consensus algorithm for the initiation and adjustment of therapy: a consensus statement from the American Diabetes Association and the European Association for the Study of Diabetes. *Diabetes Care* 29:1963–1972, 2006

Nathan DM, Davidson MB, DeFronzo RA, Heine RJ, Henry RR, Pratley R, Zinman B, American Diabetes Association: Impaired fasting glucose and impaired glucose tolerance: implications for care. *Diabetes Care* 30:753–759, 2007

National Diabetes Surveillance System: Incidence of diabetes: crude and age-adjusted incidence of diagnosed diabetes per 1,000 population aged 18-79 years, United States, 1980–2006. Available from http://www.cdc.gov/diabetes/statistics/incidence/fig2.htm, 2008. Accessed 18 August 2008

Nijpels G, Boorsma W, Dekker JM, Kostense PJ, Bouter LM, Heine RJ: A study of the effects of acarbose on glucose metabolism in patients predisposed to developing diabetes: the Dutch Acarbose Intervention Study in Persons with Impaired Glucose Tolerance (DAISI). *Diabetes Metab Res Rev* 24:611–616, 2008

Norris SL, Kansagara D, Bougatsos C, Fu R, U.S. Preventive Services Task Force: Screening adults for type 2 diabetes: a review of the evidence for the U.S. Preventive Services Task Force. *Ann Intern Med* 148:855–868, 2008

Pan XR, Li GW, Hu YH, Wang JX, Yang WY, An ZX, Hu ZX, Lin J, Xiao JZ, Cao HB, Liu PA, Jiang XG, Jiang YY, Wang JP, Zheng H, Zhang H, Bennett PH, Howard BV: Effects of diet and exercise in preventing NIDDM in people with impaired glucose tolerance: the Da Qing IGT and Diabetes Study. *Diabetes Care* 20:537–544, 1997

Ramachandran A, Snehalatha C, Mary S, Mukesh B, Bhaskar AD, Vijay V, Indian Diabetes Prevention Programme (IDPP): The Indian Diabetes Prevention Programme shows that lifestyle modification and metformin prevent type 2 diabetes in Asian Indian subjects with impaired glucose tolerance (IDPP-1). *Diabetologia* 49:289–297, 2006

Ratner R, Goldberg R, Haffner S, Marcovina S, Orchard T, Fowler S, Temprosa M, Diabetes Prevention Program Research Group: Impact of intensive lifestyle and metformin therapy on cardiovascular disease risk factors in the diabetes prevention program. *Diabetes Care* 28:888–894, 2005

Saudek CD, Herman WH, Sacks DB, Bergenstal RM, Edelman D, Davidson MB: A new look at screening and diagnosing diabetes mellitus. *J Clin Endocrinol Metab* 93:2447–2453, 2008

Selvin E, Coresh J, Shahar E, Zhang L, Steffes M, Sharrett AR: Glycaemia (haemoglobin A1c) and incident ischaemic stroke: the Atherosclerosis Risk in Communities (ARIC) Study. *Lancet Neurol* 4:821–826, 2005

Smith AG, Singleton JR: Impaired glucose tolerance and neuropathy. *Neurologist* 14:23–29, 2008

Sorkin JD, Muller DC, Fleg JL, Andres R: The relation of fasting and 2-h postch-allenge plasma glucose concentrations to mortality: data from the Baltimore Longitudinal Study of Aging with a critical review of the literature. *Diabetes Care* 28:2626–2632, 2005

Stratton IM, Adler AI, Neil HAW, Matthews DR, Manley SE, Cull CA, Hadden D, Turner RC, Holman RR, UK Prospective Diabetes Study Group: Associa-tion of glycaemia with macrovascular and microvascular complications of type 2 diabetes (UKPDS 35): prospective observational study. *BMJ* 321:405–412, 2000

Tominaga M, Eguchi H, Manaka H, Igarashi K, Kato T, Sekikawa A: Impaired glucose tolerance is a risk factor for cardiovascular disease, but not impaired fasting glucose: the Funagata Diabetes Study. *Diabetes Care* 226:920–924, 1999

Torgerson JS, Hauptman J, Boldrin MN, Sjöström L: XENical in the Prevention of Diabetes in Obese Subjects (XENDOS) study: a randomized study of orlistat as an adjunct to lifestyle changes for the prevention of type 2 diabetes in obese patients. *Diabetes Care* 27:155–161, 2004

Tuomilehto J, Lindström J, Eriksson JG, Valle TT, Hämäläinen H, Ilanne-Parikka P, Keinänen-Kiukaanniemi S, Laakso M, Louheranta A, Rastas M, Salminen V, Uusitupa M, Finnish Diabetes Prevention Study Group: Prevention of type 2 diabetes mellitus by changes in lifestyle among subjects with impaired glucose tolerance. *N Engl J Med* 344:1343–1350, 2001

Twigg SM, Kamp MC, Davis TM, Neylon EK, Flack JR, Australian Diabetes Society, Australian Diabetes Educators Association: Prediabetes: a position statement from the Australian Diabetes Society and Australian Diabetes Edu-cators Association. *Med J Aust* 186:461–465, 2007

U.K. Prospective Diabetes Study Group: U.K. Prospective Diabetes Study 16: overview of 6 years' therapy of type II diabetes: a progressive disease. *Diabetes* 44:1249–1258, 1995

U.S. Preventive Services Task Force: Screening for type 2 diabetes mellitus in adults: U.S. Preventive Services Task Force recommendation statement. *Ann Intern Med* 148:846–854, 2008

Weyer C, Bogardus C, Mott DM, Pratley RE: The natural history of insulin secretory dysfunction and insulin resistance in the pathogenesis of type 2 dia-betes mellitus. *J Clin Invest* 104:787–794, 1999

Wild S, Roglic G, Green A, Sicree R, King H: Global prevalence of diabetes: estimates for the year 2000 and projections for 2030. *Diabetes Care* 27:1047–1053, 2004

World Health Organization/International Diabetes Federation: Definition and diagnosis of diabetes mellitus and intermediate hyperglycemia: report of a

WHO/IDF consultation. Available from http://www.who.int/diabetes/publications/Definition%20and%20diagnosis%20of%20diabetes_new.pdf, 2006. Accessed 25 August 2008

Xiang AH, Peters RK, Kjos SL, Marroquin A, Goico J, Ochoa C, Kawakubo M, Buchanan TA: Effect of pioglitazone on pancreatic β-cell function and diabetes risk in Hispanic women with prior gestational diabetes. *Diabetes* 55:517–522, 2006

Dr. Aroda is a member of the MedStar Research Institute, Washington, DC. Dr. Ratner is Professor of Medicine, Georgetown University School of Medicine, Washington, DC, and a member of the MedStar Research Institute, Washington, DC.

20. Insulin Secretagogues: Sulfonylureas, Repaglinide, and Nateglinide

HAROLD E. LEBOVITZ, MD

Sulfonylurea drugs have been used in the management of hyperglycemia in patients with type 2 diabetes for >50 years. The mechanism of their anti-diabetic action is complex. They act on the β-cell to increase both basal and meal-stimulated insulin secretion. Minor effects have been attributed in some studies to various extrapancreatic actions. Chronic improvement in glycemic control by sulfonylurea treatment decreases the metabolic effects of glucose toxicity in inhibiting insulin secretion and insulin action. As a consequence of their multiple actions, sulfonylureas cause improvement in several metabolic pathways in patients with type 2 diabetes. They decrease the exaggerated overproduction of glucose by the liver, partially reverse the postreceptor defect in insulin action at the level of muscle and adipose tissue, and increase the magnitude of meal-mediated insulin secretion.

The biochemical mechanism of sulfonylurea action has been defined recently. Insulin secretion is regulated by an ATP-dependent K^+ channel located in the plasma membrane of the β-cell. Under fasting conditions, most of the channels are open, and K^+ is actively extruded from the β-cell. When the plasma glucose rises, glucose is transported into the β-cell through a specific transport molecule (GLUT2 transporter), phosphorylated by glucokinase, and metabolized in the mitochondria, where ATP is generated from ADP. High intracellular ATP and low ADP concentrations cause the ATP-dependent K^+ channel to close. K^+ accumulates within the cell membrane, thereby causing it to depolarize. A voltage-dependent Ca^{2+} channel (also located in the plasma membrane) opens, and Ca^{2+} moves from the extracellular space into the β-cell cytosol. The rising cytosolic Ca^{2+} concentration causes the insulin granule to migrate to the cell surface, where its contents are released by exocytosis.

The ATP-dependent K^+ channel consists of two subunits: one (named SUR [sulfonylurea receptor]) contains a sulfonylurea binding site (receptor) and regulates whether the channel is open or closed. The other subunit (named Kir [inwardly rectifying K^+]) comprises the channel itself. The ATP-dependent K^+ channel is functional only when its two subunits are united. The sulfonylurea receptor faces the extracellular space. When sulfonylureas bind to the ATP-dependent K^+ channel, it closes. This then causes insulin secretion. The potency of a sulfonylurea is a function of its binding affinity to the receptor. Sulfonylureas therefore potentiate glucose-mediated insulin secretion as well as stimulate basal insulin secretion.

Other tissues, such as myocardium, vascular smooth muscle, and brain, have ATP-dependent K^+ channels that contain sulfonylurea binding sites. In vascular smooth muscle and myocardial cells, the ATP-dependent K^+ channels are normally closed and opened in response to ischemia to allow potassium to be released and calcium to enter. This causes vasodilatation to occur and improves myocardial function. In experimental studies, sulfonylureas can prevent the ATP-dependent K^+ channel from opening and interfere with vasodilatation and myocardial adaptation to ischemia. A second effect of preventing the channel from opening is a decrease in K^+ flux in the myocardium, which can protect against ventricular arrhythmias. If such effects were to occur in humans with ordinary pharmacological dosing of sulfonylureas, either a detrimental or beneficial effect on the cardiovascular system may occur during ischemia. The SUR subunits of the vascular smooth muscle and myocardial cells are different isoforms than those in the β-cell. In general, they have lower binding affinities for sulfonylureas than the β-cell isoform. The only sulfonylurea shown to significantly bind to those isoforms in cardiovascular ATP-dependent K^+ channels is glyburide. Glyburide has been shown in both normal and diabetic individuals to block cardiovascular ATP-dependent channels from opening during ischemic episodes, which prevents ischemic preconditioning of the myocardium. The role of ischemic preconditioning is to render the heart less susceptible to ischemic damage. These data are worrisome because clinical data on the long-term effects of sulfonylureas on cardiovascular outcomes, including death, continue to be controversial. There are several large long-term follow-up studies of diabetic patients taking glyburide, such as the U.K. Prospective Diabetes Study (UKPDS), that have not shown an increase in adverse cardiovascular outcomes. In contrast, several recent observational studies have implicated sulfonylureas alone or in combination with metformin to increase cardiovascular clinical events and/or death. The effect of sulfonylureas, if any, on brain cells is unknown, although there is increasing evidence that the hypothalamic ATP-dependent potassium channel, which is the same isoform as the pancreatic β-cell channel, has a regulatory effect on hepatic glucose production and the adaptation to hypoglycemia.

Repaglinide, a member of the meglitinide family, is approved for clinical use and is not a sulfonylurea. It binds to a site on the SUR1 subunit of the β-cell ATP-dependent K^+ channel that is different from the binding site for sulfonylureas. Repaglinide binding leads to closure of the ATP-dependent K^+ channel with subsequent insulin release. Sulfonylureas and repaglinide seem to have similar but not identical modes of action in causing insulin release (Tables 20.1 and 20.2). Their effects are not additive.

Nateglinide is a derivative of phenylalanine and is a very rapid-acting insulin secretagogue. It binds to the sulfonylurea receptor on SUR1 but with different binding characteristics than sulfonylureas. Its rates of association and dissociation are much more rapid. It has very low binding affinity for cardiovascular ATP-dependent K^+ channels.

Several features are essential in understanding the proper use of drugs that stimulate insulin secretion. These drugs are ineffective in lowering blood glucose in patients who have a marked reduction or total loss of functioning β-cells. In contrast, hypoglycemia can be a serious consequence of their inappropriate use. For unknown reasons, not all type 2 diabetic patients respond to the antidiabetic

Table 20.1 Characteristics of Specific Insulin Secretagogues

Drug	Dose Range (mg/dl)	Peak Level (h)	Half-Life (h)	Metabolites	Excretion
Sulfonylureas					
Tolbutamide	500–3,000	3–4	4.5–6.5	Inactive	Kidney
Chlorpropamide	100–500	2–4	36	Active or unchanged	Kidney
Tolazamide	100–1,000	3–4	7	Inactive	Kidney
Glipizide	2.5–40	1–3	2–4	Inactive	Kidney 80%, feces 20%
Glipizide GITS	5–20	Constant after several days of dosing		Inactive	Kidney 80%, feces 20%
Glyburide	1.25–20	~4	10	Inactive and weakly active	Kidney 50%, feces 50%
Glyburide, micronized formulation	1.5–12	2–3	~4	Inactive and weakly active	Kidney 50%, feces 50%
Glimeperide	1–8	2–3	9	Inactive and weakly active	Kidney 60%, feces 40%
Nonsulfonylurea Insulin Secretagogues					
Repaglinide	0.5–4 with each meal	1	1	Inactive	Feces
Nateglinide	60–120 with each meal	1.8	1.4	Weakly active	Kidney 80%, feces 10%

action of sulfonylureas (primary failure), and most patients who respond very well initially may have a loss of effective antidiabetic response after several years of treatment (secondary failure). In the UKPDS, treatment with sulfonylureas (glyburide or chlorpropamide) achieved an A1C <7% in 50% of patients at 3 years, 34% at 6 years, and only 24% at 9 years.

The 6- and 9-year data from the UKPDS show that this secondary failure is a characteristic of all antidiabetic treatments and not just sulfonylureas. Little is known about repaglinide's or nateglinide's antidiabetic effects beyond 1 or 2 years of treatment. Drugs that stimulate insulin secretion do not replace dietary management of type 2 diabetes; they complement it (i.e., they are unlikely to be effective if dietary management is ignored).

Table 20.2 Comparison Between Sulfonylureas and Nonsulfonylurea Insulin Secretagogues

Sulfonylureas	Nonsulfonylurea Insulin Secretagogues
Intermediate or long duration of action	Short duration of action
Administered once or twice daily	Must be given with each meal
Major effect is a decrease in FPG	Repaglinide has the same effect in decreasing FPG as sulfonylureas. Nateglinide causes an ~20 mg/dl decrease in FPG.
Little effect of early meal-mediated insulin secretion	Increases early meal-mediated insulin secretion
Little or no effect on postprandial glucose excursion	Significant reduction in meal-mediated glucose excursion
Clinically significant hypoglycemia occurs fasting and late postprandially	Hypoglycemia (particularly nocturnal) is uncommon.
Weight gain of 2–4 kg usually occurs with treatment	Weight gain is less of a problem.
Mean decrease in A1C is ~1.5%	Mean decrease in A1C with repaglinide is equivalent to that of sulfonylureas. Mean decrease in A1C with nateglinide is ~0.8%
Inexpensive	Relatively expensive

CHOOSING AN INSULIN SECRETAGOGUE

The clinical use of a particular insulin secretagogue is determined by the characteristics described in Table 20.3. Intrinsic antidiabetic activity varies considerably and is a function of the binding affinity to the sulfonylurea receptor or the other binding sites on the ATP-dependent K^+ channel. Repaglinide, glimepiride, and glyburide are the most potent, and tolbutamide is the least potent. The intrinsic potency of each drug is important in determining the effective dose of the drug that is necessary. Clinical response in controlling hyperglycemia, however, is not

Table 20.3 Characteristics by Which to Select a Specific Insulin Secretagogue

■ Intrinsic insulin secretory potency
■ Rapidity of onset of action
■ Duration of action

■ Mode of metabolism and excretion
■ Beneficial and detrimental side effects

significantly different among the various insulin secretagogues at their effective doses except for tolbutamide and nateglinide, which are less effective than the other drugs in controlling hyperglycemia in type 2 diabetic patients.

Type 2 diabetes is characterized by both a delay and a decrease in meal-stimulated insulin secretion. The delay in insulin secretion contributes to the excessive early postprandial rise in blood glucose levels. The more rapid the onset of action of an insulin secretagogue, the shorter the delay in the rise in postprandial insulin secretion. Repaglinide and nateglinide have a rapid onset of action and, when administered at the onset of the meal, effectively restore early postprandial insulin secretion almost to normal. The interval between administration of the drug and the meal should be considered. With some sulfonylureas (glyburide and glipizide), better results are obtained if the drug is given 30 min before the meal. The ideal goal in administering an insulin secretagogue is to synchronize the peak insulin secretion with the peak postprandial glucose rise.

The duration of action of an insulin secretagogue is of considerable importance. A long-acting secretagogue is more likely to be associated with severe, prolonged, and sometimes fatal hypoglycemia in susceptible patients, i.e., those who are elderly (~70 years of age), have poor nutrition, are likely to miss meals, or have concomitant hepatic, renal, or cardiovascular disease. Shorter-acting insulin secretagogues are significantly safer in this population. The rapid-acting non-sulfonylurea secretagogues cause low rates of hypoglycemia because of their shorter duration of action.

The mode of metabolism and excretion are also important in determining the frequency and severity of hypoglycemic reactions. Insulin secretagogues that are metabolized to active metabolites are associated with more hypoglycemic reactions. Likewise, drugs or active metabolites primarily excreted by the kidney are more likely to cause hypoglycemia in patients with renal dysfunction than drugs excreted via the biliary tract.

Side effects occur that are independent of antidiabetic action. Some appear to be unique to chlorpropamide (e.g., water retention and hyponatremia). This may be the reason for the higher rate of development of hypertension and poorer risk reduction of diabetic retinopathy observed in the chlorpropamide-treated compared with the glyburide-treated patients in the UKPDS. Other side effects (e.g., alcohol-induced flushing) may occur with first-generation (low intrinsic potency) sulfonylureas such as chlorpropamide and tolbutamide but not with second-generation (high intrinsic potency) agents.

Characteristics of Specific Sulfonylurea Drugs

Table 20.1 lists the characteristics of the commonly used sulfonylurea drugs. The dose range is a function of the intrinsic potency, but the clinical effectiveness at the appropriate dose is the same for all sulfonylureas except tolbutamide. Onset and duration of action are determined by the unique pharmacokinetic properties of each agent and its specific formulation. Most sulfonylureas are metabolized in the liver to active or inactive metabolites, except chlorpropamide, which is excreted unchanged in significant quantities in the urine. Biliary excretion is significant with glyburide and glimepiride and to a lesser extent with glipizide. Major side effects other than hypoglycemia are most commonly seen with chlorpropamide.

Characteristics of Repaglinide

Repaglinide is a nonsulfonylurea insulin secretagogue. Table 20.1 lists its characteristics, and Table 20.2 compares them with those of the sulfonylureas. Repaglinide is available in 0.5-, 1.0-, and 2.0-mg doses. Its oral absorption is rapid, with peak plasma levels occurring at 1 h. Its half-life in plasma is 1 h. Its metabolites are inactive, and it is excreted mainly by the liver. The duration of action of repaglinide is ~4 h. Because of its short duration of action, it must be taken 15 min before each meal, and the incidence of hypoglycemia is low. The usual dose is 0.5–2.0 mg at the start of each meal. Repaglinide reduces both fasting plasma glucose (FPG) and postprandial glucose excursions.

Characteristics of Nateglinide

Nateglinide is a phenylalanine-derivative nonsulfonylurea insulin secretagogue. Tables 20.1 and 20.2 list its characteristics and compare them with the characteristics of sulfonylureas. Nateglinide is available as a 60- and 120-mg tablet. Its oral absorption is rapid (peak plasma level at 1.5–2.0 h). Its plasma half-life is 1.4 h. It has very rapid kinetics of both binding to and displacement from the β-cell ATP-dependent K^+ channel. It causes the most rapid release and shortest duration of release of insulin of any of the insulin secretagogues. Consequently, its effect is almost exclusively that of decreasing postprandial glucose excursions. The side effects of weight gain and hypoglycemia are less than those found with other insulin secretagogues. Nateglinide is administered as 120 mg before each meal. The dose may be reduced to 60 mg before each meal in individuals with minimal elevations in FPG.

HYPOGLYCEMIA

The most serious complication of insulin secretagogue therapy is hypoglycemia. This is best avoided or minimized by the following procedures:

1. Start insulin secretagogue therapy with the lowest possible dose, and increase the dose incrementally every 4–7 days.
2. Patients susceptible to severe and prolonged hypoglycemia should be treated with shorter-acting insulin secretagogues.
3. Sulfonylureas should be used cautiously in patients with renal dysfunction. Sulfonylureas with short duration of action, inactive metabolites, and biliary excretion are preferred. The nonsulfonylurea insulin secretagogues are particularly useful in patients with renal dysfunction.
4. Encourage patients not to skip meals after taking insulin secretagogues. Patients who frequently miss or delay meals are ideal for treatment with repaglinide or nateglinide. Those medications are only taken at the start of the meal.
5. Be careful of drug interactions.

The treatment of mild hypoglycemia in insulin secretagogue–treated patients is managed by giving food, monitoring carefully, and reducing the dosage or changing the specific agent. The treatment of severe sulfonylurea-induced hypoglycemia requires vigorous and prolonged treatment. Patients who present with gluconeuropenic symptoms and plasma glucose levels <50 mg/dl (<2.8 mmol/l) should be given 50 ml of 50% glucose intravenously followed by continuous glucose (5 or 10%) and frequent monitoring of blood glucose. Occasionally, administration of 1 mg glucagon intramuscularly or slowly intravenously may be necessary. Patients with severe intractable hypoglycemia, despite glucose administration, have been successfully treated by the addition of 50 mg octreotide administered subcutaneously every 8 h for two or three doses.

Patients with insulin secretagogue–mediated severe hypoglycemia must be monitored and treated for at least 24 h. With long-acting sulfonylureas, patients should be monitored for 72 h because recurrence of hypoglycemia is common. These patients cannot be given 50% glucose intravenously and sent home. The reason for the severe hypoglycemia must be sought and appropriate therapeutic changes made.

Repaglinide, because of its short duration of action, is associated with less frequent and less severe hypoglycemia. Nateglinide treatment is only rarely associated with significant hypoglycemia.

INDICATIONS FOR THERAPY WITH INSULIN SECRETAGOGUES

Ideal candidates for treatment with insulin secretagogues are type 2 diabetic patients who are significantly insulin deficient but still have enough β-cell function to respond to stimulation by the secretagogue. Patients likely to show good glycemic response to agents that stimulate insulin secretion

- had onset of hyperglycemia after age 30 years
- have had diagnosed hyperglycemia for <5 years
- are normal weight or obese
- are willing to follow a reasonable dietary program
- are not totally insulin deficient

There are specific indications for the use of sulfonylureas in patients who have diabetes due to insulin deficiency caused by abnormalities of ATP generation or the inability of ATP to close the β-cell ATP-dependent potassium channel. Such examples are neonatal diabetes and maturity-onset diabetes of the young (MODY) due to abnormalities of the hepatic nuclear factor-1α gene . The inability of the normal regulatory pathways to close the ATP-dependent potas-

Table 20.4 Contraindications for Insulin Secretagogue Therapy

▪ Type 1 diabetes or pancreatic diabetes ▪ Pregnancy ▪ Major surgery ▪ Severe infections, stress, or trauma ▪ History of severe adverse reaction to a sulfonylurea or similar compound (sulfa drug) (does not exclude repaglinide)	▪ Predisposition to severe hypoglycemia, e.g., patients with significant liver or kidney disease

sium channel can be bypassed by using sulfonylureas to directly close the channel by binding to the SUR receptor and restoring adequate insulin secretion.

There are also preliminary data indicating polymorphism of the *TFC7L2* gene may influence the therapeutic response to sulfonylurea in the ordinary type 2 diabetic population (individuals with a GG polymorphism have a superior response to sulfonylureas than those with a TT polymorphism).

Contraindications for insulin secretagogue therapy are given in Table 20.4.

PROPER USE OF INSULIN SECRETAGOGUES

Insulin secretagogues should be administered to type 2 diabetic patients who have been unable to adequately control their plasma glucose on a reasonable trial (4–6 weeks) of appropriate dietary therapy. When insulin secretagogue therapy is added, dietary management must continue. Patients who present with marked symptoms and random plasma glucose levels of ~300 mg/dl (16.7 mmol/l) should probably be started on dietary management and insulin secretagogue therapy together. Insulin secretagogue therapy alone is unlikely to have significant beneficial effects in an individual who has an FPG >275 mg/dl (>15.3 mmol/l) while on a reasonable dietary program.

Initiation of a newly diagnosed type 2 diabetic patient with random hyperglycemia >300 mg/dl (>16.7 mmol/l) on insulin secretagogue therapy is controversial. In general, most diabetologists are concerned that such patients are unlikely to achieve acceptable glycemic control initially because of the effects of glucose toxicity and the possibility of severe insulin deficiency. Such patients are best treated with insulin and placed on an appropriate diet. After adequate glycemic control is obtained (FPG <130 mg/dl [6.7 mmol/l]), insulin secretagogue therapy may replace insulin therapy. Peters and Davidson (1995) have disputed this approach and claim that most of their patients who present with marked symptoms and mean random plasma glucose levels of 456 mg/dl (25 mmol/l) can be well controlled by initiation of therapy with maximal doses of glyburide. Such an approach can be hazardous unless the initial evaluation shows no evidence of dehydration or acidosis and the patient is followed closely for lack of response and/or deterioration toward ketoacidosis or nonketotic hyperosmolar states. The combination of glyburide and metformin (Glucovance) has been shown to be effective in controlling initial hyperglycemia in a cohort of type 2 diabetic patients presenting with a mean FPG of 283 mg/dl and mean A1C of 10.6%. A mean daily dose of 7.9 mg glyburide and 1,571 mg metformin reduced the mean FPG and A1C to 161 mg/dl and 7.1%, respectively, after 26 weeks of treatment.

Insulin secretagogue therapy should ordinarily be instituted with a low dose and increased at 4- to 7-day intervals until the maximal benefit is achieved. Many elderly or modestly symptomatic type 2 diabetic patients may be exquisitely sensitive to insulin secretagogues, and initial institution with moderate or high doses may precipitate severe hypoglycemia. The ideal goal of therapy is to maintain preprandial plasma blood glucose levels between 90 and 130 mg/dl (5.0 and 7.2 mmol/l) and an A1C <7%. If such control is obtained and maintained, insulin secretagogue therapy might be tapered and discontinued to see whether dietary therapy alone will maintain near-normoglycemic control. There are, however, some data to suggest that long-term glycemic control is better achieved if low-dose insulin secretagogue therapy is maintained.

Chronic insulin secretagogue therapy should be continued only as long as it maintains glycemic control in the target range sought for that particular patient. Most patients will achieve the maximal benefit in improving glycemic control with one-half to two-thirds of the manufacturer's recommended maximal dose. With sulfonylurea drugs, use of the maximal recommended dose may actually be less effective than using more moderate doses. This may be the result of down-regulation or desensitization of the sulfonylurea receptor.

When target glycemic control is no longer achieved with insulin secret-agogues, a change in therapy is indicated, and this should probably be the addition of other antihyperglycemic agents alone or in combination with insulin. Recently, A Diabetes Outcome Progression Trial (ADOPT) confirmed that sulfonylurea therapy, though very effective initially in newly diagnosed type 2 diabetic patients, has a less durable effect than metformin or rosiglitazone and will require the addition of a second agent much earlier if adequate glycemic control is to be maintained.

This inability of sulfonylureas to maintain glycemic control occurs in ordinary type 2 diabetic patients in whom β-cell function continues to deteriorate with time. In the diseases in which the specific genetic abnormality is in the inability of hyperglycemia to close the ATP-dependent potassium channel, sulfonylurea effectiveness appears to be maintained.

EFFECTS OF OTHER DRUGS ON INSULIN SECRETAGOGUE ACTIONS

Many commonly used drugs can potentiate insulin secretagogue effects and precipitate hypoglycemia or antagonize insulin secretagogue effects and worsen glycemic control. Table 20.5 lists some of the more important interactions. Alcohol and aspirin interactions may provide prolonged and severe hypoglycemia.

Table 20.5 Drug Interactions with Sulfonylureas

Increase hypoglycemia

- Drugs that displace sulfonylurea from albumin-binding sites, e.g., aspirin, fibrates, trimethoprim
- Competitive inhibitors of sulfonylurea metabolism, e.g., alcohol, H^2 blockers, anticoagulants
- Inhibitors of urinary excretion of sulfonylureas, e.g., probenecid, allopurinol
- Concomitant use of drugs with hypoglycemic properties, e.g., alcohol, aspirin

- Antagonist of endogenous counterregulatory hormones, e.g., β-blockers, sympatholytic drugs

Worsen glycemic control

- Drugs that increase sulfonylurea metabolism, e.g., barbiturates, rifampin
- Agents that antagonize sulfonylurea action, e.g., β-blockers
- Inhibitors of insulin secretion or action, e.g., thiazides and loop diuretics, β-blockers, corticosteroids, estrogens, phenytoin

β-Blockers interfere with both the recognition and counterregulatory responses to hypoglycemia. Anticoagulants are competitive inhibitors of sulfonylurea metabolism, and when both classes of drugs are used, the doses of both may have to be reduced appropriately.

Any concomitant drug treatment in a patient on or to be started on insulin secretagogue therapy must be evaluated for possible drug interactions. Because sulfonylureas with high intrinsic activity are given in smaller quantities and have somewhat different binding characteristics, they are likely to have fewer drug interactions than those with low intrinsic activity.

Repaglinide metabolism may be inhibited by antifungal agents such as ketoconazole and micronazole, antibacterial agents such as erythromycin, and agents that block glucuronidation such as gemfibrozil. Drugs that increase cytochrome P_{450} enzyme system 3A4 may increase repaglinide metabolism in the liver. Such drugs include troglitazone and barbiturates. Repaglinide does not alter the metabolism of digoxin, warfarin, or theophylline. Its interactions with agents that increase hypoglycemia or worsen glycemic control are similar to those of the sulfonylureas (Table 20.5). Treating patients with repaglinide who are on other medications may require dose adjustments.

EXPECTED RESULTS

Initial treatment of patients with type 2 diabetes with either sulfonylureas or repaglinide is likely to result in a mean decrease in FPG of 60–70 mg/dl (3.3–3.8 mmol/l) and a drop in A1C of 1–2%. Nateglinide treatment primarily lowers postprandial hyperglycemia and therefore decreases mean A1C by ~0.8%. As with all pharmacological treatments in patients with type 2 diabetes, the mean improvement in glycemic control with these agents is somewhat greater when the glycemic control is poor and somewhat less when the glycemic control is only moderately abnormal.

About one-third of newly diagnosed patients will achieve their target glycemic control on treatment with an insulin secretagogue and diet. Another one-third will achieve significant improvement in glycemic control but will require additional antihyperglycemic agents if the target goal is to be achieved. The other

Table 20.6 Common Causes of Secondary Sulfonylurea Failure

Patient-related factors	Therapy-related factors
■ Overeating and weight gain	■ Inadequate drug dosage
■ Poor patient compliance	■ Desensitization to chronic sulfonylurea exposure
■ Lack of physical activity	
■ Stress	■ Impaired absorption of drug due to hyperglycemia
■ Intercurrent illnesses	
	■ Concomitant therapy with diabetogenic drugs
Disease-related factors	
■ Decreasing β-cell function	
■ Increasing insulin resistance	

one-third will have a poor response and should be put on another therapeutic regimen.

With increasing duration of type 2 diabetes, the response to sulfonylureas and probably also to repaglinide and nateglinide (although data are not available) diminishes. This decreased effectiveness is ultimately due to decreasing endogenous β-cell insulin secretory function. It is unclear whether progressive β-cell functional loss is an intrinsic characteristic of type 2 diabetes or whether it is a consequence of chronic insulin resistance and/or chronic glucose and lipid toxicity from poor control. Chronic stimulation of insulin secretion by sulfonylureas does not appear to be a cause of β-cell exhaustion. The consequence of this diminishing effect of insulin secretagogues is that modifications in therapy will be necessary.

Table 20.6 presents an extensive list of many of the factors that might contribute to diminished effectiveness of sulfonylurea therapy and probably repaglinide and nateglinide therapy. Before concluding that the diminished effectiveness is caused by decreasing β-cell function, the possibility that a correctable cause is the culprit should be excluded.

The major concerns regarding insulin secretagogue therapy are

- hypoglycemia
- weight gain
- cardiovascular disease risk

Hypoglycemia is a significant complication. The newer agents—glimepiride, repaglinide, and nateglinide—are claimed to have a significantly lower risk of hypoglycemia than the older agents. Glimepiride therapy is thought to be more effective with lower plasma insulin levels and to maintain physiological suppression of insulin secretion in response to low blood glucose levels. Repaglinide is a short-acting insulin secretagogue and is taken with each meal. Nateglinide is the shortest-acting insulin secretagogue, and it too must be taken with each meal. Additional studies are needed to quantify the degree to which these agents are associated with less clinical hypoglycemia. Glyburide treatment is noteworthy in that many studies now indicate that hypoglycemia is more common and severe with it than with other insulin secretagogue therapies.

Weight gain is noted in almost all studies involving patients with type 2 diabetes on chronic sulfonylurea therapy. In the UKPDS, this amounted to ~12.5 lb or 7% of body weight. Weight gain is lower when sulfonylureas are combined with other antihyperglycemic agents, such as acarbose or metformin. There are some data to indicate that repaglinide and especially nateglinide treatments are associated with lower weight gain than sulfonylurea treatment.

Cardiovascular disease risk associated with sulfonylurea therapy has been a concern since the University Group Diabetes Program results were published in 1970. That study suggested that tolbutamide therapy was associated with an increase in sudden death from cardiovascular disease. There has been no additional intervention study that has provided clinical validation that sulfonylureas have cardiovascular toxicity in the last 35 years. The UKPDS data were thought to settle this issue because there was no increase in macrovascular disease events in the large cohort treated with sulfonylureas for a mean of 11 years. The recent experimental studies of the myocardial and vascular smooth muscle effects of sulfonylureas, though of concern, have not been clinically validated in appropriately controlled studies. Glyburide has been shown to block ischemic preconditioning in the heart in individuals both with and without diabetes. However, there is no unequivocal clinical evidence that glyburide increases cardiovascular morbidity or mortality in patients with diabetes. Recently, several observational studies and meta-analyses have presented data that sulfonylureas alone or in combination with metformin may increase cardiovascular outcomes and death. This issue continues to be controversial and of some concern.

Studies with glimepiride, repaglinide, and nateglinide show that these agents have significantly less binding to myocardial and vascular smooth muscle ATP-dependent K^+ channels than glyburide. Glimepiride, in contrast to glyburide, does not block ischemic preconditioning. The effects of repaglinide and nateglinide on ischemic preconditioning have not been tested because their interactions with the SUR subunits in cardiovascular tissues are so weak.

BIBLIOGRAPHY

Evans JM, Ogston SA, Emslie-Smith A, Morris AD: Risk of mortality and adverse cardiovascular outcomes in type 2 diabetes: a comparison of patients treated with sulfonylureas and metformin. *Diabetologia* 49:930–936, 2006

Groop LC, Pelkonen R, Koskimies S, Bottazzo GF, Doniach D: Secondary failure to treatment with oral antidiabetic agents in non-insulin-dependent diabetes. *Diabetes Care* 9:129–133, 1986

Kahn SE, Haffner SM, Heise MA, et al.: Glycemic durability of rosiglitazone, metformin, or glyburide monotherapy. *N Engl J Med* 355:2427–2443, 2006

Lebovitz HE: Oral antidiabetic agents. In *Joslin's Diabetes Mellitus*. 14th ed. Kahn CR, Weir GC, Eds. Philadelphia, PA, Lippincott, Williams & Wilkins, 2004

Lebovitz HE: Oral therapies for diabetic hyperglycemia. *Endocrinol Metab Clin North Am* 30:909–933, 2001

Lebovitz HE, Melander A: Sulfonylureas: basic aspects and clinical uses. In *International Textbook of Diabetes Mellitus*. 3rd ed. DeFronzo RA, Ferraninni E, Keen H, Zimmet P, Eds. Colchester, U.K., Wiley, 2004

Meier JJ, Gallwitz B, Schmidt WE, et al.: Is impairment of ischaemic preconditioning by sulfonylurea drugs clinically important? *Heart* 90:9–12, 2004

Pearson ER, Flechtner I, Njolstad PR, et al.: Switching from insulin to oral sulfonylureas in patients with diabetes due to Kir6.2 mutations. *N Engl J Med* 355:467–477, 2006

Pearson ER, Donnelly LA, Kimber C, et al.: Variation in TCF7L2 influences therapeutic response to sulfonylureas. *Diabetes* 56:2178–2182, 2007

Peters AL, Davidson MB: Maximal dose glyburide therapy in markedly symptomatic patients with type 2 diabetes: a new use for an old friend. *J Clin Endocrinol Metab* 81:2423–2427, 1995

Riddle MC: Editorial: sulfonylureas differ in effects on ischemic pre-conditioning: is it time to retire glyburide? *J Clin Endocrinol Metab* 88:528–530, 2003

Rao AD, Kuhadiya N, Reynolds K, Fonseca VA: Is the combination of sulfonylureas and metformin associated with an increased risk of cardiovascular disease or all-cause mortality? *Diabetes Care* 31:1672–1678, 2008

Simpson SH, Majumdar SR, Tsuyuki RT, et al.: Dose-response relation between sulfonylurea drugs and mortality in type 2 diabetes mellitus: a population-based cohort study. *CMAJ* 174:169–174, 2006

Sperling MA: ATP-sensitive potassium channels—neonatal diabetes mellitus and beyond. *N Engl J Med* 355:507–509, 2006

Turner R, Cull C, Holman R: United Kingdom Prospective Diabetes Study 17: a 9-year update of a randomized, controlled trial on the effect of improved metabolic control on complications in non-insulin-dependent diabetes mellitus. *Ann Intern Med* 124:136–145, 1996

UK Prospective Diabetes Study 33: Intensive blood glucose control with sulfonylureas or insulin compared with conventional treatment and risk of complications in patients with type 2 diabetes. *Lancet* 352:837–853, 1998

Dr. Lebovitz is Professor of Medicine at the State University of New York Health Science Center at Brooklyn, Brooklyn, New York.

21. Metformin

Clifford J. Bailey, PhD

In 1995, metformin was introduced for the treatment of hyperglycemia in patients with type 2 diabetes in the U.S., having been used in Europe since the early 1960s. It acts to counter insulin resistance and has several potential benefits against risk factors for vascular disease that are independent of glycemic control. It may also be of use for other conditions associated with insulin resistance, such as polycystic ovarian syndrome (PCOS).

Metformin is a member the class of drugs known as biguanides, which are guanidine derivatives (Fig. 21.1). Guanidine is found in the plant *Galega officinalis* (goat's rue or French lilac), which was used in medieval Europe as a treatment for diabetes. Other biguanides, notably phenformin and buformin, were introduced for the treatment of type 2 diabetes but were withdrawn because of a significant incidence of associated lactic acidosis. Metformin does not have this risk if appropriately prescribed and is now used widely as a monotherapy and in combination with other antidiabetic agents.

MODE OF ACTION AND RATIONALE FOR USE

Key features of the therapeutic effect of metformin in patients with type 2 diabetes are as follows:

- Metformin counters insulin resistance; it does not stimulate insulin secretion.
- Metformin decreases mainly fasting (and also postprandial) hyperglycemia in type 2 diabetic patients.
- Monotherapy with metformin does not cause hypoglycemia.
- The antidiabetic action of metformin requires some circulating insulin.
- Metformin treatment does not cause weight gain and can assist modest weight loss in overweight type 2 diabetic patients.
- Metformin treatment often improves the lipid profile.
- Metformin treatment can improve other vascular risk factors (e.g., it can increase fibrinolysis).
- Metformin has been shown to reduce vascular mortality when used as initial antidiabetic therapy in overweight and obese patients with type 2 diabetes.

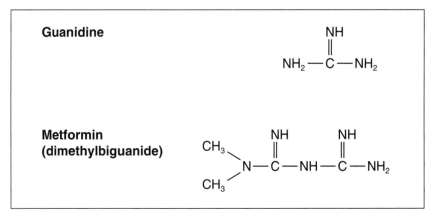

Figure 21.1. Structures of guanidine and metformin.

Blood Glucose Lowering

Metformin is an antihyperglycemic agent (rather than a hypoglycemic agent) because, when used as monotherapy, it lowers blood glucose concentrations in patients with type 2 diabetes without causing overt hypoglycemia. Also, it has little effect on blood glucose concentrations in nondiabetic individuals. Although the antihyperglycemic efficacy of metformin requires the presence of insulin, metformin does not stimulate insulin secretion. Some effects of metformin are mediated via increased insulin action (so-called insulin-sensitizing effects), and some are not directly insulin dependent.

The main blood glucose–lowering effects of metformin are summarized in Table 21.1. Fasting hyperglycemia is predominantly reduced by decreased hepatic glucose production, principally due to reduced gluconeogenesis but also through reduced glycogenolysis. At therapeutic concentrations, metformin suppresses hepatic gluconeogenesis by potentiating the effect of insulin and increasing the activity of AMP-activated protein kinase. Metformin can also reduce hepatic extraction of lactate. The rate of glycogenolysis is decreased by reducing the effect of glucagon and impeding the activity of hepatic glucose-6-phosphatase.

Insulin-mediated glucose uptake and utilization by skeletal muscle is enhanced during treatment with metformin. Euglycemic-hyperinsulinemic clamp studies in

Table 21.1 Mechanisms for the Antihyperglycemic Effect of Metformin

■ Suppression of hepatic glucose production	■ Decreased fatty acid oxidation
■ Increased insulin-mediated muscle glucose uptake	■ Increased intestinal glucose utilization

patients with type 2 diabetes have typically noted an increase in glucose uptake by ~20%, although this is not a consistent finding and appears to be influenced by the severity of the diabetic state, extent of weight reduction, and duration of therapy. Metformin increases the translocation of insulin-sensitive glucose transporters into the cell membrane and promotes the insulin- and glucose-sensitive transport properties of glucose transporters. The increased cellular uptake of glucose is associated with increased glycogen synthase activity and glycogen deposition.

Other effects of metformin that contribute to a lowering of blood glucose include an insulin-independent suppression of fatty acid oxidation and a reduction of hypertriglyceridemia. Through these effects, metformin reduces the energy supply for gluconeogenesis and improves the glucose–fatty acid (Randle) cycle. Metformin also increases glucose turnover, particularly in the splanchnic bed, which may benefit both the blood glucose–lowering and weight-stabilizing effects of the drug.

Nonglycemic Effects

In addition to its antihyperglycemic actions, metformin has been reported to counter several cardiometabolic risk factors and markers attributed to the "metabolic syndrome," as summarized in Table 21.2. While reducing insulin resistance, metformin therapy can lower fasting hyperinsulinemia, prevent weight gain,

Table 21.2 Effects of Metformin to Counter the Insulin Resistance (Metabolic) Syndrome

Features of the Insulin Resistance Syndrome	Effects of Metformin to Counter the Insulin Resistance Syndrome
Insulin resistance	Counters insulin resistance (e.g., increases insulin action to suppress hepatic glucose production and enhance muscle glucose uptake)
Hyperinsulinemia	Reduces fasting hyperinsulinemia
Abdominal obesity	Usually stabilizes body weight; reduces weight gain and can facilitate weight loss
IGT or type 2 diabetes	Reduces progression of IGT to type 2 diabetes; improves glycemic control in type 2 diabetes
Dyslipidemia ($\uparrow$VLDL-TG, $\uparrow$LDL-C, $\downarrow$HDL-C)	Modest improvement of lipid profile often seen in dyslipidemic patients
Hypertension	No significant effect on blood pressure in most studies
Procoagulant state	Some antithrombotic activity (e.g., decreases in PAI-1, fibrinogen, and platelet aggregation)
Atherosclerosis	Evidence for antiatherogenic activity from preclinical studies; no equivalent clinical studies

HDL-C, HDL cholesterol; IGT, impaired glucose tolerance; LDL-C, LDL cholesterol; VLDL-TG, very-low-density lipoprotein triglyceride.

improve the lipid profile, and decrease certain thrombotic factors. Such actions could potentially reduce vascular risk.

Circulating concentrations of triglycerides and LDL cholesterol are usually reduced by metformin in individuals with raised levels, but there is little or no effect when these parameters are already within the normal range. HDL cholesterol concentrations are slightly raised in some individuals during metformin therapy.

Several actions of metformin oppose the procoagulant state of type 2 diabetes (e.g., fibrinolytic activity is increased, sensitivity to platelet aggregating agents is decreased, and plasminogen activator inhibitor-1 [PAI-1] levels are decreased). The U.K. Prospective Diabetes Study (UKPDS) found that use of metformin as initial antidiabetic therapy in overweight patients with type 2 diabetes reduced macrovascular complications and increased survival compared with equivalent glycemic control by other agents (sulfonylureas or insulin) during a mean follow-up of 10 years.

Despite occasional claims to the contrary, most studies and clinical experience have found no significant effect of metformin on blood pressure. However, there have been preliminary reports that metformin can reduce hepatic steatosis and reduce some proinflammatory markers associated with type 2 diabetes. Initial evidence suggests that metformin is helpful in the treatment of PCOS and can reinstate menstruation and fertility.

Thus, the rationale for use of metformin to treat patients with type 2 diabetes is its antihyperglycemic efficacy and its activity against insulin resistance, with reductions in several cardiovascular risk factors. Metformin may be preferred for obese patients because it does not cause weight gain, although it shows similar antihyperglycemic efficacy in nonobese patients.

TREATMENT

Metformin (proprietary name Glucophage) is available in two tablet formulations: the standard (now called immediate-release [IR]) formulation and the extended-release (XR) formulation. The therapeutic effects of the two formulations are essentially the same, but the XR formulation is absorbed more slowly and can be given as once-daily dosing. A liquid formulation of metformin (500 mg/ml) and various generic tablet formulations of standard (IR) and extended-release (XR) metformin are available. Pharmacokinetic aspects of metformin are summarized in Table 21.3.

Indications

Metformin is indicated as monotherapy for the treatment of hyperglycemia in patients with type 2 diabetes who do not achieve appropriate target levels of glycemic control with nonpharmacological therapy, such as diet, exercise, and health education (Table 21.4). It can also be used in combination with an insulin-releasing agent (sulfonylurea, meglitinide, incretin mimetic [e.g., exenatide], or dipeptidyl peptidase [DPP] inhibitor [e.g., sitagliptin]), α-glucosidase inhibitor (acarbose or miglitol), thiazolidinedione (rosiglitazone or pioglitazone), or insulin. Metformin is helpful in patients who require weight stabilization or weight loss or who are vulnerable to hypoglycemia. Potential benefits against various

Table 21.3 Pharmacokinetic Aspects of Metformin

Variable	Comment
Bioavailability	50–60%; absorbed mainly from the small intestine; estimated time to maximal plasma concentration 0.9–2.6 h for standard (IR) formulation, 4–8 h for XR formulation
Plasma concentration	Maximal 1–2 µg/ml (~10^{-5} mol/l) 1–2 h after an oral dose of 500–1,000 mg for standard (IR) formulation; maximal concentration is ~20% lower (but area under the curve is similar) at same dose of XR formulation; negligible binding to plasma proteins
Plasma elimination half-life	~6 h
Metabolism	Not measurably metabolized
Elimination	About 90% of absorbed drug is eliminated in urine in 24 h; multiexponential pattern involving glomerular filtration and tubular secretion
Tissue distribution	Distributed in most tissues at concentrations similar to those in peripheral plasma; higher concentrations in liver and kidney; highest concentration in salivary glands and intestinal wall

atherogenic risk factors associated with insulin resistance (Table 21.2) are not specific indications but are usefully taken into account in the selection of metformin.

Elderly patients can be given metformin with appropriate adherence to the contraindications, especially renal function. Children can also receive metformin up to a maximum dose of 2,000 mg daily, although studies have not been conducted in subjects <10 years of age. Use in the elderly and in children warrants frequent monitoring.

Starting Metformin

Starting metformin therapy assumes attention to contraindications (detailed below) and appropriate monitoring of glycemic control, initially using fasting plasma glucose (FPG) and, subsequently, A1C.

Standard (IR) metformin should be taken with meals, starting with one 500- or 850-mg tablet at breakfast or other main meal. The dose can then be increased one tablet at a time at 4- to 14-day intervals, leading to two or three divided doses with the main meals, until the desired level of blood glucose control is achieved or the maximum tolerated dose is reached. A total dose of three or four 500-mg tablets or two to three 850-mg tablets is often required, with the maximum dose being 2,550 mg daily.

Gastrointestinal side effects are not uncommon during initiation of therapy. These include abdominal discomfort, diarrhea, nausea, anorexia, and a metallic

Table 21.4 Clinical Use of Metformin

Indications	As monotherapy or in combination with other oral antidiabetic agents or insulin in type 2 diabetic patients inadequately controlled by diet, exercise, and health education
Usage	500-, 850-, and 1,000-mg standard (IR) tablets: take with meals; increase dose slowly; monitor glycemic control; maximal dose 2,550 mg/day (2,000 mg/day in children)
	500- and 750-mg XR tablet: take with evening meal; increase dose slowly; monitor glycemic control; maximal dose 2,000 mg/day
Contraindications and warnings	Renal and hepatic disease; cardiac or respiratory insufficiency; any hypoxic condition; severe infection; alcohol abuse; history of lactic acidosis; temporarily discontinue during use of intravenous radiographic contrast agents; pregnancy
Side effects	Gastrointestinal symptoms and metallic taste, which improve with dose reduction; may impair absorption of vitamin B12 and folic acid
Adverse reactions	Risk of lactic acidosis in patients with a contraindication; hypoglycemia can occur when taken in combination with another antidiabetic drug or during alcohol abuse
Precautions	Check for contraindications; check hemoglobin and plasma creatinine periodically; possible interaction with cimetidine therapy

taste. These symptoms are usually transient, remit with dose reduction, and are minimized by gradual dose escalation and administration with meals.

XR metformin is usually given once daily with the evening meal or occasionally twice daily with the breakfast and evening meals. The XR tablets (500 and 750 mg) should always be taken whole so that the inner and outer polymer compartments are undisturbed and continued slow release of metformin is provided for up to 24 h. Patients may experience lesser initial gastrointestinal side effects with the XR formulation.

Contraindications and Warnings

Metformin is contraindicated in patients with impaired renal function (e.g., serum creatinine ≥1.5 mg/dl in men or ≥1.4 mg/dl in women). In older individuals, in whom serum creatinine is not a reliable measure of renal function, metformin is contraindicated if creatinine clearance is substantially impaired (e.g., <60 ml/min/1.73 m²). Renal function should be checked at least yearly during metformin therapy. It is suggested that metformin be temporarily discontinued for about 48 h during/after use of an intravascular contrast medium until normal renal function is evidently reestablished.

Any hypoxic state should be regarded as a contraindication for metformin—notably chronic congestive heart failure, acute heart failure, severe respiratory insufficiency, septicemia, and other conditions with hypoperfusion or hypoxemia. Significant liver disease, history of lactic acidosis, alcohol abuse, or other disturbances of liver function likely to prevent normal hepatic lactate metabolism should be considered as contraindications for metformin.

At present, administration of metformin is not recommended during pregnancy or lactation because of insufficient clinical data. However, animal studies and a recent large clinical trial support earlier clinical experience that metformin is not associated with increased complications in gestational diabetes compared with insulin therapy. Metformin is not teratogenic in animals, and no adverse effects on the fetus or nursing infant are apparent.

Metformin should be temporarily discontinued in favor of insulin administration during severe acute illnesses and major surgical procedures. Metformin is not effective as a primary treatment for type 1 diabetes.

Side Effects of Treatment

Lactic acidosis is a rare but serious adverse event associated with metformin therapy. Extensive worldwide experience indicates that the incidence is ~0.03 cases per 1,000 patient-years of treatment, with a mortality of ~50%. Many of these cases have occurred when the drug was inappropriately prescribed, hence the importance of adequate renal function for the drug to be eliminated and the avoidance of hypoxemia and conditions that compromise lactate metabolism. Lactic acidosis can occur in diabetic patients unrelated to metformin therapy.

The most common side effects of metformin are the gastrointestinal disturbances described above. Although these often resolve with time, dose reduction, gradual titration, and administration with meals, ~5–10% of patients do not tolerate a full therapeutic dose of metformin (e.g., 2,000 mg/day).

Long-term therapy with metformin is associated with a small decrease in the absorption of vitamin B12 and occasionally folate; however, development of anemia from this cause is rare, can be associated with poor diet, and is usually reversed by vitamin B12 supplementation.

Severe hypoglycemia is unlikely with metformin unless administered with another antidiabetic agent. In general, the blood glucose–lowering effect of metformin is additive to that of other oral antidiabetic agents while adequate β-cell function remains. Metformin usually increases the hypoglycemic effect of insulin. Use of metformin in combination with other antidiabetic agents requires appropriate adjustments of dosage based on glucose monitoring. Introduction of drugs that tend to increase blood glucose concentrations, such as corticosteroids, may also necessitate dosage adjustments.

Other clinically important drug interactions have not been identified with metformin. Metformin shows little binding to plasma proteins; it is not metabolized and is eliminated unchanged in the urine by glomerular filtration and tubular secretion. Thus, care should be taken if initiating therapies affecting renal function, such as antihypertensives, diuretics, and nonsteroidal anti-inflammatory drugs. Increased metformin levels can occur with cimetidine, which shares the same transporter in the renal tubules, and other cationic drugs could theoretically compete with metformin elimination. Minor pharmacokinetic interactions occur with furosemide and nifedipine.

EXPECTED RESULTS

The reduction of hyperglycemia and improvement in glycemic control achieved with oral antihyperglycemic drugs is influenced by many factors, including the level of initial hyperglycemia, the pathophysiological status of β-cell function and insulin resistance, and the mechanism of drug action. The therapeutic action of metformin improves sensitivity to low or moderate concentrations of insulin and therefore requires adequate remaining β-cell function.

Typically, the antihyperglycemic effect of metformin is evident throughout the range of mild to moderately severe fasting hyperglycemia (110–275 mg/dl [6.1–15.5 mmol/l] or A1C 7–12%). In clinical trials involving a broad spectrum of patients with type 2 diabetes, metformin treatment produced an average lowering of FPG by 55 mg/dl (3.1 mmol/l) and A1C by 1.5%. The absolute drop in plasma glucose and A1C will be greater at higher starting levels of hyperglycemia (e.g., FPG 275 mg/dl [15.5 mmol/l] and A1C 12%) than at lower levels (e.g., FPG 150 mg/dl [8.3 mmol/l] and A1C 8%). However, it is likely that a smaller proportion of patients will achieve target levels of glycemic control (e.g., A1C <7%) when the starting level of hyperglycemia is high.

The effect of metformin appears to be predominantly on fasting hyperglycemia, with a small effect on the meal-stimulated incremental rise in plasma glucose. A meta-analysis comparing metformin monotherapy with sulfonylurea monotherapy revealed that the two classes of drugs have comparable potency in reducing hyperglycemia and A1C.

Additional benefits ascribed to metformin therapy during trials with type 2 diabetes include a lack of weight gain or a small weight loss (mean reduction of 1–2 kg). Depending on the extent of initial dyslipidemia, there is often a small decrease in plasma LDL cholesterol and triglycerides (of ~10% in several trials) and a decrease in PAI-1. Severe episodes of hypoglycemia do not occur during metformin monotherapy, and fasting insulin concentrations are slightly reduced.

SINGLE-TABLET COMBINATIONS CONTAINING METFORMIN

Because the cellular mechanism of action of metformin is different from that of other oral antidiabetic agents, its blood glucose–lowering efficacy is generally

Table 21.5 Single-Tablet Combinations that Contain Metformin

Name	Constituents	Tablet strengths (mg)
Glucovance	Metformin + glyburide	250/1.25, 500/2.5, 500/5.0
Metaglip	Metformin + glipizide	250/2.5, 500/2.5, 500/5.0
Avandamet	Metformin + rosiglitazone	500/2, 500/4, 1,000/2, 1,000/4
Actoplus Met	Metformin + pioglitazone	500/15, 850/15
Janumet	Metformin + sitagliptin	500/50, 1,000/50

additive when combined with these agents, provided that adequate β-cell function remains. Single-tablet combinations of metformin with glyburide (Glucovance), metformin with glipizide (Metaglip), metformin with rosiglitazone (Avandamet), metformin with pioglitazone (Actoplus Met), and metformin with sitagliptin (Janumet) are now available (Table 21.5).

GLUCOVANCE

Glucovance is a single-tablet combination of metformin with the sulfonylurea glyburide. It was introduced in the U.S. in 2000. Glucovance can be used as initial antidiabetic drug therapy when substantial hyperglycemia persists after nonpharmacological interventions. Glucovance is convenient for patients transferring to a combination of metformin and glyburide because of inadequate glycemic control after monotherapy with one of these agents. Also, patients already receiving metformin and glyburide as separate tablets can be conveniently switched to Glucovance. Additionally, so-called "triple therapy" can be given using Glucovance plus a thiazolidinedione (rosiglitazone or pioglitazone).

Mode of Action and Rationale for Use

The two antidiabetic components of Glucovance, namely metformin and glyburide, act simultaneously to exert their individual blood glucose–lowering effects as described above. Provided there is adequate β-cell function, the blood glucose–lowering efficacy of the two components is approximately additive. This applies similarly whether metformin and glyburide are given as separate tablets or as Glucovance. However, there is preliminary evidence that the formulation of Glucovance may enhance the cumulative efficacy of metformin and glyburide, mainly to improve postprandial glycemic control.

Most patients with type 2 diabetes exhibit some degree of both insulin resistance and defective β-cell function. These two pathogenic facets of type 2 diabetes are addressed concurrently by Glucovance: metformin counters the insulin resistance and glyburide stimulates insulin secretion. Although the single-tablet combination of Glucovance offers the additional therapeutic benefits attributed individually to metformin and glyburide, it also carries all of the contraindications of the two compounds. When used in combination, the effects of the two compounds are not mutually exclusive (e.g., the presence of metformin will reduce the extent of weight gain associated with glyburide, but the occurrence of hypoglycemia is likely to increase).

Thus, the rationale for use of Glucovance in the treatment of type 2 diabetes is the additive blood glucose–lowering efficacy of metformin and glyburide, which act by complementary mechanisms to address insulin resistance and defective function. Glucovance enables these agents to be given simultaneously in a convenient single-tablet formulation.

Treatment

Glucovance is available at three strengths of glyburide/metformin: 1.25 mg/250 mg, 2.5/500, and 5/500. Tablets should be swallowed whole. Pharmacokinetic features are generally the same as for the two agents given in separate tablets, except that the peak circulating concentration of the glyburide component is achieved earlier (~1–3 h compared with 4–8 h) depending on food consumption (for glyburide). This result reflects the distribution of glyburide particle size in the Glucovance formulation, which includes a high proportion of small particles.

As initial antidiabetic drug therapy, Glucovance can be started if glycemic control is inadequate with nonpharmacological measures. Contraindications for both metformin and glyburide must be respected, and monitoring of FPG is required for gradual dose escalation until the desired glycemic control is achieved. It is recommended that patients begin with the lowest-strength tablet (1.25 mg glyburide/250 mg metformin). If the starting A1C level is >9%, it is usually appropriate to begin with this strength tablet twice daily with the morning and evening meals. If the starting A1C level is between 8 and 9%, begin with this strength tablet once daily with breakfast. Titrate up to twice daily, and then increase one tablet at a time to the next strength level, changing the morning tablet first. The suggested maximal daily dose is 10 mg glyburide/2,000 mg metformin in divided doses. Do not begin with the high-strength tablet (5 mg/500 mg) to reduce risk of hypoglycemia. Patients with a starting A1C <8% may be more appropriately treated with a single oral antidiabetic agent.

As second-line therapy in patients inadequately controlled on a maximally effective amount of either glyburide or metformin, it is recommended to select a starting dose of Glucovance that contains a lower amount of glyburide or metformin than is already being taken. For example, a patient inadequately controlled on 2,000 mg metformin might start Glucovance at 2.5 mg/500 mg twice daily and then increase one tablet at a time. Although a maximal suggested daily dose is 10 mg/2,000 mg, a dose of 20 mg/2,000 mg is permitted when used as second-line therapy.

In patients already taking a combination of glyburide (or another sulfonylurea) and metformin as separate tablets, it is convenient to switch to a similar dosage regimen of Glucovance, but do not exceed the daily amounts of glyburide (or equivalent of another sulfonylurea) and metformin already being taken.

For patients inadequately controlled on Glucovance, a thiazolidinedione can be added (so-called triple therapy). This addition may assist patients to achieve the desired glycemic target while there is remaining β-cell function. Patients with severe and rapidly escalating hyperglycemia, often with unintentional weight loss, should be considered for insulin therapy.

Glucovance can be used in the elderly provided there is careful and frequent monitoring, avoiding the highest doses. Glucovance has not been studied in children and is not recommended during pregnancy and lactation. It is reemphasized that the contraindications and precautions associated with the use of metformin and glyburide separately must be observed with Glucovance. Likewise, the side effects of each drug should be borne in mind when using Glucovance, and gradual dose titration with monitoring is especially important to reduce the risk of hypoglycemia.

Expected Results

In type 2 diabetes, the blood glucose–lowering effect of oral antidiabetic agents is influenced by many features of the disease process (as noted above in the metformin section of this chapter), particularly the extent of starting hyperglycemia. Previous experience with the use of metformin and glyburide in combination as separate tablets has shown that the blood glucose–lowering effect of the two agents is approximately additive.

A 26-week trial conducted for registration purposes found that initial drug therapy with Glucovance in patients with type 2 diabetes who had a starting A1C 7–11% and FPG ≤240 mg/dl reduced A1C by ~1.5% and FPG by ~40 mg/dl. The effect was generally greater among individuals with a starting hyperglycemia in the upper part of the range, and two-thirds of patients achieved a target A1C of <7%. A greater reduction in blood glucose was achieved in groups treated with Glucovance at a lower mean dose of each of the two active agents than in parallel groups treated with glyburide or metformin alone. Indeed, the Glucovance group treated with the 1.25-g/250-g strength tablets had a greater mean improvement in glycemic control than groups treated with glyburide or metformin as single therapies, and the average dosage of Glucovance contained about one-half of the dosage of glyburide or metformin as the single therapies. In particular, there was a greater improvement in the postprandial glucose excursion with Glucovance. This improvement may reflect the pharmacokinetic attribute of an initially rapid release of glyburide from the Glucovance tablet. The postprandial insulin response was greater than that with metformin alone but similar to that with glyburide alone: weight gain was greater compared with metformin alone, and there was little effect on the lipid profile. Fewer hypoglycemic symptoms were reported with the lowest strength of Glucovance than glyburide alone, but the higher strength of Glucovance was prone to more hypoglycemic symptoms, especially in patients with lower A1C levels (hence, the recommendation to initiate drug therapy with the 1.25-mg/250-mg strength of Glucovance).

An open-label study of patients with either a starting A1C >11% or FPG >240 mg/dl (>13.3 mmol/l) began with the 2.5-mg/500-mg strength Glucovance. After 26 weeks, there was a mean reduction of FPG from 283 to 161 mg/dl (15.7–8.9 mmol/l), with an average A1C of 7.1%, and this response was sustained to 52 weeks.

As second-line therapy, a 16-week study found that in patients inadequately controlled on a sulfonylurea, transfer to Glucovance and titration of the dosage enabled improvements in FPG, postprandial glucose, and A1C. For example, in patients with an A1C of ~9.5% on a maximal or near-maximal dose of glyburide, transfer to Glucovance reduced mean A1C by 1.7–1.9%, whereas continuation therapy with a sulfonylurea alone or switching to metformin alone was not effective.

Addition of the thiazolidinedione rosiglitazone to patients inadequately controlled with Glucovance (A1C ~8%) has been shown to produce an average decrease of A1C by 1% and FPG by 48 mg/dl after 24 weeks. Rosiglitazone was added at 4 mg/day and increased to 8 mg/day if target glycemic control was not achieved after 8 weeks.

METAGLIP

Metaglip is a single-tablet combination of metformin with the sulfonylurea glipizide. It was introduced in the U.S. in 2002 for use in the treatment of type 2 diabetes as initial antidiabetic drug therapy or for progression to a combination of metformin and glipizide if glycemic control is inadequate after monotherapy with metformin or glipizide (or another sulfonylurea) alone. Also, patients already taking a combination of metformin and glipizide as separate tablets can be switched to Metaglip for convenience.

Metaglip can be used in a similar manner to Glucovance (except the triple-therapy indication) and provides an appropriate combination where glipizide is already used or is preferred as the sulfonylurea to give in combination with metformin.

Mode of Action and Rationale for Use

The mode of action and rationale for use of Metaglip follow the same principles as those for Glucovance. Thus, the single-tablet combination of metformin and glipizide (Metaglip) conveniently takes advantage of the additive blood glucose–lowering efficacy of metformin and a sulfonylurea, which act by complementary mechanisms to address insulin resistance and defective β-cell function. The shorter duration of action of glipizide may be preferred in older patients or individuals more prone to hypoglycemia, although there is no specific indication for these groups, and contraindications (especially declining renal function in the elderly) must be taken into account.

Treatment

Metaglip is available at three strengths of glipizide/metformin: 2.5 mg/250 mg, 2.5/500, and 5/500. Pharmacokinetic features are generally the same as the two agents given together in separate tablets, which are also almost identical to the agents given alone.

The procedures for use of Metaglip (metformin/glipizide) are essentially the same as those of Glucovance (metformin/glyburide). Starting any oral antidiabetic drug treatment assumes that appropriate targets for glycemic control are not achieved with nonpharmacological therapy, and the nonpharmacological measures should continue to be reinforced throughout drug treatment. With Metaglip, the contraindications of both metformin and glipizide must be respected, and FPG monitoring is required for gradual dose escalation until the desired glycemic control is achieved. Gradual titration and taking the drug with meals should minimize the occurrence of gastrointestinal side effects and hypoglycemia.

As initial antidiabetic drug therapy, it is recommended to begin Metaglip with the lowest-strength tablet (2.5 mg glipizide/250 mg metformin) once daily with breakfast if the A1C level is <9% and twice daily with the morning and evening meals if the A1C level is >9%. Titrate up once daily to twice daily, and then increase one tablet at a time to the next strength level, changing the morning tablet first. In patients with type 2 diabetes who present with severe hyperglycemia, consider starting with a higher-strength tablet (2.5 mg glipizide/500 mg metformin) twice daily. The suggested maximum daily dose is 10 mg glipizide/2,000 mg metformin in divided doses (maximum permitted daily dose is 20/2,000). As with all oral antidiabetic drug therapies, provided there are no limiting adverse events or contraindications, continue dose titration until the desired glycemic control is achieved. If a titration step produces no further improvement in glycemic control, return to the previous dosage, which can be deemed the minimum dose with the maximum effect for that patient, and if the level of glycemic control is not acceptable, consider moving to the next stage of the treatment algorithm. Patients with a starting A1C <8% may be more appropriately treated with a single oral antidiabetic agent.

As second-line therapy in patients inadequately controlled on a maximally effective amount of either glipizide (or another sulfonylurea) or metformin alone, the starting dose of Metaglip should not exceed the daily dose of glipizide or metformin already being taken. This is likely to equate to Metaglip tablets of 2.5-mg/500-mg or 5-mg/500-mg strength. If glycemic control is close to target with monotherapy, it may be preferable to decrease a dosage level for the first dose of Metaglip.

In patients already taking a combination of glipizide (or another sulfonylurea) and metformin as separate tablets, a switch to Metaglip should use the nearest equivalent dosage regimen of Metaglip. Patients on a high dosage of Metaglip who are not adequately controlled and exhibit persistently severe and escalating hyperglycemia, often with unintentional weight loss, should be considered for insulin therapy.

Expected Results

Several studies in type 2 diabetes have confirmed that the blood glucose–lowering effects of metformin and a sulfonylurea are approximately additive, provided there is adequate β-cell function remaining.

Initial drug therapy with Metaglip (2.5 mg/250 mg and 2.5/500) has been studied in patients with type 2 diabetes during a 24-week trial for registration purposes. Patients had an average starting FPG of 203–210 mg/dl and A1C of ~9.1%, and Metaglip therapy produced mean decreases in FPG by 54–56 mg/dl and A1C by 2.1%. Thus, appropriate titration of the lower-strength tablets (2.5 mg/250 mg) gave similar results to the higher-strength tablets (2.5/500) in this study. These improvements in glycemic control were greater than those achieved with either glipizide alone (decreased A1C by 1.7%) or metformin alone (decreased A1C by 1.4%). Moreover, the amounts of glipizide and metformin given with the lower-strength Metaglip tablets were less than one-half of the amounts of these agents taken by the groups receiving each agent alone. The Metaglip groups also showed greater improvements in postprandial glucose excursion than groups treated with either glipizide or metformin alone. Metaglip was associated with a small decrease in body weight (by 0.4–0.5 kg), which was less than the decrease in body weight with metformin alone (by 1.9 kg). No clinically significant effects of Metaglip or its separate component drugs were observed on lipid parameters in this study. More reports of hypoglycemic symptoms and fingerstick blood glucose values ≤50 mg/dl were made by patients taking Metaglip (7.6 and 9.3% of patients taking the lower- and higher-strength tablets, respectively) compared with metformin alone (0%) and glipizide alone (2.9%). Metaglip was discontinued by 2.6% of patients because of hypoglycemic symptoms. Gastrointestinal symptoms, including diarrhea, occurred more often in the group taking metformin alone, and 1.2% of patients on Metaglip discontinued because of gastrointestinal symptoms.

As second-line therapy, an 18-week study noted that patients inadequately controlled on either a sulfonylurea or metformin alone achieved an additional decrease in mean A1C by ~1% when taking Metaglip. Improvements in FPG and postprandial glucose were also noted with Metaglip, but body weight loss was trivial (–0.3 kg) compared with metformin alone (–2.7), and there were no significant changes in lipids.

AVANDAMET

Avandamet is a single-tablet combination of metformin with the thiazolidine-dione rosiglitazone. It was introduced in the U.S. in 2002 as a second-line oral antidiabetic drug therapy for patients with type 2 diabetes. Avandamet can be used in patients who are inadequately controlled by monotherapy with metformin or rosiglitazone; patients already receiving metformin and rosiglitazone as separate tablets can switch to the single-tablet formulation if more convenient.

Mode of Action and Rationale for Use

Metformin and rosiglitazone are routinely used in combination therapy as separate tablets, and their blood glucose–lowering effects are approximately additive, provided there is adequate β-cell function. They each improve insulin sensitivity, but they do so by different and complementary mechanisms that enable their effective use in combination. Rosiglitazone stimulates the nuclear receptor peroxisome proliferator–activated receptor-γ. The blood glucose–lowering effect of metformin predominantly involves a reduction in hepatic glucose production, whereas rosiglitazone mainly causes an increase in peripheral glucose uptake. Both agents act without stimulating insulin secretion: they are antihyperglycemic and rarely cause frank hypoglycemia when used alone. Hypoglycemia can occur when these agents are used in combination, but it is usually mild. Each agent has been reported to influence certain cardiovascular risk factors associated with the "metabolic syndrome," at least in part by reducing insulin resistance.

The main rationale for use of Avandamet to treat type 2 diabetes is the convenience of single-tablet combination therapy with metformin and rosiglitazone to address insulin resistance by complementary actions with minimal risk of hypoglycemia.

Treatment

Avandamet is available at four strengths of rosiglitazone/metformin: 2 mg/500 mg, 4/500, 2/1,000, and 4/1,000. Pharmacokinetic characteristics of each agent are unaltered by the other, and the single-tablet combination shows the same characteristics as the two components coadministered as separate tablets.

Use of Avandamet in type 2 diabetes assumes that monotherapy with metformin or rosiglitazone alone does not achieve adequate glycemic control. When starting Avandamet, it is important that the contraindications and cautions are respected for both metformin and rosiglitazone. Note that rosiglitazone can cause edema and increase the risk of congestive heart failure in some patients. Data regarding the risk of myocardial ischemia with rosiglitazone are inconclusive, and long-term outcome trials with rosiglitazone are in progress. Avandamet is contraindicated in patients with New York Heart Association (NYHA) classes III or IV heart failure. Note also that Avandamet is contraindicated in patients with impaired renal function and other exclusions that apply to metformin.

Patients inadequately controlled on metformin monotherapy will typically start Avandamet at the same daily dose of metformin (up to 2,000 mg) plus 2–4 mg rosiglitazone daily, given in divided doses that correspond with the previous metformin regimen. For patients inadequately controlled on rosiglitazone monotherapy, start Avandamet with the same daily dose of rosiglitazone plus 1,000 mg metformin daily in divided doses, although it may be prudent to introduce metformin at 500 mg daily (with breakfast) for the first few days. If starting Avandamet in drug-naïve type 2 diabetic patients, begin with 2 mg/500 mg once or twice daily with meals. Titrate the dosage gradually (see advice for metformin), bearing in mind that there is a slow onset of the rosiglitazone component effect: monitor FPG and other parameters as required for each component drug.

To switch a patient from a combination of rosiglitazone and metformin as separate tablets, use the nearest equivalent daily dose of Avandamet. The maximum recommended daily dose of Avandamet is 8 mg rosiglitazone/2,000 mg metformin in divided doses.

Expected Results

Adding rosiglitazone to metformin as separate tablets has demonstrated their additive blood glucose–lowering efficacy. A 26-week trial in patients with type 2 diabetes inadequately controlled on metformin found that addition of rosiglitazone (8 mg daily) reduced A1C by 0.8% from baseline and by 1.2% compared with individuals continuing on metformin alone. Starting Avandamet in drug-naïve type 2 diabetic patients inadequately controlled by diet and exercise (baseline of A1C 8.9%) reduced A1C by 2.3% over 32 weeks with an average dose of 7.2 mg rosiglitazone/1,799 mg metformin. There was little effect on lipids except a modest reduction of triglycerides (by 18.7%). A small increase in body weight (e.g., 1–2 kg) can be expected with Avandamet in patients not previously receiving rosiglitazone, whereas significant hypoglycemia is uncommon.

During a 24-week study, addition of insulin in patients receiving Avandamet resulted in a larger reduction of A1C than in patients receiving insulin plus tablet placebo (–2.0 vs. –1.3%), despite a lower final daily insulin dose (33 vs. 59 units). A particularly rapid increase in weight on initiation of Avandamet warrants investigation for edema and any signs of heart failure. Be aware that rosiglitazone has been reported to increase the incidence of bone fractures (mainly arm, hand, and foot) after 1 year in women.

ACTOPLUS MET

Actoplus met is a single-tablet combination of metformin with the thiazolidinedione pioglitazone, introduced in the U.S. in 2005 as a second-line oral antidiabetic drug therapy for patients with type 2 diabetes. Actoplus met can be used in patients who are inadequately controlled by monotherapy with metformin or pioglitazone. Patients already receiving metformin and pioglitazone as separate tablets can switch to the single-tablet formulation if more convenient.

Mode of Action and Rationale for Use

Metformin is routinely used in combination therapy with a thiazolidinedione: the two classes of agents show approximately additive blood glucose–lowering effects when used in combination, provided there is adequate β-cell function. Each improves insulin sensitivity, but by different and complementary mechanisms. Pioglitazone stimulates the nuclear receptor peroxisome proliferator–activated receptor-γ and mainly increases peripheral glucose uptake. As described earlier in this chapter, metformin predominantly reduces hepatic glucose production. Because neither agent stimulates insulin secretion, hypoglycemia is uncommon and usually mild, even when the agents are used in combination. Each agent has been reported to influence several cardiovascular risk factors associated with the "metabolic syndrome," in part by reducing insulin resistance.

The main rationale for use of Actoplus met is convenient treatment of type 2 diabetes with a single-tablet combination of metformin and pioglitazone to address insulin resistance by complementary actions with minimal risk of hypoglycemia.

Treatment

Actoplus met is available at two strengths of pioglitazone/metformin: 15 mg/500 mg and 15/850. Pharmacokinetic characteristics of each agent are unaltered by the other, and the single-tablet combination shows similar characteristics to the individual components coadministered as separate tablets.

Actoplus met is normally used to treat type 2 diabetes when monotherapy with metformin or pioglitazone alone does not achieve adequate glycemic control. When starting Actoplus met, it is important to respect the contraindications and cautions for both metformin and pioglitazone. Because pioglitazone can cause edema and increase the risk of congestive heart failure in some patients, Actoplus met is contraindicated in patients with NYHA classes III or IV heart failure. Actoplus met is also contraindicated in patients with impaired renal function and other exclusions that apply to metformin.

Patients inadequately controlled on metformin monotherapy will typically start Actoplus met at a similar daily dose of metformin plus 15–30 mg pioglitazone daily, given in divided doses that coincide where possible with the previous metformin regimen. For patients inadequately controlled on pioglitazone monotherapy, start Actoplus met with a similar daily dose of pioglitazone plus 1,000 mg metformin daily in divided doses, although it may be prudent to introduce metformin at 500 mg daily (with breakfast) for the first few days. If starting Actoplus met in drug-naïve type 2 patients, begin with 15 mg/500 mg once or twice daily with meals. Titrate the dosage gradually (see advice for metformin earlier), bearing in mind that there is a slow onset of the pioglitazone component effect: monitor FPG and other parameters as required for each component drug.

To switch a patient from a combination of pioglitazone and metformin as separate tablets, use the nearest equivalent daily dose of Actoplus met. The maximum recommended daily dose of Actoplus met is 45 mg pioglitazone/2,550 mg metformin in divided doses.

Expected Results

Adding pioglitazone to metformin as separate tablets has demonstrated their additive blood glucose–lowering efficacy. A 24-week trial in patients with type 2 diabetes inadequately controlled on metformin found that addition of pioglitazone at 30 or 45 mg daily reduced A1C by 0.8 and 1.0%, respectively, from baseline. There is little peer-reviewed published evidence regarding use of the single-tablet combination of pioglitazone and metformin (Actoplus met), and use of the combination is largely based on experience gained using the separate tablets. In addition to its glucose-lowering effect without risk of significant hypoglycemia, introduction of the combination is likely to cause a small increase in body weight (e.g., 1–2 kg) in patients who have not previously received pioglitazone. These patients may also show a modest reduction of triglycerides and free fatty acids.

Note that a particularly rapid increase in weight on initiation of Actoplus met warrants investigation for edema and any signs of heart failure. Pioglitazone has been reported to increase the incidence of nonverbebral bone fractures in women.

JANUMET

Janumet is a single-tablet combination of metformin with the DPP-4 inhibitor sitagliptin. It was introduced in the U.S. in 2007 to treat type 2 diabetic patients with inadequate glycemic control after monotherapy with metformin or sitagliptin alone. Also, patients already taking a combination of metformin and sitagliptin can be switched to Janumet for convenience.

Janumet can be used in a similar manner to the metformin-sulfonylurea combinations of Glucovance or Metaglip, but Janumet is unlikely to cause significant hypoglycemia or weight gain.

Mode of Action and Rationale for Use

Janumet conveniently exploits the additive blood glucose–lowering efficacy of metformin and sitagliptin, which act by complementary mechanisms. Metformin counters insulin resistance (described earlier), and sitagliptin acts primarily to address defective islet function. Sitagliptin selectively inhibits activity of the circulating and cell-surface enzyme DPP-4. DPP-4 normally causes rapid degradation of the incretin hormones glucagon-like peptide (GLP)-1 and glucose-dependent insulinotropic polypeptide (GIP). Thus, inhibition of DPP-4 activity with sitagliptin prevents the rapid degradation of GLP-1 and GIP, thereby enhancing endogenous incretin activity. This is associated with increased glucose-induced insulin secretion. The raised circulating concentrations of active GLP-1 also suppress glucagon secretion and may slow the rate of gastric emptying and exert a small satiety effect. There is preliminary evidence that metformin might facilitate an increase in GLP-1 concentrations.

Because the effects of sitagliptin on insulin and glucagon secretion are glucose dependent, there is low risk of significant hypoglycemia, and the potential effects on satiety and gastric emptying may contribute to weight neutrality. Thus, the two active components of Janumet (metformin and sitagliptin) lower blood glucose with nominal risk of serious hypoglycemia or weight gain. Moreover, metformin substantially lowers basal glycemia, whereas sitagliptin particularly reduces prandial glucose excursions.

Because both sitagliptin and metformin are eliminated unchanged in the urine (sitagliptin mainly through tubular secretion, and metformin by filtration and secretion), Janumet is contraindicated in patients with renal impairment. Like metformin, sitagliptin is not extensively protein bound and has little effect on P450 isoenzymes. Although attention is drawn to coadministration with drugs that affect renal function or share the same renal secretion mechanism as sitagliptin, Janumet does not appear to have significant drug interactions based on available data.

Treatment

Janumet is available at two strengths of sitagliptin/metformin: 50 mg/500 mg and 50/1,000. When sitagliptin and metformin are coadministered, their pharmacokinetic features remain similar to the agents given alone.

Starting Janumet normally assumes that appropriate targets for glycemic control are not achieved with nonpharmacological therapy or with one antidiabetic agent (metformin or sitagliptin) alone. Nonpharmacological measures should continue to be reinforced throughout any program of diabetes management. With Janumet, the contraindications of both metformin and sitagliptin must be respected, and FPG monitoring is required for gradual dose escalation until the desired glycemic control is achieved. Introduction and titration of Janumet follows the general principles set out for metformin earlier.

In patients inadequately controlled on a maximally effective amount of metformin or sitagliptin alone, the starting dose of Janumet should equate where possible (but not exceed) the daily dose of either metformin or sitagliptin already being taken. In patients already taking metformin, this is likely to be Janumet tablets of 50-mg/500-mg or 50-mg/1,000-mg strength once or twice daily with the main meals. In patients already taking sitagliptin, start with the 50-mg/500-mg strength initially once daily and titrate up as indicated for metformin. The maximum recommended daily dose is 100 mg sitagliptin and 2,000 mg metformin.

For patients already taking a combination of sitagliptin and metformin as separate tablets, a switch to Janumet should use the nearest equivalent dosage regimen of Janumet. Patients aiming for tight glycemic control who are close to an A1C target of ~7% can be given Janumet with little risk of serious hypoglycemia. Patients susceptible to or experiencing episodes of hypoglycemia with a sulfonylurea or meglitinide combined with metformin may be at less risk of hypoglycemia with Janumet. Switching such patients to Janumet should use the nearest equivalent dose of metformin. Patients exhibiting persistently severe and escalating hyperglycemia, often with unintentional weight loss, should be considered for insulin therapy.

Expected Results

Evidence for the blood glucose–lowering efficacy of Janumet is mostly based on studies with metformin and sitagliptin as separate tablets. In type 2 diabetic patients inadequately controlled (A1C ~8.5%) with metformin, addition of sitagliptin (100 mg/day) for 24 weeks reduced A1C by a mean of 0.7%. The 2-h postprandial glucose concentration was reduced by 51 mg/dl (2.8 mmol/l). Several further randomized prospective trials in patients inadequately controlled (A1C ~8%) with metformin have noted that addition of sitagliptin (100 mg/day) for 24 weeks typically reduced A1C by ~0.65–0.8%.

A 24-week randomized study in which drug-naïve type 2 diabetic patients with an A1C ~8.8% received initial antidiabetic drug therapy with sitagliptin/metformin at either 100 mg/1,000 mg or 100/2,000 found reductions in A1C of ~1.5 and 2.0%, respectively. In each of the studies involving a sitagliptin-metformin combination, there has been a low incidence of hypoglycemia and no weight gain or sometimes a small weight loss. The incidence of gastrointestinal side effects was similar for the combination as for the respective dose of metformin monotherapy.

BIBLIOGRAPHY

Bailey CJ: Treating insulin resistance in type 2 diabetes with metformin and thiazolidinediones. *Diabetes Obesity Metab* 7:675–691, 2005

Bailey CJ, Turner RC: Drug therapy: metformin. *N Engl J Med* 334:574–579, 1996

Cusi K, DeFronzo RA: Metformin: a review of its metabolic effects. *Diabetes Rev* 6:89–130, 1998

DeFronzo RA, Goodman AM, Multicenter Metformin Study Group: Efficacy of metformin in patients with non-insulin-dependent diabetes mellitus. *N Engl J Med* 333:541–549, 1995

Fonseca V, Rosenstock J, Patwardhan R, Salzman A: Effect of metformin and rosiglitazone combination therapy in patients with type 2 diabetes mellitus. *JAMA* 283:1695–1702, 2000

Garber AJ, Larsen J, Schneider SH, Piper BA, Henry D: Simultaneous glyburide/metformin therapy is superior to component monotherapy as an initial pharmacological treatment for type 2 diabetes. *Diabetes Obes Metab* 4:201–208, 2002

Goldstein BJ, Feinglos MN, Lunceford JK, Johnson J, Williams-Herman DE: Effect of initial combination therapy with sitagliptin, a dipeptidyl peptidase-4 inhibitor, and metformin on glycemic control in patients with type 2 diabetes. *Diabetes Care* 30:1979–1987, 2007

Howlett HCS, Bailey CJ: A risk-benefit assessment of metformin in type 2 diabetes mellitus. *Drug Safety* 20:489–503, 1999

Krentz AJ, Bailey CJ: Oral antidiabetic agents: current role in type 2 diabetes mellitus. *Drugs* 65:385–411, 2005

Misbin RI, Green L, Stadel BV, Gueriguian JL, Gubbi A, Fleming GA: Lactic acidosis in patients with diabetes treated with metformin. *N Engl J Med* 338:285–286, 1997

U.K. Prospective Diabetes Study Group: Effect of intensive blood-glucose control with metformin on complications in overweight patients with type 2 diabetes (UKPDS 34). *Lancet* 352:854–865, 1998

Dr. Bailey is Professor of Clinical Science and Head of Diabetes Research at Aston University, Birmingham, U.K.

22. α-Glucosidase Inhibitors in the Treatment of Hyperglycemia

Rémi Rabasa-Lhoret, MD, PhD, and Jean-Louis Chiasson, MD

Dietary intervention remains the cornerstone of treatment strategies for patients with type 2 diabetes. Although the focus of dietary intervention is frequently on weight reduction, dietary intervention also has a direct effect on hyperglycemia. When diet and exercise fail, oral antidiabetic medications such as sulfonylureas, biguanides, or thiazolidinediones are added. These agents have been shown to decrease fasting plasma blood glucose, but in >60% of patients, postprandial hyperglycemia persists and probably accounts for the sustained increase in A1C levels. Such postprandial glycemic excursion contributes to the development of diabetes-specific complications (e.g., retinopathy and nephropathy) and could be involved in the development of macrovascular complications. Slowly absorbed carbohydrates and a high-fiber diet blunt the postprandial elevation of plasma glucose and insulin levels, but most patients find these regimens difficult to follow long term. Pharmacological agents (α-glucosidase inhibitors) have been developed to delay the digestion of complex carbohydrate. By their original mechanism of action, they significantly reduce postprandial glycemic and insulinemic excursion, regardless of the current therapy in place and the type of diabetes (type 1 or type 2).

MECHANISM OF ACTION

α-Glucosidase inhibitors are competitive suppressants of small intestine brush border α-glucosidases, which are essential to hydrolyze disaccharides, oligosaccharides, and polysaccharides to monosaccharides. Normally, carbohydrates are primarily and rapidly absorbed in the first part of the small intestine. With α-glucosidase inhibitors, carbohydrate absorption and digestion are delayed and prolonged throughout the small intestine, resulting in a reduction of the postprandial plasma glucose elevation in both type 1 and type 2 diabetes. Acarbose, the principal medication of this class, is a pseudotetrasaccharide of microbial origin, structurally analogous to an oligosaccharide derived from starch digestion. It has a high affinity for the carbohydrate-binding site of various α-glucosidase enzymes, exceeding the affinity (10- to 100,000-fold) of regular oligosaccharides from nutritional carbohydrates. Because of its structure, acarbose cannot be cleaved, and therefore enzymatic hydrolysis is blocked. Despite its high affinity for these enzymes, acarbose binding is reversible after 4–6 h. Owing to its specificity for α-glucosidases, β-glucosidases (e.g., lactases) are not inhibited by acarbose; therefore, the digestion and absorption of lactose are not affected by acarbose treatment. Oral glucose administration is also not affected by the drug. Acarbose is poorly absorbed, and <1–2% of the active compound appears in the plasma.

The delay of carbohydrate digestion and absorption in the small bowel can increase the amount of fermentable carbohydrates reaching the colon. This results in gastrointestinal (GI) symptoms (i.e., flatulence and diarrhea) but does not interfere with the use of the energy content of carbohydrates, which are metabolized by colonic microflora to short-chain fatty acids and then absorbed.

α-Glucosidase inhibitors also modify the secretion of GI peptides: gastric inhibitory peptide and glucagon-like peptide-1. These two peptides, also called incretins, have an important role to increase insulin secretion in a glucose-dependent fashion and to inhibit glucagon secretion. When an α-glucosidase inhibitor is taken with a meal rich in carbohydrates, gastric inhibitory peptide secretion is decreased, whereas glucagon-like peptide-1 is markedly increased, particularly in the late postprandial period. It is unclear whether such modifications in the secretion of these important incretins play a role in the overall beneficial effect of α-glucosidase inhibitors.

CLINICAL USE

Three α-glucosidase inhibitors have been developed: acarbose, miglitol, and voglibose. Their pharmacological profiles are very similar, and acarbose is the most widely tested, available, and used.

Because of their mechanism of action, α-glucosidase inhibitors should be taken within the first 15 min of each of the three major meals. The mechanism of action also explains the necessity of initiating treatment at a low dose and increasing it slowly to minimize GI side effects. α-Glucosidase content in the small intestine is high in the upper jejunum and low in the distal jejunum and ileum. When initiating treatment at a low dose, the small amount of carbohydrates reaching the distal part of the small intestine will induce α-glucosidase synthesis, thus minimizing the carbohydrate load reaching the large intestine, which is responsible for the side effects. It is recommended to start at a low dose (i.e., 25 or 50 mg o.d. for 1 week) and then slowly increase by 25–50 mg in each subsequent week based on GI tolerance and clinical efficacy.

Titration should be based on 1- or 2-h postprandial plasma glucose and GI tolerance. If GI side effects become significant during titration, the dose should be reduced for some time because these side effects decrease with time. Treatment efficacy is seen from the first week and is maintained over the long term. Maximal efficacy is obtained between 50 and 100 mg t.i.d. Some studies, though not all, suggest that the maximal benefit–to–side effect ratio is obtained at 50 mg t.i.d.

INDICATIONS FOR α-GLUCOSIDASE INHIBITOR THERAPY

When diet and exercise fail to maintain optimal blood glucose control, prescription of α-glucosidase inhibitors should be considered in patients with diabetes in the following situations:

- As primary therapy for
  - ☐ Patients with normal fasting blood glucose and postprandial hyperglycemia
  - ☐ Patients with type 2 diabetes with mild to moderate hyperglycemia (<180 mg/dl [10 mmol/l])
  - ☐ Patients with type 2 diabetes as an alternative when other oral hypoglycemic agents are contraindicated (e.g., existing or significant risk of hypoglycemia with sulfonylurea, risk of lactic acidosis with biguanides). Elderly patients with mild diabetes represent an important population for this indication.
- As an adjunct therapy for
  - ☐ Patients with inadequate glycemic control under other oral agents, particularly with postprandial hyperglycemia
  - ☐ Patients using insulin to reduce insulin requirement, decrease postprandial glycemic excursion, and lessen hypoglycemia

EFFICACY

Most published studies have shown a moderate but constant decline of A1C. This decrease is maintained long term and is mostly related to postprandial glycemic reduction because the fasting plasma glucose fall is generally not significant.

In Combination with Diet Therapy

In controlled trials compared with placebo, acarbose elicited a significant reduction of postprandial hyperglycemia (approximately –54 mg/dl [–3 mmol/l]) along with a mean 0.8% decrease of A1C (Table 22.1). Studies with miglitol gave comparable results.

In Comparison with Other Oral Hypoglycemic Agents

When compared in the same study with sulfonylurea and biguanides, α-glucosidase inhibitors showed a comparable reduction of A1C (~1%) in four of five trials. In the remaining study, miglitol was less efficient than glibenclamide.

In Association with Other Oral Hypoglycemic Agents

Because the mechanism of action of acarbose is different from that of other oral hypoglycemic agents, an additive benefit can be expected with coadministration. This additive effect has been confirmed in seven different trials. When acarbose is added to ongoing suboptimal treatment with sulfonylureas or biguanides, a mean 0.75% decrease of A1C can be expected (Table 22.1). Several small studies comparing the effect of adding either acarbose or metformin to existing sulfonylurea therapy have found the two drugs to be equivalent as adjunctive treatment. There is only one published comparison of thiazolidinediones and acarbose. In that small study, the addition of troglitazone to patients previously treated with acarbose produced significant glycemic improvement.

In Association with Insulin

In patients with type 2 diabetes, adding acarbose to insulin treatment evoked a mean 0.6% reduction of A1C in three different studies (Table 22.1). In patients

Table 22.1 Mean Reduction of A1C and Fasting and Postprandial Plasma Glucose When Acarbose Is Added to Previous Antidiabetic Therapeutics

Treatment already in place (numbers of studies/ numbers of subjects)	A1C (%)	Plasma glucose mg/dl (mmol/l)	
		Fasting*†	Postprandial
Diet (30/2,831)	−0.80	−19.8 (−1.1)	−41.4 (−2.3)
Diet + sulfonylurea (6/342)	0.78	−10.2 (−0.57)	−54.4 (−3.02)
Diet + biguanides (2/148)	−0.72	−10.2 (−0.57)	−63.1 (−3.5)
Diet + insulin (4/338)	−0.59	−11.0 (−0.61)	−48.0 (−2.66)

*Mean of studies from which this information was available.
†In most studies, this reduction is not significant.

with type 1 diabetes, a similar decrease of A1C was reported, with no increase of hypoglycemic risk. Small studies have also suggested that acarbose could reduce the risk of nocturnal or exercise-induced hypoglycemia.

Long-Term Effect

Only two studies lasted ≥1 year. The results from these works support the hypothesis that the glucose-lowering effect of acarbose is maintained long term. In the U.K. Prospective Diabetes Study, a 3-year trial tested the addition of acarbose to other forms of antidiabetic treatment. Patients remaining on acarbose at the end of the trial benefited by a 0.5% reduction of A1C, but the dropout rate was extremely high. In a study by Chiasson et al. (1994), significant benefit was proven after 1 year of treatment, regardless of the previous therapy in place.

For Type 2 Diabetes Prevention

In obese subjects with impaired glucose tolerance, lifestyle modification is highly effective in preventing or delaying the development of type 2 diabetes. In two important intervention trials, a 5–7% weight reduction and physical activity >150 min/week produced a reduction of nearly 60% of new cases of diabetes over 3 years. Pharmacological interventions using metformin, rosiglitazone, or orlistat have also been shown to be effective. Compared with placebo, acarbose resulted in a 35.6% risk reduction of new cases of diabetes. Although these new data offer potential new applications for α-glucosidase inhibitors, and even though it is accepted for diabetes prevention in >25 countries, there is no FDA indication in the U.S. for pharmacological interventions in patients with impaired glucose tolerance.

TOLERABILITY

As monotherapy, α-glucosidase inhibitors are safe agents that do not induce hypoglycemia and have a neutral effect on weight. However, they may potentiate the hypoglycemic action of sulfonylureas and insulin. A reduction in the dosage of concomitant hypoglycemic agents may be necessary when α-glucosidase inhibitor treatment is introduced. If a patient given acarbose experiences hypoglycemia, the hypoglycemia should be treated with glucose because the absorption of sucrose and complex carbohydrates is delayed by the drug. Patients should be well educated on this potential occurrence.

The main side effects of α-glucosidase inhibitors are GI symptoms consisting of abdominal distention, flatulence, diarrhea, and borborygmus in ~50% of patients. Safety studies have shown no deleterious effects on digestive tract morphology. The side effects are related to intracolonic fermentation and consequent gas production of carbohydrates not absorbed in the small bowel. The symptoms are dose dependent and tend to decrease with continued treatment. The best strategy to minimize the GI side effects is to use a "start low and go slow" dosage policy. It is estimated that ~5% of patients are unable to tolerate acarbose, a rate comparable to that of biguanides. Despite these frequent GI symptoms, the quality of life of patients on acarbose has been shown to be as good as with sulfonylurea or insulin therapy.

An elevation of liver enzymes has been reported on rare occasions in patients on high doses of acarbose (300 mg t.i.d.); it was moderate and always returned to normal after cessation of the drug. There are a few reports of ileus associated with acarbose treatment in Japanese patients.

Concurrent administration of antacids, bile acid resins, intestinal absorbents, or digestive enzyme preparations may reduce the effect of α-glucosidase inhibitors. Rare interaction with digoxin has also been reported, resulting in decreased drug absorption with acarbose.

Formal contraindications to α-glucosidase inhibitor therapy are intestinal malabsorption syndromes, inflammatory bowel disease, intestinal obstruction, and hepatic disease. However, small studies have suggested that acarbose is safe for patients with severe hepatic impairment. It is also contraindicated in cases of severe renal impairment (creatinine clearance <25 ml/min), in pregnant or lactating women, and in children aged <12 years because of a lack of data in these patient groups.

CONCLUSION

α-Glucosidase inhibitors significantly decrease postprandial plasma glucose and insulin, resulting in a reduction of A1C regardless of the therapeutic regimen already in place. This decline of A1C is sufficient to be associated with a long-term fall in microvascular complications. Recent data indicate that α-glucosidase inhibitors could be an option in the treatment of impaired glucose tolerance to prevent the development of diabetes. Although α-glucosidase inhibitors are safe agents, frequency of GI side effects may limit their use. It is thus recommended to initiate treatment with a low dose and to titrate upward slowly.

BIBLIOGRAPHY

van de Laar FA, Lucassen PL, Akkermans RP, van de Lisdonk EH, Rutten GE, van Weel C: α-Glucosidase inhibitors for patients with type 2 diabetes: results from a Cochrane systematic review and meta-analysis. *Diabetes Care* 28:154–163, 2005

Chiasson J-L, Josse RG, Gomis R, Hanefeld M, Karasik A, Laakso M: Acarbose for prevention of type 2 diabetes mellitus: the STOP-NIDDM randomised trial. *Lancet* 359:2072–2077, 2002

Chiasson J-L, Josse RG, Hunt JA, Palmason C, Rodger NW, Ross SA, et al.: The efficacy of acarbose in the treatment of patients with non-insulin-dependent diabetes mellitus. *Ann Intern Med* 121:928–935, 1994

Holman RR, Cull C, Turner RC, UKPDS Study Group: A randomized double-blind trial of acarbose in type 2 diabetes shows improved glycemic control over 3 years (UKPDS 44). *Diabetes Care* 22:960–964, 1999

Lebovitz H: α-Glucosidase inhibitors as agents in the treatment of diabetes. *Diabetes Reviews* 6:132–145, 1998

Tattersall R: Alpha-glucosidase inhibition as an adjunct to the treatment of type 1 diabetes. *Diabet Med* 10:688–693, 1993

Dr. Rabasa-Lhoret is Assistant Professor of Medicine, Department of Medicine Nutrition, Université de Montréal, Montréal, Canada. Dr. Chiasson is Professor of Medicine, Department of Medicine, Université de Montréal, Montréal, Canada. Both authors are from the Research Group on Diabetes and Metabolic Regulation, Université de Montréal, and members of the Montreal Diabetes Research Center, Montréal, Canada.

23. Thiazolidinediones

HAROLD E. LEBOVITZ, MD

The thiazolidinediones are a class of antihyperglycemic agents whose primary action is to decrease peripheral insulin resistance. Clinical and laboratory studies have revealed that they also have dramatic actions in improving many of the components of the metabolic (insulin resistance) syndrome. Several thiazolidinediones have been developed and were approved for use in clinical practice for the treatment of type 2 diabetes. Troglitazone was the first member of the thiazolidinedione family to be approved in 1997. It was very effective in improving insulin resistance and glycemic control; however, a rare complication of hepatic toxicity, leading to hepatic failure and death, caused its removal from the market in March 2000. Two other thiazolidinediones (i.e., pioglitazone and rosiglitazone) have been approved for the treatment of type 2 diabetes since 1999. Extensive clinical trials and clinical use in millions of patients have shown these drugs to be highly effective in the management of hyperglycemia and insulin resistance in patients with type 2 diabetes and not to have significant hepatotoxicity. However, other adverse side effects that appear to be common to all thiazolidinediones have been observed, and clinicians need to evaluate appropriate risk/benefit considerations when prescribing a thiazolidinedione.

MECHANISM OF ACTION

Thiazolidinediones exert their primary effects through activation of specific nuclear receptors named peroxisome proliferator–activated receptors (PPARs). There are three subtypes of these receptors: PPAR-α, -γ, and -δ. Most data suggest that the antidiabetic effects of thiazolidinediones are closely related to their ability to bind to and activate the PPAR-γ subtype receptor. PPARs, when activated, increase transcription of genes that have recognition sites for the specific PPAR subtype that was activated. Some of the gene products that are activated by PPAR-γ are important regulators of adipocyte differentiation, lipid homeostasis, and insulin action.

In type 2 diabetic patients, the intracellular insulin action pathway appears to be blocked at the level of the phosphoinositide-3 kinase molecule. This decrease in activity results when fatty acid products and cytokines are released from adipose tissue and enter the muscle and liver, which causes an activation of serine and threonine phosphorylases and puts phosphate groups on the insulin receptor sub-

Table 23.1 Clinically Relevant Metabolic Effects of Thiazolidinediones

Glycemic effects
- Increase insulin-mediated glucose uptake and utilization
- Decrease hyperglycemia in insulin-resistant type 2 diabetic patients

Nonglycemic effects
- Lipids
  - ☐ Convert small, dense LDL particles to large, buoyant LDL particles
  - ☐ Increase plasma HDL cholesterol
  - ☐ Decrease plasma triglycerides if they are elevated (>200 mg/dl)
  - ☐ Increase adipogenesis
  - ☐ Decrease plasma free fatty acids
- Vascular
  - ☐ Improve endothelial dysfunction
  - ☐ Reduce vascular peripheral resistance with 4-mmHg decreases in 24-h mean systolic and diastolic blood pressure
  - ☐ Improve procoagulant state by decreasing plasma fibrinogen and PAI-1
  - ☐ Decrease noninfective inflammation as measured by decreases in markers such as CRP
  - ☐ Decrease carotid artery intimal and medial thickness
  - ☐ Decrease neo-intimal proliferation after coronary stent implantation
  - ☐ Reduce microalbuminuria
- Pancreatic β-cells
  - ☐ Slow the rate of loss of β-cell insulin secretory function

strate-1 and -2 molecules in muscle and liver, respectively. This renders the molecules unable to transmit the insulin signal downstream to molecules that increase glucose transport in muscle, increase glycogen synthesis in liver, and generate nitric oxide in vascular endothelium. Thiazolidinediones decrease the release of free fatty acids and cytokines and increase adiponectin release from adipose tissue, and this reduces their inhibitory effects on phosphoinositide-3 kinase activity.

The in vivo effects of thiazolidinediones in humans (Table 23.1) have been studied extensively and can be divided into effects that regulate insulin action on glucose metabolism through their effects on adipose tissue and effects that alter the nonglycemic components of the metabolic syndrome. With the exception of their effects on plasma lipids, pioglitazone and rosiglitazone appear to have very similar actions. In head-to-head studies in a selected hypertriglyceridemic type 2 diabetic population, pioglitazone had a small effect in decreasing plasma triglycerides, whereas rosiglitazone did not. Both raised plasma LDL cholesterol levels, with rosiglitazone causing a somewhat greater rise, and both raised HDL cholesterol, with pioglitazone raising somewhat more.

Effects on Insulin Action and Glucose Metabolism

The effects of thiazolidinediones on glucose metabolism in type 2 diabetic patients have been elucidated using isotopic techniques that measure hepatic glucose production, insulin-mediated peripheral glucose uptake, and lipid metabolism as well as the standard parameters of glycemic control and lipoprotein homeostasis. Because thiazolidinediones act largely through activating gene transcription, their metabolic effects are not maximal until 3–6 weeks after initiating treatment.

The effect of thiazolidinediones in decreasing hepatic glucose production in type 2 diabetic patients appears moderate because they reduce fasting hyperglycemia by a mean of 50–70 mg/dl. The mechanism by which thiazolidinediones improve fasting hyperglycemia differs from that of metformin, and their effects in suppressing hepatic glucose production and fasting hyperglycemia are additive to those of metformin.

Both pioglitazone and rosiglitazone dramatically improve insulin sensitivity in patients with type 2 diabetes and insulin resistance. The magnitude of improvement depends on the baseline state and can vary from 35 to 70%. The improvement in insulin sensitivity has been demonstrated using the euglycemic-hyperinsulinemic clamp, the frequently sampled intravenous glucose tolerance test (analyzed by Bergman's minimal model), and the homeostasis model assessment for insulin resistance (HOMA-IR) model of Matthews.

The improvement in postprandial hyperglycemia is in large part the consequence of an increase in muscle responsiveness to insulin. The thiazolidinedione improvement in insulin action is thought to be secondary to their effects on adipose tissue metabolism. Insulin resistance in the ordinary type 2 diabetic patient is the result of diminished transmission of the intracellular insulin signal cascade in muscle as well as liver. The thiazolidinediones partially correct the adipose tissue–mediated abnormalities mentioned previously and thereby improve the intracellular transmission of the insulin signal.

Nonglycemic Actions of Thiazolidinediones

Thiazolidinediones are PPAR-γ agonists. PPAR-γ nuclear receptors are present in many tissues, including adipose tissue, endothelial cells, macrophages, vascular smooth muscle cells, skeletal muscle, and proximal tubular cells of the kidney. Treatment with thiazolidinediones improves many of the components of the metabolic syndrome.

- Insulin resistance dyslipidemia

  The dyslipidemia of insulin resistance is characterized by an increase in plasma free fatty acids and triglycerides, a decrease in plasma HDL cholesterol, and a shift in the LDL cholesterol particle pattern from predominately large, buoyant particles to predominately small, dense particles. Treatment with thiazolidinediones decreases plasma free fatty acids 20–30%; increases plasma HDL cholesterol levels between 10 and 20%; converts LDL cholesterol particles from small, dense particles to large, buoyant particles; and modestly reduces plasma triglycerides if they are >200 mg/dl (effects of rosiglitazone on plasma triglycerides are inconsistent). They also significantly decrease hepatic steatosis by as much as 50%.

- Endothelial dysfunction

  Normal endothelium maintains the balance between vasoconstriction and vasodilatation, prevents platelets and inflammatory cells from attaching, prevents vascular smooth muscle cell and fibroblast proliferation, and impedes lipid deposits. Insulin resistance shifts the pattern of endothelial function from the antiatherosclerotic profile above to a proatherosclerotic one. Treatment with thiazolidinediones restores arterial vasodilatation with mean decreases in 24-h ambulatory systolic and diastolic blood pressures of 3–5 mmHg. These PPAR-γ agonists decrease the production of adhesion molecules and growth factors and decrease vascular smooth muscle cell and fibroblast proliferation.

- Procoagulant state
  Insulin resistance leads to increases in serum fibrinogen and an increase in plasminogen activator inhibitor type 1 (PAI-1) production by adipose tissue and endothelial cells. PAI-1 is a known risk factor for clinical cardiovascular events. Treatment of insulin resistance with thiazolidinediones decreases the elevated levels of PAI-1.
- Inflammation
  Insulin resistance is associated with a noninfective inflammatory state. Various cytokines, such as tumor necrosis factor (TNF)-α and interleukin-1 and -6, and markers of inflammation, such as C-reactive protein (CRP), serum amyloid A, and fibrinogen, are increased in insulin resistance. Inflammatory markers have been shown to be risk factors for myocardial infarction. Thiazolidinedione treatment of insulin-resistant patients decreases these markers (TNF-α and CRP), suggesting that the inflammatory process is being reduced.

CLINICAL USE

The primary beneficial effect of thiazolidinedione treatment in type 2 diabetic patients is improving insulin-mediated effects on glucose metabolism in insulin-resistant individuals (Table 23.2). This result improves glycemic control and reduces insulin requirements. Secondary benefits are a reduction in plasma free fatty acids, a decrease in hepatic triglyceride content, an improvement in lipid profile, a return of endothelial function toward normal, a decrease in blood pressure, a lessening of the procoagulant state, and a reduction in the inflammatory response. These secondary benefits, which are reductions in cardiovascular risk factors, have been demonstrated with all thiazolidinediones and suggest that therapy with thiazolidinediones should have the potential to decrease clinical cardiovascular events. Somewhat surprisingly, recent clinical trials have not convincingly demonstrated such effects. An important secondary benefit of thiazolidinedione therapy that has been shown in several studies is a preservation of pancreatic β-cell function. All three thiazolidinediones—troglitazone, rosiglitazone, and pioglitazone—decrease the progression of pre-diabetes to diabetes by ~60% over a 3- to 4-year period. A Diabetes Outcome Progression Trial (ADOPT) showed greater durability of glycemic effectiveness with rosiglitazone compared to glyburide or metformin over a period of 5 years.

For thiazolidinediones to be effective in improving glycemia, insulin resistance must exist, and adequate amounts of circulating endogenous or exogenous insulin must be present.

Table 23.2 Reported Results of Rosiglitazone and Pioglitazone Treatment on Glycemic Control in Type 2 Diabetic Patients

	A1C (%)		Fasting Plasma Glucose (mg/dl)	
	Baseline	Decrease	Baseline	Decrease
Monotherapy				
Pioglitazone	10.3	1.6	276	65
Rosiglitazone	8.8	1.5	220	76
Combination with metformin				
Pioglitazone	9.9	0.8	252	38
Rosiglitazone	8.9	1.2	219	53
Combination with insulin secretogogues				
Pioglitazone	9.9	1.3	239	58
Rosiglitazone	9.2	1.0	205	44
Combination with insulin				
Pioglitazone	9.8	1.0	229	49
Rosiglitazone	9.0	1.3	209	47

Pioglitazone dose was 45 mg/day in monotherapy and 30 mg/day when added to metformin, sulfonylureas, and insulin. Rosiglitazone dose was 8 mg/day in monotherapy and when added to metformin and insulin and 4 mg/day when added to sulfonylureas.

Pioglitazone should be taken once daily without regard to meals. The usual starting dose for monotherapy is 15–30 mg/day, which may be increased to 45 mg/day if necessary. For patients not responding to monotherapy, combination therapy should be considered. In combination with metformin, sulfonylureas, or insulin, the recommended dose is 15–30 mg/day. The dose of pioglitazone should not exceed 45 mg/day in monotherapy or in combination therapy.

Rosiglitazone should be started at 4 mg/day or 2 mg twice daily without regard to meals. In monotherapy or in combination with metformin, the dose can be increased to 8 mg/day as a single dose or divided in two daily doses. It is recommended that the maximal daily dose when combined with sulfonylureas be limited to 4 mg/day. Coadministration of rosiglitazone and insulin is not recommended. Use of rosiglitazone with nitrates is not recommended.

Monotherapy with thiazolidinediones is indicated in type 2 diabetic patients who are not adequately controlled with diet and increased physical activity. The glycemic responses to pioglitazone and rosiglitazone are listed in Table 23.2. As monotherapy, thiazolidinediones should not replace sulfonylurea or metformin treatment because they have not been shown to be more effective than the other agents, although rosiglitazone has been shown to have a more durable effect on glycemic control. The glycemic response to thiazolidinediones as measured by blood glucose levels develops slowly over a period of 6–8 weeks. The maximal decrease in A1C occurs after 12–14 weeks.

A more effective glycemic response to thiazolidinediones is seen when they are combined with either insulin secretogogues or insulin treatment in patients with type 2 diabetes. These combinations make more insulin available to be sensitized by the thiazolidinediones. Combination therapy of thiazolidinediones with metformin also has increased effectiveness in improving glycemic control because the two classes of sensitizers have different mechanisms of action and their insulin-sensitizing effects are additive.

Table 23.2 lists the effects of treatment of type 2 diabetic patients with thiazolidinediones on the parameters of glycemic control. Because it is known that the absolute magnitude of the glycemic response to oral antidiabetic agents is a function of the baseline level of glycemia, it is difficult to compare the therapy-mediated decrease in A1C in type 2 diabetic patients whose baseline A1C levels are different. In monotherapy, both pioglitazone and rosiglitazone decrease mean A1C 1.5% in type 2 diabetic patients whose mean baseline A1C is ~9.0%. With rosiglitazone, 30% of that cohort achieved an A1C ≤7.0%. The addition of thiazolidinediones to patients inadequately controlled with metformin, sulfonylureas, or insulin results in further decreases in A1C of 0.8–1.3% (Table 23.2). Combination therapy of thiazolidinediones with metformin generally carries very little risk of hypoglycemia. However, when thiazolidinediones are added to sulfonylurea or insulin therapy, blood glucose must be closely monitored because the dose of the insulin-providing drug frequently needs to be decreased to avoid significant hypoglycemia.

Rosiglitazone (Avandia) is available in 2-, 4-, and 8-mg tablets. The combination of rosiglitazone plus metformin is available as a combination tablet (Avandamet) at doses of 2 mg/500 mg, 4/500, 2/1,000, and 4/1,000. A combination of rosiglitazone plus glimepiride is available in tablets of 4 mg/1 mg, 4/2, 4/4, 8/2, and 8/4. Pioglitazone (Actos) is available in 15-, 30-, and 45-mg tablets. A combination of pioglitazone plus metformin is available in 15-mg/500-mg and 15-mg/850-mg tablets. A combination pioglitazone plus glimepiride is available in 30-mg/2-mg and 30-mg/4-mg tablets.

Rosiglitazone metabolism is deceased by gemfibrozil and increased by rifampin, and the dose may have to be adjusted accordingly. Pioglitazone interactions with gemfibrozil and rifampin are similar to those of rosiglitazone. Pioglitazone may potentially interact with oral contraceptives through their common metabolism by cytochrome CYP 3A4. Ketoconazole may affect the metabolism of pioglitazone, and their combined use requires careful monitoring of pioglitazone's effects.

EFFECTS OF THIAZOLIDINEDIONES ON CLINICAL CARDIOVASCULAR EVENTS

Because of the effects of thiazolidinediones in decreasing insulin resistance, improving diabetic dyslipidemia, decreasing the inflammatory cascade, improving endothelial dysfunction, decreasing the prothrombotic state, decreasing the progression of carotid artery intima-media thickening, and reducing coronary artery stent re-stenosis, it was expected that chronic thiazolidinedione therapy would decrease clinical cardiovascular events. Surprisingly, two major long-term clinical trials to evaluate the effects of thiazolidinedione therapy on clinical cardiovascular outcomes, PROactive with pioglitazone and RECORD with rosiglitazone, have failed to show unequivocal benefits. PROactive was a prospective, randomized, controlled trial of 5,238 patients with type 2 diabetes who had evidence of macrovascular disease. They received glucose-lowering drugs with either placebo or pioglitazone. After an average observation time of 34.5 months, there was no significant difference in the primary composite cardiovascular end points between the two treatment groups. A composite secondary end point, which was defined only 12 days before locking the database and included all-cause mortality, nonfatal myocardial infarction (excluding silent infarction), and stroke, showed a 16% reduction with pioglitazone ($P < 0.027$). An analysis of the individual clinical end points (i.e., death; nonfatal myocardial infarction, including silent myocardial infarction; stroke; leg amputation; and acute coronary syndrome) as prespecified in the initial design of the study showed no significant differences between the two groups.

Several issues with the design and analyses of the data raise controversy about the interpretation of the data. The genesis of the secondary composite end point 12 days before locking the data is unusual. The exclusion of silent myocardial infarction in the composite secondary end point has not been justified. The low rate of statin use in the study is no longer the standard of care, and the secondary analysis shown at the presentation of the data indicated that those patients who were receiving statin therapy appeared to have no benefit in cardiovascular risk reduction from the addition of pioglitazone. A separate analysis of the subset of patients entering the study with a previous myocardial infarction also showed equivocal results. An interim (3.75-year follow-up) analysis of the RECORD study, which is a cardiovascular outcome study in 4,447 type 2 diabetic patients randomized to rosiglitazone with either metformin or sulfonylurea or to metformin with a sulfonylurea, showed no significant difference in any cardiovascular outcome due to rosiglitazone other than a 2.15-fold increase in congestive heart failure.

In contrast to a benefit in cardiovascular outcomes, a meta-analysis of clinical trial data from rosiglitazone studies reported in the *New England Journal of Medicine* in May 2007 suggested that rosiglitazone increases ischemic cardiovascular events in type 2 diabetic patients. This study has been heavily criticized; however, analyses from several groups, including the U.S. Food and Drug Administration (FDA) indicate that meta-analyses of clinical trials in which the end point was glycemic control and in which adverse events were not adjudicated do suggest a weak signal when rosiglitazone is compared to placebo but not with active comparators. The FDA found no signal for death or myocardial infarction but only to possible angina symptoms. A subsequent examination of all of the large, randomized, controlled long-term clinical trials involving rosiglitazone treatment, such as ADOPT, DREAM, RECORD, ACCORD, and the Veterans Administration Diabetes Trial have not shown any significant effect of rosiglitazone on clinical cardiovascular events other than congestive heart failure. Nonetheless, the FDA black box warning for rosiglitazone includes the following statement:

"A meta-analysis of 42 clinical studies (mean duration 6 months, 14,237 total patients), most of which compared Avandia to placebo, showed Avandia to be associated with an increased risk of myocardial ischemic events such as angina or myocardial infarction. Three other studies (mean duration 41 months, 14,067 total patients) comparing Avandia to some other approved oral antidiabetic agent or placebo have not confirmed or excluded this risk. In their entirety, the available data on the risk of myocardial ischemia are inconclusive."

SIDE EFFECTS

1. Hepatic

Troglitazone, the first thiazolidinedione to be approved and marketed, was associated with a rare idiosyncratic hepatotoxicity that led to liver failure and death. This condition led to the removal of troglitazone from the market in March 2000. There was an initial concern that liver toxicity might be a class effect of all thiazolidinediones. During its clinical trials, troglitazone treatment caused a threefold increase in the number of patients developing significant elevations of alanine aminotransferase (ALT) levels compared with placebo treatment, and two patients developed jaundice. During the clinical trials with pioglitazone and rosiglitazone, there was no increase in the number of patients developing significantly elevated ALT levels compared with placebo treatment, and no cases of drug-related jaundice occurred. In the decade that pioglitazone and rosiglitazone have been on the market, there has been no indication of significant drug-related hepatotoxicity. Despite this, it is still recommended that pioglitazone and rosiglitazone not be given to individuals with baseline ALT levels >2.5 times the upper limit of the normal range. Patients on thiazolidinediones should have liver function tests at baseline and periodically thereafter. In the event that liver enzymes rise to more than three times the upper limit of the normal range, the thiazolidinedione should be discontinued.

Several studies, including a 48-week trial of rosiglitazone therapy, have shown some improvement in the clinical and pathological features of patients with hepatic steatosis and nonalcoholic steatohepatitis treated with thiazolidinediones. This use has not been evaluated or approved by the FDA.

2. Weight Gain

Weight gain has been a constant feature of therapy with all of the thiazolidinediones. The weight gain is due to both an increase in body fat and fluid retention. PPAR-γ agonists play a key role in the differentiation of precursor cells into fat cells. During treatment of type 2 diabetic patients, thiazolidinediones increase subcutaneous adiposity but cause no significant change in visceral adiposity. The increase in total body fat averages ~1.5 kg at low doses and 3.5–4.0 kg at the maximal doses. The weight gain is somewhat greater when thiazolidinediones are combined with sulfonylureas and greatest with combination therapy with insulin (~4–5.4 kg). The increase in weight reflects increases in subcutaneous fat because visceral fat mass is generally unchanged or slightly reduced. A rare individual can gain as much as 5–30 kg. It is unclear as to what is different about these rare individuals.

3. Fluid Retention

Fluid retention is also seen during treatment with all thiazolidinediones. Hemoglobin and hematocrit are decreased on average ≤1 g/dl and ≤3.3%, respectively. These changes occur during the first 12 weeks of therapy and reflect increases in plasma volume because red blood cell mass is unchanged. Mild to moderate peripheral edema is observed in 4–5% of patients on thiazolidinedione monotherapy. This increases to 6–8% on thiazolidinedione and sulfonylurea combination therapy and 15% on thiazolidinedione and insulin combination treatment. The fluid retention is mediated by activation of PPAR-γ receptors in the proximal tubule of the nephron, which facilitate increased reabsorption of sodium in the proximal tubule. The fluid retention is poorly responsive to loop diuretics because they act predominately at the distal tubule. Indirect studies suggest that aldosterone antagonists may be the best agents with which to attempt to treat the thiazolidinedione-mediated fluid retention. The magnitude of fluid retention is ordinarily modest, although a rare patient may experience >5 kg of fluid retention. Discontinuation of the thiazolidinedione in such patients results in excretion of the retained fluid.

4. Congestive Heart Failure

The development of congestive heart failure in type 2 diabetic patients treated with thiazolidinediones has been an uncommon but consistent finding. This is likely a manifestation of excess fluid retention in individuals who have an increased susceptibility to develop heart failure. Most reported cases were in individuals given the maximum dose of the thiazolidinedione. Risk factors included combination therapy with insulin, female sex, and predisposing conditions such as chronic renal failure or prior cardiovascular disease. Thiazolidinedione-precipitated serious heart failure was reported in 5.7 % of the PROactive patients (type 2 diabetes with previous cardiovascular disease) treated with pioglitazone as compared with 4.1% of the control population. In the DREAM study with a population of patients with pre-diabetes, congestive heart failure occurred in 0.5% of the rosiglitazone-treated patients and only 0.1% of the placebo-treated patients. In the ADOPT study, which recruited new-onset type 2 diabetic patients, congestive heart failure occurred in 1.5% of the rosiglitazone-treated patients, 1.3% of the metformin-treated patients, and only 0.6% of the glyburide-treated patients. In the RECORD study, heart failure occurred in 1.7% of rosiglitazone-treated patients and in 0.8% of patients treated with metformin and sulfonylureas. Heart failure that can be attributed to thiazolidinedione therapy usually occurs within the first several months of treatment. In patients at risk, therapy with thiazolidinediones should be initiated with the lowest dose (15 mg pioglitazone daily or 2 mg rosiglitazone daily) and gradually titrated up with careful observation of weight gain and evidence of fluid retention. The maximal dose of the thiazolidinedione is to be avoided if possible, particularly when combined with insulin. Excessive weight gain during the first several weeks of thiazolidinedione therapy is indicative of excessive fluid retention and, if not reduced by diuretic therapy, indicates that thiazolidinedione therapy should be discontinued.

The FDA has placed a black box warning about congestive heart failure on the labeling of both pioglitazone and rosiglitazone.

- "Thiazolidinediones cause or exacerbate congestive heart failure in some patients. After initiation of Avandia (Actos), and after dose increases, observe patients carefully for signs and symptoms of heart failure (including excessive, rapid weight gain, dyspnea, and/or edema). If these signs and symptoms develop, the heart failure should be managed according to the current standards of care. Furthermore, discontinuation or dose reduction of Avandia (Actos) must be considered."

- "Avandia (Actos) is not recommended in patients with symptomatic heart failure. Initiation of Avandia (Actos) in patients with established NYHA (New York Heart Association) class III or IV heart failure is contraindicated."

5. Bone Fractures

In the ADOPT study, bone fractures were reported as an adverse event. Data from 1,840 women and 2,511 men randomly assigned to rosiglitazone, metformin, or glyburide for a median of 4 years were examined with respect to the occurrence of bone fractures. In men, fracture rates did not differ between treatment groups. In women, bone fractures had occurred in 9.3% of the patients on rosiglitazone, 5.1% of those on metformin, and 3.5% of those on glyburide. The increase in fractures with rosiglitazone occurred in pre- and postmenopausal women, and fractures occurred predominately in the lower and upper extremities. Subsequently, increased fracture risk has been noted with pioglitazone in the PROactive study population, the Periscope population, and in a polycystic ovary syndrome population. An analysis of 1,020 cases of low-trauma fractures in the large U.K. General Practice Research Database found that both chronic rosiglitazone and pioglitazone treatment (more than eight prescriptions corresponding to 12–18 months of therapy) increased the occurrence of bone fractures 2.43-fold compared with not using the treatment. Fractures were predominately in the hip and wrist and were independent of sex and age. Patients taking other antidiabetic agents had no increase in fractures.

The mechanisms for the thiazolidinedione-associated increased risk of bone fractures appears to be an increase in bone marrow stem cells differentiating into adipocytes and a decrease in bone formation from osteoblasts.

CONTRAINDICATIONS

Thiazolidinediones are not effective in the treatment of patients with type 1 diabetes (Table 23.3). Their effects on fetal development are unknown, and they should not be used during pregnancy. As noted above, thiazolidinediones are not recommended for treatment of diabetes in individuals with active liver disease. Initiation of thiazolidinedione therapy in patients with established NYHA class III or IV heart failure is contraindicated.

EXPECTED RESULTS

Thiazolidinedione treatment decreases insulin resistance and improves insulin sensitivity to physiological levels of insulin by 35–70%. These improvements can be measured by sophisticated techniques, such as the euglycemic-hyperinsulinemic clamp or the frequently sampled intravenous glucose tolerance test, or by simpler and more clinically available procedures, such as the HOMA-IR.

In the average type 2 diabetic patient with a mean A1C of 8.5–9.0%, monotherapy with a thiazolidinedione will achieve a target A1C of ≤7.0% in ~30% of patients. The ADOPT study showed that monotherapy with rosiglitazone is able

Table 23.3 Thiazolidinedione Therapy

Indications/FDA-approved

■ Treatment of hyperglycemia in insulin-resistant type 2 diabetic patients
  ☐ Monotherapy
  ☐ Combination with sulfonylureas, metformin, or insulin

Pending further study and approval

■ Treatment of androgen excess and anovulation in polycystic ovarian syndrome
■ Prevention of progression of impaired glucose tolerance to type 2 diabetes

Contraindications

■ Type 1 diabetes
■ Patients with clinical liver abnormalities
■ Pregnant patients

to sustain somewhat better long-term glycemic control (as measured by A1C in newly diagnosed type 2 diabetic patients) than metformin and very much better than glyburide. This greater durability of thiazolidinedione's glycemic effect is the result of its β-cell–protective effects. Although the ADOPT data might indicate that thiazolidinediones should be considered as the drug of choice for first-line treatment, this is obviated by their much greater side-effect profile and higher cost as compared to metformin, and most algorithms would place them as second- or third-line treatment options. Early use of combination rosiglitazone plus glipizide was able to achieve an A1C ≤7.0% in 56% of patients and an A1C ≤6.5% in 34% of patients in a recent study in which glipizide alone was able to achieve an A1C ≤7% in only 22% of the recently diagnosed type 2 diabetic patients. Early use of a combination of rosiglitazone and metformin achieved target goals of A1C ≤7.0 and ≤6.5% in 55 and 35%, respectively, of recently diagnosed type 2 diabetic patients. Similar combination data exist for pioglitazone. The data indicate that early use of combination therapy with thiazolidinediones plus either metformin or an insulin secretogogue is highly effective in improving glycemic control. As noted in Table 23.2, addition of a thiazolidinedione to patients not achieving adequate glycemic control on metformin, insulin secretogogues, or insulin is highly effective in improving glycemic control at the appropriate stage of type 2 diabetes.

Several nonglycemic effects of thiazolidinedione therapy are to be expected. These include improvement of the endothelial dysfunction of insulin resistance and other aspects of the metabolic syndrome, as described in Table 23.1. The clinical significance of these benefits are unclear.

Both rosiglitazone (DREAM trial) and pioglitazone (ACT NOW trial) have been shown to reduce the progression of pre-diabetes to diabetes by >60% over a median period of ~3 years. Because of their side-effect profiles, the role of these agents in treating individuals with pre-diabetes is unclear. Neither agent has been approved by the FDA for the treatment of pre-diabetes.

Thiazolidinediones decrease hyperinsulinemia in women with polycystic ovarian disease. This results in reduction in androgen secretion and, in some anovulatory women, restoration of ovulation. Such diabetic patients may be at risk of becoming pregnant during thiazolidinedione treatment. Thiazolidinediones should not be administered during pregnancy because of the potential increase in fetal mortality and growth retardation that have been demonstrated during mid-gestation and late gestation in laboratory animals.

The only differences demonstrated between rosiglitazone and pioglitazone in head-to-head studies were the small differences in lipid profiles achieved in a set of hypertriglyceridemic patients who were not on any lipid-lowering agents. Several studies have shown that the lipid profile effects of thiazolidinediones are minor in patients on statin therapy. Thus, in practical terms pioglitazone and rosiglitazone have very similar effects in type 2 diabetic patients on statin therapy.

Patients who are potentially at high risk for congestive heart failure or bone fractures should be carefully evaluated before initiating thiazolidinedione therapy and should receive periodic careful follow-up while on therapy.

BIBLIOGRAPHY

Aronoff S, Rosenblatt S, Braithwaite S, Egan JW, Mathisen AL, Schneider RL: Pioglitazone hydrochloride monotherapy improves glycemic control in the treatment of patients with type 2 diabetes. *Diabetes Care* 23:1605–1611, 2000

Bilous RW: Rosiglitazone and myocardial infarction: cause for concern or misleading meta-analysis. *Diabet Med* 24:931–933, 2007

Dormandy JA, Charbonnel B, Eckland DJ, et al. : Secondary prevention of macrovascular events in patients with type 2 diabetes in the PROactive Study: a randomized controlled trial. *Lancet* 366:1279–1289, 2005

Eurich DT, McAlister FA, Blackburn DF, et al.: Benefits and harms of antidiabetic agents in patients with diabetes and heart failure: systemic review. *BMJ* 335:497, 2007

Fonseca VA, Rosenstock J, Patwardhan R, Salzman A: Effect of metformin and rosiglitazone combination therapy in patients with type 2 diabetes mellitus. *JAMA* 283:1695–1702, 2000

Forst T, Pfutzner A, Lubben G, et al.: Effect of simvistatin and/or pioglitazone on insulin resistance, insulin secretion, adiponectin and proinsulin levels in non-diabetic patients at cardiovascular risk-the PROSTAT study. *Metabolism* 56:491–496, 2007

Glintborg D, Andersen M, Hagen C, et al.: Association of pioglitazone treatment with decreased bone mineral density in obese premenopausal patients with polycystic ovary syndrome: a randomized, placebo-controlled trial. *J Clin Endocrinol Metab* 93:1696–1701, 2008

Home PD, Pocock SJ, Beck-Nielsen H, et al.: Rosiglitazone evaluated for cardiovascular outcomes—an interim analysis. *N Engl J Med* 357:28–38, 2007

Kahn SE, Haffner SM, Heise MA, et al.: Glycemic durability of rosiglitazone, metformin, or glyburide monotherapy. *N Engl J Med* 355:2427–2443, 2006

Kahn SE, Zinman B, Lachin JM, et al.: Rosiglitazone-associated fractures in type 2 diabetes: an analysis from ADOPT. *Diabetes Care* 31:845–851, 2008

Lebovitz HE: *Clinician's Manual on Insulin Resistance.* London, Science Press, 2002

Lebovitz HE, Banerji MA: Insulin resistance and its treatment by thiazolidinediones. *Recent Prog Horm Res* 56:265–294, 2001

Lebovitz HE, Dole JF, Patwardhan R, Rappaport EB, Freed MI: Rosiglitazone monotherapy is effective in patients with type 2 diabetes. *J Clin Endocrinol Metab* 86:280–288, 2001

Lebovitz HE, Kreider M, Freed MI: Evaluation of liver function in type 2 diabetic patients during clinical trials: evidence that rosiglitazone does not cause hepatic dysfunction. *Diabetes Care* 25:815–821, 2002

Leier CV, Haas GJ: Diabetes and heart failure: the role of thiazolidinediones in managing these partners in crime. *J Amer Coll Cardiol* 50:37–39, 2007

Meier C, Kraenzlin ME, Bodmer M, et al.: Use of thiazolidinediones and fracture risk. *Arch Intern Med* 168:820–825, 2008

Mudaliar S, Chang AR, Henry RR: Thiazolidinediones, peripheral edema, and type 2 diabetes: incidence, pathophysiology, and clinical implications. *Endocr Pract* 9:406–416, 2003

Mulrow CD, Cornell JE, Localio AR: Rosiglitazone: a thunderstorm from scarce and fragile data. *Ann Intern Med* 147:585–587, 2007

Nissen SE, Wolski K: Effect of rosiglitazone on the risk of myocardial infarction and death from cardiovascular causes. *N Engl J Med* 356:2457–2471, 2007

Parulkar AA, Pendergrass ML, Granda-Ayala R, Lee TR, Fonseca VA: Non-hypoglycemic effects of thiazolidinediones. *Ann Intern Med* 134:61–71, 2001

Raskin P, Rendell M, Riddle MC, Dole JF, Freed MI, Rosenstock J: A randomized trial of rosiglitazone therapy in patients with inadequately controlled insulin-treated type 2 diabetes. *Diabetes Care* 24:1226–1232, 2001

Solomon DH, Winkelmayer WC: Cardiovascular risk and the thiazolidinediones: déjà vu all over again. *JAMA* 298:1216–1218, 2007

Westerbacka J: PROactive in patients with type 2 diabetes and previous myocardial infarction. *J Amer Coll Cardiol* 49:1781–1782, 2007

Dr. Lebovitz is Professor of Medicine at the State University of New York Health Science Center at Brooklyn, Brooklyn, NY.

24. Insulin Treatment

Jay S. Skyler, MD, MACP

Insulin was isolated and became available for clinical use in the early 1920s. It revolutionized the treatment of diabetes. Today, essentially all patients with type 1 diabetes and many patients with type 2 diabetes require insulin therapy. Although insulin has been available for nearly 90 years, major advances have been made over the past three decades in the way insulin therapy is used in clinical practice. Much of the progress is a consequence of three factors:

1. The introduction of self-monitoring of blood glucose (SMBG) into routine practice.
2. A change in the philosophy of diabetes management, such that patient self-management and flexibility in lifestyle have come to drive contemporary treatment approaches.
3. The development of insulin analogs that have time-action profiles aligned with physiological insulin secretion—both meal-related insulin secretion and basal insulin secretion.

This chapter emphasizes these changing practices. Because of major differences in both pathophysiology and treatment strategy, type 1 and type 2 diabetes are considered separately.

GENERAL CONSIDERATIONS

Types of Insulin

There are four major characteristics of insulin preparations:

1. Time course of action
2. Degree of purity
3. Concentration
4. Species of origin

The time course of action falls into four general categories:

1. Rapid-acting, including the genetically engineered insulin analogs insulin lispro, insulin aspart, and insulin glulisine.
2. Short-acting, specifically regular insulin (also known as soluble insulin).

3. Intermediate-acting, including NPH insulin (also known as isophane insulin) and lente insulin (also known as insulin zinc suspension; lente insulin is no longer available in the U.S.).
4. Long-acting, including the insulin analogs insulin glargine and insulin detemir, and ultralente insulin (also known as extended insulin zinc suspension; ultralente insulin is no longer available in the U.S.).

There are preparations of mixtures of regular and NPH insulins, including a human insulin mixture containing 70% NPH and 30% regular insulin (called "70/30") and a human insulin mixture containing 50% NPH and 50% regular insulin (called "50/50"). There are also preparations of mixtures of insulins based on insulin analogs—two formulations of insulin lispro (one containing 75% intermediate-acting and 25% rapid-acting insulin, called "lispro 75/25" and the other containing 50% intermediate-acting and 50% rapid-acting insulin, called "lispro 50/50") and one formulation of insulin aspart (containing 70% intermediate-acting and 30% rapid-acting insulin, called "aspart 70/30"). The action profiles of the various insulin preparations are summarized in Table 24.1.

Table 24.1 Time Course of Action of Human Insulin Preparations

Insulin Preparation	Onset of Action	Peak Action	Effective Duration of Action
Rapid-acting insulin analogs			
Insulin lispro	5–15 min	30–90 min	3–5 h
Insulin aspart	5–15 min	30–90 min	3–5 h
Insulin glulisine*	5–15 min	30–90 min	3–5 h
Short-acting insulin			
Regular	30–60 min	2–3 h	5–8 h
Intermediate-acting insulins			
NPH	2–4 h	4–10 h	10–16 h
Lente*	3–4 h	4–12 h	12–18 h
Long-acting insulins			
Ultralente*	6–10 h	10–16 h	18–24 h
Insulin glargine	2–4 h	Peakless	20–24 h
Insulin detemir	2–4 h	6–14 h	16–20 h
Insulin mixtures			
70/30 human mix (70% NPH, 30% regular)	30–60 min	Dual	10–16 h
75/25 lispro analog mix (75% intermediate, 25% lispro)	5–15 min	Dual	12–20 h
70/30 aspart analog mix (70% intermediate, 30% aspart)	5–15 min	Dual	12–20 h
50/50 human mix (50% NPH, 50% regular)	30–60 min	Dual	10–16 h
50/50 lispro analog mix (50% intermediate, 50%lispro)	5–15 min	Dual	12–20 h

* No longer available in the U.S.

Purity of insulin preparations generally is reflected by the amount of noninsulin proteins in the preparation. Insulins are defined as purified when they contain <10 ppm of noninsulin proteins and highly purified when they contain <1 ppm of noninsulin proteins. All insulin preparations sold in the U.S. and most Western countries are highly purified.

Insulin potency is measured in units. Originally, units were based on biological activity, but more recently, 1 mg insulin was defined to have 27.5 units of activity. In the U.S. (and most other countries), insulin preparations contain 100 units/ml and are known as U-100 insulin. For patients needing large doses of insulin, highly concentrated U-500 short-acting (regular) insulin (500 units/ml) is available. In some parts of the world, insulin preparations contain 40 units/ml and are known as U-40 insulin.

For many years, insulin was derived by extraction from bovine and porcine pancreas (mostly either a mixture of beef and pork insulin or only of pork origin). Today, most insulin is commercially produced by recombinant DNA technology. Preparations may be of the same amino acid sequence as native human insulin and thus are called "human insulin." The amino acid sequence may be intentionally altered to produce insulin analogs with altered pharmacological profiles—both rapid-acting analogs (insulin lispro, insulin aspart, and insulin glulisine) and long-acting basal analogs (insulin glargine and insulin detemir). Recombinant insulin preparations (both insulin and analogs) are less immunogenic than animal extracts.

Adverse Effects of Insulin Therapy

The major potential problem with insulin therapy is the risk of hypoglycemia. Other problems are cutaneous reactions to insulin and immunological reactions to insulin, leading to insulin allergy and insulin resistance.

THERAPY FOR TYPE 1 DIABETES

Insulin Secretion

There are two types of physiological insulin secretion:

1. Continuous basal insulin secretion
2. Incremental prandial insulin secretion, controlling meal-related glucose excursions

This is schematically depicted in Fig. 24.1. Basal insulin secretion restrains hepatic glucose production, keeping it in equilibrium with basal glucose utilization by brain and other tissues that are obligate glucose consumers. After meals, meal-related prandial insulin secretion stimulates glucose utilization and storage while inhibiting hepatic glucose output. Patients with type 1 diabetes lack both basal and meal-related prandial insulin secretion.

Flexible Insulin Programs

Contemporary insulin regimens for type 1 diabetes have multiple components that attempt to mimic the two normal types of endogenous physiological insulin secretion:

1. By providing components that give meal-related prandial insulin every time the person eats
2. By providing a separate insulin component to provide basal insulinemia overnight and between meals

Meal-related prandial insulin therapy. Prandial incremental insulin secretion is best duplicated by giving preprandial injections of a rapid-onset insulin analog (insulin lispro, insulin aspart, or insulin glulisine) before each meal by syringe, pen, or pump. Each preprandial insulin dose is adjusted individually to provide meal insulinemia appropriate to the size of the meal. Thus, the size of the premeal insulin dose parallels the size of the meal, ideally by relating the dose of insulin to the composition of the meal, particularly the carbohydrate content. In addition, the timing of meals need not be fixed, and meals may be omitted along with the accompanying preprandial insulin dose. The use of preprandial insulin doses permits total flexibility in meal timing. Patients may consume any number of meals per day— one, two, three, or more—taking meal-related prandial insulin with each meal, the dose determined by the meal content.

Rapid-onset insulin analogs (insulin lispro, insulin aspart, and insulin glulisine) are usually given immediately before eating a meal. In contrast, short-acting regular insulin administered subcutaneously has an onset of action that is not immediate, and prandial injections of regular insulin are best given at least 20–40 min before eating a given meal in an attempt to have prandial insulinemia parallel meal-related glycemic excursions. Moreover, its profile is less optimal than that of the rapid-onset analogs in that it has sustained action for a number of hours and thus may lead to postprandial hypoglycemia.

Basal insulin therapy. Basal insulinemia is best duplicated by giving one or two daily injections of a long-acting insulin analog (insulin glargine or insulin detemir). These long-acting insulin analogs are peakless and provide optimal basal insulinemia. Although insulin glargine and insulin detemir may have action up to 24 h and thus may be given once daily, as a consequence of their waning insulin effect at ~24 h, it may be desirable to divide these long-acting insulins into two doses, particularly in patients who do not have any endogenous insulin. In fact, by dividing these basal insulins into two doses—half on awakening and half on retiring—there may be greater flexibility in lifestyle, facilitating such things as varying times of going to bed and sleeping late some days.

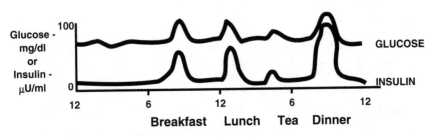

Figure 24.1 Twenty-four-hour plasma glucose and insulin profiles in a hypothetical nondiabetic individual.

Basal insulin replacement may be attempted with intermediate-acting insulin (NPH insulin) at bedtime and in a small morning dose, but this is far less optimal because NPH insulin does not have a flat insulin profile, but rather it has a clear peak of activity. NPH insulin has onset of action ~2 h after injection and has peak insulin levels ~8–10 h after injection, with action often not sustained beyond 12 or 14 h. When used, bedtime NPH insulin is given to provide overnight basal insulinemia, with peak serum insulin levels before breakfast, the time of relative insulin resistance known as the dawn phenomenon. Bedtime administration of NPH insulin also minimizes its nocturnal peak of insulin action, reducing the risk of nocturnal hypoglycemia. A small morning dose of intermediate-acting insulin provides basal insulinemia during the day. It is essential to include a morning dose of intermediate-acting insulin in patients using rapid-acting insulin analogs to ensure adequate basal insulinemia during the day, but this may be obviated if regular insulin is used for meals because of the prolonged "tail" of insulin action with regular insulin. Indeed, some patients may need a little intermediate-acting insulin with the predinner injection of a rapid-acting insulin analog if there is a long interval until bedtime and bedtime hyperglycemia occurs as a consequence of the waning effect of predinner rapid-acting insulin. In fact, a group in Perugia, Italy, used multiple small doses (four to six per day) of NPH insulin to replicate basal insulinemia by allowing curves to run together and create flat insulinemia at steady state.

Blood glucose targets. Blood glucose targets must be individualized for each patient. Targets must be explicitly defined if they are to be achieved. For healthy young patients, who readily recognize hypoglycemic symptoms and spontaneously recover from hypoglycemia, such targets may nearly approximate the levels of glycemia seen in nondiabetic individuals (Table 24.2). Targets are lower during pregnancy and should be raised in subjects who have difficulty perceiving hypoglycemic symptoms, who do not spontaneously recover from hypoglycemia, or in whom hypoglycemia might be particularly dangerous (e.g., patients with angina pectoris or transient ischemic attacks). In motivated patients, realistic targets are achievable 70–80% of the time.

Insulin programs. Basal/meal-related insulin programs are schematically depicted in Fig. 24.2. The multiple-dose premeal insulin plus basal insulin regimen has become increasingly popular in recent years and is the preferred approach to insulin therapy in type 1 diabetes. It offers flexibility in meal size and timing. It is

Table 24.2 Representative Target Blood Glucose Levels Suitable for a Young, Otherwise Healthy Patient with Type 1 Diabetes

	mg/dl	mmol/l
Preprandial	70–130	3.9–7.2
1-h postprandial	100–180	5.6–10.0
2-h postprandial	80–150	4.4–8.3
2:00 to 4:00 a.m.	100–140	5.6–7.8

straightforward and easy to both understand and implement. Moreover, the introduction of insulin pens has stimulated its popularity.

Initial insulin doses and distribution. The insulin dosage required for meticulous glycemic control in typical patients with type 1 diabetes within 20% of their ideal body weight, in the absence of intercurrent infections or other periods of instability, is ~0.5–1.0 units/kg body wt/day. During the relative remission (honeymoon period) early in the course of the disease, insulin requirements generally are less. During intercurrent illness, dosage requirements may increase markedly. Dosage also increases during the adolescent growth spurt, and some adolescents may have a sustained increased dose requirement.

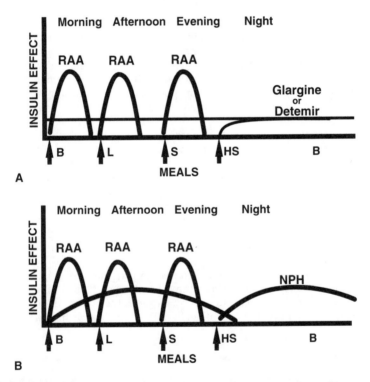

Figure 24.2 Idealized insulin effect provided by flexible multiple-dose regimens separately providing basal insulin and prandial insulin. *A:* Prandial injections of a rapid-acting insulin analog (insulin lispro, insulin aspart, or insulin glulisine) and basal insulin as a bedtime injection of insulin glargine or insulin detemir. *B:* Prandial injections of a rapid-acting insulin analog (insulin lispro, insulin aspart, or insulin glulisine) and basal insulin as an intermediate-acting NPH insulin at bedtime and before breakfast.

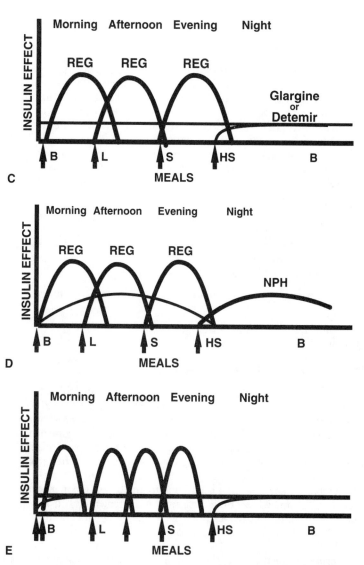

Figure 24.2 (Continued) *C:* Prandial injections of short-acting regular insulin and basal insulin as a bedtime injection of insulin glargine or detemir. *D:* Prandial injections of short-acting regular insulin and basal insulin as intermediate-acting NPH insulin at bedtime and before breakfast. *E:* Example of an insulin program involving four prandial injections of a rapid-acting insulin analog before meals and before an afternoon snack and basal insulin in which insulin glargine or insulin detemir is administered at one-half of daily dose on arising and one-half of daily dose on retiring, giving greater flexibility in sleeping hours. *Abbreviations:* B, breakfast; L, lunch; S, supper; HS, bedtime snack; RAA, rapid-acting insulin analog; Arrow, time of insulin injection.

About 50% of the total daily insulin dose is used to provide basal insulinemia. The remainder is divided among the meals either empirically, proportionate to the carbohydrate content of the meals, or by giving ~1.0–1.5 units insulin per 10 g carbohydrate consumed.

Dose alteration. Patients are provided with an action plan to alter their therapy to achieve individual defined blood glucose targets. These actions are guided by SMBG determinations and daily records. For prandial doses, the action taken may depend on the answers to several questions the patient needs to ask before any premeal insulin injection:

- What is my blood glucose level now?
- What do I plan to eat now (i.e., usual-size meal, large meal, or small meal; how much carbohydrate)?
- What do I plan to do after eating (i.e., usual activity, increased activity, decreased activity)?
- What has happened under these circumstances previously?

The answers dictate the treatment response. The intervention actions may include altering

- food intake (size or content of food)
- activity
- insulin dosage
- timing of insulin injections in relation to meals

An example of an action plan for dose alteration is given in Table 24.3. The plan assumes that the preprandial and bedtime blood glucose targets are 70–130 mg/dl (3.9–7.2 mmol/l). The plan should also call for separate action in response to a pattern of glycemia over several days. An example of such a pattern control action plan is given in Table 24.4. Such actions presuppose that the patient has a relatively stable pattern of meals and activities, has no intercurrent illness, and is free from unusual stress.

Considerable patient education is required to implement the management plan. Moreover, the patient needs continued access to and interaction with an expert multidisciplinary diabetes management team if successful management is to be achieved.

Other Insulin Programs

Considering prandial and basal insulin needs separately permits flexibility in eating and activity. Yet such an approach requires a motivated, educated patient who carefully monitors blood glucose several (usually four or more) times daily. In the absence of motivation, education, or frequent blood glucose monitoring, an alternative approach is to maintain day-to-day consistency both of activity and of timing and quantity of food intake and thus permit prescription of a relatively constant insulin dose. This permits use of either *1*) twice-daily administration of mixtures of short- or rapid-acting insulin plus intermediate-acting insulin (NPH), the so-called "split-mixed" insulin regimen, or *2*) morning administration of a mixture of short- or rapid-acting insulin plus intermediate-acting insulin, with predinner short- or rapid-acting insulin and bedtime intermediate-acting insulin—an approach used to minimize nocturnal hypoglycemia and counteract the

Table 24.3 Sample Plan for Premeal Rapid-Acting Insulin Dosing

Once insulin dosage is stable, use the following scheme for premeal alteration of dosage of rapid-acting insulin (insulin lispro, insulin aspart, or insulin glulisine):

BG <50 mg/dl (<2.8 mmol/l)
– Reduce premeal dose by 2–3 units.
– Delay injection until 10–15 min after starting to eat.
– Include ≥10 g rapidly available carbohydrate in the meal.

BG 50–70 mg/dl (2.8–3.9 mmol/l)
– Reduce premeal dose by 1–2 units.
– Delay injection until after starting to eat.

BG 70–130 mg/dl (3.9–7.2 mmol/l)
– Take prescribed premeal dose.

BG 130–150 mg/dl (7.2–8.3 mmol/l)
– Increase premeal dose by 1 unit.

BG 150–200 mg/dl (8.3–11.1 mmol/l)
– Increase premeal dose by 2 units.

BG 200–250 mg/dl (11.1–13.9 mmol/l)
– Increase premeal dose by 3 units.

BG 250–300 mg/dl (13.9–16.7 mmol/l)
– Increase premeal dose by 4 units.
– Consider delaying meal to 10–20 min after injection.

BG 300–350 mg/dl (16.7–19.4 mmol/l)
– Increase premeal dose by 5 units.
– Delay meal to 15–20 min after injection.
– Check urine ketones. If moderate to high, increase fluid intake, consider extra insulin (1–2 units). Recheck BG and urine ketones in 2–3 h.

BG 350–400 mg/dl (19.4–22.2 mmol/l)
– Increase premeal dose by 6 units.
– Delay meal to 20–30 min after injection.
– Check urine ketones. If moderate to high, increase fluid intake, consider extra insulin (1–2 units). Recheck BG and urine ketones in 2–3 h.

BG >400 mg/dl (>22.2 mmol/l)
– Increase premeal dose by 7 units.
– Delay meal to ~30 min after injection.
– Check urine ketones. If moderate to high, increase fluid intake, consider extra insulin (1–2 units). Recheck BG and urine ketones in 2–3 h.

Planned meal is larger than usual
– Increase dose by 1–2 units.

Planned meal is smaller than usual
– Decrease dose by 1–2 units.

Plan to be unusually active after eating
– Eat extra carbohydrate and/or decrease dose by 1–2 units.

Plan to be unusually sedentary after eating
– Consider increasing dose by 1–2 units.

Plan assumes target goals in Table 24.2 and should be individualized for each patient. BG, blood glucose.

dawn phenomenon. It must be emphasized that these are suboptimal insulin programs. They are schematically depicted in Fig. 24.3.

Generally, it is not possible to adequately control glycemia in type 1 diabetes using one or two injections of intermediate-acting insulin alone. The exception may be early in the course of the disease when some endogenous insulin secretion remains.

Table 24.4 Sample Pattern Adjustment Action Plan

This Action Plan assumes that the preprandial blood glucose targets are 70–130 mg/dl (3.9–7.2 mmol/l) and that the patient is measuring preprandial and bedtime glucose on a regular basis. Plans must be individualized for each patient.

Assumptions
– Basal insulin (bedtime glargine, detemir, or NPH, or basal rate of insulin pump CSII) is the major insulin acting overnight. Its effect is reflected in the results of blood glucose tests during the middle of the night and on arising the next morning.
– Prebreakfast rapid-acting insulin (lispro, aspart, or glulisine) has major action between breakfast and lunch. Its effect is primarily reflected in the results of blood glucose tests after breakfast and before lunch.
– Prelunch rapid-acting insulin (lispro, aspart, or glulisine) has major action between lunch and supper. Its effect is primarily reflected in the results of blood glucose tests after lunch and before supper.
– Presupper rapid-acting insulin (lispro, aspart, or glulisine) has major action between supper and bedtime. Its effect is primarily reflected in the results of blood glucose tests after supper and at bedtime.

Hyperglycemia not explained by unusual diet/exercise/insulin
– If prebreakfast blood glucose is >130 mg/dl for 3–5 days in a row, increase basal insulin (bedtime glargine, detemir, or NPH) by 1 or 2 units (0.05–0.1 units/h for CSII). [Before making such changes, verify that the blood glucose nadir, usually around 3–4 a.m., is not <70 mg/dl.]
– If prelunch blood glucose is >130 mg/dl for 3–5 days in a row, increase prebreakfast shorter-acting insulin (lispro, aspart, or glulisine) by 1 or 2 units.
– If presupper blood glucose is >130 mg/dl for 3–5 days in a row, increase prelunch shorter-acting insulin (lispro, aspart, or glulisine) by 1 or 2 units.
– If bedtime blood glucose is >130 mg/dl for 3–5 days in a row, increase presupper shorter-acting insulin (lispro, aspart, or glulisine) by 1 or 2 units.
– Only increase one insulin component at a time, starting with the one affecting the earliest blood glucose during the day.

Hypoglycemia not explained by unusual diet/exercise/insulin
– If prebreakfast blood glucose is <70 mg/dl, or if there is evidence of hypoglycemic reactions occurring during the night, reduce basal insulin (bedtime glargine, detemir, or NPH) by 1 or 2 units (0.05-0.1 units/h for CSII).
– If prelunch blood glucose is <70 mg/dl, or if you have a hypoglycemic reaction between breakfast and lunch, reduce prebreakfast shorter-acting insulin (lispro, aspart, or glulisine) by 1 or 2 units.
– If presupper blood glucose is <70 mg/dl, or if you have a hypoglycemic reaction between lunch and supper, reduce prelunch shorter-acting insulin (lispro, aspart, or glulisine) by 1 or 2 units.
– If bedtime blood glucose is <70 mg/dl, or if you have a hypoglycemic reaction between supper and bedtime, reduce presupper shorter-acting insulin (lispro, aspart, or glulisine) by 1 or 2 units.
– Verify hypoglycemic symptoms with blood glucose measurements. Treat hypoglycemic reactions with 10–15 g of rapidly absorbed simple sugar.

CSII, continuous subcutaneous insulin infusion.

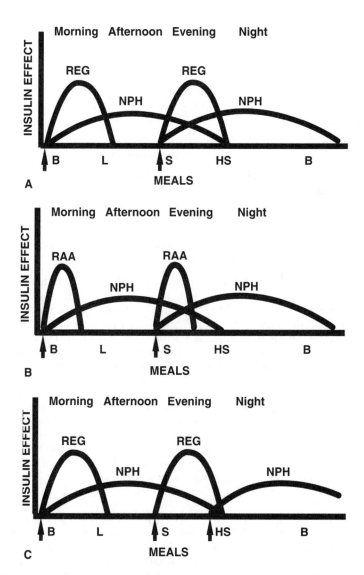

Figure 24.3 Idealized insulin effect provided by split-mixed insulin regimens. *A:* Two daily injections of short-acting regular insulin and intermediate-acting NPH insulin before breakfast and before supper. *B:* Two daily injections of a rapid-acting insulin analog (insulin lispro, insulin aspart, or insulin glulisine) and an intermediate-acting NPH insulin before breakfast and before supper. *C:* Regimen consisting of a morning injection of short-acting regular insulin and intermediate-acting NPH insulin, a presupper injection of short-acting regular insulin, and a bedtime injection of intermediate-acting NPH insulin. *Abbreviations:* B, breakfast; L, lunch; S, supper; HS, bedtime snack; RAA, rapid-acting insulin analog; Arrow, time of insulin injection.

THERAPY FOR TYPE 2 DIABETES

Pathophysiological Defects

Patients with type 2 diabetes have defects in both insulin secretion and insulin action. The impairments in insulin secretion are manifested in at least three ways:

1. Blunted or absent first-phase insulin response to glucose, so that insulin secretion is delayed and fails to restore prandial glycemic excursions in a timely manner.
2. Decreased sensitivity of insulin response to glucose, such that hyperglycemia may fail to trigger an appropriate insulin response.
3. Decreased overall insulin secretory capacity, progressive in nature with more prolonged and therefore more severe type 2 diabetes.

This impairment in insulin secretory response is not static but dynamic, such that chronic hyperglycemia may itself aggravate the impairment in insulin secretion, a phenomenon known as glucose toxicity. Thus, with decompensation of glycemic control in type 2 diabetes, there is concomitant deterioration in insulin secretory response. Moreover, and most important, when there is correction of hyperglycemia, there is some reversal of the impairment in endogenous insulin response to a meal challenge (i.e., a demonstrable improvement in insulin secretion). Thus, attainment of glucose control facilitates maintenance of glucose control.

Patients with type 2 diabetes also have impaired insulin action (insulin resistance) at target cells. This increases the overall insulin requirement. Like the defect in insulin secretion, this impairment in insulin action is not static but dynamic. Chronic hyperglycemia may aggravate the impairment of insulin action, another manifestation of glucose toxicity. Thus, with decompensation of glycemic control, insulin action is diminished. Moreover, when hyperglycemia is corrected, some reversal in the impairment of insulin action occurs.

Insulin Programs for Type 2 Diabetes

Recommended blood glucose targets for patients with type 2 diabetes are summarized in Table 24.5. When patients have been placed on a stable diet and activity program, they can be divided by degree of severity into four groups—mild, moderate, severe, and very severe—based on their level of fasting glycemia and ability to restore postprandial glycemia to basal levels (as a measure of intactness of prandial insulin secretion).

Table 24.5 Blood Glucose Targets for Type 2 Diabetes

	Goal	
	mg/dl	mmol/l
Fasting and preprandial	70–100	3.9–5.6
Postprandial	100–180	5.6–10.0
Bedtime	100–140	5.6–7.8

Mild type 2 diabetes. Insulin therapy usually is not used for patients with mild type 2 diabetes, i.e., individuals with fasting plasma glucose <110 mg/dl (<6.1 mmol/l).

Moderate type 2 diabetes. For patients with moderate type 2 diabetes, i.e., individuals with fasting plasma glucose 110–180 mg/dl (6.1–10.0 mmol/l), basal insulin therapy alone is often sufficient, with endogenous insulin secretion (perhaps facilitated by oral agents) being adequate to control meal-related prandial glucose excursions. Basal insulinemia may be initiated by long-acting (or NPH) insulin at bedtime. This is schematically depicted in Fig. 24.4. Required doses are generally in the range of 0.3–0.4 units/kg per day, but may be initiated with either 10 units or 0.2 units/kg at bedtime and increasing the dose based on prevailing fasting glucose, such as every week as outlined in Table 24.6, or every 3 days as outlined in Table 24.7. Basal insulin therapy serves to supplement the patient's endogenous

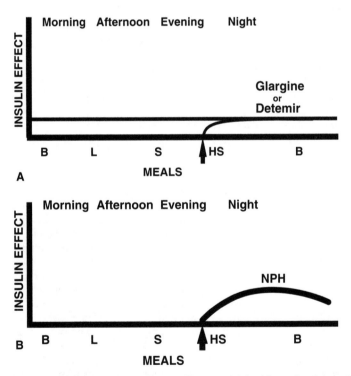

Figure 24.4 Idealized basal insulin effect provided by a bedtime injection. *A:* Bedtime injection of long-acting insulin glargine or insulin detemir. *B:* Bedtime injection of intermediate-acting NPH insulin. *Abbreviations:* B, breakfast; L, lunch; S, supper; HS, bedtime snack; Arrow, time of insulin injection.

Table 24.6 Sample Plan for Bedtime Basal Insulin Dosing in Type 2 Diabetes

This action plan assumes that the FBG target is 70–100 mg/dl (3.9–5.6 mmol/l). Plans should be individualized for each patient.

Start with 10 units at bedtime of basal insulin (insulin glargine, insulin detemir, or NPH insulin). Adjust the dose weekly based on the following guidelines:

If mean FBG during the previous 4 days is >180 mg/dl (>10.0 mmol/l):
■ Increase bedtime basal insulin dose by 8 units.

If mean FBG during the previous 4 days is 140–180 mg/dl (7.8–10.0 mmol/l):
■ Increase bedtime basal insulin dose by 6 units.

If mean FBG during the previous 4 days is 120–140 mg/dl (6.7–7.8 mmol/l):
■ Increase bedtime basal insulin dose by 4 units.

If mean FBG during the previous 4 days is 100–120 mg/dl (5.6–6.7 mmol/l):
■ Increase bedtime basal insulin dose by 2 units.

If mean FBG during the previous 4 days is 70–100 mg/dl (3.9–5.6 mmol/l):
■ Maintain current bedtime basal insulin dose.

If any FBG during the previous week is <70 mg/dl (<3.9 mmol/l):
■ Return to previous bedtime basal insulin dose

If any FBG during the previous week is <56 mg/dl (<3.1 mmol/l) or if there is any episode of severe hypoglycemia:
■ Reduce the bedtime basal insulin dose by 2–4 units.

FBG, fasting blood glucose.

insulin secretion and provides sufficient insulin to overcome the prevailing insulin resistance.

Severe type 2 diabetes. For patients with severe type 2 diabetes, i.e., individuals with fasting plasma glucose >180 mg/dl (>10.0 mmol/l), around-the-clock insulinization is necessary (bedtime NPH alone cannot be used). Most patients in this category require the addition of rapid-acting or short-acting insulin to attain adequate glucose control. Total daily doses required are generally in the range of 0.5–1.2 units/kg per day. However, large doses, even >1.5 units/kg per day, may be required at least initially to overcome prevailing insulin resistance. Such high-dose therapy may be necessary only to attain control, with subsequent control maintained on lower doses, on a basal insulin program, or even with oral hypoglycemic agents. Often, insulin therapy is continued at doses in the range of 0.3–1.0 units/kg per day. Premixed insulin may be used.

Very severe type 2 diabetes. The last category is patients with very severe type 2 diabetes, i.e., individuals with non-intact endogenous insulin response to meals, such that postprandial glycemia is not restored to basal levels within 5 h of meal consumption. In such individuals, fasting plasma glucose is usually quite elevated as well, i.e., >200–300 mg/dl (>11.1–16.7 mmol/l), but this category may include individuals with lesser degrees of fasting hyperglycemia. The insulin deficiency is

Table 24.7 Alternative Sample Plan for Bedtime Basal Insulin Dosing in Type 2 Diabetes

This action plan assumes that the FBG target is 80–110 mg/dl (4.4–6.1 mmol/l).

Start with 10 units at bedtime of basal insulin (insulin glargine, insulin detemir, or NPH insulin). Adjust the dose every 3 days based on the following guidelines:

If mean FBG during the previous 3 days is <80 mg/dl (<4.4 mmol/l):
■ Decrease bedtime basal insulin dose by 3 units.

If mean FBG during the previous 3 days is 80–110 mg/dl (4.4–6.1 mmol/l):
■ Maintain current bedtime basal insulin dose.

If mean FBG during the previous 3 days is >110 mg/dl (>6.1 mmol/l):
■ Increase bedtime basal insulin dose by 3 units.

FBG, fasting blood glucose.

so profound that, initially, these patients may be difficult to distinguish from patients with type 1 diabetes, although they generally do not manifest ketosis. Indeed, because of their similarity to type 1 diabetic patients, they are best treated like type 1 diabetic patients initially.

In all patients with type 2 diabetes, pathophysiological defects improve as glycemic control is attained and maintained. This facilitates control and may permit patients initially treated with insulin to be maintained with oral hypoglycemic agents or even on a diet and activity program alone.

Most patients with type 2 diabetes can be controlled with insulin if adequate doses are given and if the patient follows an appropriate meal and exercise program. The latter facilitates insulin action. Failure to follow a diet may countermand the effects of insulin and lead to a vicious cycle of progressively increasing insulin doses with failure to control glycemia.

TEMPORARY INSULIN THERAPY

One important use of insulin is as temporary therapy

- to initially attain glycemic control in patients with severe type 2 diabetes
- to overcome glucose toxicity
- to re-regulate decompensated patients

Indeed, type 2 diabetes may be considered a disease of periodic decompensation with the need for re-regulation, usually with insulin. For this reason, all patients with type 2 diabetes should learn insulin administration techniques and be prepared to initiate insulin therapy in the face of expected periodic decompensation, which occurs both spontaneously and with intercurrent illness or stress. Unfortunately, however, the temporary use of insulin is one of the more neglected principles of management of type 2 diabetes.

The hypothesis that short-term insulin therapy may induce long-lasting metabolic improvements in patients with type 2 diabetes has been tested. The degree of success varies depending on the stage of the disease. This approach works extraordinarily well early in the disease to initially attain glycemic control and to re-regulate decompensated patients with intercurrent illness or stress. When used in long-standing patients in whom other therapy has failed to achieve adequate glycemic control, results with temporary insulin therapy are variable. These patients probably have progressive pancreatic β-cell failure.

When using insulin to initially attain glycemic control, vigorous insulin therapy is needed to overcome insulin resistance and glucose toxicity. The plan here is a program of "sequential therapy" in which insulin is used initially to attain glycemic control, with subsequent control maintained by oral agents, diet and exercise, or basal insulin therapy.

When using insulin to re-regulate decompensated patients with intercurrent illness, it is often possible to merely add the insulin to existing oral therapy. As such, insulin may be used for a few days to a few weeks. Dosage may be either as supplemental insulin based on the prevailing level of preprandial glycemia (e.g., 1–2 units rapid-acting or short-acting insulin for every 50 mg/dl [2.7 mmol/l] above the preprandial glucose target) or as a relatively small total dose (e.g., 0.2–0.3 units/kg per day) added to the existing therapy, either as basal insulin or a combination of prandial and basal insulin.

INSULIN PROGRAMS FOR ELDERLY PATIENTS

Insulin therapy is often used in the elderly as a last resort—after failure of dietary management and maximum doses of oral hypoglycemic agents. The aim of therapy in the elderly is to relieve symptoms and prevent both hypoglycemia and acute complications of uncontrolled diabetes (e.g., hyperosmolar states). Schedules for the injection of insulin should be kept as simple as possible because self-administration may be difficult and dosage errors are not uncommon. Either long-acting basal insulin or premixed insulin may be used.

BIBLIOGRAPHY

Bretzel RG, Nuber U, Landgraf W, Owens DR, Bradley C, Linn T: Once-daily basal insulin glargine versus thrice-daily prandial insulin lispro in people with type 2 diabetes on oral hypoglycaemic agents (APOLLO): an open randomised controlled trial. *Lancet* 371:1073–1084, 2008

DeWitt DE, Dugdale DC: Using new insulin strategies in the outpatient treatment of diabetes mellitus: clinical applications. *JAMA* 289:2265–2269, 2003

DeWitt DE, Hirsch IB: Outpatient insulin treatment in type 1 and type 2 diabetes mellitus: scientific review. *JAMA* 289:2254–2264, 2003

Gerich JE: Novel insulins: expanding options in diabetes management. *Am J Med* 113:308–316, 2002

Hirsch IB, Farkas-Hirsch R, Skyler JS: Intensive insulin therapy for treatment of type 1 diabetes. *Diabetes Care* 13:1265–1283, 1990

Holman RR, Thorne KI, Farmer AJ, Davies MJ, Keenan JF, Paul S, Levy JC, 4-T Study Group: Addition of biphasic, prandial, or basal insulin to oral therapy in type 2 diabetes. *N Engl J Med* 357:1716–1730, 2007

Nathan DM, Buse JB, Davidson MB, Ferrannini E, Holman RR, Sherwin R, Zinman B, American Diabetes Association, European Association for the Study of Diabetes: Medical management of hyperglycemia in type 2 diabetes: a consensus algorithm for the initiation and adjustment of therapy: a consensus statement of the American Diabetes Association and the European Association for the Study of Diabetes. *Diabetes Care* 32:193–203, 2009

Porcellati F, Rossetti P, Pampanelli S, Fanelli CG, Torlone E, Scionti L, Perriello G, Bolli GB: Better long-term glycemic control with the basal insulin glargine as compared to NPH in patients with type 1 diabetes mellitus given mealtime lispro insulin. *Diabet Med* 21:1213–1220, 2004

Riddle MC: Starting and advancing insulin for type 2 diabetes: algorithms and individualized methods are both necessary. *J Clin Endocrinol Metab* 93:372–374, 2008

Riddle MC, Rosenstock J, Gerich J, the Insulin Glargine 4002 Study Investigators: The Treat-to-Target Trial: randomized addition of glargine or human NPH insulin to oral therapy of type 2 diabetic patients. *Diabetes Care* 26:3080–3086, 2003

Schade DS, Santiago JV, Skyler JS, Rizza R: *Intensive Insulin Therapy.* Princeton, NJ, Excerpta Med, 1983

Skyler JS: Insulin pharmacology. *Med Clin North Am* 72:1337–1354, 1988

Skyler JS: Insulin therapy in type II diabetes: who needs it, how much of it, and for how long? *Postgrad Med* 101:85–90, 92–94, 96, 1997

Skyler JS: Insulin therapy in type 1 diabetes mellitus. In *Current Therapy of Diabetes Mellitus.* DeFronzo RA, Ed. St. Louis, MO, Mosby, 1998, p. 36–49

Skyler JS: Insulin therapy in type 2 diabetes mellitus. In *Current Therapy of Diabetes Mellitus.* DeFronzo RA, Ed. St. Louis, MO, Mosby, 1998, p. 108–116

Zinman B: The physiologic replacement of insulin. *N Engl J Med* 321:363–370, 1989

Dr. Skyler is Professor of Medicine, Pediatrics and Psychology, and Associate Director of the Diabetes Research Institute at the University of Miami, Miami, Florida.

25. Incretin Mimetic and Incretin-Enhancing Therapies

Sunder Mudaliar, MD, and Robert R. Henry, MD

INTRODUCTION

The ingestion of food results in the release of a number of gastrointestinal (GI) enzymes and hormones that facilitate the absorption and metabolism of nutrients. Among these hormones are the incretins, which are produced by the GI tract in response to nutrient entry and play a major role in glucose homeostasis by stimulating insulin secretion, suppressing glucagon secretion, inhibiting gastric emptying, and reducing appetite and food intake. The observation that enteral nutrition provokes a more potent insulinotropic response than a similar load of glucose delivered intravenously led to the development of the incretin concept (Fig. 25.1). The first incretin to be identified was glucose-dependent insulinotropic polypeptide (GIP), which is synthesized in the K-cells in the proximal small bowel. Later, a second incretin hormone, glucagon-like peptide-1 (GLP-1) was identified, which is mainly produced in the enteroendocrine L-cells in the distal ileum and colon. The circulating levels of intact GLP-1 and GIP decrease rapidly following secretion into the circulation because of enzymatic inactivation, mainly by dipeptidyl peptidase-4 (DPP-4). There are currently two mechanisms by which the therapeutic potential of the incretin hormones can be exploited: through the incretin mimetics, such as the GLP-1 analogs (liraglutide) and exenatide (synthetic exendin-4), which are potent DPP-4 degradation–resistant GLP-1R agonists, and the DPP-4 inhibitors, which potentiate the incretin hormones by competitively inhibiting the enzyme responsible for their degradation. Clinical trials with the incretin mimetics and the DPP-4 inhibitors have demonstrated that these agents are effective in the management of hyperglycemia in patients with type 2 diabetes and may also possess other potential beneficial nonglycemic effects.

MECHANISM OF ACTION

Incretin Mimetics/Incretin Agonists

The endogenous incretin hormones GIP and GLP-1 exert their actions through interaction with G-protein–coupled receptors. The GIP receptor is mainly expressed on pancreatic β-cells, whereas the GLP-1 receptor (GLP-1R) is

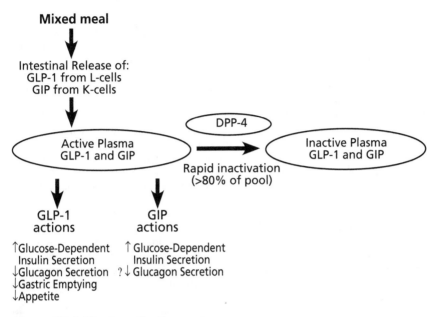

Figure 25.1 The Incretin Concept.

more widely expressed in the α- and β-cells in the islets and also in peripheral tissues, including the central and peripheral nervous systems, heart, kidney, lung, and GI tract. Activation of GLP-1R and GIP receptor in rodent and human islet cells leads to glucose-dependent insulin secretion and also an antiapoptotic effect with enhanced β-cell survival. In addition, GLP-1R activation leads to inhibition of glucagon secretion, gastric emptying, and decreased appetite/increased satiety. Of note, although GLP-1 effects on glucagon secretion, like those on insulin secretory responses, are glucose dependent, the counterregulatory release of glucagon in response to hypoglycemia is fully preserved even in the presence of pharmacological concentrations of GLP-1.

In patients with type 2 diabetes, the effect of the incretins to enhance insulin secretion is reduced or even absent due to a small but significant reduction in meal-stimulated levels of GLP-1 and an attenuation of the insulinotropic effect of GIP (despite near-normal levels). Because GLP-1 action (unlike GIP action) is preserved in patients with type 2 diabetes, therapeutic efforts have been focused on the development of GLP-1R agonists.

Exenatide is the first GLP-1 mimetic approved by the U.S. Food and Drug Administration (FDA) for use in patients with type 2 diabetes. Exenatide is a synthetic version of exendin-4, a 39–amino acid peptide that was originally purified from the saliva of the Gila monster (*Heloderma suspectum*). Exenatide shares ~50% amino acid sequence identity with human GLP-1 and is a potent agonist at the GLP-1R. Exenatide improves glucose control by multiple mechanisms. It augments insulin release in a glucose-dependent manner, suppresses glucagon secretion, slows gastric emptying, reduces food intake, reduces weight, and may preserve or restore β-cell function and/or mass. A prominent feature of type 2 diabetes is an absence of first-phase insulin secretion (the insulin normally secreted by pancreatic β-cells within 10 min after a sudden rise in plasma glucose concentrations). This early insulin response appears to be lost in the early stages of the disease, even when fasting glucose concentrations are only slightly elevated above normal. In one study, exenatide-treated patients with type 2 diabetes had an insulin secretory pattern similar to that of healthy subjects in both first (0–10 min) and second (10–180 min) phases after glucose challenge, in contrast to saline-treated diabetic subjects.

It should be noted that the enhancement of insulin secretion and glucagon suppression by exenatide is glucose dependent. This means that as glucose concentrations fall to the normal range, the insulinotropic and antiglucagon effects decrease. More importantly, exenatide administration does not impair normal counterregulatory hormone responses to hypoglycemia.

Because exenatide is resistant to DPP-4 inactivation, it has a long duration of action after subcutaneous administration, reaching peak plasma concentrations in ~2 h with a half-life of ~2.4 h. The drug is pharmacologically active for ~6–8 h and is predominantly eliminated by glomerular filtration. In in vitro models and animal models, exenatide has been shown to promote pancreatic β-cell proliferation and islet neogenesis from precursor cells. Currently, it is not clear whether these effects can be replicated in humans.

Liraglutide is another GLP-1 analog that is currently in phase-III studies in the U.S. This molecule is a GLP-1(7-37) analog combined with palmitic acid. With the addition of this fatty acid, the GLP-1 complex binds to serum albumin, and this increases the duration of action of liraglutide relative to native GLP-1. Albumin-bound GLP-1 is also less susceptible to degradation by DPP-4, and it has reduced renal clearance. Liraglutide has a half-life of ~10–14 h after subcutaneous administration in humans and can be given as a once-daily injection. Similar to GLP-1 and exenatide, liraglutide administration lowers postprandial glucose excursions, at least partly, by enhancing increased meal-stimulated insulin secretion, suppressing glucagon release, and delaying gastric emptying. Also similar to GLP-1 and exenatide, chronic administration of liraglutide to diabetic mice increases β-cell proliferation and β-cell mass.

Incretin-Enhancing DPP-4 Inhibitors

The endogenous incretin hormones GIP and GLP-1 are rapidly inactivated within minutes by DPP-4. Inhibition of DPP-4 prevents the inactivation of GLP-1 and thereby enhances and prolongs the action of endogenously released incretin hormones. Sitagliptin (Januvia) is the first compound in this class to be approved by the FDA for use in patients with type 2 diabetes. Another compound—vildagliptin—is currently undergoing late phase-III studies. Both drugs are orally active, rapidly absorbed, and efficiently inhibit plasma DPP-4 activity. Plasma DPP-4 activity is inhibited by almost 100% at 15–30 min after oral administration, and >80% inhibition is present for >16 h.

Several clinical studies in humans have demonstrated increases in active GLP-1 concentrations after administration of sitagliptin and vildagliptin. It has also been noted that DPP-4 inhibition increases not only prandial but also fasting levels of active GLP-1. Indeed, DPP-4 inhibition results in an overall increase in

GLP-1 levels with preserved circadian rhythm throughout the day. Because DPP-4 also inactivates the other incretin hormone, GIP, the concentrations of active GIP are also increased throughout a 24-h period after DPP-4 inhibition. This, however, is probably of less importance for the antidiabetic action of DPP-4 inhibition because, as mentioned earlier, GIP's insulinotropic action is attenuated in patients with diabetes. The increase in GLP-1 after DPP-4 inhibition stimulates insulin secretion, and studies have shown improved acute β-cell function with DPP-4 inhibition. Sitagliptin has been shown to increase homeostasis model assessment-B (HOMA-B) index, a marker for insulin secretion, and to reduce proinsulin-to-insulin ratio (a marker for β-cell function). Vildagliptin has also been shown to increase the insulin response in relation to glucose increase after meal ingestion. In animal studies, increased β-cell mass has been observed after DPP-4 inhibition. However, so far, this has not been demonstrated in humans.

Similar to the GLP-1 analogs, inhibition of glucagon secretion is another important mechanism for improved glycemic control by DPP-4 inhibition. However, in contrast to the GLP-1 analogs exenatide and liraglutide, the DPP-4 inhibitors are weight neutral and do not seem to affect gastric emptying, satiety, or appetite.

CLINICAL USE

Incretin Mimetics/Incretin Agonists

As discussed above, the incretin mimetics are effective in lowering blood glucose through their effects on the GLP-1R, which results in enhancement of glucose-dependent insulin secretion, glucose-dependent suppression of inappropriately high glucagon secretion, slowing of gastric emptying, and reduction of food intake.

The only incretin mimetic currently approved for use in the U.S. is exenatide, which is approved for use as adjunctive therapy to improve glycemic control in patients with type 2 diabetes who are taking a thiazolidinedione, metformin, a sulfonylurea, or a combination of metformin and a sulfonylurea and have not achieved adequate glycemic control (Table 25.1). The recommended starting dosage is 5 μg subcutaneously twice daily (in the thigh, upper arm, or abdomen) 0–60 min before the morning and evening meals (at least 6 h apart), and this dosage can be increased to 10 μg twice daily after 1 month of therapy if well tolerated. Exenatide should not be administered after a meal, and if a dose is missed, the treatment regimen should be resumed as prescribed with the next scheduled dose. Exenatide is supplied in prefilled pen injectors with fixed 5- and 10-μg doses, and the pen is prefilled with 60 doses (enough for a 30-day, twice-daily regimen).

In large, placebo-controlled trials in patients with type 2 diabetes who did not achieve glycemic control with maximally effective doses of oral antidiabetic agents (metformin, sulphonylureas, a combination of both, or thiazolidinediones), treatment with 10 μg exenatide b.i.d. resulted in mean A1C reductions of 0.8–1% over 30 weeks, with either prevention of weight gain or modest weight loss of 1.5–3 kg. Of note, patients continuing in the open-label extension of these studies not only maintained their glycemic control, but also lost more weight, with the total weight loss reaching 4–5 kg after 80 weeks. The most common adverse events with exenatide were GI (nausea, or more rarely vomiting or diarrhea). However, exenatide was rarely discontinued because of side effects. Of note, an increased number of mild to moderate hypoglycemic events was noted in patients given exenatide and sulphonylureas, but not in those given exenatide and metformin, despite a similar reduction in glycemia. Although the glucose-dependent insulino-tropic effects of exenatide should have prevented the occurrence of hypoglycemia, these effects are overridden by the concurrent administration of exogenous glu-cose-independent secretagogues (sulfonylureas or exogenous insulin).

Exenatide has also been compared with insulin glargine as adjunctive treat-ment for diabetic patients not achieving effective glucose control on metformin and a sulphonylurea. In a 6-month, open-label study, fasting glucose concentra-tions were reduced more in patients receiving insulin glargine, whereas postpran-dial glucose reduction was greater with exenatide (especially after breakfast and dinner). Both exenatide and insulin glargine reduced A1C by 1.1%. Of note, there was no significant difference in the overall rate of hypoglycemia, although noctur-nal hypoglycemia occurred more frequently with glargine administered at night, and daytime hypoglycemia was more common in patients given premeal exenatide. As expected, GI side effects (nausea, vomiting, and diarrhea) were more often reported with exenatide, and the dropout rate (19.4 vs. 9.7%) was also higher in the exenatide-treated cohort. The major benefit in the exenatide group was a

Table 25.1 Effectiveness of Exenatide and Sitagliptiin on A1C and Fasting Plasma Glucose

	A1C (%)		Fasting Plasma Glucose (mg/dl)	
	Base-line	Decrease	Base-line	Decrease
Initial Monotherapy				
Exenatide	NA*	NA	NA	NA
Sitagliptin	8.0	0.8	171	13
Initial Combination: sitagliptin + metformin	8.8	1.9	197	64
Combination with Metformin				
Exenatide	8.2	0.8	168	11
Sitagliptin	8.0	0.7	169	16
Combination with Sulfonylurea				
Exenatide	8.6	0.9	178	11
Sitagliptin	8.4	0.3	181	01
Combination with Thiazolidinedione				
Exenatide	7.9	0.9	164	29
Sitagliptin	8.0	0.8	168	17
Combination with Sulfonylurea and Metformin				
Exenatide	8.5	0.8	178	11
Sitagliptin	8.4	0.6	179	08

*Exenatide is currently not approved for use as monotherapy.

2.3-kg weight loss versus a gain of 1.8 kg in the glargine group. A major limitation of the study was that only 21.6% of the insulin glargine group and 8.6% of the exenatide group achieved the target level for fasting plasma glucose of <100 mg/dl. It must be mentioned here that exenatide is currently not approved for use in combination with insulin. Interestingly, a recent analysis found that despite an additional daily injection and a higher rate of GI adverse events, treatment satisfaction with exenatide injection twice daily was comparable with that of patients receiving glargine once daily (possibly because of weight reduction with exenatide). However, detailed cost-benefit analyses remain to be performed.

Of note, ~40–50% of patients receiving exenatide develop antibodies with weak binding affinity and low titers. So far, antibody formation has not been associated with any attenuation of the glucose-lowering effect of exenatide. However, the clinical significance of this finding remains to be clarified in longer-term studies.

Exenatide injection needs to be given twice a day because a subcutaneous injection of exenatide only produces effective glucose lowering for ~6–8 h. This may be a deterrent for some patients who may not prefer multiple daily injections. Thus, there is considerable interest in the development of exenatide long-acting release (LAR), which is a polylactide-glycolide microsphere suspension containing 3% exendin-4. In one small study in 45 patients with type 2 diabetes, 0.8 and 2 mg exenatide LAR given weekly decreased A1C by 1.4 and 1.7%, respectively, after 15 weeks, along with no weight gain in the 0.8-mg group and a weight loss of 3.8 kg in the 2 mg group. Exenatide LAR is currently being assessed in phase-III studies.

Liraglutide is another incretin mimetic that is in advanced phase-III clinical studies in humans, and like exenatide, liraglutide also effectively improves glycemic control in patients with type 2 diabetes, with preliminary data showing a decrease in A1C of 1.14% and weight loss of ~3 kg from baseline with the highest dose of liraglutide.

Incretin-Enhancing DPP-4 Inhibitors

DPP-4 inhibitors enhance levels of the active incretin hormones GLP-1 and GIP after the ingestion of a meal by preventing their degradation by the enzyme DPP-4. In the presence of elevated glucose concentrations, both GLP-1 and GIP increase insulin release, and GLP-1 lowers glucagon secretion, thereby decreasing the postmeal rise in glucose concentration and reducing fasting glucose concentrations. Sitagliptin (Januvia) is the first oral, once-daily, potent, and highly selective DPP-4 inhibitor approved for the treatment of type 2 diabetes (Table 25.1). Sitagliptin 100 mg inhibits plasma DPP-4 activity by 80% over 24 h, and this inhibition results in a two- to threefold increase in active GLP-1 and GIP levels, an increase in insulin and C-peptide levels, lower plasma glucagon levels, and lower glycemic excursion after an oral glucose tolerance test.

Currently, sitagliptin is indicated as monotherapy, as an adjunct to diet and exercise, to improve glycemic control in adult patients with type 2 diabetes; as initial therapy in combination with metformin; and as add-on therapy to metformin, a sulfonylurea, or the combination of a sulfonylurea and metformin when these oral agents do not provide adequate glycemic control. The recommended dose of sitagliptin is 100 mg once daily, with or without food, for all approved indications. No dosage adjustment is needed for patients with mild to moderate hepatic insufficiency or in patients with mild renal insufficiency (creatinine clearance ≥50 ml/min). For patients with moderate renal insufficiency (creatinine clearance ≥30 to <50 ml/min), the dose of sitagliptin is 50 mg once daily. For patients with severe renal insufficiency (creatinine clearance <30 ml/min) or in individuals with end-stage renal disease requiring dialysis, the dose of sitagliptin is 25 mg once daily. Because dosage adjustments are made on the basis of renal function, assessment of renal function is recommended prior to initiation of treatment with sitagliptin and periodically thereafter.

As with the incretin mimetics, when sitagliptin is used in combination with insulin secretagogues, such as sulfonylureas, the incidence of hypoglycemia is increased and should be closely monitored when sitagliptin is used in combination with a sulfonylurea. A lower dose of the sulfonylurea may be needed to reduce the risk of hypoglycemia.

Apart from sitagliptin, the other DPP-4 inhibitors undergoing late phase-III clinical studies include vildagliptin (LAF237; Galvus), saxagliptin (BMS-477118), and alogliptin (Syr-322; Takeda), and these should come before the FDA for approval in the near future.

SIDE EFFECTS

Incretin Mimetics/Incretin Agonists

The main side effects of incretin-mimetic therapy are GI in nature and include nausea, vomiting, and diarrhea. Of these, nausea is the most common GI side effect and in the clinical studies has occurred in up to 57% of patients treated with exenatide versus ~13% in those treated with placebo or comparable agents. Vomiting and diarrhea occur less commonly, in up to 17 and 13% of exenatide-treated patients versus up to 4 and 6% in those treated with comparator drugs, respectively. With continued therapy, the frequency and severity of nausea decreases over time in most of the patients who initially experience it. In some studies, up to 5% of subjects have discontinued due to the nausea and other GI side effects. Compared with exenatide, fewer data are available for liraglutide, the other incretin-mimetic in clinical studies. However, the available data suggest that the incidence of GI side effects may be lower than that seen with exenatide.

Recently, several postmarketing cases of acute pancreatitis have been reported in patients treated with exenatide. If pancreatitis is suspected, Byetta and other potentially suspect drugs should be discontinued, confirmatory tests performed, and appropriate treatment initiated. Resuming treatment with exenatide is not recommended if pancreatitis is confirmed and an alternative etiology for the pancreatitis has not been identified.

Because exenatide slows gastric emptying, it may delay the absorption and onset of action of concomitantly administered oral medications. For medications that are dependent on threshold concentrations for efficacy, such as contraceptives and antibiotics, or medications that require rapid GI absorption for a rapid onset of action (e.g., sildenafil or analgesics), patients should be advised to take the medication at least 1 h before exenatide administration. If such drugs are to be administered with food, patients should be advised to take them with a meal or snack when exenatide is not administered. Since exenatide has been on the market, there have been some spontaneously reported cases of increased INR (International Normalized Ratio) with concomitant use of warfarin and exenatide, sometimes associated with bleeding. Thus, INR should be closely monitored for a while when exenatide is started or the dose is changed.

Incretin-Enhancing DPP-4 Inhibitors

Unlike the incretin mimetics, which have predominant GI adverse effects, the DPP-4 inhibitors have a side-effect profile that is comparable to that of placebo except for a slightly increased risk of infection (nasopharyngitis and urinary tract infection) and headache. The exact significance of this is at present unclear. Of note, the FDA adverse-event reporting system recently reported 10 cases of angioedema during the first 8 months of postmarketing sitagliptin exposure. The proinflammatory peptides bradykinin and substance P have been implicated in the pathogenesis of angioedema. Substance P is sequentially truncated by DPP-4 into less potent molecules, and it is possible that DPP-4 inhibition might play a role in the pathogenesis of angioedema. Currently, this does not seem to be a problem, but patients should be monitored for any unexpected side effects. Recently, cases of pancreatitis and cutaneous vasculitis have been reported in postmarketing surveillance reports. Because these events are voluntarily reported from a population of uncertain size, it is not always possible to reliably estimate their frequency or establish a causal relationship to drug exposure.

CONTRAINDICATIONS

Incretin Mimetics/Incretin Agonists

Exenatide is contraindicated in patients with known hypersensitivity to the drug or to any of the product components. Exenatide is also not recommended for use in patients with end-stage renal disease or severe renal impairment (creatinine clearance <30 ml/min), children, and lactating/pregnant women. There are also no data on the use of exenatide in patients with type 1 diabetes.

Incretin-Enhancing DPP-4 Inhibitors

Sitagliptin is contraindicated in those patients with a history of a serious hypersensitivity reaction to sitagliptin, such as anaphylaxis or angioedema.

EXPECTED RESULTS

Incretin Mimetics/Incretin Agonists

Glucose control. In randomized clinical studies, the addition of exenatide in patients with type 2 diabetes with a mean A1C of ~8.5% resulted in mean reductions in A1C of ~1.0% and FPG of ~30 mg/dl. In these studies, ~45% of patients achieved an A1C <7.0%, and the dropout rate varied from 10 to 31%, primarily due to GI side effects (especially nausea), which tended to subside with time. Modest improvements in insulin sensitivity (as measured by HOMA) have also been reported.

Weight loss. In addition to improving glycemia, a notable advantage of the GLP-1 analogs is that they concurrently reduce body weight, independent of GI side effects. In the clinical studies, over 2 years, exenatide use resulted in a mean weight loss of 1.4 kg when compared to placebo and 4.8 kg when compared to insulin.

Lipid/blood pressure effects. In open-label extension studies, subset completer analysis revealed some improvements in lipid and blood pressure with exenatide therapy as compared to placebo. These include significant decreases in triglycerides (12%) and LDL cholesterol (6%) and an increase in HDL cholesterol (24%). The blood pressure changes include a mean decrease in systolic and diastolic blood pressure of 2.6 ± 0.9 and 1.9 ± 0.5 mmHg, respectively.

β-Cell function and β-cell regeneration. As discussed above, in rodent models and cultured β-cells, GLP-1R agonists not only lower blood glucose but also stimulate β-cell signaling pathways, which lead to β-cell replication/proliferation, inhibition of β-cell apoptosis, and an expansion of β-cell mass. Whether similar changes occur in humans is not known, but in clinical studies, exenatide has been shown to improve surrogate measures of β-cell function.

Incretin-Enhancing DPP-4 Inhibitors

Glucose control. In clinical studies, sitagliptin, the only currently FDA-approved DPP-4 inhibitor, lowered A1C by ~0.7% in patients with type 2 diabetes and a mean A1C of ~8.0%. The mean reduction in FPG with sitagliptin was ~20 mg/dl, and ~40% of subjects achieved an A1C goal of <7%. However, in one study when sitagliptin was used in combination with metformin as initial treatment in patients with type 2 diabetes (mean A1C 8.8%), greater reductions in A1C of 1.9% and FPG of 64 mg/dl were observed, suggesting that the greater benefit of this combination may be due to the complementary actions of these two agents. In human studies, metformin has been shown to significantly increase circulating GLP-1 partly by the inhibition of peptide degradation (possibly through a direct effect on DPP-4).

The above glycemic improvements were achieved without any major side effects. So far, the use of the DPP-4 inhibitors does not appear to improve measures of insulin sensitivity.

Weight loss. In contrast to the GLP-1R analogs, the use of DPP-4 inhibitors is not associated with any weight loss. In the clinical studies, sitagliptin has been weight neutral.

Lipid/blood pressure effects. Unlike GLP-1R analogs, use of the DPP-4 inhibitors has not been shown to have any effects on lipid or blood pressure parameters.

β-Cell function and β-cell regeneration. Measures of β-cell function have been measured in some of the clinical studies with sitagliptin, and these have shown only modest improvements in β-cell function as measured by the HOMA method and some favorable changes in the proinsulin-to-insulin ratio.

Table 25.2 Summary of Exenatide and Sitagliptin in Incretin Therapy

Indications/FDA approved
- Exenatide: In combination with
  - sulfonylureas
  - metformin
  - sulfonylureas + metformin
  - thiazolidinediones
- Sitagliptin: As initial monotherapy
  As initial combination therapy with metformin
  In combination with
  - sulfonylureas
  - metformin

Dose
- Exenatide: Initially 5 µg b.i.d. before morning and evening meals for 30 days and then titrated to 10 µg b.i.d. Exenatide is not recommended for use in patients with end-stage renal disease or severe renal impairment (creatinine clearance <30 ml/min).
- Sitagliptin: 100 mg once daily, with or without food
  - In patients with moderate renal insufficiency (creatinine clearance ≥30 to <50 ml/min): 50 mg once daily
  - In patients with severe renal insufficiency (creatinine clearance <30 ml/min) and in those with end-stage renal disease requiring dialysis: 25 mg once daily

Side effects
- Exenatide: GI (mainly nausea that tends to decrease with time)
- Sitagliptin: Side-effect profile comparable to placebo

Contraindications
- Exenatide: Known hypersensitivity to the drug. Caution in renal failure and type 1 diabetes (no data available)
- Sitagliptin: History of a serious hypersensitivity reaction to sitagliptin, such as anaphylaxis or angioedema

BIBLIOGRAPHY

Ahrén B: Dipeptidyl peptidase-4 inhibitors: clinical data and clinical implications. *Diabetes Care* 30:1344–1350, 2007

Amori RE, Lau J, Pittas AG: Efficacy and safety of incretin therapy in type 2 diabetes: systematic review and meta-analysis. *JAMA* 298:194–206, 2007

Drucker DJ, Nauck MA: The incretin system: glucagon-like peptide-1 receptor agonists and dipeptidyl peptidase-4 inhibitors in type 2 diabetes. *Lancet* 368:1696–1705, 2006

Garber A, Henry R, Ratner R, Garcia-Hernandez PA, Rodriguez-Pattzi H, Olvera-Alvarez I, Hale PM, Zdravkovic M, Bode B, LEAD-3 (Mono) Study Group: Liragludtide versus glimepiride monotherapy for type 2 diabetes (LEAD-3 Mono): a randomised, 52-week, phase III, double-blind, parallel-treatment trial. *Lancet* 373:473–481, 2009

Hermansen K, Kipnes M, Luo E, Fanurik D, Khatami H, Stein P, Sitagliptin Study 035 Group: Efficacy and safety of the dipeptidyl peptidase-4 inhibitor, sitagliptin, in patients with type 2 diabetes mellitus inadequately controlled on glimepiride alone or on glimepiride and metformin. *Diabetes Obes Metab* 9:733–745, 2007

Klonoff DC, Buse JB, Nielsen LL, Guan X, Bowlus CL, Holcombe JH, Wintle ME, Maggs DG: Exenatide effects on diabetes, obesity, cardiovascular risk factors and hepatic biomarkers in patients with type 2 diabetes treated for at least 3 years. *Curr Med Res Opin* 24:275–286, 2008

Mari A, Sallas WM, He YL, Watson C, Ligueros-Seylan M, Dunning BE, Deacon CF, Holst JJ, Foley JE: Vildagliptin, a dipeptidyl peptidase-IV inhibitor, improves model-assessed beta-cell function in patients with type 2 diabetes. *J Clin Endocrinol Metab* 90:4888–4894, 2005

Vilsbøll T, Zdravkovic M, Le-Thi T, Krarup T, Schmitz O, Courrèges JP, Verhoeven R, Bugánová I, Madsbad S: Liraglutide, a long-acting human glucagon-like peptide-1 analog, given as monotherapy significantly improves glycemic control and lowers body weight without risk of hypoglycemia in patients with type 2 diabetes. *Diabetes Care* 30:1608–1610, 2007

Dr. Mudaliar is Staff Physician, Section of Diabetes/Metabolism, VA San Diego HealthCare System, and Associate Clinical Professor of Medicine, University of California at San Diego, San Diego, California. Dr. Henry is Chief, Section of Diabetes/ Metabolism, VA San Diego HealthCare System, and Professor of Medicine, University of California at San Diego, San Diego, California.

26. Hyperglycemia in the Hospital Setting

SUSAN SHAPIRO BRAITHWAITE, MD, FACP, FACE

Hyperglycemia in the hospital setting occurs commonly and correlates with mortality and length of stay for patients with or without a previous history of diabetes (1,2). The medical and surgical outcomes of hospitalized patients depend in part on prevention or control of hyperglycemia in the hospital (3–10). The morbidities associated with hospitalization and the conditions of hospital routine increase the risk for spontaneous and iatrogenic hypoglycemia (11–17). Management strategies do not invariably succeed in meeting present-day glycemic targets (18).

The fundamental problem is the need to control hyperglycemia in the hospital setting for a vulnerable population without introducing morbidity or mortality due to hypoglycemia. Insulin resistance fluctuates in relation to the nature and severity of the underlying medical condition, comorbidities, nutritional status, and organ dysfunction. Concomitant treatment of the patient, including medications and carbohydrate exposure, frequently change. Preestablished ambulatory therapies are not necessarily efficacious or safe. The factors responsible for hyperglycemia, including stress and mediators, and the pathogenesis of harms induced by hyperglycemia in the hospital setting or of the benefits conferred by insulin therapy are incompletely understood. There is proof of inferiority of sliding-scale management compared to scheduled subcutaneous insulin and intravenous insulin infusion (19,20). Within either category of preferred management, however, scheduled subcutaneous insulin therapy or intravenous insulin infusion, there is lack of proof of superiority of any particular published approach. The ideal glycemic targets remain controversial and might differ according to factors that include patient population, diagnoses, and setting within the hospital.

A second problem is the need to work within the constraints of complex institutional care. Successful management requires coordination of blood glucose monitoring, nutrition, and administration of medication. Handoffs by providers, shift changes of nurses, and patient relocations between the emergency department or the preadmitting office, holding areas, the operating room, the critical-care setting, general wards, and home all require communication strategies. Important to patient safety is the protection of two competing principles, individualization of patient care and institutional standardization of procedures to excellence. To achieve individualization according to patient characteristics, the necessary complexity can be embedded in a branching pathway that permits selections and standardizes components of care to excellence (Table 26.1).

A third problem is the need for institutional self-evaluation (21–23). Measurement of glucose as an analyte yields differing results depending on methodology, site of sampling, and patient factors. No simple laboratory analytical method comparable with measurement of A1C can capture the results of short-term average glycemic control at the patient level under conditions of hospitalization. The analysis of institutional aggregate data presents challenges. Glycemic outcomes may be reported by using as the unit of observation the blood glucose, the time-weighted area under the curve for the entire patient stay, an average for the individual patient for a critical time frame, the patient day, the aggregate blood glucose average for various hospital wards or services, the count of hyperglycemic or hypoglycemic events, or other measure. Evaluation methods that assess only central tendency and variability of a large number of blood glucose measurements may obscure the impact of isolated severe episodes of hypoglycemia. Analysis of hypoglycemia requires isolation of severe episodes and evaluation of the clinical impact of nonfatal events (16).

DISCUSSION

Preexisting diabetes and newly recognized hospital hyperglycemia are treated with insulin to achieve target range control during admission. Treatment with oral antihyperglycemic agents is generally interrupted during admission and is replaced with insulin therapy. From the time of preadmission and preprocedure planning to the time of discharge, and during transitions between treatment modalities and hospital sites, therapeutic strategies and insulin dose requirements undergo modification. Potentially both subcutaneous insulin injection therapy and intravenous

---

Table 26.1 Elements of a Glycemic Management Pathway

- Preadmission instructions
- A1C
- Nutrition orders
- Nursing orders
  —point-of-care glucose monitoring
  —call parameters
  —nursing assessment of needs
- Pharmacy-scheduled insulin orders
  —subcutaneous insulin
  —intravenous insulin infusion
  —insulin for patient self-management

- Pharmacy "PRN" orders
  —subcutaneous insulin correction doses
  —dextrose 50% in water
  —glucagon
- Cancellation of conflicting orders
- Consultations as needed
  —nutritionist
  —nurse educator
  —endocrinologist, diabetes specialist, or hospitalist
  —other providers
- Patient education
- Discharge planning

PRN, as needed.

insulin infusion may be utilized at different times during hospitalization, together with transitioning strategies (19,20,24–39). Some experienced patients are candidates for self-management with insulin (21,36).

Through multidisciplinary effort and consensus, a standardized set of hospital-wide, ward-based, or service-based policies, protocols, and procedures are developed for inpatient management with appropriate subroutines, defining roles for the provider, nurse, pharmacist, laboratory staff, nutrition personnel, diabetes specialist, and patient. Hospital staff receive in-servicing on components of the pathway. Elements of the pathway are selected and ordered by the provider (Table 26.1). The content of the pathway includes preadmission planning, dietary options with menu display of carbohydrate content, hypoglycemia treatment and prevention, display of pharmacy orders, charting tools for display of the results of blood glucose monitoring and insulin administration, standardized templates for provider-directed insulin management and periprocedure modifications, a program for diabetes hospital patient self-management, provision for consultations, options for patient education, and discharge planning. Paper or computerized order sets are completed by checking boxes, entering numbers, and providing additional directions. Order sets are designed to offer several appropriate patterns of insulin use and glucose monitoring appropriate to common patterns of carbohydrate exposure and to facilitate daily insulin dose and pattern revisions.

The insulin requirement may be considered to have basal and nutritional components. The basal requirement is the amount of insulin necessary to prevent unchecked gluconeogenesis and ketogenesis. The basal amount is necessary and sufficient to maintain euglycemia in the absence of carbohydrate exposure under current conditions of comorbidity and medication. The nutritional insulin requirement is the amount of insulin above the basal insulin dose that is necessary to maintain euglycemia during normal meals, infusion of maintenance fluids containing dextrose, or administration of intravenous or enteral nutritional support. Nutritional insulin used to cover discrete meals is called prandial insulin. During subcutaneous insulin therapy, the principal determinant of the types of insulin used and pattern of administration is the pattern of carbohydrate exposure. Correction dose therapy refers to the use of supplemental doses of rapid-acting insulin analog or short-acting insulin added to scheduled subcutaneous therapy in order to achieve rapid correction of hyperglycemia.

Expert opinion has been offered in support of management principles and specific glycemic targets (40,41). With recognition that hospital hyperglycemia may be discovered among patients not known to have diabetes, glucose monitoring appropriate to patient condition should be ordered upon admission. For patients not known to have diabetes, a determination that scheduled insulin is required usually is based on hospital, ward, and service glycemic thresholds for intervention appropriate to patient condition. The targets and strategy endorsed by the American Diabetes Association (ADA) are evolving to reflect results of clinical research (41). Revisions of glycemic targets may be anticipated in response to new evidence.

TREATMENT

For all dosing guidelines, individualization is appropriate when general guidelines do not match the characteristics of the patient.

The term "total daily dose of insulin" (TDDI) means total number of units of any type of insulin taken per 24 h, viewed retrospectively. The term "24-h dose of basal insulin" will be used to mean the total number of units of NPH or long-acting insulin analog administered per 24 h to patients who also use prandial therapy with rapid-acting insulin analogs or regular insulin. Once the TDDI has been corrected to eliminate hypoglycemia, if any, then empirically the reassigned 24-h basal insulin dose for NPO status may be computed with reference to the TDDI. The "reassigned 24-h dose of basal insulin for NPO status" for type 1 diabetes is estimated at 50% of the TDDI or the total daily amount of NPH or long-acting insulin analog (if either of these is used), whichever is the smaller amount. The "reassigned 24-h dose of basal insulin for NPO status" for type 2 diabetes, if basal insulin is required at all, is estimated at 25% of the TDDI or 0.15 units/kg body wt, whichever is the smaller amount.

Preadmission Planning for Elective Procedures

Before elective surgical procedures, to assess adequacy of glycemic control of patients with known diabetes, the provider should review the history of symptoms of hypoglycemia or hyperglycemia and the results self-monitoring of blood glucose and should measure A1C. If insulin is used and hypoglycemia is reported, preoperative or preprocedure reduction of the TDDI by 10–20% should occur. Uncontrolled hyperglycemic patients should postpone elective procedures while intensification of glycemic management is attempted.

If a procedure is planned for the morning of admission, the patient is instructed on oral intake and antihyperglycemic mediation. In general oral antihyperglycemic agents and scheduled doses of regular insulin or rapid-acting insulin analog should be withheld starting the night before surgery. There may be a perioperative requirement for exogenous basal insulin, but the patient may not be equipped with the ideal insulin preparation at home to deliver preoperative basal insulin. For patients treated with premixed insulin or biphasic insulin analog preparations, the last preoperative dose of premixed insulin or biphasic insulin analog is taken at supper on the day before surgery, possibly reduced by 10–20% for type 1 diabetes according to history of hypoglycemia and generally reduced to an amount ≤50% of the usual dose for type 2 diabetes.

For patients with access to NPH or long-acting insulin analog at home, basal insulin is provided preoperatively, starting at bedtime on the night before surgery, by continuing the use of NPH or long-acting insulin analog until arrival, divided into morning and evening fractions in the pattern to which the patient is accustomed, in a daily amount equaling the reassigned 24-h dose of basal insulin for NPO status or by replacement of subcutaneous insulin on the morning of surgery with intravenous insulin infusion, initiated upon arrival. For some patients with type 2 diabetes, home basal insulin may be withheld beginning the night before or morning of surgery.

Upon arrival for a procedure to be followed by hospitalization, subcutaneous correction doses of regular insulin or rapid-acting analog for blood glucose >180 mg/dl or intravenous insulin infusion for blood glucose >140 mg/dl are ordered prior to induction of anesthesia. Patients who have withheld the morning component of the reassigned 24-h dose of basal insulin for NPO status for the day of surgery, but who were candidates for subcutaneous management, may be given the omitted dose of NPH or long-acting insulin analog upon arrival. The decision to use intravenous insulin infusion depends on the anticipated duration and complexity of surgery, expected hemodynamic stability, the results of blood glucose monitoring, and the classification of diabetes. In all cases, patients with type 1 diabetes must either have active effect from previously administered subcutaneous insulin on board or must receive intravenous insulin infusion. Intraoperative monitoring is required for procedures that are prolonged >1 h or are complex. In case of intraoperative destabilization of the patient or rising blood glucose, an initial decision to rely upon subcutaneous insulin may be revised in favor of intravenous infusion.

Nutrition

Nutrition orders include meal plans; dextrose-containing maintenance intravenous fluids; oral nutritional supplements; enteral continuous, overnight, or bolus tube feedings; or total parenteral nutrition (TPN). The glycemic management pathway includes subroutines that link delivery of nutrition to a pattern of point-of-care glucose monitoring and insulin administration. Consultative involvement of nutrition specialists often is advantageous for inpatient care and patient education. Some facilities use carbohydrate counting to assign prandial doses of rapid-acting insulin analog for patients who are eating. During normal dietary intake, for patients or staff inexperienced in use of the skills of advanced carbohydrate counting, a consistent carbohydrate meal plan is advocated (40). Dietary options should be developed by the institutions, with menu display of carbohydrate content.

Hypoglycemia Treatment and Prevention

A nursing hypoglycemia protocol not only outlines use of oral carbohydrate, concentrated intravenous dextrose, or glucagon for treatment of hypoglycemia, but also describes measures to prevent hypoglycemia. A pharmacy order may be required in advance to make intravenous concentrated dextrose or glucagon available as needed for treatment of hypoglycemia under the nursing protocol. For patients receiving scheduled antihyperglycemic therapy, the preventive component of the protocol either specifies an action or requires a call to the provider in case of sudden interruption of enteral carbohydrate exposure. The provider receiving such as call may interrupt or revise nutritional insulin orders, increase the frequency of blood glucose monitoring, and/or order infusion of dextrose in saline or water at a concentration and infusion rate that the patient would require and tolerate and for a duration necessary to cover the action of insulin already given.

Subcutaneous Insulin Therapy

Standardized paper or computerized templates are recommended for entry of orders for blood glucose monitoring and for scheduled and correction insulin doses, with times, frequency, additional directions, priority, and other components of orders associated with insulin therapy (Fig. 26.1). The additional directions should appear in the display of pharmacy orders. The ideal bedside glycemic management flowsheet should chart times, results of blood glucose monitoring, and insulin administered.

Assignment of scheduled total daily dose of subcutaneous insulin. After a determination has been made that subcutaneous insulin is required in the hospital, the first task for the prescriber is to determine the initial daily dose that will be scheduled. The method of dose assignment differs for the patient naïve to insulin and eating discrete meals, the patient who had used insulin in the ambulatory setting and is eating, the patient with negligible oral energy intake, and the patient at the point of transition from intravenous insulin therapy. Analysis of comorbidities, concomitant medications, and classification of diabetes contributes to initial dose assignment and to the allocation of the dose to components of therapy (20,24,31,32).

For the patient naïve to insulin in the ambulatory setting but manifesting hyperglycemia in the hospital and eating discrete meals, estimates of insulin requirement are based on body weight. For type 2 diabetes, the initial total daily dose using various published methods may be estimated conservatively at 0.3 units/kg/day (26), 0.4 units/kg/day for blood glucose 140–200 mg/dl and 0.5 units/kg/day for blood glucose 201–400 mg/dl (20), or 0.5–0.7 units/kg/day (32), or with a range of 0.4–1.0 units/kg/day (24). For the patient with newly diagnosed type 1 diabetes, the initial estimate may be 0.5 units/kg/day (26) or the range may be 0.5–0.7 or 0.3–0.5 units/kg/day (24,32). For diabetes of unknown classification, an initial total daily dose of 0.3–0.5 units/kg/day may be used (32). In the RABBIT-2 trial of basal-prandial-correction therapy versus sliding scale for type 2 diabetic patients on a general medical ward, the group receiving basal-bolus therapy had a mean daily dose of 22 ± 2 units of basal insulin glargine and

Subcutaneous scheduled daily insulin. Check appropriate times or meal times to right, and fill in insulin doses below.	☐ 0600 or ☐ Breakfast	☐ 1200 or ☐ Lunch	☐ 1800 or ☐ Supper	☐ 2400 or ☐ Bedtime
Rapid-acting insulin analog	_____ units	_____ units	_____ units	_____ units
Short-acting regular insulin	_____ units	_____ units	_____ units	_____ units
Intermediate-acting NPH insulin	_____ units	_____ units	_____ units	_____ units
Long-acting insulin analog	_____ units			_____ units
Other insulin: _____	_____ units	_____ units	_____ units	_____ units

Figure 26.1 Part of a Diabetes Order Set, specifying scheduled insulin, completed by checking boxes and entering numbers.

20 ± 1 units of glulisine (20). The actual individual requirement is quickly established through the addition of correction doses to the initial scheduled total daily dose and by daily revision of scheduled therapy.

For the patient who used insulin in the ambulatory setting and who is eating, the caregiver should determine the preadmission TDDI, which may be appraised as an average taken over 3–7 days immediately prior to admission. If unexplained hypoglycemia has been occurring, a 10–20% decrement of the TDDI is appropriate, targeting for reduction the components of therapy judged responsible for the hypoglycemia.

For the patient with negligible oral energy intake and requiring insulin therapy, the reassigned 24-h dose of basal insulin for NPO status is computed. Some patients with type 2 diabetes treated with discontinuous carbohydrate exposure, such as overnight enteral tube feedings, may have negligible basal requirements for exogenous insulin but may require nutritional insulin. The nutritional insulin required over a future time interval is applicable to the time interval during which carbohydrate exposure will occur and is estimated initially as 1 unit/10 g carbohydrate which will be infused over that interval. The daily dose of scheduled insulin consists of the combined amounts of basal and nutritional insulin.

For the patient who is transitioning from intravenous to subcutaneous therapy, insulin requirements can be inferred from the average hourly infusion rate during intravenous insulin infusion. For evaluation of basal requirements, a 6- to 8-h time segment is identified during which intravenous infusion of dextrose was negligible or <40 cc/h of fluids containing 5% dextrose in water were administered, often between midnight and 0600 or 0800 h. In the U.S., this condition is commonly met after cardiothoracic surgery. The average hourly amount is projected to a 24-h requirement. The initial subcutaneous daily dose estimated to meet basal requirements is taken to be ≤80% of the estimated 24-h amount. When the 80% rule was used after cardiothoracic surgery for transitioning to glargine after 26.6 ± 22.6 h of postoperative intravenous insulin infusion therapy, the mean glargine dose was 57.6 ± 30.4 units (34). Prandial doses of rapid-acting insulin analog are introduced at a starting amount of 3–6 units and gradually increased, depending on oral intake. Thereafter, depending on the condition of the patient, a daily dose reduction of basal insulin is made and the doses of prandial insulin are gradually increased, so that the relative proportions gradually approach 50% basal and 50% prandial insulin (26,29,31,32,34,38).

Correction doses of subcutaneous insulin. Correction doses of rapid-acting insulin analog may be given before meals; before meals and at bedtime; or before meals, at bedtime, and at 0300 h (Fig. 26.2). The decision to use bedtime and 0300 h correction doses depends on a risk-benefit analysis related to insulin sensitivity and the urgency of control of hyperglycemia. Alternatively, for patients not eating, correction doses of rapid-acting analog or regular insulin may be given every 6 h.

Daily revisions of dose of subcutaneous insulin therapy. The TDDI each day in the hospital is reappraised as the total amount of insulin of any type, scheduled plus correction, actually given over the previous 24 h. The computation includes the correction doses that were administered and excludes insulin doses that were withheld. Doses of each component of subcutaneous insulin therapy may require adjustment once or twice daily. For patients experiencing hypoglycemia (blood glucose <70 mg/dl), a 20% reduction of the TDDI may be indicated (20). Reductions are made to the components of therapy that were judged responsible for the hypoglycemia, or the insulin is reapportioned in the previously established pattern to give the newly assigned daily dose of scheduled insulin. If new development of

---

Correction dose insulin orders:
Route subcutaneous, priority PRN for range of blood glucose elevation, at the following times:

      before meals
      before meals, at bedtime
      before meals, at bedtime, at 0300 h
      every 6 h

For ALGORITHM assignment, preferred criterion = TDDI, adding all scheduled components.
For ALGORITHM assignment, alternative criterion = body weight.

Algorithm may be selected or revised according to clinical judgment and response to previous therapy. Freetext entries may be substituted.

ALGORITHM 1	ALGORITHM 2	ALGORITHM 3	ALGORITHM 4	ALGORITHM 5	ALGORITHM 6
SUBCUTANE-OUS INSULIN	SUBCUTANE-OUS INSULIN	SUBCUTANE-OUS INSULIN	SUBCUTANE-OUS INSULIN	SUBCUTANE-OUS INSULIN	SUBCUTANE-OUS INSULIN
☐ Rapid-acting insulin analog	☐ Rapid-acting insulin analog	☐ Rapid-acting insulin analog	☐ Rapid-acting insulin analog	☐ Rapid-acting insulin analog	☐ Rapid-acting insulin analog
[TDDI ≈ 24 (<28) units or wt <56 kg]	[TDDI ≈ 30 (28–36) units, or wt 56–73.9 kg]	[TDDI ≈ 45 (37–55) units, or wt 74–111.9 kg]	[TDDI ≈ 72 (56–90) units, or wt 112–181.9 kg]	[TDDI ≈ 120 (91–144) units or wt ≥182 kg]	[TDDI ≈ 180 (>144) units]
☐ Regular insulin	☐ Regular insulin	☐ Regular insulin	☐ Regular insulin	☐ Regular insulin	☐ Regular insulin
[TDDI ≈ 20 (<23) units, or wt <46 kg]	[TDDI ≈ 25 (23–30) units, or wt 46–61.9 kg]	[TDDI ≈ 37.5 (31–46) units, or wt 62–93.9 kg]	[TDDI ≈ 60 (47–75) units, or wt 94–151.9 kg]	[TDDI ≈ 100 (76–120) units or wt ≥152 kg]	[TDDI ≈ 150 (>120) units]
CBG units	**CBG units**	**CBG units**	**CBG units**	**CBG units**	**CBG units**
150–224 1	150–209 1	150–189 1	150–199 2	150–209 4	150–199 5
225–299 2	210–269 2	190–229 2	200–249 4	210–269 8	200–249 10
300–374 3	270–329 3	230–269 3	250–299 6	270–329 12	250–299 15
375–449 4	330–389 4	270–309 4	300–349 8	330–389 16	300–349 20
≥450 5	≥390 5	310–349 5	350–399 10	≥390 20	≥350 25
		350–389 6	≥400 12		
		≥390 7			

Figure 26.2 Correction dose insulin PRN hyperglycemia. PRN, as needed; CBG, capillary blood glucose.

renal, hepatic, or cardiac failure occurs, insulin requirements may decline, such that a downward trend of blood glucose monitoring during euglycemia may signal the need for an anticipatory reduction of some components of scheduled insulin therapy. Conversely, medical and surgical stress, intravenous dextrose, nutritional support, or medication may result in an increase of insulin requirement. Upward adjustments of scheduled insulin necessitated by hyperglycemia during subcutaneous therapy often are made by increments of ~10% to the TDDI. The increments are apportioned among the components of therapy or are applied to the components of therapy judged most likely to correct the pattern of hyperglycemia.

Pattern assignment according to carbohydrate exposure. There are six common patterns of carbohydrate exposure in the hospital: discrete meals, continuous exposure or no carbohydrate exposure, overnight enteral tube feeds, daytime grazing, bolus tube feedings (37), and peritoneal dialysis. To prevent hypoglycemia by timing the effect of subcutaneous insulin appropriately and to optimize protection against unexpected interruption of nutrition, the pattern of blood glucose monitoring, types of insulin, timing of insulin doses, and additional directions concerning insulin must match the dominant pattern of carbohydrate exposure (Table 26.2). For patients who formerly used insulin, the ambulatory pattern of administration of insulin may have to be changed. For example, for a patient who is eating in the hospital, the use of glargine as insulin monotherapy combined with oral agents, or twice-daily use of biphasic insulin, requires revision.

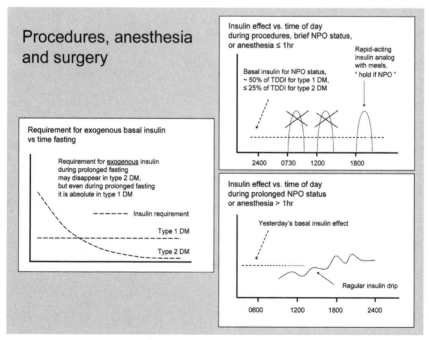

Figure 26.3 Procedures: anesthesia and surgery.

For patients who are eating, the most appropriate prescribing style in the hospital is basal-prandial-correction therapy. The virtue of basal-prandial-correction therapy for a population at risk of meal schedule interruption is that prandial doses of rapid-acting insulin analog can be interrupted without compromise to the basal component of insulin therapy. Long-acting insulin analog glargine or detemir or twice-daily injection of intermediate-acting NPH insulin is used to provide basal coverage. The daily dose of long-acting insulin analog is divided

Table 26.2 Subcutaneous Insulin Therapy

Dominant Pattern of Carbohydrate Exposure	Point-of-Care Monitoring of Blood Glucose (Nursing Orders)	Scheduled Insulin (Pharmacy Orders)	Additional Directions to Insulin Orders
discrete meals	before meals and at bedtime (ACHS) *or* before meals, at bedtime, and 0300 h (ACHS and 0300 h)	basal insulin† glargine once daily or twice daily, at bedtime (qHS) and/or 0800 h, *or* detemir or NPH twice daily at 0800 and 2200 h	"do not withhold" for type 1 diabetes *or* "reduce 50% if NPO" for type 2 diabetes *or* "hold if NPO" for type 2 diabetes
		prandial insulin§ lispro with meals *or* aspart with meals *or* glulisine with meals	"hold if NPO" (recommended) *and* "hold if blood glucose <80–100 mg/dl (specify)" *and* "hold until 50% of tray taken" (optional, not recommended once oral intake is secure)
continuous carbohydrate exposure *or* no carbohydrate exposure	every 6 h	NPH every 6 h *	"hold if tube feeds stop," *and* "hold for 6 h before tube feeds stop"
		scheduled regular insulin every 6 h *	"hold if tube feeds stop," *and* "hold for 6 h before tube feeds stop," *and* "hold if blood glucose <100 mg/dl"

(continued on page 311)

into two parts by some patients or providers. Rapid-acting insulin analog lispro, aspart, or glulisine or short-acting regular insulin is given three times daily before meals to provide prandial coverage. When oral intake is not assured, additional directions may be provided allowing observation of actual intake prior to administration of prandial insulin ("hold until 50% of tray taken"), but the dose of rapid-acting analog should not be delayed >20 min from the beginning of a meal. As soon as oral intake is assured, the doses are delivered preprandially.

Normally, the 24-h dose of basal insulin should not exceed 50% of the TDDI during basal-prandial-correction therapy in the hospital. For many patients using insulin prior to admission, it is appropriate to reapportion the TDDI so that basal insulin does not exceed 50% of the total daily dose, and prandial insulin is prescribed as the other 50%. Medical comorbidities or medications may alter the usual

Table 26.2 Subcutaneous Insulin Therapy *(continued)*

Dominant Pattern of Carbohydrate Exposure	Point-of-Care Monitoring of Blood Glucose (Nursing Orders)	Scheduled Insulin (Pharmacy Orders)	Additional Directions to Insulin Orders
"grazing" on meals and nutritional supplements	before meals and at bedtime (ACHS) *or* before meals, at bedtime, and 0300 h (ACHS and 0300 h)	mixed NPH and scheduled regular insulin at breakfast* *and either* mixed NPH and scheduled regular insulin at supper* *or* scheduled regular insulin at supper and NPH at bedtime*	"hold if NPO"
overnight enteral tube feedings with daytime oral "grazing"	before meals, at bedtime, and 0300 h (ACHS and 0300 h)	70/30 NPH/regular insulin every evening as premedication to tube feeds*	"hold if no tube feeds"
bolus tube feedings	before feedings and at bedtime		

*Dose of NPH insulin is approximately twice the dose of regular insulin; in type 1 diabetes, these components of therapy are added to basal insulin, which may be prescribed as once-daily glargine and is ordered with the additional direction "do not withhold." †Usually ~50% of TDDI (higher immediately after heart surgery), but 33% of TDDI or less in renal failure, hepatic failure, or conditions involving malnutrition such as cystic fibrosis, and during corticosteroid therapy. §Usually ~50% of TDDI (lower immediately after heart surgery), but 67% of TDDI or higher in renal failure, hepatic failure, or conditions involving malnutrition such as cystic fibrosis, and during corticosteroid therapy.

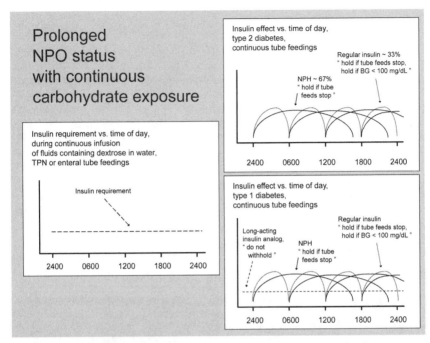

Figure 26.4 Prolonged NPO status with continuous carbohydrate exposure. BG, blood glucose.

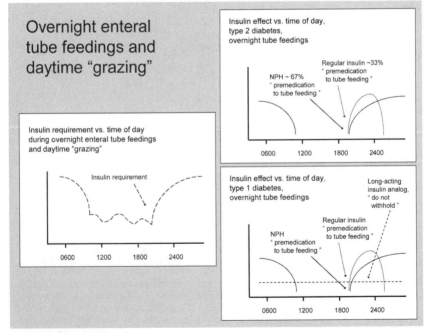

Figure 26.5 Overnight enteral tube feedings and daytime "grazing."

ratio of basal to prandial insulin. The existence of comorbidities, such as renal failure, hepatic failure, congestive heart failure, and malnutrition, as with cystic fibrosis, or the use of corticosteroid therapy, tend to be associated with a lower ratio of basal to prandial insulin requirement, sometimes ~33% basal and ~67% prandial. The immediate postoperative recovery period after major procedures, such as coronary bypass surgery, may be associated with a higher basal relative to prandial requirement, such that basal insulin exceeds 50% of the total daily dose.

For type 2 diabetes, the 24-h dose requirement for basal insulin is dependent on energy intake and may disappear during prolonged fasting, such that the caregiver may establish a reassigned 24-h dose of basal insulin for NPO status as an amount considered safe and necessary for intervals of reduced oral intake. For type 1 diabetes, the reassigned 24-h dose of basal insulin for NPO status tends to be invariant, despite reduced oral intake. To prevent unchecked gluconeogenesis and ketogenesis, the dose should be provided regardless of reduction of oral intake.

For patients receiving continuous carbohydrate exposure or no carbohydrate exposure who require subcutaneous insulin, mixtures of NPH and regular insulin are provided every 6 h. The situation occurs during NPO status with or without maintenance dextrose-containing intravenous fluids, TPN, or continuous enteral feedings. The amount of NPH is ~67% of the TDDI and regular insulin ~33%. Additional directions specify that both components of scheduled subcutaneous insulin therapy are withheld in case of interruption of carbohydrate exposure. Monitoring of blood glucose occurs at 6-h intervals. Regular insulin is withheld in case blood glucose results are below a given threshold, such as 100 mg/dl. The threshold depends on patient characteristics. Correction doses of regular insulin are given at 6-h intervals, as needed. The prescribing style provides for deliberate overlap of the effect of scheduled insulin doses, such that a relatively flat line of insulin effect is achieved. Each dose is small enough that risks of hypoglycemia are minimized in case of unexpected interruption of carbohydrate exposure. During enteral feedings, orders for long-acting insulin analog should be added for patients with type 1 diabetes to provide the basal part of the TDDI, tagged with the additional direction "do not withhold."

Overnight enteral feedings may be covered with a premedication order for a mixture of NPH and regular insulin to be given daily at the time the enteral feedings begin. Monitoring of blood glucose occurs before meals, at bedtime, and at 0300 h. Some patients have sufficient daytime oral intake that a morning mixed dose of NPH and regular insulin is required.

Daytime grazing sometimes is best met with mixtures of NPH and regular insulin given before breakfast and before supper. Monitoring of blood glucose is ordered before meals, at bedtime, and possibly at 0300 h.

Bolus enteral feedings may be treated with rapid-acting insulin analog combined with basal insulin (37).

Blood glucose monitoring must be appropriately timed to match the pattern of carbohydrate exposure.

Intravenous Insulin Infusion Therapy

Hyperglycemic patients in the intensive care unit (ICU) generally should be treated with intravenous insulin infusion. Some hospitals have introduced intravenous insulin infusion outside of the ICU setting. Safety and effectiveness is achieved both by use of a dose-defining algorithm that does not require computation or subjective interpretation by nursing staff, and by staff education.

The medical outcome advantages that first were identified in the care of cardiac surgery patients and surgical ICU patients were achieved with the use of manual insulin infusion algorithms that targeted the insulin infusion rate for adjustments (6,7). When such algorithms incorporate rate of change of blood glucose, distance of blood glucose from target, and previous insulin infusion rate to determine the next insulin infusion rate, excellent glycemic results are obtained (28).

Ease of use, safety, and excellent glycemic results also are achieved with the use of dose-defining insulin infusion algorithms with an alternative design that targets the maintenance rate of insulin infusion, column assignment, or multiplier for adjustments. Under this second type of algorithm design, the revision to the maintenance rate or multiplier is derived from the previous rate of change or fractional change of blood glucose and the previous insulin infusion rate or multiplier. The distance of blood glucose from target or from a given low value (such as 60 mg/dl) together with the reassigned maintenance rate, column assignment, or multiplier determine the next insulin infusion rate. At a given blood glucose, the change of the insulin infusion rate with respect to blood glucose is a continuous and increasing function of the maintenance rate or multiplier. Algorithms targeting adjustment of maintenance rate, column assignment or multiplier may be displayed in tabular form by rounding off the output of the underlying equations.

Two examples of column-based tabular algorithms are shown, having the limitation that the target range is predefined (Figs. 26.6 and 26.7) (25,30). The rate of change of blood glucose determines the need for column reassignment. Computerization of algorithms targeting adjustment of a multiplier may improve glycemic results compared with alternative manual methods (27). The algorithms mentioned target blood glucose ranges lower than those advocated for the initial treatment of diabetic ketoacidosis or hyperglycemic hyperosmolar state.

Algorithms in common use in the U.S. reactively adapt to changes in insulin resistance or carbohydrate exposure, such that oscillations of blood glucose are inevitable. Utilization of additional input data, especially information about carbohydrate exposure, and model predictive engineering principles are likely to improve these designs (33,35,39).

For patients receiving prolonged intravenous insulin therapy who are hemodynamically stable and who do not require pressors, administration of scheduled subcutaneous insulin is possible well in advance of anticipated independence from intravenous infusion. For patients who are eating, early introduction of subcutaneous basal insulin and prandial doses of rapid-acting insulin analog may stabilize blood glucose and insulin infusion rates. For patients receiving continuous carbohydrate exposure and experiencing prolonged NPO (nothing by mouth) status while receiving intravenous insulin infusion, mixtures of NPH and regular insulin at 6-h intervals may be used concomitantly with insulin infusion.

Transitioning to independence from intravenous insulin requires hemodynamic stability and freedom from pressors and generally should not occur prior to transfer out of the ICU. An exception would be a patient with prolonged ICU care who is independent of pressors, whose insulin requirement and comorbidities are stable, and who is expected to have a predictable pattern of carbohydrate exposure and requirement for concomitant medications that might affect blood glucose. Ventilator-dependent patients receiving continuous enteral feedings sometimes are transitioned to scheduled subcutaneous therapy in the medical ICU, and patients receiving TPN sometimes are transitioned to combinations of subcutaneous therapy and insulin in the TPN bag. For patients requiring >0.5 units/h of intravenous insulin infusion and for patients with type 1 diabetes, subcutaneous insulin is introduced ≥2 h before interruption of intravenous insulin infusion. At the time of transitioning to subcutaneous therapy, if the intravenous

Column 1		Column 2		Column 3		Column 4		Column 5		Column 6	
BG	U/h	BG	U/h	BG	U/h	BG	U/h	BG	U/h	BG	U/h
<70	Off	<70	Off	<70	Off	<70	Off	<70	Off	<70	Off
70-79	Off	70-79	Off	70-79	Off	70-79	Off	70-79	0.5	70-79	1
80-89	Off	80-89	Off	80-89	Off	80-89	0.5	80-89	1	80-89	1.5
90-99	Off	90-99	Off	90-99	0.5	90-99	1	90-99	1.5	90-99	2
100-109	**Off**	**100-109**	**0.5**	**100-109**	**1**	**100-109**	**1.5**	**100-109**	**2**	**100-109**	**3**
110-129	**0.5**	**110-129**	**1**	**110-129**	**1.5**	**110-129**	**2**	**110-129**	**3**	**110-129**	**4**
130-149	**1**	**130-149**	**1.5**	**130-149**	**2**	**130-149**	**3**	**130-149**	**4**	**130-149**	**6**
150-179	1.5	150-169	2	150-179	3	150-169	4	150-179	6	150-169	8
		170-189	2.5			170-189	5			170-189	10
180-209	2	190-209	3	180-209	4	190-209	6	180-209	8	190-209	12
210-269	3	210-254	4	210-239	5	210-229	7	210-239	10	210-229	14
				240-269	6	230-269	8	240-269	12	230-249	16
270-329	4	255-299	5	270-299	7	270-309	10	270-299	14	250-269	18
		300-345	6	300-329	8	310-349	12	300-329	16	270-309	20
330-389	5			330-359	9			330-359	18	310-349	24
		346-389	7	360-389	10	350-389	14	360-389	20	350-389	28
≥390	6	≥390	8	≥390	11	≥390	16	≥390	22	≥390	32

*BG = blood glucose (mg/dL). Boldface entries denote target range.

†Note: Target BG range is 100 to 150 mg/dL. Each column represents a different insulin requirement for maintenance of target BG range. Each column shows BG and corresponding intravenous insulin infusion rate. Testing is done hourly until the patient meets criteria for stability, at which time testing is done every 2 h. The default instruction to nursing staff is to begin with column 2, with use of a priming bolus of insulin in amount dependent on glucose concentration. The staff is instructed under protocol to switch to the next higher column under the following circumstances:
- BG ≥200 mg/dL for 1 h and decreasing <30 mg/dL during past 1 h
- BG ≥150 mg/dL for 2 h and decreasing <60 mg/dL during past 2 h

The staff tests BG every 1 h if drip is turned off by protocol. After drip interruption for low BG, the staff resumes the insulin infusion when BG >109 mg/dL. The staff switches to the next lower column in either of the following circumstances:
- The infusion was interrupted for low BG but now is resuming   *or*
- The patient has been on column 4, 5, or 6 for past 8 h, with BG within target range.

Figure 26.6 Algorithm for intravenous insulin infusion: protocol of Braithwaite et al. (25); reprinted with permission.

insulin infusion will be interrupted prior to the time when the first dose of scheduled insulin comes due, a bridging dose of regular or NPH insulin may be used.

Patient Self-Management in the Hospital

A hospital patient diabetes self-management program is achieved by developing policy, protocols, procedures, and educational materials for patients and staff to allow experienced patients to continue insulin self-management in the hospital.

Column 1		Column 2		Column 3		Column 4		Column 5		Column 6	
BG	U/h	BG	U/h	BG	U/h	BG	U/h	BG	U/h	BG	U/h
<70	0.05	<70	0.05	<70	0.05	<70	0.05	<70	0.05		
70–74	0.1	70–74	0.1	70–74	0.1	70–74	0.1	70–74	0.1		
75–79	0.1	75–79	0.2	75–79	0.2	75–79	0.2	75–79	0.2		
80–84	0.2	80–84	0.2	80–84	0.3	80–84	0.3	80–84	0.3	80–84	0.3
85–89	0.3	85–89	0.4	85–89	0.4	85–89	0.5	85–89	0.6	85–89	0.6
90–94	0.4	90–94	0.6	90–94	0.7	90–94	0.8	90–94	1.0	90–94	1.2
95–99	0.5	95–99	0.8	95–99	1.1	95–99	1.4	95–99	1.9	95–99	2.3
100–104	0.7	100–104	1.3	100–104	1.8	100–104	2.4	100–104	3.3	100–104	4.3
105–109	1	105–109	2	105–109	3	105–109	4	105–109	6	105–109	8
110–127	1.2	110–121	2.3	110–122	3.5	110–127	5	110–122	7	110–127	10
128–144	1.5	122–133	2.6	123–134	4	128–144	6	123–134	8	128–144	12
145–162	1.7	134–144	3	135–147	4.5	145–179	8	135–159	10	145–162	14
163–179	2	145–162	3.5	148–159	5	180–214	10	160–184	12	163–179	16
180–249	3	163–179	4	160–209	7	215–249	12	185–209	14	180–214	20
250–319	4	180–249	6	210–259	9	250–319	16	210–259	18	215–249	24
320–389	5	250–319	8	260–309	11	320–389	20	260–309	22	250–319	32
≥390	6	≥320	10	≥310	13	≥390	24	≥310	26	≥320	40

BG is given in units of mg/dL. Partial instructions are:
• Start insulin drip assigned to Column 2 and adjust drip rate according to Column 2.
• If BG ≥180 for 2 h, AND NOT FALLING at least 30 mg/dL each hour, go to next higher column.
• If BG ≥110 at every test time for past 8 h on the current column, go to the next higher column.
• If BG ≥110 now, but if some BG <110 in past 8 h, do not change column.
• If 80 ≤ BG <110 now, and if at least one BG ≥110 during past 8 h, do not change column.
• If on Column 2–6 for past 8 h, AND BG 110 at all times for past 8 h, go to next lower column.
• If BG <80 now, and on Column 2–6, go to next lower column, and check BG every 1 h until BG 80.
• If BG <70, treat according to hypoglycemia protocol (not shown) and go to next lower column.
• Initially, or after any reassignment to a higher column, test BG every 1 h.
• If on same column for 4 h, may change frequency of BG testing to every 2 h.
  Record insulin drip rate changes on ICU flow sheet. Record column assignments on ICU flow sheet and on the medication administration record.
  Request new glycemic management plan 2 h before discontinuing drip.

Figure 26.7 Insulin infusion protocol table and partial instructions. Reprinted with permission from Braithwaite et al. (30).

The program aims at patient satisfaction and enablement to determine appropriate timing and dosing of prandial and correction doses of insulin and, for users of continuous subcutaneous insulin infusion by pump, to deliver variable basal rates. Such a program may be of greatest interest to insulin-sensitive patients but may be made available to any experienced insulin user. The details of the program ensure safety and compliance with regulatory requirements. A protocol outlines initial determination of patient candidacy, the process of obtaining patient agreement to self-management, conditions of altered competency or comorbidity preventing or requiring suspension of self-management, authorization of staff to interrupt self-management, conditions of insulin storage, method of chart documentation of glucose monitoring and insulin administration, and specific procedures to be followed during and after brief general anesthesia or conscious sedation. By ordering patient participation in a self-management program, the provider is not relieved of the duty to monitor and treat the patient. The hospital monitors the program (21,36).

Discharge Planning

The need for intensification of preadmission therapy of known diabetes may be recognized by the discovery of elevated A1C. The likelihood that patients without known diabetes may be confirmed to have diabetes by venous plasma glucose standards is predicted by the A1C (19,42). Hospitalization often represents the "teachable moment" such that multidisciplinary educational intervention should be initiated. At discharge, outpatient follow-up is planned for classification of hyperglycemia or treatment of diabetes and continuation of patient education.

OUTCOME

Morbidity and mortality are recognized complications of iatrogenic hypoglycemia (15,16). Hypoglycemia may result in part from comorbidities, reflecting the severity of illness (12). Hypoglycemia often is iatrogenic, and in the ICU setting it may independently predict mortality (15). A large international trial found that both hypoglycemia and mortality in the ICU setting were increased by a policy of targeting blood glucose <110 mg/dl as compared with a conventional policy targeting blood glucose <180 mg/dl using intravenous insulin infusion (43). In consequence of safety concerns regarding hypoglycemia, definition of the ideal glycemic target range for hospitalized patients under various conditions of illness and observation is undergoing revision. Fear of hypoglycemia, however, need not prevent caregivers from using validated strategies designed to prevent hypoglycemia while seeking target range control.

Observational data suggest that a link exists between patient outcomes and hyperglycemia in the hospital and/or before admission. In comparison to historical controls, intravenous infusion of insulin for the first 3 days after heart surgery reduced the rate of deep sternal wound infection and mortality among diabetic patients (4,7). A randomized trial of glucose-insulin-potassium infusion sufficient to improve hyperglycemia, followed by subcutaneous insulin therapy in the ambulatory setting, reduced long-term mortality after myocardial infarction (3). A randomized trial of strict glycemic control in the surgical ICU showed that targeting blood glucose 80–110 mg/dl reduced mortality, duration of ventilator dependency, transfusion requirement, new-onset renal failure, length of stay, neuropathy, sepsis, and mortality (6). Intensification of glycemic management in a mixed ICU resulted in mortality reduction and estimated cost reduction (8).

A relationship to hyperglycemia has been observationally demonstrated across a wide variety of surgical procedures with respect to postoperative infection rate and postoperative mortality (1,10). It has been suggested that specific outcomes, such as mortality from pneumonia, stroke expansion, remission after induction chemotherapy for leukemia, mortality for trauma patients, atrial fibrillation after heart surgery, and acute rejection after kidney transplantation, are related to the presence of diabetes or to glycemic control. The length of stay and hospital mortality on general wards is correlated with detection of hyperglycemia among patients not previously known to have had diabetes (2). While awaiting proof of a causal relationship between hyperglycemia and outcomes from the results of randomized prospective trials, the strategies outlined in this chapter attempt to define a safe and effective approach to attainment of ADA targets in the general and ICU hospital setting.

BIBLIOGRAPHY

1. Clement S, Braithwaite SS, Magee MF, et al.: Management of diabetes and hyperglycemia in hospitals. *Diabetes Care* 27:553–591, 2004

2. Umpierrez GE, Isaacs SD, Bazargan N, You X, Thaler LM, Kitabchi AE: Hyperglycemia: an independent marker of in-hospital mortality in patients with undiagnosed diabetes. *J Clin Endocrinol Metab* 87:978–982, 2002

3. Malmberg K, Ryden L, Efendic S, et al.: Randomized trial of insulin-glucose infusion followed by subcutaneous insulin treatment in diabetic patients with acute myocardial infarction (DIGAMI study): effects on mortality at 1 year. *J Am Coll Cardiol* 26:57–65, 1995

4. Zerr KJ, Furnary AP, Grunkemeier GL: Glucose control lowers the risk of wound infection in diabetics after open heart operations. *Ann Thorac Surg* 63:356–361, 1997

5. Pomposelli JJ, Baxter JK, Babineau TJ, et al.: Early postoperative glucose control predicts nosocomial infection rate in diabetic patients. *J Parenteral & Enteral Nutr* 22:77–81, 1998

6. Van den Berghe G, Wouters P, Weekers F, et al.: Intensive insulin therapy in critically ill patients. *N Engl J Med* 345:1359–1367, 2001

7. Furnary AP, Gao G, Grunkemeier GL, et al.: Continuous insulin infusion reduces mortality in patients with diabetes undergoing coronary artery bypass grafting. *J Thorac Cardiovasc Surg* 125:1007–1021, 2003

8. Krinsley JS: Effect of an intensive glucose management protocol on the mortality of critically ill adult patients. *Mayo Clin Proc* 79:992–1000, 2004

9. Van den Berghe G, Wilmer A, Hermans G, et al.: Intensive insulin therapy in the medical ICU. *N Engl J Med* 354:449–461, 2006

10. Braithwaite SS: Defining the benefits of euglycemia in the hospitalized patient. *J Hosp Med* 2 (Suppl. 1):5–12, 2007

11. Fischer KF, Lees JA, Newman JH: Hypoglycemia in hospitalized patients. *N Engl J Med* 315:1245–1250, 1986

12. Kagansky N, Levy S, Rimon E, et al.: Hypoglycemia as a predictor of mortality in hospitalized elderly patients. *Arch Intern Med* 163:1825–1829, 2003

13. Van den Berghe G, Wilmer A, Milants I, et al.: Intensive insulin therapy in mixed medical/surgical intensive care units: benefit versus harm. *Diabetes* 55:3151–3159, 2006

14. Vriesendorp TM, van Santen S, DeVries JH, et al.: Predisposing factors for hypoglycemia in the intensive care unit. *Crit Care Med* 34:96–101, 2006

15. Krinsley JS, Grover A: Severe hypoglycemia in critically ill patients: risk factors and outcomes. *Crit Care Med* 35:2262–2267, 2007

16. Varghese P, Gleason V, Sorokin R, Senholzi C, Jabbour S, Gottlieb JE: Hypoglycemia in hospitalized patients treated with antihyperglycemic agents. *J Hosp Med* 2:234–240, 2007

17. Brunkhorst FM, Engel C, Bloos F, et al.: Intensive insulin therapy and pentastarch resuscitation in severe sepsis. *N Engl J Med* 358:125–139, 2008

18. Wexler DJ, Meigs JB, Cagliero E, Nathan DM, Grant RW: Prevalence of hyper- and hypoglycemia among inpatients with diabetes: a national survey of 44 U.S. hospitals. *Diabetes Care* 30:367–369, 2007

19. Baldwin D, Villanueva G, McNutt R, Bhatnagar S: Eliminating inpatient sliding-scale insulin: a reeducation project with medical house staff. *Diabetes Care* 28:1008–1011, 2005

20. Umpierrez GE, Smiley D, Zisman A, et al.: Randomized study of basal-bolus insulin therapy in the inpatient management of patients with type 2 diabetes (RABBIT 2 trial). *Diabetes Care* 30:2181–2186, 2007

21. Cook CB, Boyle ME, Cisar NS, et al.: Use of continuous subcutaneous insulin infusion (insulin pump) therapy in the hospital setting: proposed guidelines and outcome measures. *Diabetes Educ* 31:849–857, 2005

22. Goldberg PA, Bozzo JE, Thomas PG, et al.: "Glucometrics"—assessing the quality of inpatient glucose management. *Diabetes Technol Ther* 8:560–569, 2006

23. Hoofnagle AN, Peterson G, Kelly J, Sayre C, Chou D, Hirsch IB: Utilization of serum and plasma glucose measurements as a benchmark for improved hospital-wide glycemic control. *Endocrine Pract* 14: 556–563, 2008

24. Trence DL, Kelly JL, Hirsch IB: The rationale and management of hyperglycemia for in-patients with cardiovascular disease: time for change. *J Clin Endocrinol Metab* 88:2430–2437, 2003

25. Bode BW, Braithwaite SS, Steed RD, Davidson PC: Intravenous insulin infusion therapy: indications, methods, and transition to subcutaneous insulin therapy. *Endocr Pract* 10 (Suppl. 2):71–80, 2004

26. Campbell KB, Braithwaite SS: Hospital management of hyperglycemia. *Clin Diabetes* 22:81–88, 2004

27. Davidson PC, Steed RD, Bode BW: Glucommander: a computer-directed intravenous insulin system shown to be safe, simple, and effective in 120,618 h of operation. *Diabetes Care* 28:2418–2423, 2005

28. Goldberg PA, Roussel MG, Inzucchi SE: Clinical results of an updated insulin infusion protocol in critically ill patients. *Diabetes Spectrum* 18:188–191, 2005

29. Thompson CL, Dunn KC, Menon MC, Kearns LE, Braithwaite SS: Hyperglycemia in the hospital. *Diabetes Spectrum* 18:20–27, 2005

30. Braithwaite SS, Edkins R, Macgregor KL, et al.: Performance of a dose-defining insulin infusion protocol among trauma service intensive care unit admissions. *Diabetes Technol Ther* 8:476–488, 2006

31. Braithwaite SS: The transition from insulin infusions to long-term diabetes therapy: the argument for insulin analogs. *Semin Thorac Cardiovasc Surg* 18:366–378, 2006

32. DeSantis AJ, Schmeltz LR, Schmidt K, et al.: Inpatient management of hyperglycemia: the Northwestern experience. *Endocr Pract* 12:491–505, 2006

33. Plank J, Blaha J, Cordingley J, et al.: Multicentric, randomized, controlled trial to evaluate blood glucose control by the model predictive control algorithm versus routine glucose management protocols in intensive care unit patients. *Diabetes Care* 29:271–276, 2006

34. Schmeltz LR, DeSantis AJ, Schmidt K, et al.: Conversion of intravenous insulin infusions to subcutaneously administered insulin glargine in patients with hyperglycemia. *Endocr Pract* 12:641–650, 2006

35. Boulkina LS, Braithwaite SS: Practical aspects of intensive insulinization in the intensive care unit. *Curr Opin Clin Nutr Metab Care* 10:197–205, 2007

36. Braithwaite SS, Mehrotra HP, Robertson B, McElveen LM, Thompson CL: Managing hyperglycemia in hospitalized patients. *Clin Cornerstone* 8:44–57, 2007

37. Grainger A, Eiden K, Kemper J, Reeds D: A pilot study to evaluate the effectiveness of glargine and multiple injections of lispro in patients with type 2 diabetes receiving tube feedings in a cardiovascular intensive care unit. *Nutr Clin Pract* 22:545–552, 2007

38. Schmeltz LR, DeSantis AJ, Thiyagarajan V, et al.: Reduction of surgical mortality and morbidity in diabetic patients undergoing cardiac surgery with a combined intravenous and subcutaneous insulin glucose management strategy. *Diabetes Care* 30:823–828, 2007

39. Wilson M, Weinreb J, Hoo GW: Intensive insulin therapy in critical care: a review of 12 protocols. *Diabetes Care* 30:1005–1011, 2007

40. Schafer RG, Bohannon B, Franz MJ, et al.: Translation of the diabetes nutrition recommendations for health care institutions. *Diabetes Care* 26 (Suppl. 1):S70–S72, 2003

41. American Diabetes Association: Standards of medical care in diabetes—2009. *Diabetes Care* 32 (Suppl. 1):S13–S61, 2009

42. Greci LS, Kailasam M, Malkani S, et al.: Utility of HbA$_{1c}$ levels for diabetes case finding in hospitalized patients with hyperglycemia. *Diabetes Care* 26:1064–1068, 2003

43. NICE-SUGAR Study Investigators: Intensive versus conventional glucose control in critically ill patients. *N Engl J Med* 360:1283–1297, 2009

Dr. Braithwaite is Visiting Clinical Professor at the University of Illinois at Chicago, Chicago, Illinois.

27. Insulin Pump Therapy

Jennifer Sherr, MD, William Tamborlane, MD, and Bruce Bode, MD

Since the discovery of insulin almost a century ago, the goal of curing diabetes has remained elusive. Yet, various methods to improve the care of those living with the condition have occurred. In the late 1970s, the use of continuous subcutaneous insulin infusion (CSII) pump therapy was introduced. Diabetes care subsequently improved as self-monitoring of blood glucose (SMBG), A1C assays, and purified insulins were made available. With the findings of the Diabetes Control and Complications Trial (DCCT) demonstrating the association of intensive therapy with fewer complications, a renewed interest in pump therapy was sparked. As pump therapy has evolved, its use has grown more widespread. Herein the benefits of pump therapy as compared to multiple daily injection (MDI) therapy will be discussed along with the selection of suitable candidates for pump use and how to initiate such therapy. Finally, the advent of continuous glucose monitoring (CGM) with the goal of the development of an artificial pancreas will be covered.

CSII EXPERIENCE

In 1993, the findings of the DCCT were published and showed that the benefits achieved from intensive therapy in regard to the development and progression of complications outweighed the associated two- to threefold increase in the risk of severe hypoglycemia. Beneficial effects were also demonstrated in the subgroup analysis in the small number of adolescents who participated in the trial. Almost one-half of the intensively treated group (42%) used insulin pump therapy during the last full year of the study. DCCT investigators observed a 0.2–0.4% decrease in A1C using CSII, as well as an improvement in lifestyle flexibility. The ability to translate intensive therapy with CSII therapy into clinical use remained a question, as did the willingness of physicians, nurse practioners, and patients to accept this therapy. Thus, further studies exploring the benefits of CSII were undertaken.

Glycemic control has been shown to improve in adults and children who have type 1 diabetes when they use pump therapy for insulin delivery. In large nonrandomized and randomized studies, the average A1C has decreased from 0.2 to >1%, with the average being between 0.4 and 0.6%. These trials have also shown that despite initial concerns of increased frequency of hypoglycemia in patients utilizing CSII therapy, the frequency of clinically important hypoglycemia was reduced. Concerns over weight gain associated with CSII therapy were also proven wrong in studies of children and adolescents, because BMI Z-scores did not increase after switching from injection to pump therapy. A meta-analysis of 11 studies with a parallel design published in 2003 showed a weighted summary mean difference in A1C between CSII and MDI/conventional therapy was 0.95%, with a 95% CI of 0.8–1.1%. In 2002, a meta-analysis of 12 randomized controlled trials comparing CSII therapy versus MDI therapy also showed a reduction of 0.44% in A1C (95% CI 0.20–0.69) and a ~14% drop in total daily insulin dose in patients using CSII.

Critics of these meta-analyses point out that many of these studies used NPH rather than long-acting insulin analogs for comparison in the MDI groups. However, studies comparing use of long-acting insulin analogs have shown similar or lower A1C levels, decreased glucose variability, and increased treatment satisfaction in patients on CSII therapy versus glargine-based MDI therapy.

Experience with CSII in patients with type 2 diabetes is limited but encouraging. Glycemic control has been shown to be as good as or better than MDI, with better fasting and postbreakfast glucose values. Quality of life has been reported to be improved with CSII therapy in patients with type 2 diabetes.

ADVANTAGES OF CSII

A multitude of factors are likely to play a role in the improved glycemic control seen in patients with diabetes using CSII. In the initial studies of pump therapy, including the DCCT, regular insulin was used. In contrast to regular insulin, rapid-acting insulin analogs (lispro, aspart, and glulisine) have earlier and sharper peaks and a much shorter duration of action. Lispro and aspart insulin have been shown to provide better control of postprandial hyperglycemia and to decrease the risk of late postprandial hypoglycemia in comparison to regular insulin in CSII-treated patients. Early pump studies demonstrated that CSII therapy led to decreased variability in absorption of subcutaneously delivered insulin. Even the time-action profiles of long-acting insulin analogs (glargine and detemir) have been shown to vary from 27 to 48% in the same individual, which contributes to the risk of nocturnal hypoglycemia. In contrast, the short-acting insulins that are used in CSII vary in absorption by <3% on a daily basis. Although the ability to mimic endogenous insulin peak and duration remains elusive due to delays in absorption from the subcutaneous infusion site, rapid-acting analogs are the best approximation currently available, and this class of insulin is the mainstay for CSII therapy.

Other advantages of insulin pump therapy include a reduction in the occurrence of severe hypoglycemia. On average, adults with type 1 diabetes on MDI therapy have rates of severe hypoglycemia requiring assistance ranging anywhere from 20 to 50 episodes per 100 patient-years, and hypoglycemia rates are even higher in youth with type 1 diabetes. In contrast, adults and children on CSII have rates of hypoglycemia ranging from 15 to 30 per 100 patient-years. These results have remained true for even the youngest children on CSII therapy, with many randomized and nonrandomized studies demonstrating a lower incidence of hypoglycemia after initiation of CSII. Fear of hypoglycemia remains a major obstacle to successful intensive management, regardless of the method of insulin administration.

Titration of basal insulin replacement through CSII therapy has proven to be beneficial in decreasing both the frequency and severity of hypoglycemia. Instead of administering one or two fixed doses of long-acting insulin analogs whose time-action curves cannot be altered, CSII-treated patients can program anywhere between 12 and 48 basal rates, and the basal infusion can be acutely lowered or suspended. Studies completed by the Diabetes Research in Children Network (DirecNet) have shown that the risk of hypoglycemia is increased both during exercise and on the night after a 75-min period of moderate-intensity aerobic exercise in patients on fixed insulin dosing. A randomized crossover study subsequently demonstrated that suspending basal rates for those on CSII therapy decreased the risk of hypoglycemia, defined as blood glucose <70 mg/dl, from 43 to 16%. The use of variable basal rates, temporary basal rates, and the ability to suspend basal insulin delivery aid in achieving normoglycemia and decreasing episodes of hypoglycemia.

Along with variable basal rates, new "smart" pumps have been preprogrammed with correction factors and carbohydrate ratios, allowing patients to enter their blood glucose and expected carbohydrate intake and allow the pump to determine the bolus dose of insulin to be delivered. Doses of insulin can be delivered in smaller increments via pump therapy as compared to MDI therapy. The "insulin-on-board" function of current pumps is intended to reduce stacking of correction boluses by decreasing the amount of insulin recommended to correct elevated glucose levels given the amount of insulin that is likely still pharmacologically active from the previous bolus. The bolus history function is also beneficial to practitioners, who can utilize this tool to determine whether their patients are bolusing as prescribed and whether they are using the bolus calculator function. Cross-sectional studies have shown that patients who missed <1 bolus per week versus those who missed ≥1 mealtime bolus had better A1C (8.0 vs. 8.8%, respectively). Mealtime alarms, which remind patients to monitor their blood glucose and to change the infusion set, can also be programmed.

Lower insulin requirements and frequency of hypoglycemia may reduce the risk of excessive weight in insulin pump patients. However, as a result of the greater flexibility in taking insulin to cover any type of food, patients must be cautioned that any excess calorie intake, with improving glycemic control, can result in weight gain.

Another important advantage of CSII over MDI therapy is that it allows patients to lead more normal lives and simplifies irregular meal schedules and other unplanned activities. Patients can eat, snack, work, exercise, and sleep based on their own personal schedules and needs rather than on the peaks of insulin given many hours earlier. Whereas basal-bolus therapy with glargine or detemir and a rapid-acting insulin analog can provide similar freedom in terms of lifestyle, randomized and nonrandomized trials have shown improved quality of life scores measured via different scales and higher treatment satisfaction in patients treated with CSII. Three randomized studies have shown a great proportion (>95%) of subjects decided to continue on CSII after study completion. This explains why >60% of the members of the American Diabetes Association and the American Association of Diabetes Educators who are health care providers with type 1 diabetes were using insulin pump therapy when surveyed in a cross-sectional study in 2000.

Although there are many advantages to CSII therapy, some risks exist. Because of the absence of a depot of long-acting insulin, patients using CSII are at greater risk of developing diabetic ketoacidosis (DKA) than individuals using MDI therapy. However, with appropriate training and troubleshooting of high blood glucose values, the CSII rates of DKA have only been slightly higher than the rates seen with MDI treatment. Providing patients with specific instructions to treat high blood glucose levels has resulted in minimizing the risk of DKA. Some adolescents who are prone to recurrent episodes of ketoacidosis because of missed insulin injections can have a reduction in DKA and hospitalizations when switched to CSII.

IMPLEMENTING PUMP THERAPY

In 2006, an international consensus conference was convened in Berlin to review the evidence supporting the use of CSII in youth with type 1 diabetes. The consensus statement from that conference provides indications for use of this technology, which can be applied to the adult patients as well (Table 27.1). The consensus statement deemed CSII to be the most physiological method currently available for the delivery of insulin. Benefits of this therapy over MDI stemmed from the increased flexibility it provides patients and the more precise insulin delivery that is available (dose of 0.05 units instead of 0.5 units). However, despite the varied indications for CSII and advantages of its use, appropriate candidates for CSII therapy need to be selected by the treatment teams.

Some patients view pump therapy as a "cure," not realizing that work is required to make CSII a valuable treatment tool that can aid in successful management of diabetes. It is the job of the treatment team to identify patients who would best be suited to using this therapy. To be considered for CSII in the Yale Pediatric Diabetes Clinic, patients must be performing at least four blood glucose measurements per day and recording these numbers in a logbook or electronic spreadsheet, be consistently attending follow-up visits, be committed to the goal

Table 27.1 Indications for Use of CSII in Pediatrics

Conditions under which CSII should be considered
1. Recurrent severe hypoglycemia
2. Wide fluctuations in blood glucose levels, regardless of A1C
3. Suboptimal diabetes control (i.e., A1C exceeds target range for age)
4. Microvascular complications and/or risk factors for macrovascular complications
5. Good metabolic control but insulin regimen that compromises lifestyle

Circumstances in which CSII may be beneficial
1. Young children and especially infants and neonates
2. Adolescents with eating disorders
3. Children and adolescents with a pronounced dawn phenomenon
4. Children with needle phobia
5. Pregnant adolescents, ideally preconception
6. Ketosis-prone individuals
7. Competitive athletes

Adapted from Phillip et al. (2007).

of intensive insulin therapy, have a solid understanding of diabetes management (including carbohydrate counting), and have at least fair control (i.e., A1C ≤8.5%). However, some patients with poor control on MDI therapy may be very successful with CSII. These are often patients who have become frustrated and discouraged on MDI therapy as a result of inadequate success in achieving their goals because of the limitations of MDI therapy.

Once a patient is deemed appropriate for CSII therapy, selection of a pump is necessary. Table 27.2 reviews various pumps currently available for use and some of the features of these pumps. All of these pumps are considered "smart" and calculate the dose of insulin required for carbohydrate coverage or correction dose of insulin. Selecting an appropriate pump is done on an individual basis, with patients identifying features they feel are important and multidisciplinary teams giving guidance.

Starting Insulin Dose on CSII

After a pump is selected and an order placed, patients and their families are encouraged to review educational materials, DVDs, and computer programs that

Table 27.2 Pump Options and Features

Pump	Insulin Reservoir Capacity, (units)	Minimal Basal Rate Increments, (units/h)	Minimal Bous Dose Increments, (units)	Other features
Animas Ping	200	0.025	0.05	• Smallest pump • Largest display screen • 500-food individualized database • Wireless delivery of bolus from One Touch meter
Deltec Cozmo	300	0.05	0.05	• Integrated Freestyle meter • Enhanced meal maker • Basal rates by day of week • Replacement of basal rate after disconnecting pump
Disetronic Spirit	315	0.1	0.1	• Reversible display • Menu display customization option
Medtronic Paradigm 522/722	180 or 300	0.05	0.1	• Only available pump with real-time CGM on market • Optional remote control for bolus dosing • CareLink Personal Therapy management tool
Insulet Omnipod	200	0.05	0.05	• No tubing • 1,000 common foods in PDA • Freestyle Meter in PDA component

are shipped with the pump. Pump trainers then arrange for a ~60–90 min outpatient visit to initiate CSII therapy. Most commonly, the starting dose of insulin for CSII is based on the current total daily dose (TDD) of insulin a patient is receiving on MDI therapy. Often, this TDD is reduced by 10–25%; however, if a patient is not at target in regard to glycemic control (i.e., A1C >8.5%), minimal to no reduction may be necessary. Alternatively, the dose of insulin can be calculated based on the patient's weight (i.e., weight in kg × 0.5). Rapid-acting insulin analogs (such as lispro, aspart, and glulisine) are typically used in CSII, but regular insulin may also be used.

Once the starting dose of insulin to be used is determined, ~50% is given as basal insulin. The basal dose is initially divided by 24 to get the units per hour, given often as a single basal rate. For example, if a patient was to get a total of 40 units/day when they start CSII, then 20 units would be the total daily basal insulin dosage, and this would be given as 0.8 units/h. Bolus doses of insulin compromise the other half of the insulin to be supplied via CSII. There are two types of boluses that can be given, a correction bolus or a meal bolus. Correction factors (or insulin sensitivity factors) represent how many milligrams per deciliter 1 unit of rapid-acting insulin will drop the blood glucose. Carbohydrate ratios determine how many grams of carbohydrates 1 unit of rapid-acting insulin will cover. There are many ways to determine these bolus doses of insulin. If a patient is on basal-bolus therapy with glargine or detemir prior to CSII, then the factors used on MDI therapy can be programmed into the pump. Alternatively, carbohydrate ratios can be calculated by dividing 500 or 450 by the TDD of insulin. Similarly, a correction factor can be derived by dividing 1,800 by the TDD. An even simpler approach used in the pediatric population is to determine the carbohydrate ratio and correction factor based on the patient's age (Table 27.3).

After initiation of CSII, patients are advised to check their blood glucose frequently, so appropriate adjustments to basal rates, carbohydrates ratios, and correction factors can be made. Basal and bolus doses are adjusted based on monitoring of the patient's blood glucose before meals, 2 h after eating, and at bedtime, midnight, and 3:00 A.M. Patients then contact the clinic as needed for dose adjustments either by calling or faxing blood glucose logs for review. If a patient is noted to have

Table 27.3 Correction Factors and Carbohydrate Ratio Based on Age for Initial Pump Settings

Age (years)	Correction factor (mg/dl)	Carbohydrate ratio (g)*
<3	225	45
4–5	200	40
5–7	150	30
8–11	125	20
Prepubertal and/or <13	75	15
Pubertal and/or >13	50	10

*Often a lower carbohydrate ratio is needed for breakfast (–2 g for breakfast carbohydrate ratio). For example, for children aged <3 years, start breakfast carbohydrate ratio at 43 g.

high blood glucose 2 h postmeal, then the carbohydrate ratio is adjusted. Correction factors are adjusted if the correction boluses fail to return blood glucose levels to the target range. Basal rates are adjusted based on premeal and overnight blood glucose levels. Basal rate change should be implemented 2–3 h prior to time of high or low glucose values in order to correct the problem. To guide daytime basal rate adjustments, some clinicians instruct their patients to delay or skip a meal and monitor blood glucose levels every 2 h in the fasting state.

Very young children on CSII may need more basal insulin given in the evening and early morning hours (between 9:00 P.M. and 3:00 A.M.), which is in marked contrast to adolescents and adults, who often need more basal insulin in the early dawn hours between 3:00 A.M. and breakfast. Such changes can be made by frequent monitoring of bedtime and overnight glucose readings.

Guidelines for prevention and treatment of hypoglycemia and hyperglycemia must be provided. Patients are encouraged to treat all low blood glucose values with a set amount of carbohydrate (specifically rapid-acting glucose in the form of glucose tablets, glucose gel, or juice). Patients are taught to adjust both their bolus and basal doses to avoid hypoglycemia. Instruction on the use of temporary basal rates is also provided to allow patients to decrease basal insulin, as needed; for example, both during physical activity and on nights after increased activity, as required.

Hyperglycemia troubleshooting and prevention, as well as sick-day management, is taught upon initiation of pump therapy and reviewed at each follow-up visit. Patients must be able to understand that they are only using short-acting insulin with no long-acting insulin depot. If they experience hyperglycemia, blood glucose >250 mg/dl (>13.9 mmol/l), they should troubleshoot this accordingly by taking a correction bolus dose. If the blood glucose does not return to target 2 h after a correction bolus dose is given or if they are nauseated or feel sick, patients should check their urine for ketones. If ketones are positive or patients have persistent hyperglycemia, despite administering a correction bolus, they should give a correction bolus by manual insulin injection, change their insulin infusion set line, and repeat delivery of correction bolus doses by injection until glucose levels are back within normal range. Patients are taught to troubleshoot hyperglycemia by not only inspecting the infusion site area, but also by inspecting the infusion site line, luerlock, and basal/bolus doses set in the pump memory. Such meticulous attention to troubleshooting hyperglycemia should prevent DKA; however, hyperglycemic crisis can still occur because of crimping of the infusion set cannula, leakage of insulin from the insulin syringe or luerlock, air in the insulin tubing, dislodgement of the soft cannula from underneath the skin, and other potential problems, including not giving the insulin dose, no insulin in the syringe, and no basal delivery.

The patients should wear the pump continuously, but they can usually disconnect for periods of up to 2 h without any adverse consequences. If the pump is suspended for >2 h, supplemental insulin may need to be given to cover the basal rate, along with bolus insulin to cover food intake. Some patients who are disconnected for >2 h on a routine basis for athletic activities (e.g., swimming, football) may want to consider giving a portion of their basal dose as a long-acting analog every morning, with appropriate reduction in the pump basal dose. If patients desire a pump holiday or they must return to MDI for a period of >24 h, they should take insulin glargine or detemir at a dose equal to their CSII basal rate daily, along with meal and correction dose injections of a rapid-acting insulin analog until they return to CSII.

INSULIN PUMP THERAPY FOLLOW-UP

Clinical follow-up of patients on insulin pump therapy is similar to follow-up of individuals on other forms of intensive diabetes management with MDI therapy. Patients are encouraged to continue monitoring their glucose at least four times a day and log their blood glucose values. Follow-up with the health care team (a physician or nurse practitioner) is done 2 weeks after starting pump therapy.

Once glucose levels are stabilized, visits are done on a quarterly basis. Pump memories are checked in addition to reviewing the patient's logbook to determine the TDD of insulin, current pump settings, and adequacy of these settings. Adjustment of the basal rate, bolus doses, carbohydrate-to-insulin ratio, and correction boluses should be done to obtain the glycemic targets set for that individual patient. Hypoglycemia, hyperglycemia, DKA prevention, troubleshooting, and sick-day management should be reviewed. Follow-up with a registered dietitian is done as needed to review carbohydrate counting practices, guidelines for normal nutrition, and weight management.

When the patient's A1C is above goal, it is important to note the frequency of SMBG, the number of bolus doses given, and the individual's record-keeping habits. Diet and knowledge of food intake should be examined, as should bolusing practices with food and snacks. The memory features on blood glucose meters and on insulin pumps are helpful in verifying the patient's record of glucose monitoring and bolus frequency. Infusion site areas should be examined for atrophy, hypertrophy, and inflammation. Appropriate rotation of sites should be encouraged. If evidence of infection exists, appropriate use of antistaphylococcal soap should be used before insertion of the infusion set, along with eradication of the staph-carrier state by using mupirocin calcium cream 2% (Bactroban) or another antistaphylococcal ointment in the nares of the nose. Other factors affecting glycemic control, such as marked fear of hypoglycemia or overtreatment of low blood glucose values, need to be explored if glycemic targets are not met.

If the A1C goal is still not met, the patient's satisfaction with pump therapy needs to be re-assessed. If the patient is motivated and committed to CSII then more frequent contact with the health care team to review blood glucose levels and fine tune therapy may help to bring the A1C into target range. With the advent of continuous glucose monitors (for continuous glucose monitoring [CGM]), greater fine-tuning of the patient's regimen may be possible. However, if a patient is not satisfied with his/her current regimen, transitioning back to injection therapy must be considered.

CGM

CGM devices were first approved by the FDA in 2006. Currently, three units are commercially available to patients, the Minimed Paradigm REAL-Time System,

DexCom Seven, and Abbott FreeStyle Navigator. In comparison to SMBG, which gives the patient only brief "snapshots" as to where the blood glucose lies at the time of the test, CGM provides the opportunity to look at not only the current glucose reading, but also where the glucose has been and what rate and direction the glucose reading may be heading. Based on this real-time glucose data and retrospective analysis, appropriate changes in insulin dosage and nutritional intake and activity may be made. The need for such technology was evidenced by a study of 54 youth with type 1 diabetes that was conducted in 2001. That study used CGM and demonstrated that 90% of patients had a peak postprandial glucose level of >180 mg/dl after every meal, and 70% of patients had a sensor glucose value <60 mg/dl on one of the three nights of monitoring. The real-time CGM devices that are currently available are more accurate and user-friendly than the first generation of devices, and early studies have suggested beneficial effects of these systems in the management of patients with type 1 diabetes. A large-scale randomized trial of all three systems demonstrated that A1C levels could be reduced by 0.5% in patients who were aged ≥25 years. Similar results were obtained in 8- to 24-year-olds who used the device with similar frequency as adults.

Newer applications of CGM include the hopes of developing a closed-loop system. Automated closed-loop insulin delivery systems combining external insulin pumps with current real-time CGM devices are already being studied. With these advances, the dream of an artificial pancreas as a viable treatment option for patients with type 1 diabetes may be possible in the not-too-distant future.

CONCLUSION

Technological advances, like CSII, have drastically altered the way that patients are able to manage their diabetes. Randomized and nonrandomized studies have shown the efficacy of CSII across all age-groups; quality-of-life surveys have revealed increased patient satisfaction when using this therapy as compared to MDI therapy. Newer technologies like CGM and the goal of an artificial pancreas will continue to alter the way that patients, and health care providers, are able to care for diabetes.

BIBLIOGRAPHY

Bode BW, Steed RD, Davidson PC: Reduction in severe hypoglycemia with long-term continuous subcutaneous insulin infusion in type I diabetes. *Diabetes Care* 19:324–327, 1996

Bode BW, Tamborlane WV, Davidson PC: Insulin pump therapy in the 21st century: strategies for successful use in adults, adolescents, and children with diabetes. *Postgrad Med* 111:69–77, 2002

Boland E, Monsod T, Delucia M, Brandt C, Fernando S, Tamborlane W: Limitations of conventional methods of self-monitoring of blood glucose: lessons learned from 3 days of continuous glucose sensing in pediatric patients with type 1 diabetes. *Diabetes Care* 24:1858–1862, 2001

Diabetes Research in Children Network Study Group: Prevention of hypoglycemia during exercise in children with type 1 diabetes by suspending basal insulin. *Diabetes Care* 29:2200–2204, 2006

Juvenile Diabetes Research Foundation Continuous Glucose Monitoring Study Group: Continuous glucose monitoring and intensive treatment of type 1 diabetes. *N Engl J Med* 359:1464–1476, 2008

Phillip M, Battelino T, Rodriguez H, Danne T, Kaufman F: Use of insulin pump therapy in pediatric age-group: consensus statement from the European Society for Paediatric Endocrinology, the Lawson Wilkins Pediatric Endocrine Society, and the International Society for Pediatric and Adolescent Diabetes, endorsed by the American Diabetes Association and the European Association for the Study of Diabetes. *Diabetes Care* 30:1653–1662, 2007

Tamborlane WV, Swan K, Sikes KA, Steffen AT, Weinzimer SA: The renaissance of insulin pump treatment in childhood type 1 diabetes. *Rev Endocr Metab Disord* 7:205–213, 2006

Weinzimer SA, Tamborlane WV: Sensor-augmented pump therapy in type 1 diabetes. *Curr Op Endocr Diabetes Obes* 15:118–122, 2008

Dr. Sherr is a Pediatric Endocrinology Fellow at Yale School of Medicine, New Haven, Connecticut. Dr. Tamborlane is Professor and Chief of Pediatric Endocrinology at Yale School of Medicine, and is the Deputy Director for the Yale Center for Clinical Investigation, New Haven, Connecticut. Dr. Bode is Medical Director at the Diabetes Resource Center of Atlanta, Atlanta Diabetes Associates, Atlanta, Georgia.

28. Combination Therapies with Oral Agents or Oral Agents and Insulin

MATTHEW C. RIDDLE, MD

Conclusive evidence that appropriate glycemic control can reduce microvascular complications justifies striving for glycemic control that achieves A1C levels ≤7%, unless long duration of diabetes and high cardiovascular risk, or other factors, suggest a higher A1C target is more appropriate. Recent large clinical trials show that treating patients with type 2 diabetes with lifestyle intervention and a single pharmacological agent is unlikely to achieve and sustain such glycemic control. What strategies should be used to maintain A1C at or below the 7% target when therapy with a single antihyperglycemic agent is not successful? The possibilities are to combine oral agents with different mechanisms of action, to combine insulin with one or more oral agents, to use multiple injections of insulin without oral agents, or to use one of these approaches together with one of the new injectable therapies based on gastrointestinal peptide hormones. This chapter focuses on the rationale and use of the first two options above, the various combinations of oral agents or oral agents with insulin, for controlling hyperglycemia in patients with type 2 diabetes.

RATIONALE FOR COMBINATION THERAPY

Factors influencing glucose metabolism are as follows:

- glucose balance (production versus uptake) across the liver
- insulin and glucagon secretory rates
- rate of gastrointestinal absorption of carbohydrate
- rate of peripheral (muscle and adipose tissue) glucose uptake and utilization

These processes are all abnormally regulated in type 2 diabetes, and all can be modified by the antihyperglycemic agents now available. Table 28.1 highlights the primary actions of currently available agents. Judicious use of combinations of oral agents or combinations of insulin with oral antihyperglycemic agents takes advantage of these different modes of action.

Two main kinds of combinations can be distinguished. First, an agent that enhances the availability of insulin can be combined with one that improves the effectiveness of insulin. Second, an agent that is most effective in controlling basal

Table 28.1 Currently Available Classes of Antidiabetic Agents

Class/drug	Primary Mode of Action				Primary Effect on Glycemia	
	Decrease hepatic glucose production	Increase insulin secretion	Delay carbo-hydrate absorption	Increase peripheral glucose uptake	Decrease fasting plasma glucose	Decrease postprandial plasma glucose
Sulfonylurea						
Glimepiride	+++	+++	0	++	+++	+
Glipizide	+++	+++	0	++	+++	+
Glyburide	+++	+++	0	++	+++	+
Nonsulfonylurea secretagogues						
Nateglinide	++	+++	0	+++	++	++
Repaglinide	++	+++	0	+++	++	++
DPP-4 inhibitor						
Sitagliptin	++	++	0	++	++	+
Biguanide						
Metformin	+++	0	0	+	+++	+
Thiazolidinediones						
Pioglitazone	++	0	0	+++	++	++
Rosiglitazone	++	0	0	+++	++	++
α-Glucosidase inhibitor	+++	0	+	0	+	+++
Acarbose	+	0	+++	0	+	+++
Miglitol	+	0	+++	0	+	+++
Basal insulin						
NPH	+++	+++	0	+	+++	+
Glargine	+++	+++	0	+	+++	+
Detemir	+++	+++	0	+	+++	+
Prandial insulin						
Regular	+++	+++	0	+++	++	++
Aspart	+++	+++	0	+++	+	+++
Glulisine	+++	+++	0	+++	+	+++
Lispro	+++	+++	0	+++	+	+++

0, no effect; +, small effect; ++, moderate effect; +++, marked effect.

(fasting and preprandial) hyperglycemia can be combined with one that has its main effect on postprandial increases of glucose. The combination of basal insulin with short- or rapid-acting insulin most clearly illustrates this tactic, but oral combinations can use this approach as well. Also, the nonglycemic effects of combinations can improve other aspects of the metabolic derangements seen with type 2 diabetes. A good example is the ability of metformin to prevent weight gain caused by insulin when the two are used together to improve glycemic control.

Table 28.2 Combinations of Oral Agents Used to Treat Type 2 Diabetes

	A1C change (%) versus first agent alone	Weight change (lb) versus first agent alone
Widely used, values from systematic meta-analysis		
Metformin added to sulfonylurea	−1.0 (11)	~0 (5)
Sulfonylurea added to metformin	−1.0 (11)	+5 (9)
Thiazolidinedione added to sulfonylurea	−1.0 (4)	Increase
Thiazolidinedione added to metformin	−0.6 (4)	Increase
Less often used, values from limited studies		
Nateglinide added to metformin	−0.4 to 0.7	Increase
Repaglinide added to metformin	1.1	Increase
Acarbose added to metformin	−0.7 to −0.8	~0
Acarbose added to sulfonylurea	−0.8 to −0.9	~0
Sitagliptin added to metformin	−0.7	~0
Sitagliptin added to thiazolidinedione	−0.7	~0

The meta-analysis from which the upper part of this table is adapted is by Bolen et al. (2007). The numbers in parentheses show the number of studies in each category included in the meta-analysis.

COMBINATIONS OF ORAL ANTIDIABETIC AGENTS

Table 28.2 lists combinations of oral antihyperglycemic agents that have been used to treat patients with type 2 diabetes. Combinations of agents that increase insulin secretion, e.g., sulfonylureas, repaglinide, or nateglinide, with agents that decrease insulin requirements, e.g., metformin, α-glucosidase inhibitors (acarbose and miglitol), and thiazolidinediones (pioglitazone and rosiglitazone), have been well studied and their effects validated; hence, they are approved by the U.S. Food and Drug Administration (FDA). The effects expected are the mean data reported from large and rigorous clinical trials. The combinations of α-glucosidase inhibitors, such as acarbose, with insulin secretagogues or insulin sensitizers are useful when additional effects in specifically lowering postprandial hyperglycemia are desired. The thiazolidinediones and metformin improve insulin sensitivity by different mechanisms and seem to preferentially affect different organs (metformin affects the liver and thiazolidinediones the skeletal muscle). Combination therapy with these two classes of insulin sensitizers has added benefits in improving insulin sensitivity and achieving glycemic control. In contrast, sulfonylureas and the non-sulfonylurea secretagogues (repaglinide and nateglinide) have very similar mechanisms of action and do not have additive effects. The combination of sitagliptin, which potentiates insulin secretion and also suppresses glucagon secretion, with metformin provides moderate additional reduction of glucose.

All of the combinations discussed above are effective only when endogenous insulin capacity is adequate to support their effects. As endogenous insulin secretion continues to decrease with increasing duration of type 2 diabetes, combinations of oral agents are progressively less effective.

Table 28.3 Combinations of Insulin and Oral Agents Used to Treat Type 2 Diabetes

	A1C change (%) versus first prior treatment alone	Weight change (lb) per 1% A1C reduction versus first prior treatment alone
Widely used, values from systematic meta-analysis		
Basal insulin added to metformin	−2.5 (1)	+1 (1)
Basal insulin added to sulfonylurea	−2.1 (7)	+5 (4)
Basal insulin added to sulfonylurea and metformin	−1.9 (4)	+3 (6)
Less often used, values from systematic meta-analysis		
Metformin added to insulin	−1.9 (4)	−1 (4)
Sulfonylurea added to insulin	−1.4 (7)	+3 (9)
Thiazolidinedione added to insulin	−1.3 (2)	+8 (3)
Less often used, values from limited studies		
α-Glucosidase inhibitor added to insulin	−0.6	~0
DPP-IV inhibitor (vildagliptin) added to insulin	−0.3	+1

The meta-analysis from which the upper parts of this table is adapted is by Yki-Jarvinen (2001). The numbers in parentheses show the number of studies in each category included in the meta-analysis .

COMBINATIONS OF ORAL ANTIDIABETIC AGENTS WITH INSULIN

In the later stages of type 2 diabetes, results of treatment can be improved by combining the oral agents with insulin. Different mechanisms underlie the benefits of different combinations. Metformin and the thiazolidinediones both increase tissue sensitivity to endogenous and injected insulin and thereby maximize the effectiveness of the remaining endogenous insulin while permitting smaller dosages of injected insulin to be effective. α-Glucosidase inhibitors delay the absorption of dietary carbohydrates, making the reduced and delayed secretion of endogenous insulin more effective and potentially extending the time when basal insulin without prandial injections can be successful. Oral agents that potentiate the secretion of endogenous insulin can provide a more physiological insulin response when combined with exogenous insulin, allowing improved glycemic control without increased risk of hypoglycemia.

Table 28.3 lists combinations of oral antidiabetic agents and insulin for which there are sufficient data to evaluate their effects. Several recent studies have evaluated the effect of combining insulin treatment with metformin. These studies show a mean decrease in A1C of 0.7–2.5%, depending partly on whether insulin dosage was simultaneously adjusted. Hypoglycemia can occur, but generally this combination reduces the risk of insulin-induced hypoglycemia at any given level of glycemic control. Moreover, concurrent use of metformin largely prevents the weight gain frequently seen during insulin use.

The combination of a sulfonylurea with insulin has been controversial. This combination can reduce A1C by 0.3–2.3%, depending on whether insulin dosage is adjusted. However, the frequency of hypoglycemia relative to that expected with insulin therapy alone differs between studies, and improvement in glycemic control is less consistent than with other insulin and oral agent combinations. One contributor to problems with hypoglycemia in earlier studies was the use of glyburide, an agent more likely to cause hypoglycemia than other sulfonylureas. The glycemic benefits of a later-generation sulfonylurea combined with insulin often become apparent when the sulfonylurea is discontinued and A1C increases.

Adding pioglitazone or rosiglitazone to insulin therapy can improve glycemic control in insulin-resistant type 2 diabetic patients who are inadequately controlled, especially those taking substantial doses (e.g., ≥70 units/day) of insulin. The improvement in glycemic control is accompanied by variable (15–50%) decreases of mean insulin requirements. Care must be exercised when adding a thiazolidinedione to the regimen for patients already taking insulin. One concern is that the added effect of a thiazolidinedione may develop over ≥3 months and lead to unanticipated hypoglycemia. Also, this combination can cause significant fluid retention. Mild to moderate edema is quite common (10–20%), and congestive heart failure can occur, even in patients without previously recognized heart disease. Because of these concerns, FDA recommendations for use of thiazolidinediones have become more conservative, especially for rosiglitazone, which is no longer recommended for combination with insulin. Patients at risk for heart failure should not use either thiazolidinedione, and patients adding pioglitazone to insulin should begin with a low dosage, increase dosage slowly, and be carefully observed.

Less information is available about combining acarbose or sitagliptin with insulin. Adding acarbose to insulin can limit postprandial glycemic increases, modestly improve A1C (~0.5%), and perhaps reduce episodes of hypoglycemia.

Table 28.4 Scheme for Adding Basal or Intermediate-Acting Insulin to Oral Agents

Start with 10 units of basal (glargine) or intermediate-acting (NPH) insulin at bedtime (~10:00 P.M.). Adjust insulin dose weekly according to the following guidelines:

Self-monitored FPG (mg/dl)	Increase in insulin dose (units/day)
≥180	8
≥140 but <180	6
≥120 but <140	4
≥100 but <120	2
Treat-to-target FPG ≤100 mg/dl	

Do not increase insulin dose if FPG is <72 mg/dl on 2 days. Decrease insulin dose 2–4 units/day if FPG is <56 mg/dl or clinically significant hypoglycemia occurs.

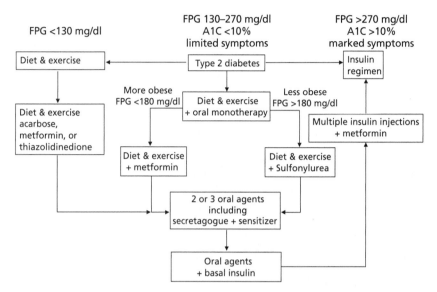

Figure 28.1 An approach to the management of hyperglycemia in patients with type 2 diabetes.

Although many studies have examined addition of oral agents to insulin, the usual setting for this combination in clinical practice is when oral therapies are no longer successful alone and insulin is added. Adding a basal insulin dose at night to oral medications during the day is a simple approach that improves glycemic control by reducing overnight hepatic glucose production. The goal is to give enough basal insulin to achieve a fasting plasma glucose (FPG) level between 100 and 130 mg/dl (5.9 and 7.2 mmol/l). Table 28.4 provides the titration scheme that was used in a recent treat-to-target study that added either NPH or glargine insulin at bedtime to the regimen of type 2 diabetic patients who were not well controlled on one or more oral agents.

WHEN AND HOW TO INSTITUTE COMBINATION THERAPY

Fig. 28.1 is a general guide to combination therapy. Individuals with little elevation of FPG (<130 mg.dl [>8.3 mmol/l]) often show improved A1C with diet and increased physical activity. Some, however, will require the addition of monotherapy with metformin, a thiazolidinedione, or an α-glucosidase inhibitor, agents that have little risk of causing hypoglycemia, to achieve an A1C between 6.0 and 7.0%. At the other end of the scale of glycemic control, patients with severe and symptomatic hyperglycemia (usually FPG >270 mg/dl [>15 mmol/l] and A1C >10%) are best treated initially with insulin. Most type 2 diabetic patients fall between these extremes (FPG 130–270 mg/dl [7.2–15 mmol/l] and A1C <10.0%)

Table 28.5 Recommended Dosing Schedules for Combination Therapy

α-Glucosidase inhibitors	
Acarbose	25–100 mg with each meal
Miglitol	25–100 mg with each meal
Metformin	500–1,000 mg twice daily before meals
Sulfonylureas	
Glipizide, conventional	5–10 mg twice daily
Glipizide extended-release	5 mg once daily
Glimepiride	4 mg once daily
Glyburide	5 mg twice daily
Nonsulfonylurea secretogogues	
Nateglinide	60–120 mg with each meal
Repaglinide	1–2 mg with each meal
Thiazolidinediones	
Rosiglitazone	2–4 mg once daily
Pioglitazone	15–30 mg once daily
Basal insulins	
Detemir, NPH, or glargine	Start with 5–10 units daily, usually at bedtime
	Increase on a regular schedule
	e.g., 1–2 units every 3 days or 2–4 units weekly
	Goal is FPG between 110 and 130 mg/dl
	(6.1–7.2 mmol/l)
Multiple insulin doses	Dosages are very variable and must be individualized

and should be started on lifestyle intervention accompanied by monotherapy with an oral antihyperglycemic agent. A detailed scheme for managing this group of patients, taking into consideration the results of medical outcome studies, has recently been published (Nathan 2009).

Those who are predominantly insulin resistant (with central and/or generalized obesity) might best be treated with an agent that decreases insulin resistance (usually metformin). Those who are more insulin deficient and have relatively high glucose levels (less obese individuals with FPG >180 mg/dl [<10.0 mmol/l]) might be better candidates for an agent that increases insulin secretion (usually a sulfonylurea).

Most patients will not achieve their target glycemic control on monotherapy either initially or after several years of treatment. These individuals require combination therapy. Typical dosages used in various regimens are given in Table 28.5. Because of long experience, low cost, and convincing evidence for medical benefits, the combination of metformin and a sulfonylurea is most widely used.

Combination oral agent therapy will lose its effectiveness when insulin secretion becomes markedly deficient. At that stage, endogenous insulin capacity is so depleted that overnight hepatic glucose production is unrestrained and marked fasting hyperglycemia ensues. This can be ameliorated by administering intermediate-acting or long-acting (basal) insulin at bedtime (~10:00 P.M.) and continuing oral agents during the day. Introducing insulin this way is most appropriate when one or two oral agents are incompletely successful. At this stage of diabetes, this method is generally as effective as multiple injections of insulin and causes less weight gain and hypoglycemia.

If endogenous secretory capacity declines even further and little or no insulin secretion occurs with meals, then oral antihyperglycemic agents become ineffective and a multiple insulin injection regimen becomes necessary. Frequently, this can be a regimen combining intermediate-acting and short-acting insulin before breakfast, short-acting insulin before the evening meal, and intermediate-acting insulin at bedtime. An alternative is to give basal insulin (such as glargine) once daily or NPH or detemir twice daily and to precede each meal with a rapid-acting insulin analog (lispro, aspart, or glulisine). Also available, though limited by the difficulty in matching insulin action to mealtime requirements, is twice-daily premixed insulin (70/30 or 75/25). Because many type 2 diabetic patients are severely insulin resistant, it may be necessary to treat them with very large doses of insulin (>100 units/day), and in this situation better glycemic control at lower doses of insulin may be achieved by continuing or adding pioglitazone or metformin to the insulin regimen.

USEFUL HINTS FOR COMBINATION THERAPY IN TYPE 2 DIABETIC PATIENTS

The following are useful guidelines when contemplating combination therapy in patients with type 2 diabetes:

1. About 5–10% of patients who develop diabetes as adults, and seem to have type 2 diabetes, actually have slowly evolving type 1 diabetes (latent autoimmune diabetes in adults [LADA]). These individuals tend to be younger and leaner than typical patients with type 2 diabetes and often lack a family history of diabetes. They usually require insulin therapy within the first 6 years after diagnosis. Measurement of GAD (glutamic acid decarboxylase) antibodies can confirm this diagnosis in potential cases.

2. Laboratory confirmation of insulin resistance at diagnosis of diabetes is seldom necessary because clinical features (central obesity, acanthosis nigricans, hypertension, hypertriglyceridemia, decreased plasma HDL cholesterol) are usually sufficient. In selected cases, demonstration of elevated plasma C-peptide, fasting or after a meal challenge, can verify the presence of severe insulin resistance.

3. Most oral antidiabetic agents achieve near-maximal effects at one-half to two-thirds of the maximal dose recommended by the manufacturer. Giving maximal dosage of a single agent before adding a second agent is usually not effective and can increase side effects.

4. If one oral antidiabetic agent does not lower glycemia to the target range, changing to a different oral agent rarely achieves better glycemic control. However, combining two oral agents with different modes of action will result in improved glycemic control.

5. The use of three different oral antidiabetic agents, although theoretically appealing, has few clinical data to validate it and may not be cost-effective.

The data that are available indicate that adding the third oral agent rarely lowers the A1C to <7% if the A1C before adding the third agent is much higher than 8%.

6. Bedtime insulin and oral agents taken during the day are frequently as effective in achieving glycemic control as multiple injections of insulin in patients with earlier type 2 diabetes or in those for whom oral agents have initially failed.

BIBLIOGRAPHY

Aviles-Santa L, Sinding J, Raskin P: Effects of metformin in patients with poorly controlled, insulin-treated type 2 diabetes mellitus: a randomized, double-blind, placebo-controlled trial. *Ann Intern Med* 131:182–188, 1999

Bolen S, Feldman L, Vassy J, Wilson L, Yeh H-C, Marinopoulos S, Wiley C, Selvin E, Wilson R, Bass EB, Brancati FL: Systematic review: comparative effectiveness and safety of oral medications for type 2 diabetes mellitus. *Ann Intern Med* 147:383–399, 2007

Chiasson J-L, Josse RG, Hunt JA, Palmason C, Rodger NW, Ross SA, Ryan EA, Tan MH, Wolever TMS: The efficacy of acarbose in the treatment of patients with non-insulin-dependent diabetes mellitus. *Ann Intern Med* 121:928–935, 1994

DeFronzo RA, Goodman AM: Efficacy of metformin in patients with non-insulin-dependent diabetes mellitus: the Multicenter Metformin Study Group. *N Engl J Med* 333:541–549, 1995

Fonseca V, Rosenstock J, Patwardhan R, Salzman A: Effect of metformin and rosiglitazone combination therapy in patients with type 2 diabetes mellitus: a randomized controlled trial. *JAMA* 283:1695–1702, 2000

Goldstein BJ, Feinglos MN, Lunceford JK, Johnson J, Williams-Herma DE, Sitagliptin 036 Study Group: Effect of initial combination therapy with sitagliptin, a dipeptidyl peptidase-4 inhibitor, and metformin on glycemic control in patients with type 2 diabetes. *Diabetes Care* 30:1979–1987, 2007

Holman RR, Thorne DI, Farmer AJ, Davies MJ, Keenan JF, Paul S, Levy JC, 4-T Study Group: Addition of biphasic, prandial, or basal insulin to oral therapy in type 2 diabetes. *N Engl J Med* 357:1716–1730, 2007

Inzucchi SE: Oral antihyperglycemic therapy for type 2 diabetes: scientific review. *JAMA* 287:360–372, 2002

Lebovitz HE: Oral therapies for diabetic hyperglycemia. *Endocrinol Metab Clin North Am* 30:909–933, 2001

Nathan DM, Buse JB, Davidson MB, Ferrannini E, Holman RR, Sherwin R, Zinman B, American Diabetes Association, European Association for the Study of Diabetes: Medical management of hyperglycemia in type 2 diabetes: a consensus algorithm for the initiation and adjustment of therapy: a consensus statement of the American Diabetes Association and the European Association for the Study of Diabetes. *Diabetes Care* 32:193–203, 2009

Raskin P, Rendell M, Riddle MC, Dole JF, Freed MI, Rosenstock J, Rosiglitazone Clinical Trials Study Group: A randomized trial of rosiglitazone therapy in patients with inadequately controlled insulin-treated type 2 diabetes. *Diabetes Care* 24:1226–1232, 2001

Riddle MC, Rosenstock J, Gerich J, Insulin Glargine 4002 Study Investigators: The Treat-to-Target Trial: randomized addition of glargine or human NPH insulin to oral therapy of type 2 diabetic patients. *Diabetes Care* 26:3080–3086, 2003

Riddle MC: Glycemic management of type 2 diabetes: an emerging strategy with oral agents, insulins, and combinations. *Endocrinol Metab Clin North Am* 34:77–98, 2005

U.K. Prospective Diabetes Study Group: United Kingdom Prospective Diabetes Study 24: a 6-year, randomized, controlled trial comparing sulfonylurea, insulin and metformin therapy in patients with newly diagnosed type 2 diabetes that could not be controlled with diet therapy. *Ann Intern Med* 128:165–175, 1998

Wright AW, Burden ACF, Paisey RB, Cull C, Holman RR, U.K. Prospective Diabetes Study Group: Sulfonylurea inadequacy: Efficacy of addition of insulin over 6 years in patients with type 2 diabetes in the U.K. Prospective Diabetes Stud (UKPDS 57). *Diabetes Care* 25:330–336, 2002

Wulffele MG, Kooy A, Lehert P, Bets D, Ogterop JC, van der Berg BB, Donker AJM, Stehouwer CDA: Combination of insulin and metformin in the treatment of type 2 diabetes. *Diabetes Care* 25:2133–2140, 2002

Yki-Jarvinen H: Combination therapies with insulin in type 2 diabetes. *Diabetes Care* 24:758–767, 2001

Yki-Jarvinen H, Ryysy L, Nikkila K, Tulokas T, Vanamo R, Heikkila M: Comparison of bedtime insulin regimens in patients with type 2 diabetes mellitus: a randomized, controlled trial. *Ann Intern Med* 130:389–396, 1999

Dr. Riddle is Professor of Medicine at Oregon Health & Science University, Portland, Oregon.

29. Glycemic Control and Chronic Diabetes Complications

HAROLD E. LEBOVITZ, MD

O ur understanding of the relationship between chronic glycemic control and the vascular complications of diabetes was greatly enhanced by the results of several large, randomized, controlled intervention studies that were completed in the 1990s. Those studies demonstrated that microvascular complications are highly correlated with mean glycemic control, as measured by A1C, and that improvement in glycemic control results in reduction in all microvascular complications. In contrast, those same studies failed to show a significant reduction in macrovascular complications with improved glycemic control. The effects of intensive glycemic control on clinical cardiovascular events were the focus of several large intervention trials completed and reported in 2008. The patient populations recruited in those trials did not show significant risk reduction in cardiovascular events with intensive glycemic control.

An unexpected result of the extensions of some of the intervention studies is the remarkable finding that initial glycemic control influences vascular complication rates and severity for many years beyond the time that the glycemic control occurred. These observations suggest that vascular tissues are imprinted with glycemic effects that persist for many years and that those effects continue to influence the rate of development of complications for many years.

Table 29.1 lists the more noteworthy earlier studies that have been the basis for our knowledge about chronic glycemic control and the development of diabetic vascular complications.

INTERVENTION STUDIES

The Diabetes Control and Complications Trial (DCCT) was both a primary and secondary intervention trial in patients with type 1 diabetes that tested the effects of intensive glycemic control versus ordinary glycemic control on the development or progression of microvascular and neuropathic complications. For the study, 1,441 patients were recruited and treated for an average of 6.5 years. Intensive treatment involved insulin injections three or four times per day or insulin pump therapy. Ordinary treatment was insulin injections one or two times per day. The glycemic control for the ordinary-treatment group over the 6.5 years of the study was a mean A1C of 9.1% and a daily average plasma glucose of 231 mg/dl (12.8 mmol/l) (nondiabetic values: A1C ≤6%, plasma glucose 110 mg/dl [6.1

Table 29.1 Studies Demonstrating the Relationship Between Glycemic Control and Chronic Complications

	Diabetic Patients (*n*)	Data Reported
Intervention studies		
DCCT	1,441 type 1	1993
EDIC (follow-up of the DCCT)	1,229 type 1	2002 to present
Kumamoto study	110 Japanese type 2	1995
UKPDS	5,102 newly diagnosed type 2	1998
Epidemiological studies		
Wisconsin	1,516	1994
Steno 1—type 2 diabetes	328	1995
Finnish elderly study	229	1994

---

mmol/l]). The intensively treated group maintained an average A1C of 7.2% and a daily average plasma glucose of 155 mg/dl (8.6 mmol/l). The results of both the primary and secondary intervention arms showed that this degree of difference in glycemic control resulted in risk reductions of 63% for retinopathy, 60% for neuropathy, and 54% for nephropathy. Specific details of the results of this remarkable study are given in Tables 29.2 and 29.3. Intensive glycemic control was associated with a greater than threefold increase in severe hypoglycemia (62 vs. 19 episodes/100 patient-years) and a remarkable increase in body weight.

The Kumamoto study, a much smaller study carried out in 110 thin Japanese type 2 diabetic patients with essentially the same protocol as the DCCT, showed similar results. Their ordinary-treatment group maintained an A1C of 9.4% and a fasting plasma glucose (FPG) of 164 mg/dl (9.1 mmol/l), and the intensively treated patients had a mean A1C of 7.1% and a mean FPG of 126 mg/dl (7 mmol/l). The intensive-treatment patients had a risk reduction of 69% for retinopathy and 70% for nephropathy compared with the ordinary-treatment group.

Table 29.2 Results of Primary Prevention Study (DCCT)

Complication	Conventional Therapy (rate/100 patient-yr)	Intensive Therapy (rate/100 patient-yr)	Risk Reduction (%)
≥3-step sustained retinopathy	4.7	1.2	76
Urinary albumin excretion ≥40 mg/24 h	3.4	2.3	34
Clinical neuropathy at 5 yr	9.8	3.1	69

Table 29.3 Results of Secondary Intervention Study (DCCT)

Complication	Conventional Therapy (rate/100 patient-yr)	Intensive Therapy (rate/100 patient-yr)	Risk Reduction (%)
Laser treatment	2.3	0.9	56
Urinary albumin excretion ≥300 mg/24 h	1.4	0.6	56
Clinical neuropathy at 5 yr	16.1	7.0	57

The U.K. Prospective Diabetes Study (UKPDS) was primarily designed to assess the chronic effects of intensive glycemic control on the development of clinical microvascular and macrovascular complications in newly diagnosed type 2 diabetic patients. A secondary goal was to compare the outcomes of treatment with a first-generation sulfonylurea (chlorpropamide), a second-generation sulfo-nylurea (glyburide), and insulin to that of conventional (diet and exercise) treatment in nonoverweight patients and those same treatments as well as metformin treatment in overweight patients. A total of 5,102 newly diagnosed type 2 diabetic patients were recruited and initially treated for 3 months with a diet and an increased physical activity program. The 4,209 patients who were symptom free and had an FPG between 108 and 270 mg/dl (6.0 and 15 mmol/l, respectively) after the 3-month run-in were randomized to the various treatments. The mean duration of treatment was 11 years. The target glycemic goal was an FPG of 108 mg/dl (6.0 mmol/l). However, to evaluate both the individual treatments as well as intensive glycemic control, the researchers did not add additional therapies to the treatment regimens of the individual patients until the patients became symptomatic or the FPG exceeded 270 mg/dl (15 mmol/l). This conflict frequently interfered with the principle of obtaining early intensive glycemic management. Despite this shortcoming, the intensively treated patients (insulin and sulfonylurea treatments) had a median A1C during the study of 7.0%, and the conventionally treated group had a median A1C of 7.9%. The 0.9% difference in the intensively treated patients resulted in a significant reduction in microvascular complications (Table 29.4).

Thus, it can be extrapolated from the intervention studies in both type 1 and type 2 diabetic patients that a 1% decrease in A1C reduces the risk of microvascular complications by ~30%.

Neither the DCCT nor the Kumamoto study had enough macrovascular events to determine the effects of glycemic control on the development or progression of macrovascular disease. Whereas the UKPDS had a 16% reduction in the risk of myocardial infarctions in the intensively treated group, this failed to achieve statistical significance. Therefore, both studies failed to demonstrate a clear benefit of intensive glycemic control in reducing macrovascular complications.

Table 29.4 Results of Intensive Glycemic Control in the UKPDS

Complication	Risk Reduction (%)	Statistical Significance (*P*)
Any diabetes-related end point	↓ 12	0.029
Myocardial infarction	↓ 16	0.052
Microvascular end points	↓ 25	0.0099
Retinal photocoagulation	↓ 29	0.0031
Cataract extraction	↓ 24	0.046
Microalbuminuria at 12 yr	↓ 33	<0.001

EPIDEMIOLOGICAL STUDIES

Several epidemiological studies suggest that glycemic control does influence both the number and severity of macrovascular events. For 10 years, the Wisconsin epidemiology study followed 682 individuals who had developed diabetes before age 30 years and 834 who developed diabetes after age 30 years.

The data showed that there was a progressive increase in mortality, development of ischemic heart disease, development of proteinuria, and progression of retinopathy in both groups of diabetic patients as the patients' A1C values went from the lowest fourth (5.4–8.5%) to the highest fourth (11.6–20.8%) of the population. In 328 white type 2 diabetic patients followed for 5 years at Steno hospital in Denmark, cardiovascular mortality was two- to threefold greater in individuals who maintained an A1C >7.8% compared with those who maintained an A1C <7.8%. Similarly, in the Finnish elderly study reported by Kuusisto et al. (1994), cardiovascular events and mortality during a 3.5-year follow-up were five- to eightfold greater in type 2 diabetic patients who had an A1C >7% compared with those with an A1C <7%.

An analysis of the epidemiological data from the UKPDS indicated that each 1% decrease in mean A1C of the entire study population was associated with a statistically significant 14% decrease in myocardial infarctions.

From currently available data, it is reasonable to conclude that microvascular and probably macrovascular complications in both type 1 and type 2 diabetic patients will increase as glycemic control worsens. Complications can be minimized at an A1C level <7%. Our current criteria for the goals of glycemic control are based on the results of studies such as those discussed here.

ADDITIONAL KEY FINDINGS FROM THE INTERVENTION STUDIES

Metformin Reduces Macrovascular Disease

An additional important finding in the UKPDS in the overweight cohort was that treatment with metformin significantly reduced myocardial infarctions and diabetes-related deaths (Table 29.5). These effects were not observed with insulin or sulfonylurea treatments, which gave the same reduction in A1C when com-

Table 29.5 Effects of Metformin Treatment in the UKPDS Overweight Type 2 Diabetes Cohort

Complication	Risk Reduction (%)	Statistical Significance (*P*)
Any diabetes-related end point	↓ 32	0.0023
Diabetes-related deaths	↓ 42	0.017
All-cause mortality	↓ 36	0.011
Myocardial infarction	↓ 39	0.01

pared with conventional treatment (0.6%) as metformin. These observations suggest that it is the effects of metformin on the metabolic syndrome that account for its benefits on macrovascular disease.

Glycemic Control Imprints Vascular Tissues and Determines the Development of Diabetic Vascular Complications for Many Additional Years

In both the DCCT and the UKPDS, there was a long lag time between the establishment of intensive glycemic control and the observed decrease in microvascular complications. This time lag was 3–3.5 years in the DCCT and ~9 years in the UKPDS. The corollary of the concept that the effects of poor glycemic control persist even after good control is established is that early intensive glycemic control protects the microvascular and macrovascular systems against poor glycemic control for many years, and this is being demonstrated in the ongoing Epidemiology of Diabetes Interventions and Complications (EDIC) study. The EDIC study is the long-term follow-up of DCCT cohort subjects after they return to community health providers. As of 2005, 93% of the original cohort was included in EDIC. Within the first year or two of returning to the community-based health care system, the glycemic control of the previously intensively treated cohort worsened from a mean A1C of 7.2 to 7.9%. The previous control group improved their A1C from 9.1 to 8.3%. For the 8 years of follow-up, the previously intensively treated patients had a mean A1C of 8.0%, whereas the conventional control group had a mean A1C of 8.2%. Despite the slight difference in mean A1C, the previously intensively treated cohort developed retinopathy and nephropathy at statistically significantly lower rates than the previous conventional control cohort (Table 29.6), indicating that the protective effect of early intensive glycemic control as well as the detrimental effects of poor glycemic control last for many years.

A critical observation arising from the EDIC study was the demonstration that early intensive glycemic control for only a mean of 6.5 years resulted in a significant reduction in cardiovascular complications during a mean follow-up of 17 years. Forty-six cardiovascular events occurred in 31 patients who had received intensive glycemic control, and 98 events occurred in 52 patients who had received conventional treatment. The risk of nonfatal myocardial infarction, stroke, or death from cardiovascular disease was reduced by 57% (*P* = 0.02) in the cohort that had previously received intensive glycemic control. These data show that intensive glycemic control in type 1 diabetic patients does reduce cardiovascular complications. They further point out that the glucose intervention must start early in the course of diabetes and that the benefits are only seen after many years.

Table 29.6 Renal Disease at Years 7 and 8 of Follow-up in 1,298 Subjects in the EDIC Study

	Conventional Therapy	Intensive Therapy
Development of new microalbuminuria		
7–8 yr	15.8	6.8
	Risk reduction = 49	
Development of new albuminuria		
7–8 yr	9.4	1.4
	Risk reduction = 78	
Aggregate end points		
Serum creatinine >2 mg/dl	19 (2.8)	5 (0.7)
Chronic dialysis or kidney transplant	7 (1.0)	4 (0.6)
Hypertension prevalence	40.3	29.9

Data are % and *n* (%).

These observations emphasize that aggressive early treatment of glycemia in patients with diabetes provides the maximal protection against chronic microvascular and macrovascular complications.

RECENT INTERVENTION STUDIES FOCUSING ON GLYCEMIC CONTROL AND CLINICAL CARDIOVASCULAR OUTCOMES IN TYPE 2 DIABETIC PATIENTS

To attempt to determine whether intensive glycemic control reduces cardiovascular events in patients with type 2 diabetes, three intervention studies (Action to Control Cardiovascular Risk in Diabetes [ACCORD], Action in Diabetes and Vascular Disease: Preterax and Diamicron-MR Controlled Evaluation [ADVANCE], and the Veterans Administration Diabetes Trial [VADT]) were designed and implemented during the 2000s. The results of these studies were reported in June 2008 at the Scientific Sessions of the American Diabetes Association. Each study had as its primary end point the time to first cardiovascular end point in patients randomized to intensive glycemic control or conventional glycemic control. The clinical end point for ACCORD and ADVANCE was a composite of death due to cardiovascular disease, nonfatal myocardial infarction, and stroke. The VADT had a composite end point that also included acute coronary syndrome and coronary revascularization. The salient features of the studies are listed in Table 29.7. Intensive glycemic control had no significant benefit in reducing cardiovascular complications in any of the trials (hazard ratios: ACCORD, 0.90 [$P = 0.16$]; ADVANCE, 0.94 [$P = 0.32$]; and VADT, 0.87 [$P = 0.12$]).

As noted in Table 29.7, the type 2 diabetic populations in all three trials had had diabetes for many years and at entry had had previous cardiovascular events or very high cardiovascular risk. Thus, the conclusion that can be drawn from these results is that intensive glycemic control initiated in type 2 diabetic patients with far advanced cardiovascular disease is not beneficial in reducing additional cardiovascular events. Such results are not surprising as intensive glycemic control

Table 29.7 Key Features of the ACCORD, ADVANCE, and VADT Studies

	ACCORD	ADVANCE	VADT
Baseline characteristics of patient populations			
n	10,251	11,400	1,791
Mean age (years)	62.2	66	60.4
Mean BMI (kg/m²)	32.2	28.5	31.3
Mean diabetes duration (years)	10	8.0	11.5
Previous cardiovascular event (%)	35.2	32.2	31.3
Mean A1C (%)	8.3	7.5	9.4
Median A1C during study (%)			
Intensive control	6.4	6.3	6.9
Conventional control	7.5	7.0	8.6

decreases the onset and progression of retinopathy, nephropathy, and neuropathy but has little or no beneficial effects on proliferative retinopathy, diabetic nephropathy with decreasing glomerular filtration rate, or diabetic neuropathy after the neurons are degenerated.

Several additional points came out of these studies. ADVANCE showed that intensive glycemic treatment did decrease the development and progression of nephropathy by 20%. ACCORD showed that overly aggressive strategies to control glycemia were associated with an increase in mortality, markedly excessive weight gain, and a high prevalence of severe hypoglycemia. ACCORD subanalyses showed that individuals with no preexisting cardiovascular disease or those who at study entry had A1C ≤8.0% did have a statistically significant reduction in cardiovascular events with intensive glycemic control. VADT presented secondary analyses and a substudy measuring coronary artery calcification that suggest that intensive glycemic control may reduce cardiovascular complications if started early in the course of type 2 diabetes and in patients who initially have early cardiovascular changes.

SUMMARY

Intensive glycemic control prevents and delays the development of microvascular complications. The earlier the intensive control is initiated, the more likely the benefit. Intensive glycemic control is not of benefit in reducing subsequent cardiovascular events in patients who have clinical cardiovascular disease but may be of benefit if initiated early in the course of diabetes before significant cardiovascular disease is already established.

BIBLIOGRAPHY

ACCORD Study Group: Effects of intensive glucose lowering in type 2 diabetes. *N Engl J Med* 358:2545–2559, 2008

ADVANCE collaborative group: Intensive blood glucose control and vascular outcomes in patients with type 2 diabetes. *N Engl J Med* 358:2560–2572, 2008

DCCT Research Group: The effect of intensive treatment of diabetes on the development and progression of long-term complications in IDDM. *N Engl J Med* 329:977–986, 1993

DCCT Research Group: Effect of intensive therapy on the microvascular complications of type 1 diabetes mellitus. *JAMA* 287:2563–2567, 2002

DCCT/EDIC Research Group: Sustained effect of intensive insulin treatment of type 1 diabetes mellitus on development and progression of diabetic nephropathy. *JAMA* 290:2159–2167, 2003

DCCT/EDIC Research Group: Intensive diabetes treatment and cardiovascular disease in patients with type 1 diabetes. *N Engl J Med* 353:2643–2653, 2005

Gall MA, Borch-Johnsen K, Hougaard R, Nielsen FS, Parving HH: Albuminuria and poor glycemic control predict mortality in NIDDM. *Diabetes* 44:1303–1309, 1995

Klein R: Hyperglycemia and microvascular and macrovascular disease in diabetes. *Diabetes Care* 18:258–268, 1995

Kuusisto J, Mykkanen L, Pyorala K, Laakso M: NIDDM and its metabolic control predict coronary heart disease in elderly subjects. *Diabetes* 43:960–967, 1994

Ohkubo Y, Kishikawa H, Araki E, Mirata T, Isami S, Motoyoshi S, Kojima Y, Furuyoshi N, Shichiri M: Intensive insulin therapy prevents the progression of diabetic microvascular complications in Japanese patients with non-insulin-dependent diabetes mellitus: a randomized prospective 6-year study. *Diabetes Res Clin Pract* 28:103–117, 1995

Turner R, Cull C, Holman R: United Kingdom Prospective Diabetes Study 17: a 9-year update of a randomized, controlled trial on the effect of improved metabolic control on complications in non-insulin-dependent diabetes mellitus. *Ann Intern Med* 124:136–145, 1996

U.K. Prospective Diabetes Study Group: Intensive blood-glucose control with sulphonylureas or insulin compared with conventional treatment and risk of complications in patients with type 2 diabetes (UKPDS 33). *Lancet* 352:837–853, 1998

U.K. Prospective Diabetes Study Group: Effect of intensive blood glucose control with metformin on complications in overweight patients with type 2 diabetes (UKPDS 34). *Lancet* 352:854–865, 1998

Veterans Administration: Veterans Administration Diabetes Trial data. Presentation at the 68th Scientific Sessions of the American Diabetes Association, June 2008, San Francisco, California.

Dr. Lebovitz is Professor of Medicine at the State University of New York Health Science Center at Brooklyn, Brooklyn, New York.

30. Management of Surgery and Anesthesia

Ildiko Lingvay, MD, MPH, Larissa Avilés-Santa, MD, MPH, and Philip Raskin, MD

Approximately 50% of all patients with diabetes will undergo surgery at least once in their lifetime. The types of surgery performed are usually influenced by the presence of long-term diabetes complications, including amputations, ulcer debridement, and renal transplantation. However, patients with diabetes are also subject to the same types of surgery performed on patients without diabetes, such as cardiothoracic, peripheral vascular, and ophthalmologic procedures. Approximately 17% of all patients with diabetes who undergo surgery will have some type of complication, the most common being postsurgical infections and cardiovascular complications (Table 30.1). Therefore, a thorough assessment of the patient's actual metabolic status and glycemic control, cardiovascular status, and the presence of underlying complications related to diabetes (e.g., neuropathy and nephropathy) in the preoperative period is necessary to predict or prevent certain adverse events.

PATHOPHYSIOLOGY

Several factors that predispose patients with diabetes to metabolic decompensation include the patient's insulin reserve, endocrine response to surgical stress, volume status (particularly dehydration), and the need to be fasting.

During anesthesia and surgery, there is an increase in the plasma concentration of counterregulatory hormones. An elevation in the levels of glucagon, catecholamines, cortisol, and growth hormone is observed in individuals with and without diabetes. Increased secretion of these hormones leads to a marked increase in hepatic glucose production (due to both glycogenolysis and gluconeogenesis), a decrease in insulin-mediated glucose uptake, increased lipolysis with elevated levels of nonesterified fatty acids, and decreased insulin secretion. In nondiabetic individuals, major surgery is frequently associated with elevations in blood glucose into the range of 150–200 mg/dl (8.3–11.1 mmol/l). In individuals with diabetes, insulin secretion is impaired; thus, in the presence of a major surgical stress, severe hyperglycemia with or without ketosis can occur unless adequate insulin replacement is provided. The severity of the metabolic abnormality is proportional to the extent and duration of the surgical procedure and the impairment of insulin secretion. Because surgical patients are usually fasting, administration of insulin will cause hypoglycemia if an adequate and constant source of carbohydrate is not available.

Table 30.1 Complications of Diabetes During Surgery, Anesthesia, and Postoperative Periods

Metabolic
  Diabetic ketoacidosis
  Nonketotic hyperosmolar states
  Hypoglycemia
  Hyperkalemia
  Hypokalemia
  Cardiovascular complications
  Hypotension (related to autonomic diabetic neuropathy)

Arrhythmia
  Postoperative myocardial infarction
  Other thrombotic phenomena

Renal
  Acute kidney failure
  Volume overload

Infections

Other perioperative complications often faced by patients with diabetes include myocardial ischemia and infarction, cerebrovascular accidents, fluid and electrolytic abnormalities, hemodynamic abnormalities during anesthesia, and impaired healing and infection of surgical wounds.

Depending on the surgical procedure and its duration, life-support measures and instrumentation, and the type of anesthesia and anesthetic agent used, cardiac output and peripheral vascular resistance will temporarily change. This can lead to blood pressure and heart rate changes, which could precipitate or aggravate underlying myocardial and/or coronary disease that is sometimes occult or asymptomatic in individuals with diabetes. The risks of postoperative cardiovascular complications become more evident in individuals with known coronary or peripheral arterial disease and cardiomyopathy. Autonomic neuropathy can cause severe hypotension during the induction of anesthesia, and its presence should be evaluated before any procedure involving general and/or spinal anesthesia. The anesthesiologist must be informed about the findings of the autonomic nervous system evaluation.

Intravascular and extravascular fluid status will influence the sudden shifts in volume status and electrolytic changes experienced during acute stress associated with surgery. Hyperglycemia, whether chronic or acute, is almost always associated with intravascular fluid depletion, which in turn can alter cardiac output and peripheral vascular resistance. If not corrected, volume depletion can contribute to increased morbidity during the perioperative period. Diabetic nephropathy, with or without proteinuria, makes fluid and electrolyte management difficult, and the use of intravenous fluids, vasopressors, vasodilators, and diuretics must be carefully planned.

Chronic hyperglycemia has been associated with delayed wound healing as a consequence of inadequate collagen repair and remodeling. In addition, because of impaired leukocyte chemotaxis and defective immune defense mechanisms, infections at surgical sites are common. This picture becomes more complicated by underlying poor nutrition, which further impairs healing.

EVALUATION OF PATIENTS WITH DIABETES BEFORE SURGERY

Metabolic Control

The degree of metabolic control should be evaluated before surgery, and attempts should be made to improve poor control on an outpatient basis before elective procedures. Chronically hyperglycemic patients are frequently dehydrated. Dehydration can be accompanied by electrolytic abnormalities, particularly sodium and potassium loss, and by intravascular volume depletion, with subsequent hemodynamic imbalance. Admission to the hospital to optimize metabolic control 12–16 h before elective procedures is recommended for all patients with type 1 diabetes and those with type 2 diabetes who have inadequate metabolic control. A stabilization period of 12–16 h is also recommended for semiurgent procedures if severe hyperglycemia is present. In patients with severe metabolic derangements (diabetic ketoacidosis or hyperosmolar nonketotic states) who need urgent surgical intervention, 6–8 h of intensive treatment usually improves the general condition of the patient. This period also allows clarification of the diagnosis in cases of acute abdominal pain that could be the consequence of diabetic ketoacidosis rather than a surgical abdomen.

Correction of chronic hyperglycemia and assessment of nutritional status before surgery or immediately after surgery is recommended. Increased protein and caloric intake was shown to improve collagen formation and healing. In addition, depending on other coexistent medical conditions (e.g., obstructive pulmonary disease or chronic renal insufficiency), specific nutritional needs may have to be addressed.

Cardiovascular Status

Atherosclerotic heart disease is highly prevalent in the diabetic population. Long-standing diabetes is often accompanied by arterial hypertension and dyslipidemia, increasing the risk of atherosclerosis, leading to ischemia, myocardial infarction, and cerebrovascular accidents during the perioperative period. A preoperative assessment and evaluation of risk factors for coronary artery disease is crucial, even in asymptomatic patients, because the risk of silent ischemia is considerable.

The risk of cardiovascular complications should be stratified depending on the urgency (elective versus emergent) and type of procedure (cardiac versus noncardiac) to determine the need for preoperative testing. Recent cardiovascular history, physical examination, and electrocardiographic findings generally provide sufficient information to determine risks. Further tests to estimate functional capacity and rule out (and treat) coronary disease may be needed in individuals with a positive cardiovascular review of systems and unstable coronary syndromes.

Well-controlled hypertension does not pose a major risk to surgery, but patients receiving β-blockers may develop hypoglycemia without warning symptoms and should be monitored accordingly. Type 1 diabetic patients receiving β-blockers are also at a greater risk for prolonged episodes of insulin-induced hypoglycemia.

Diabetic patients have increased thrombotic risk. Antithrombotic therapy (including unfractionated or low-weight heparin, antiembolic graduated pressure stockings, and ambulation) should be considered unless specifically contraindicated during the period the patient is confined to bed.

The use of vasopressors for the treatment of severe hypotension associated with sepsis or extreme intravascular volume loss has been associated with remarkable peripheral vasoconstriction. Patients with poor peripheral pulses and who require high doses of vasopressors during the course of a critical illness are at risk of gangrene of the digits. Vasopressors, however, should not be restricted or halted if their benefits outweigh the risk of amputation.

Neurological Status

Disordered gastrointestinal motility may increase the risk of aspiration and may delay the resumption of enteral feeding. In addition, general anesthesia may cause nausea and vomiting. Bladder dysfunction may lead to urinary retention and subsequent obstructive uropathy and fluid overload. Urinary retention due to decreased bladder contractility has been observed with the use of narcotics for pain management. Therefore, if a patient has evidence of either gastrointestinal dysmotility or bladder dysfunction with the use of antiemetic and/or narcotic analgesic agents, careful monitoring of fluid intake and urinary output should be addressed before and after surgery. As mentioned before, the anesthesiologist should be alerted to the presence of orthostatic blood pressure changes associated with advanced neuropathy to predict possible hemodynamic changes during anesthesia induction.

Renal Function

Measurement of blood urea nitrogen, serum creatinine, electrolytes, and proteinuria should be performed before surgery. Azotemic patients may have problems with fluid management, and monitoring of central venous or pulmonary artery wedge pressure may be necessary. Hyperkalemia with or without hyponatremia is often seen in patients with mild to moderate renal insufficiency, and hyperkalemia can precipitate an acute cardiac arrhythmia. This metabolic finding often results from diabetic autonomic neuropathy and hyporeninemic hypoaldosteronism. Hypokalemia may be present, and insulin and glucose infusion therapy may aggravate this condition. Proteinuria, with resulting hypoalbuminemia, can cause extravasation of fluid to the interstitial space, therefore potentiating problems with intravascular volume, cardiac output, and alveolar oxygen exchange. Depending on the severity of proteinuria, a combination of diuretics, fluid restriction, hemodialysis, or ultrafiltration will be necessary for stabilization of intravascular volume status.

METABOLIC MANAGEMENT AND MONITORING

Insulin and Glucose Administration During Surgery

The use of an insulin and glucose infusion is recommended for all patients with type 1 diabetes, patients with insulin-treated type 2 diabetes, and patients with poorly controlled drug- or diet-treated type 2 diabetes who are undergoing general anesthesia, regardless of the planned duration of the surgical procedure.

Several methods of insulin administration during the perioperative period are in use. Most of the protocols include the intravenous administration of short-acting insulin (regular human insulin) and 5–10% glucose solution. Subcutaneous administration of insulin is associated with unpredictable absorption and variable plasma insulin levels and is not recommended for surgical patients except for those undergoing minor procedures. In some of the protocols with intravenous insulin, the glucose and insulin are contained in the same infusion mixture. The theoretical advantage of this approach is that if the glucose infusion is accidentally disconnected or obstructed, then so is the insulin infusion, avoiding the risk of hypoglycemia. The disadvantage of this method is that no flexibility is allowed for changes in the delivery rate of either insulin or glucose infusion.

Another approach is to administer insulin and glucose in separate bags but through the same vein, i.e., to "piggyback" the insulin infusion onto the glucose infusion. This allows independent adjustments to each infusion according to the levels of hourly capillary blood glucose measurements. An example of such a protocol is shown in Table 30.2. With this protocol, a blood glucose level in the range of 100–125 mg/dl (5.6–6.9 mmol/l) is easily maintained during the entire perioperative period. As with every therapeutic protocol, clinical judgment must be used. Depending on the individual patient, increases or decreases in the rate of insulin or glucose infusion for a given capillary blood glucose range may be necessary.

Electrolyte solutions are administered as needed into the glucose infusion or with a separate infusion. In patients with azotemia or other problems with fluid management or those receiving large amounts of other solutions, 10% dextrose

Table 30.2 Representative Protocol for Insulin-Glucose Infusion for Perioperative Periods

1. Discontinue all subcutaneous insulin after initiation of glucose-insulin infusion.
2. Measure capillary blood glucose levels at 1-h intervals.
3. Infuse 5% dextrose (D_5W) intravenously via infusion pump.
4. Make insulin solution using regular insulin to a concentration of 1 unit/cc. Give piggyback using an infusion pump into the 5% dextrose infusion.
5. Based on hourly blood glucose determination, adjust each infusion according to the following schedule:

Blood Glucose		Insulin Infusion		
mg/dl	mmol/l	ml/h	units/h	D_5W Infusion (ml/h)
<71*	<3.9	0.5	0.5	150
71–100	3.9–5.6	1.0	1.0	125
101–150	5.6–8.3	2.0	2.0	100
151–200	8.3–11.1	3.0	3.0	50
201–250	11.1–13.9	4.0	4.0	0
251–300	13.9–16.7	6.0	6.0	0
≥300	≥16.7	10.0	10.0	0

In use at the Diabetes Treatment Center at Parkland Memorial Hospital, Dallas, Texas.
*Give 20 ml $D_{50}W$ intravenously and repeat blood glucose measurement 15 min later.

(D_{10}W) can be substituted for the 5% dextrose (D_5W) solution. If D_{10}W is not available, it can be made by adding 100 g 50% dextrose (D_{50}W) to 1,000 ml D_5W.

Patients with severe fluid management problems, e.g., those with congestive heart failure or end-stage renal disease, may not tolerate the amounts of fluids administered with either a D_5W or D_{10}W infusion. Thus, to provide an adequate carbohydrate supply, D_{50}W must be administered through a central venous line. Table 30.3 shows a protocol for diabetic patients who are at high risk for fluid overload. Again, clinical judgment dictates individual changes in the protocol as necessary.

Patients undergoing coronary artery bypass graft surgery and/or cardiopulmonary bypass often require higher doses of insulin to achieve glycemic control during the perioperative period. Intensive glycemic control using intravenous insulin and dextrose solution during the perioperative period and during the subacute phase of myocardial infarction has been shown to improve cardiovascular morbidity and mortality as well as general postoperative outcome in diabetic patients. Therefore, its use should be encouraged both during and after surgery, and treatment goals should approach blood glucose levels of 100–125 mg/dl (5.6–6.9 mmol/l).

The blood glucose level must be monitored at hourly intervals. Capillary blood glucose measurements taken in the operating and recovery rooms with bedside glucose monitoring devices are adequate for perioperative management. Hourly measurements are necessary to keep the blood glucose level between 100

Table 30.3 Protocol for Insulin-Glucose Infusion for Perioperative Patients at Risk of Volume Overload

1. Discontinue all subcutaneous insulin after initiation of glucose-insulin infusion.
2. Measure capillary blood glucose levels at 1-h intervals.
3. Infuse 50% dextrose (D_{50}W) intravenously into central venous line via infusion pump.
4. Make insulin solution using regular insulin to a concentration of 1 unit/cc. Give piggyback via infusion pump into D_{50}W infusion.
5. Based on hourly blood glucose determination, adjust each infusion according to the following schedule:

Blood Glucose		Insulin Infusion		
mg/dl	mmol/l	ml/h	units/h	D_{50}W Infusion (ml/h)
<71*	<3.9	0.5	0.5	25
71–100	3.9–5.6	1.0	1.0	20
101–150	5.6–8.3	2.0	2.0	15
151–200	8.3–11.1	3.0	3.0	10
201–250	11.1–13.9	4.0	4.0	0
251–300	13.9–16.7	6.0	6.0	0
≥300	≥16.7	10.0	10.0	0

In use at University Diabetes Treatment Center at Parkland Memorial Hospital, Dallas, Texas.
*Give 20 ml D_{50}W intravenously and repeat blood glucose measurement 15 min later.

and 125 mg/dl (5.6 and 6.9 mmol/l) and to ensure safety should the glucose infusion inadvertently be discontinued.

The management of stable diabetic patients undergoing minor procedures (e.g., endoscopic techniques or surgery performed under local anesthesia) involves withholding the morning dose of insulin or oral agent if the patient is going to be fasting and measuring capillary blood glucose every 2–4 h. Type 1 diabetic patients should not have insulin withheld. Depending on the individual, taking either one-third or one-half of the intermediate-acting insulin usually taken in the morning is a potential alternative. Also, supplemental subcutaneous short-acting insulin can be administered following a variable insulin schedule, and the patient's usual insulin dosage or oral agent can be resumed after surgery when the patient can eat (Table 30.4). However, if the period of time that the patient must wait to go to surgery is unknown, then it would be prudent to use the insulin-glucose infusion instead. In critically ill patients or those who have undergone emergency surgery, insulin therapy can be continued after surgery for better stabilization of glucose levels.

Postoperative Metabolic Management

The glucose and insulin infusion should be continued until the metabolic condition is stable and the patient is able to tolerate oral feeding. The insulin and glucose infusions should not be stopped until 1–2 h after the administration of subcutaneous insulin. After major surgery, the glucose and insulin infusions

---

Table 30.4 Diabetes Management During Minor Surgical Procedures

Day of procedure (if patient NPO)
1. Withhold morning dose of insulin or oral agent.
2. Measure capillary blood glucose level before procedure and every 2–4 h.
3. Give short- or fast-acting insulin subcutaneously every 2–4 h as follows:

Blood Glucose		Short- or Fast-Acting Insulin (units)
mg/dl	mmol/l	
<151	<5.6	0
151–200	5.6–11.1	2
201–250	11.1–13.9	3
251–300	13.9–16.7	5
≥300	≥16.7	6

4. Give usual afternoon insulin or oral agent dose.

Day of procedure (if breakfast allowed)
1. Give normal morning dose of insulin or oral agent.
2. Measure blood glucose levels before and after procedure.
3. Give supplemental 4 units of short- or fast-acting insulin subcutaneously if blood glucose >250 mg/dl.
4. Give usual afternoon insulin or oral agent dose.

Modified from Rosenstock and Raskin (1987). NPO, nothing by mouth.

should be continued until the patient is able to eat solid food without difficulty. In these patients, the use of multiple subcutaneous injections of short-acting insulin before meals and intermediate- or long-acting basal insulin at bedtime is recommended during the first 24–48 h after the insulin and glucose infusions are stopped and before the patient's usual insulin regimen is resumed. Table 30.5 shows an example of such an insulin injection schedule. If a patient had been taking a long-acting insulin (such as insulin glargine) before surgery, we recommend stopping the insulin-glucose infusion 1–2 h after resuming the long-acting insulin to avoid hyperglycemia due to a lack of basal insulin.

Depending on the type of procedure, some patients will require continuous enteral nutrition. In these cases, we recommend multiple short-acting insulin injections, for example, every 4–6 h. Because the patient is receiving food continuously, the risk of hypoglycemia is low. Intermediate- or long-acting insulin should be used with caution because hypoglycemia may take place in the case of sudden or inadvertent removal of the enteral tube.

The use of total parenteral nutrition (TPN) is occasionally required in the postoperative period. Diabetic patients can develop serious metabolic derangements with TPN. A variable insulin infusion schedule (similar to that shown in Table 30.2) with hourly determinations of blood glucose is also recommended under these circumstances, but additional glucose infusion is not required because it is contained within the TPN solution. Initially, the insulin should be given as a

Table 30.5 Postoperative Diabetes Management When Patient Tolerates Solid Food

1. Do not discontinue intravenous insulin-glucose infusion until after first subcutaneous insulin dose is administered.
2. Measure capillary blood glucose before meals, at 10:00 P.M., and at 3:00 A.M.*
3. Provide three meals and three snacks (20–30 kcal/kg per day).
4. Administer preprandial short- or fast-acting insulin subcutaneously according to the following variable insulin dosage schedule:

Blood Glucose		Short- or Fast-Acting Insulin (units)			
mg/dl	mmol/l	Breakfast	Lunch	Dinner	10:00 P.M.
<71	<3.9	3	2	2	0
71–100	3.9–5.6	4	3	3	0
101–150	5.6–8.3	6	4	4	0
151–200	8.3–11.1	8	6	6	0
201–250	11.1–13.9	10	8	8	1
251–300	13.9–16.7	12	10	10	2
≥300	≥16.7	14	12	12	3

5. Administer intermediate- or long-acting basal insulin 10–20 units subcutaneously at 10:00 P.M.

Modified from Rosenstock and Raskin (1987). *If hypoglycemia is present at 3:00 A.M., reduce the 10:00 P.M. intermediate-acting insulin dose.

continuous infusion separate from the TPN solution. Once a stable dose of insulin is ascertained (often within 12–24 h), the total amount of insulin required over 24 h can be added to the TPN bag, and the frequency of the capillary blood glucose measurements can be reduced to every 2–4 h. The doses of insulin needed during TPN can be high and are often >100 units in 24 h, depending on the patient's metabolic status and insulin sensitivity.

Electrolytes should be closely monitored in the perioperative period and adequately replaced. Severe hypokalemia and hypophosphatemia may occur, especially if an intravenous insulin infusion is used.

Postoperative Cardiovascular Evaluation

Serial postoperative electrocardiograms are recommended for older diabetic patients, patients with long-standing type 1 diabetes, and patients with known heart disease. Postoperative myocardial infarction may be silent and has a high mortality.

Intravascular fluid and wedge pressure monitoring after surgery might be necessary in some patients with cardiomyopathy, depending on the procedure performed.

When ambulation of the patient begins, attention must be paid to the possibility of orthostatic hypotension. Evaluation and reevaluation of the mental and neurological status will help to assess changes associated with possible embolism of unstable carotid or aortic plaques after instrumentation during heart surgery.

Early ambulation should be encouraged, depending on the type of surgical procedure. If ambulation is not allowed or is not possible, antithrombotic measures should be instituted soon after surgery.

Postoperative Renal Evaluation

Careful monitoring of blood urea nitrogen and serum creatinine levels will help to detect acute kidney failure that may occur, especially after procedures with iodinated contrast material. If contrast material is to be used, the patient should be well hydrated before and after the procedure. Patients on metformin should be advised to withhold this medication the morning before receiving intravenous contrast and resume metformin 48 h after the test is performed if renal function has not worsened.

Postoperative Infection

Wound infections are common among diabetic patients with poor metabolic control. Fever may not always be present, so warning signs can be subtle, followed by a precipitous course. Impaired granulocyte function due to hyperglycemia may predispose the patient to bacterial infections. Poor circulation due to macroangiopathy or microangiopathy can also contribute to postoperative infection. Tight metabolic control during the perioperative period can decrease the risk of postoperative infection and improve the postoperative outcome.

Wound infections in individuals with diabetes are usually caused by mixed flora, and antibiotic coverage must include coverage for anaerobic bacteria, gram-negative enteric bacteria, and *Staphylococcus aureus*. If surgical debridement and drainage is needed, it should be performed early. Cultures should be obtained during drainage procedures and before antibiotic therapy is started. In patients with severe infections that are not responding to antibiotic therapy, *Candida* species or other fungal species should be suspected.

In addition to surgical wounds, other sources of infection during the postoperative period include intravenous catheter insertion sites, pressure and decubitus ulcers, nasopharynx (due to nasotracheal or orotracheal tubes for ventilatory support or nasotracheal tubes for feeding purposes), and urinary catheterization. Blood and urine cultures, chest radiography, removal or replacement of intravenous catheters, and cultures of the catheter tips should be performed if the infection focus cannot be easily identified. Guidelines for prevention of decubitus ulcers and replacement of intravenous lines should be followed to prevent infections in those sites.

The elderly and poorly nourished patients of all ages are at a higher risk of developing pressure ulcers after just a few hours of bed confinement. Prevention of pressure ulcers and maintenance of skin integrity should be established as soon as possible.

Other Considerations

Any hospitalization of a patient with diabetes is an opportunity to assess effectiveness of lifestyle and pharmacological interventions, reevaluate the plan of care, perform the recommended periodic evaluations (including A1C, lipid profile, evaluation of microalbuminuria, foot exam, neurological exam, and ophthalmologic exam), and update routine vaccinations (tetanus, pneumonia, and influenza). The postoperative recovery period can often be used to educate the patient about diabetes, its complications, and the importance of glycemic control for prevention of long-term complications. Prior to discharge, a customized plan of care with appropriate follow-up should be established for each patient.

SUMMARY

Cardiovascular complications and infections are the most common complications patients with diabetes experience after surgery. A thorough history and physical evaluation will help to determine the presence of potential long-term diabetes complications that could influence the postoperative outcome. Glycemic, metabolic, and nutritional status and cardiovascular, neurological, and renal function should be evaluated and optimized, if possible, before surgery. Cardiovascular, hemodynamic, and intravascular volume status should be carefully monitored during and after surgery, and normoglycemia should be achieved and maintained during surgery and recovery. Depending on the procedure and coexistent physical conditions, further guidelines for prevention of infections and other postoperative complications should be addressed.

BIBLIOGRAPHY

ACE/ADA Task Force on Inpatient Diabetes: American College of Endocrinology and American Diabetes Association consensus statement on inpatient diabetes and glycemic control. *Diabetes Care* 29:1955–1962, 2006

American Diabetes Association: Standards of medical care in diabetes—2009. *Diabetes Care* 32 (Suppl. 1):S13–S61, 2009

Burgos LG, Ebert TJ, Asiddas C, Turner LA, Pattison CZ, Wang-Cheng R, Kamysine JP: Increased intraoperative cardiovascular morbidity in diabetics with autonomic neuropathy. *Anesthesiology* 70:591–597, 1989

Furnary AP, Zerr KJ, Grunkemeier GL, Starr A: Continuous intravenous insulin infusion reduces the incidence of deep sternal wound infection in diabetic patients after cardiac surgical procedures. *Ann Thorac Surg* 67:352–362, 1999

Hollenberg SM: Preoperative cardiac risk assessment. *Chest* 115:51S–57S, 1999

Ingels C, Debaveye Y, Milants I, Buelens E, Peeraer A, Devriendt Y, Vanhoutte T, Van Damme A, Schetz M, Wouters PJ, Van den Berghe G: Strict blood glucose control with insulin during intensive care after cardiac surgery: impact on 4-years survival, dependency on medical care, and quality-of-life. *Eur Heart J* 27:2716–2724, 2006

Jeejeebhoy KN: Total parenteral nutrition: potion or poison? *Am J Clin Nutr* 74:160–163, 2001

John R, Choudhri AF, Weinberg AD, Ting W, Rose EA, Smith CR, Oz MC: Multicenter review of preoperative risk factors for stroke after coronary artery bypass grafting. *Ann Thorac Surg* 69:30–36, 2000

Lazar HL, Fitzgerald C, Gross C, Heeren T, Aldea GS, Shemin RJ: Determinants of length of stay after coronary artery bypass graft surgery. *Circulation* 92 (Suppl. 9):II20–II24, 1995

Malmberg K: Prospective randomized study of intensive insulin treatment on long term survival after acute myocardial infarction in patients with diabetes mellitus. *Br Med J* 314:1512–1515, 1997

Malmberg K, Norhammar A, Wedel H, Rydén L: Glycometabolic state at admission: important risk marker of mortality in conventionally treated patients with diabetes mellitus and acute myocardial infarction: long term results from the Diabetes and Insulin-Glucose Infusion in Acute Myocardial Infarction (DIGAMI) study. *Circulation* 99:2626–2632, 1999

Malmberg K, Rydén L, Hamsten A, Herlitz J, Waldenstrom A, Wedel H: Mortality prediction in diabetic patients with myocardial infarction: experiences from the DIGAMI study. *Cardiovasc Res* 34:248–253, 1997

Malmberg K, Rydén L, Wedel H, Birkeland K, Bootsma A, Dickstein K, Efendic S, Fisher M, Hamsten A, Herlitz J, Hildebrandt P, MacLeod K, Laakso M, Torp-Pedersen C, Waldenström A, DIGAMI 2 Investigators: Intense metabolic control by means of insulin in patients with diabetes mellitus and acute myocardial infarction (DIGAMI 2): effects on mortality and morbidity. *Eur Heart J* 26:650–661, 2005

Rosenstock J, Raskin P: Surgery! Practical guidelines for diabetes management. *Clinical Diabetes* 5:49–61, 1987

Rydén L, Standl E, Bartnik M, Van den Berghe G, Betteridge J, de Boer MJ, Cosentino F, Jönsson B, Laakso M, Malmberg K, Priori S, Ostergren J, Tuomilehto J, Thrainsdottir I, Vanhorebeek I, Stramba-Badiale M, Lindgren P, Qiao Q, Priori SG, Blanc JJ, Budaj A, Camm J, Dean V, Deckers J, Dickstein K, Lekakis J, McGregor K, Metra M, Morais J, Osterspey A, Tamargo J, Zamorano JL, Deckers JW, Bertrand M, Charbonnel B, Erdmann E, Ferrannini E, Flyvbjerg A, Gohlke H, Juanatey JR, Graham I, Monteiro PF, Parhofer K, Pyörälä K, Raz I, Schernthaner G, Volpe M, Wood D, Task Force on Diabetes and Cardiovascular Diseases of the European Society of Cardiology (ESC), European Association for the Study of Diabetes (EASD): Guidelines on diabetes, pre-diabetes, and cardiovascular diseases: executive summary: the Task Force on Diabetes and Cardiovascular Diseases of the European Society of Cardiology (ESC) and of the European Association for the Study of Diabetes (EASD). *Eur Heart J* 28:88–136, 2007

Van den Berghe G, Wilmer A, Milants I, Wouters PJ, Bouckaert B, Bruyninckx F, Bouillon R, Schetz M: Intensive insulin therapy in mixed medical/surgical intensive care units: benefit versus harm. *Diabetes* 55:3151–3159, 2006

van den Berghe G, Wouters P, Weekers F, Verwaest C, Bruyninckx F, Schetz M, Vlasselaers D, Ferdinande P, Lauwers P, Bouillon R: Intensive insulin therapy in critically ill patients. *N Engl J Med* 345:1359–1367, 2001

Zerr KJ, Furnary AP, Grunkemeier GL, Bookin S, Kanhere V, Starr A: Glucose control lowers the risk of wound infection in diabetics after open heart operations. *Ann Thorac Surg* 63:356–361, 1997

Dr. Lingvay is Assistant Professor of Internal Medicine and Dr. Raskin is Professor of Internal Medicine at the University of Texas Southwestern Medical Center at Dallas, Dallas, Texas. Dr. Avilés-Santa is a Medical Officer at the National Heart, Lung, and Blood Institute at the National Institutes of Health.

31. Diabetes in Older Adults

Jeffrey B. Halter, MD

Diabetes is an important health problem among the elderly population. The dramatic age-related increase in the prevalence rate of diabetes is demonstrated in Fig. 31.1, indicating that >20% of people in the U.S. aged >60 years have been diagnosed with diabetes, and the total prevalence rate of diabetes in older adults is ~23%. The rapid growth of the U.S. aging population suggests that there will be continued growth in the number of older adults with diabetes. Hyperglycemia in older adults is not a benign condition because it is associated with risk for long-term diabetes complications. Thus, the management of hyperglycemia in an older adult with diabetes should be considered seriously. Findings from the Diabetes Prevention Program (DPP) and other studies indicate that progression to type 2 diabetes can be slowed, including in older adults. An intensive lifestyle intervention was particularly effective to reduce progression in people aged >60 years in the DPP.

PATHOPHYSIOLOGY AND RATIONALE FOR TREATMENT

Most older adults with diabetes have type 2 diabetes. The pathogenesis of type 2 diabetes in this group is similar to that in other age-groups. Many factors may contribute to the high rate of development of type 2 diabetes in older adults (Fig. 31.2). Age-related impairments of both pancreatic β-cell function and insulin action appear to be important factors in the pathophysiology of hyperglycemia in older adults with diabetes. An age-related increase in body adiposity and a decrease in physical activity both contribute to the insulin resistance during aging. In addition, the prevalence of coexisting illnesses and use of various drugs may contribute to the development of hyperglycemia.

The short-term risks of poor diabetes control for older adults merit intervention. Marked hyperglycemia associated with glucosuria and weight loss is a catabolic state that predisposes the patient with diabetes to various acute illnesses, particularly infections. The most extreme example of poor diabetes control among older adults is the hyperglycemic hyperosmolar nonketotic syndrome, which is associated with a high mortality rate and requires aggressive intervention.

Elderly diabetic patients are also at risk for many long-term complications and have higher rates of disability than nondiabetic older adults. This risk may not be simply a function of known duration of diabetes, because the patient is likely to

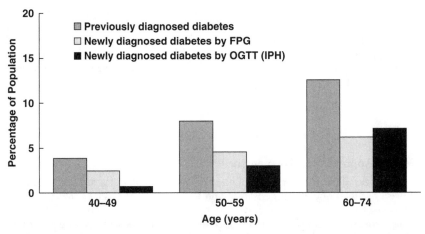

Figure 31.1 Prevalence of type 2 diabetes among older adults according to age and American Diabetes Association diagnostic criteria (the Third National Health and Nutrition Examination Survey). FPG, fasting plasma glucose; IPH, isolated postchallenge hyperglycemia; OGTT, oral glucose tolerance test. Adapted from Harris et al. (1998) and Resnick et al. (2000).

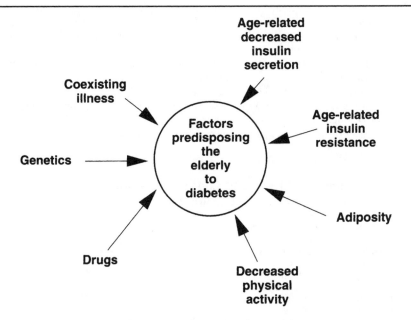

Figure 31.2 Factors predisposing older adults to the development of diabetes. From Halter (1990).

have had asymptomatic undetected hyperglycemia for years before the initial diagnosis was made. Older patients with diabetes have an approximately twofold increased risk for myocardial infarction, stroke, and renal insufficiency compared with people of the same age without diabetes. The risk for amputation in an older adult with diabetes is increased ~10-fold. The overall cardiovascular risk in people with diabetes has been estimated to be equivalent to aging 15 years.

THERAPY

General Approach to Management

The overall treatment goals of a basic diabetes care plan for an older adult are to prevent metabolic decompensation and to control other factors that may contribute to the high risk of cardiovascular complications in such a patient. This chapter focuses on control of hyperglycemia, a goal that should be one part of an overall strategy of risk reduction. Such a strategy must also include intensive effort at identifying and controlling hypertension, lipid disorders, and cigarette smoking. Thus, a complex, multifaceted treatment program may be needed for many older adults with diabetes.

Severe symptomatic hyperglycemia must be treated to control excessive fatty acid mobilization and oxidation, excessive protein catabolism and muscle wasting, excessive glucose production, and urinary loss of calories in the form of glucose. Development of a rational long-term treatment plan for hyperglycemia in an older diabetic patient must take into consideration *1*) remaining life expectancy, *2*) presence of diabetes complications, *3*) presence of coexisting medical or neuropsychiatric disorders, and *4*) the patient's ability and willingness to comply with the proposed diabetes treatment program (Table 31.1). Because the decision-making process for an older adult may be complex, diabetic patients aged >75 years are often excluded from national and local diabetes quality-care programs. However, such quality measures may be appropriate for many older adults. For example, for an otherwise healthy 75-year-old patient without other major medical problems or diabetes complications in whom a reasonable remaining life expectancy

Table 31.1 Important Factors to Consider for Diabetes Management in Older Adults

- The patient's remaining life expectancy
- Patient commitment
- Availability of support services
- Economic issues
- Coexisting health problems
  - ☐ Psychiatric or cognitive disorder
  - ☐ Other medical problems
  - ☐ Diabetes complications
  - ☐ Major limitation of diabetes functional status
- Complexity of medical regimen

(≥10–15 years) is anticipated, it seems reasonable to strive for a fasting glucose level of 100–130 mg/dl (5.6–7.2 mmol/l), postprandial glucose levels <180 mg/dl (<10 mmol/l), and A1C <7%.

In older diabetic patients with advanced microvascular complications (especially diabetic nephropathy and retinopathy), the likelihood of ameliorating their progression may be less. Therefore, more conservative therapeutic targets (e.g., fasting glucose <140 mg/dl [<7.8 mmol/l] and an A1C of <7.5 or <8%) may be more prudent. Older diabetic patients with serious associated medical problems, especially cardiovascular or cerebrovascular problems, should be treated in a manner similar to patients with advanced diabetes complications. A less aggressive approach is also advocated in patients with a major cognitive disorder, neuropsychiatric disorders, or a demonstrated inability to comply with the proposed therapeutic regimen.

Once a therapeutic goal for glycemic control has been established, an orderly approach to treatment, including diet, exercise, oral agents, and insulin, should be developed.

Nutrition Therapy

Dietary intervention as a primary mode of diabetes management should be considered first for an overweight older adult because of the potential effectiveness of weight reduction and its relative safety. Even a modest amount of weight reduction in an obese older adult can lead to a marked improvement in the degree of hyperglycemia, presumably by reducing resistance to insulin.

Substantial barriers may limit the effectiveness of a weight-reducing diet in an older adult. Lifelong dietary habits, often based on long-standing cultural traditions, may be particularly challenging to modify. Many older adults have changes in taste, vision, or smell that may lead to difficulties with food preparation. Arthritis or other neurological or muscular disorders may limit the patient's access to the most appropriate kinds of foods, and financial factors may also be important. Because of these complexities, the skills of an experienced dietitian and the help of family may be of considerable importance in instituting and maintaining an appropriate dietary regimen.

Exercise

A carefully developed exercise program can benefit older adults with diabetes. The same principles that guide the choice of exercise program in younger patients with diabetes apply to older adults. It is important to recognize that the intensity of physical training must be commensurate with the patient's degree of physical fitness. Because of the high incidence of clinically silent coronary artery disease among older adults with diabetes, any physical training program should be based on an appropriate exercise tolerance test and carried out with careful supervision. A foot injury resulting from an exercise program could have devastating effects in an older adult who is at a high risk for infection and amputation. Therefore, choice of appropriate footwear is critical. As with any exercise program, the risk of hypoglycemia should be minimized.

Hypoglycemic Drugs Other than Insulin

If the defined treatment goal is not achieved with a program of diet and exercise, it is appropriate to consider the use of one or more oral drugs or injectables other than insulin. The dosage, mechanism of action, efficacy, and specific side effects of available glucose-lowering drugs are discussed in other chapters. Although no major differences in the clinical pharmacology of these drugs in older patients have been defined, a prudent approach to their use in this population is to start with a relatively small dose and increase slowly, while observing the patient's response. Use of a combination of two or more drugs with different mechanisms of action may be attractive for a given patient, although there is limited information on the use of such combinations in older adults. The potential benefits of a multiple drug regimen for control of hyperglycemia must be carefully weighed against the potential risks and adherence problems. For an older diabetic patient who may have multiple coexisting comorbidities, such as hypertension, heart disease, osteoporosis, and chronic obstructive pulmonary disease, the overall drug regimen may easily exceed 10 medications.

Oral drug regimens can cause hypoglycemia in older adults. Because of the importance of the kidneys and liver for drug elimination and the importance of the liver for glucose counterregulation, both renal and hepatic insufficiency are substantial risk factors for the development of severe hypoglycemia during sulfonylurea therapy or multiple drug regimens. An age-related decline in renal function would contribute to this susceptibility. Despite the potential for hypoglycemia with use of sulfonylurea drugs, the risk appears to be small in older adults who have good nutrition status and who do not have major problems with renal or hepatic insufficiency. When hypoglycemia does occur, patients need to be carefully observed for a considerable period, particularly with some of the longer-acting agents. Chlorpropamide and glyburide should be avoided in older adults because of the concern for prolonged hypoglycemia.

Metformin should be avoided in older adults with renal or hepatic insufficiency, decompensated heart failure, or during any severe acute illness because of the potential risk for these coexisting conditions to predispose a patient to the development of lactic acidosis. The gastrointestinal side effects associated with use of α-glucosidase inhibitors may limit their utility in older adults who have an underlying gastrointestinal disorder or for whom adequate calorie intake and maintenance of body weight is a coexisting health problem. Thiazolidinediones should not be used in older adults with heart failure. Drugs related to glucagon-like peptide may be relatively safe in older adults, although more data are needed in this population.

Insulin

When the treatment goal for a patient has not been met by use of a weight-reduction diet, exercise, and use of other glucose-lowering drugs, insulin therapy should be considered. For some older diabetic patients with a modest goal for hyperglycemia management, a relatively simple insulin regimen may be preferable to a more complex multiple drug program.

Insulin does not have any major drug interactions, and there are virtually no contraindications to its use. It is important to emphasize, however, that the use of insulin requires that the patient or care provider be trained in self-monitoring of blood glucose (SMBG). Skills required for independence in insulin administration

---

Table 31.2 Potential Risk Factors for Hypoglycemia in Older Diabetic Patients

- Impaired autonomic nervous system function
- Impaired counterregulatory responses
- Poor or irregular nutrition
- Cognitive disorder
- Use of alcohol or other sedating agent
- Polypharmacy
- Kidney or liver failure

---

and SMBG that must be evaluated in older individuals with diabetes include the following:

- sufficient cognitive function to manage a complex regimen
- adequate vision to read labels, syringes, pens, and glucose monitoring equipment
- fine motor control to draw up and use insulin

Limitations in some of these areas can be overcome. Family members and home health aides can help with administering insulin. Insulin pens may overcome problems with manual dexterity or vision. The developing technology of SMBG can make up for limitations in vision and some of the fine motor skills.

The major risk associated with insulin administration in older adults is the development of hypoglycemia. Risk factors that may increase the likelihood of a hypoglycemic reaction in older adults are described in Table 31.2. Whereas age-related changes in hypoglycemia counterregulatory mechanisms have been described, the changes are subtle in otherwise healthy older adults and are unlikely to result in greater risk of hypoglycemia during insulin therapy.

BIBLIOGRAPHY

Abrahamson MJ: A 74-year old woman with diabetes. *JAMA* 297:196–204, 2007

Booth GL, Kapral MK, Fung K, Tu JV: Relation between age and cardiovascular disease in men and women with diabetes compared with non-diabetic people: a population-based retrospective cohort study. *Lancet* 368:29–36, 2006

California Health Foundation/American Geriatrics Society Panel on Improving Care for Elders with Diabetes: Guidelines for improving the care of the older person with diabetes mellitus. *J Am Geriatr Soc* 51:S265–S280, 2003

Caruso LB, Silliman RA, Demissie S, Greenfield S, Wagner EH: What can we do to improve physical function in older persons with type 2 diabetes? *J Gerontol Med Sci* 55A:M372–M377, 2000

Chang AM, Halter JB: Aging and insulin secretion. *Am J Physiol Endocrinol Metab* 284:E7–E12, 2003

Diabetes Prevention Program Research Group: Reduction in the incidence of type 2 diabetes with lifestyle intervention or metformin. *N Engl J Med* 346:393–403, 2002

Halter JB: *Diabetes Update: Elderly Patients With Non-Insulin-Dependent Diabetes Mellitus.* Kalamazoo, MI, Upjohn, 1990

Harris MI, Flegal KM, Cowie CC, Eberhardt MS, Goldstein DE, Little RR, et al.: Prevalence of diabetes, impaired fasting glucose, and impaired glucose tolerance in U.S. adults. *Diabetes Care* 21:518–524, 1998

Holman RR, Thorne KI, Farmer AJ, Davies MJ, Keenan JF, Paul S, Levy JC: Addition of biphasic, prandial, or basal insulin to oral therapy in type 2 diabetes. *N Engl J Med* 357:1716–1730, 2007

Resnick HE, Harris MI, Brock DB, Harris TB: American Diabetes Association diabetes diagnostic criteria, advancing age, and cardiovascular disease risk profiles: results from the Third National Health and Nutrition Examination Survey. *Diabetes Care* 23:176–180, 2000

Resnick HE, Foster GL, Bardsley J, Ratner RE: Achievement of American Diabetes Association clinical practice recommendations among U.S. adults with diabetes, 1999-2002: the National Health and Nutrition Examination Survey. *Diabetes Care* 29:531–537, 2006

Resnick HE, Heineman J, Stone R, Shorr RI: Diabetes in U.S. nursing homes, 2004. *Diabetes Care* 31:287–288, 2008

Selvin E, Coresh J, Brancati FL: The burden and treatment of diabetes in elderly individuals in the U.S. *Diabetes Care* 29:2415– 2419, 2006

Shorr RI, Ray WA, Daugherty JR, Griffin MR: Incidence and risk factors for serious hypoglycemia in older persons using insulin or sulfonylureas. *Arch Intern Med* 157:1681–1686, 1997

Sinclair AJ, Conroy SP, Bayer AJ: Impact of diabetes on physical function in older people. *Diabetes Care* 31:233–235, 2008

Wray LA, Ofstedal MB, Langa KM, Blaum CS: The effect of diabetes on disability in middle-aged and older adults. *J Gerontol A Med Sci* 60:1206–1211, 2005

Dr. Halter is Professor of Internal Medicine, Chief of the Division of Geriatric Medicine, and Director of the Geriatrics Center and the Institute of Gerontology, University of Michigan, Ann Arbor, Michigan.

32. Hypoglycemia in Patients with Type 1 Diabetes

STEPHANIE A. AMIEL, BSc, MD, FRCP

Hypoglycemia is the most common acute complication of insulin therapy for diabetes. Exogenous insulin can cause blood glucose to fall to levels too low to support normal brain function. Fear of hypoglycemia is common and causes as much anxiety as the fear of developing long-term complications. In health, blood glucose concentrations are normally maintained between very narrow limits, despite huge variations in the rate of glucose use by the body (exercise vs. rest) and the rate of entry of glucose from outside (eating vs. not eating). Insulin, which suppresses glucose production from the liver and drives glucose uptake by muscle and fat, is the major regulator of circulating glucose concentrations. Insulin delivery is normally directly into the liver, and its secretion is precisely controlled by complex central and local mechanisms. These result in a very large variation in circulating insulin concentrations during the day that achieves very stable blood glucose concentrations.

Replacing endogenous insulin secretion with exogenous insulin, which is delivered to the peripheral circulation by erratic and relatively slow absorption from the subcutaneous injection site in doses that are at best intelligent estimations, sometimes results in hypoglycemia. Other defects in the normal mechanisms of glucose regulation follow the failure of the pancreatic β-cell to make insulin, further increasing the risk. Hypoglycemia and fear of hypoglycemia are major barriers to achieving the glycemic goals required to prevent long-term diabetes complications.

Every patient using insulin is at risk of hypoglycemia and should be instructed in how to recognize, treat, and avoid it. Education in the principles of insulin action and replacement and the factors that influence insulin requirement, backed up by self-monitoring of blood glucose, allows patients to become comfortable adjusting their insulin dosage according to glucose level, food intake, and physical activity and thus achieve truly good diabetes control—a near-normal A1C with no problematic hypoglycemia.

DEFINITIONS

For such a common complication of insulin therapy, hypoglycemia is surprisingly hard to define. The precise definition of "low blood glucose" remains controversial. Whipple defined hypoglycemia clinically, requiring three factors to be present: *1*) symptoms attributable to low blood glucose, *2*) a measurably low blood glucose concentration, and *3*) recovery on restoration of the blood glucose concentration to normal levels. This triad remains the mainstay of diagnosis, but there are two further considerations. One is the potential for hypoglycemia to be asymptomatic—in other words, the person experiencing the hypoglycemia has no subjective awareness of the falling glucose and presents only with signs perceptible to another person. Such hypoglycemia unawareness affects perhaps 25% of people with type 1 diabetes at any time. Whipple's triad is easily adjusted to deal with this by adding the words "and/or signs" to the first statement. More difficult is agreeing on the biochemical definition of the lower limit of a normal blood glucose concentration. A 2005 American Diabetes Association (ADA) consensus statement suggested that any blood glucose <72 mg/dl (<4 mmol/l) should be considered hypoglycemia, primarily on the basis that *1*) counterregulatory changes in body chemistry, especially a reduction in the secretion of endogenous insulin and an increase in release of pancreatic glucagon, may be detectable at this level, and *2*) exposure to arterialized plasma glucose of only slightly <72 mg/dl (<4 mmol/l) has been shown to induce a defect in glucagon and adrenergic responses to subsequent hypoglycemia, at least temporarily. However, blood glucose is often <72 mg/dl (<4 mmol/l) in health. The glucose concentration associated with the onset of counterregulatory responses is variable, changing particularly according to the recent glucose experience of the individual, and neither insulin nor glucagon can be the major defense against hypoglycemia in people with insulin deficiency.

Although using 72 mg/dl (4 mmol/l)—or even 81 mg/dl (4.5 mmol/l)—as an appropriate lower limit for the desirable glucose range a patient with diabetes may wish to achieve is certainly appropriate, to consider anything lower than this as pathological leads to significant overdiagnosis of hypoglycemia, to an extent that is likely to impair attempts to achieve normoglycemia and inappropriate therapeutic decisions. The European Medical Advisory Agency has used 54 mg/dl (3 mmol/l) to define hypoglycemia in a way that has relevance in assessing the safety of new diabetes therapies. It is associated with the onset of measurable cognitive impairment during hypoglycemia, and avoidance of exposure to blood glucose concentrations <54 mg/dl (<3 mmol/l) allows restoration of symptomatic responses to hypoglycemia in people with defective hypoglycemia awareness. However, such a definition would allow patients very easily to slip into more serious hypoglycemia with clinically important cognitive deficiency, and in routine clinical practice, a compromise definition that hypoglycemia means blood glucose <63 mg/dl (<3.5 mmol/l) is usual.

Other important definitions are used to describe the severity of an individual episode of hypoglycemia. Conventionally, mild hypoglycemia is an episode that the patient perceives (i.e., has symptoms of hypoglycemia) and can self-treat. In contrast, severe hypoglycemia is that in which the patient is unable to self-treat, because of the cognitive impairment associated with the failure of brain glucose supplies, and has to be rescued by someone else. Severe hypoglycemia may be subdivided to define episodes associated with coma or seizure or those that require parenteral therapy (intramuscular glucagon or intravenous glucose). Some authorities also refer to moderate hypoglycemia as episodes that are self-managed but very disruptive; however, the lack of precision of this definition makes this a cumbersome category to use.

The normal response to a falling blood glucose concentration is cessation of endogenous insulin secretion and increase of pancreatic glucagon release, the latter driven not just by the falling blood glucose concentration but also by the reduction in activity of neighboring β-cells. These first defenses against hypoglycemia normally start at plasma glucose concentrations just below 72 mg/dl (4 mmol/l). Glucagon and epinephrine (beginning at between 54 and 63 mg/dl [3 and 3.5 mmol/l] in health) are the most rapid-acting counterregulatory hormones, with effects on plasma glucose measurable in minutes. Activation of the sympathetic nervous system in response to hypoglycemia is also fast. The other stress hormones, cortisol and growth hormone, are slower to respond, and their effects become apparent a few hours after the hypoglycemic episode and may persist for hours after that. α-Adrenergic stimulation results in insulin suppression, and β-stimulation results in glucagon secretion with inhibition of glucose utilization and increased glucose production. Together, these processes will normally limit a fall in plasma glucose and maintain sufficient glucose in the circulation to maintain cerebral function (>54 mg/dl [>3 mmol/l]).

Furthermore, the counterregulatory stress responses are accompanied by generation of symptoms, sometimes classified into autonomic symptoms (sweating, shakiness, anxiety, warmth, palpitation, and tingling), attributed to the autonomic stress response, and neuroglycopenic symptoms (dizziness, irritability, difficulty in speaking, confusion, lack of energy, drowsiness, and poor concentration), attributed to the failure of adequate glucose supplies to the cerebral cortex. In children too young to express themselves and in the elderly, these categories may be different—behavioral cues become more relevant in the former and neurological symptoms in the latter. Hunger, an essential element of the natural defense against hypoglycemia because it prompts corrective food ingestion, and blurred vision do not fit neatly with either category. Nevertheless, the nature of the symptom is less important than the fact that the person experiencing the hypoglycemia recognizes it for what it is at a time when cognitive function is not too impaired for an appropriate response. With the inevitable failures of the normal counterregulatory processes implicit in insulin deficiency and replacement, subjective awareness and the ability to treat by eating is the insulin-deficient person's best defense against severe hypoglycemia.

Symptoms of hypoglycemia that occur before the onset of significant confusion provide the diabetic patient's best defense against severe hypoglycemia. Loss of the ability to generate or perceive such symptoms is called hypoglycemia unawareness and is associated with a threefold increase in the risk of severe hypoglycemia. Unawareness is due to additional defects (additional to the unresponsiveness of injected insulin to ambient glucose and the failure of glucagon response from the otherwise healthy α-cell) in the normal glucose counterregulatory mechanisms, in which the onset of the catecholamine and autonomic stress response and their associated symptoms is delayed to a lower glucose concentration than normal and is diminished at any given glucose concentration. Because even a small degree of hypoglycemia can result in detectable cognitive impairment, confusion precedes any potentially symptomatic warning in hypoglycemia unawareness, so the patient has no opportunity to self-treat and stop the glucose fall.

The syndrome of counterregulatory failure and hypoglycemia unawareness is inducible by prior exposure to hypoglycemia, and symptoms can be restored by scrupulous avoidance of further exposure to blood glucose concentrations of <54 mg/dl (<3 mmol/l). It is important to realize that this does not mean simply losing control of the glucose, as will be discussed below. Hypoglycemia unawareness can occur in anyone with diabetes but is most frequent in patients with diabetes of >15 years' duration, of whom 25% of patients report unawareness, and in some regimens of intensive insulin management.

ASSESSING THE PATIENT FOR HYPOGLYCEMIA

As with any medical problem, the first step in managing hypoglycemia is diagnosis. Some patients may present complaining of hypoglycemia problems, but all patients on insulin are at risk, and hypoglycemia should always be discussed. An assessment should be made of the occurrence and frequency for all grades of hypoglycemia: severe, mild, asymptomatic, and biochemical. Asymptomatic hypoglycemia is best assessed by asking whether other people have to tell the patient that he or she is low. It is also important to ask close relatives or friends as well as the patient. Biochemical hypoglycemia is defined as that detected unexpectedly on a routine home blood glucose monitoring test. Awareness status can be quantified using simple questionnaires, such as the Clarke or Gold scores. Where a problem with hypoglycemia is suspected, it is helpful to document the patient's usual daily timetable, noting the usual times of food intake, insulin administration, and activity, and to inspect the blood glucose log to relate hypoglycemia to activity levels, days of the week, and other behavioral predictors.

CAUSES AND PREVENTION OF HYPOGLYCEMIA

The cause of hypoglycemia in insulin-treated people is primarily the insulin. Conditions of relative or absolute insulin excess can occur when:

- the insulin taken is more than is required, or the timing of its absorption does not match need
- access to exogenous glucose is decreased (e.g., during the night, when a meal is delayed or missed, or the meal has insufficient carbohydrates for the dose of insulin taken); gastric emptying is delayed because of high-fat content in a meal or if there is coincidental hyperglycemia (gastroparesis in autonomic neuropathy is thought to increase risk of hypoglycemia, although the evidence that this occurs is surprisingly lacking); or food absorption is delayed by intercurrent gastrointestinal disease, such as gastroenteritis or celiac disease
- glucose utilization is increased during and after exercise. Note that unusually prolonged or vigorous (relative to the individual's usual routine) exercise will continue to lower blood glucose as the muscle and liver glycogen stores used during the exercise are restored—a process that can take >18 h.
- insulin sensitivity is increased (e.g., at night time, in early pregnancy, recovery from infections, lactation, menopause, or intercurrent abnormalities of

counterregulatory mechanisms, such as adrenal failure or pituitary hormone insufficiency)
- hepatic glucose production is decreased (e.g., because of inhibited gluconeogenesis caused by excessive alcohol intake)
- insulin clearance is decreased, as in renal failure, hypothyroidism, high concentrations of circulating insulin-binding antibodies, or liver failure

Other causes of temporary insulin excess include variations in insulin absorption from the subcutaneous sites. There may be a 20–30% variation in the rate of absorption of insulin, depending on body or ambient temperature, blood flow, anatomical site, or depth of injection, among other factors. There is less variability with analog insulins.

Relative or Absolute Insulin Excess

1. At Night. Insulin action should be considered in two categories—basal insulin secretion, which acts to control endogenous glucose production, and meal-related or prandial insulin. The former is continuous and requires only modest amounts—the "mean" dose for the "typical" adult person is ~1 unit/h. The requirement is not flat, with the human body being most insulin sensitive ~2–4 A.M., followed by a variable rise in insulin requirement to a peak at ~7–9 A.M. The tendency of blood glucose to rise in the morning is exacerbated in diabetes, when the overnight background insulin may start to run out. Attempts to improve the prebreakfast blood glucose by increasing the dose of the overnight insulin may increase the risk of hypoglycemia in the earlier part of the night. Close to 50% of severe hypoglycemia episodes occurs during sleep, when the individual cannot perceive symptoms or is not alert enough to respond to the symptoms and when, in deep sleep, the normal protective hormonal responses to hypoglycemia are very significantly less than when awake. Nighttime hypoglycemia may be enough to cause reduced awareness of any hypoglycemia the next day. Both the overnight basal insulin replacement and the tail end of the insulin taken for the evening meal may contribute to hypoglycemia in the night, as may exercise or alcohol taken the day before.

Nocturnal hypoglycemia is now probably best detected by continuous glucose monitoring, although the duration of an individual episode may be overestimated. Although the traditional blood glucose check is at 3:00 A.M., the expected time of maximal insulin sensitivity and peak action of a conventional intermediate-acting insulin injected in the evening, failure to detect hypoglycemia at this time does not rule out nocturnal hypoglycemia that is earlier or later. The ability of the prebedtime blood glucose to predict nocturnal hypoglycemia is controversial, perhaps because this is primarily controlled by the pre–evening meal insulin, but a low-normal fasting glucose is increasingly recognized as associated with subnormal glucose in the night. Inexplicable fluctuations in fasting glucose, or even consistently low-normal fasting blood glucose concentrations, should encourage a search for nocturnal hypoglycemia, and continuous glucose monitoring may be helpful for this.

Strategies demonstrated to reduce nocturnal hypoglycemia start by suspecting it is there. Using continuous glucose monitoring may be helpful in demonstrating the phenomenon to the patient. Otherwise, conventional blood glucose monitoring at bedtime and between 2:00 and 4:00 A.M. and between 6:00 and 7:00 A.M. for three consecutive nights every few months may be useful, and a 2:00–4:00 A.M. test should always be done before increasing overnight basal insulin to improve fasting glucose. Monitoring blood glucose levels during the night should also be done after days of intense physical activity, after changes in work shifts, when staying up unusually late, and when changing time zones. The blood glucose nadir should be >63 mg/dl (>3.5 mmol/l) or 72 mg/dl (4 mmol/l), where there is considered to be high risk of nocturnal hypoglycemia.

Taking the evening dose of background insulin at bedtime rather than with the evening meal and the use of both rapid- and long-acting insulin analogs have been shown to be effective in reducing nocturnal hypoglycemia without loss of control of the fasting glucose. The efficacy of rapid-acting analogs to reduce nocturnal hypoglycemia confirm the contribution of the tail end of the evening meal's short-acting regular insulin (which can also be offset by a bedtime snack) but may be associated with "escape" from the insulin action between the end of the rapid-acting analog and the onset of action of a bedtime background insulin, especially in children eating early in the evening—and perhaps rising late. This can cause hyperglycemia that can affect A1C. For those patients still taking conventional nocturnal background NPH insulin before the evening meal, a bedtime snack is also essential, and incorporating protein in the snack may extend the effect a little and enhance glucagon levels. The long-acting analogs also are associated with reduced nocturnal hypoglycemia, presumably because of their flatter, and more reproducible, action profiles. Such analogs can overcome quite substantial dawn phenomenon. Although recent meta-analyses fail to confirm major impact of analog use on diabetes control in general, there are enough data on their reduced risk of nocturnal hypoglycemia to support their use in patients experiencing problems with nocturnal hypoglycemia or hypoglycemia unawareness. There is a report showing that when using insulin glargine as background, less nocturnal hypoglycemia occurs when it is given at the beginning rather than at the end of the day, but this is at the cost of a higher prebreakfast glucose level.

A continuous infusion of rapid-acting insulin to provide background insulinization in insulin pump therapy, which can be programmed to provide higher infusion rates in the early morning, dictated by blood glucose measurements, can be very useful where there is difficulty controlling the prebreakfast blood glucose without nocturnal hypoglycemia. Such insulin pump therapy has been clearly demonstrated to reduce severe hypoglycemia rates, although the role of reeducation in insulin adjustment strategies is not always clear in the published literature. Nevertheless, in experienced hands, continuous infusion is a good way of replacing background insulin and can produce significant improvements in hypoglycemia experience.

2. Day. Meal-related insulin is usually given in the form of a regular insulin or rapid-acting analog injected ideally ~30 min before eating in the first case or 10 min to immediately before eating in the case of fast-acting analogs. Mismatch between the absorption of the insulin and of the meal is common. Continuous glucose monitoring confirms the difficulties in getting perfect postprandial glucose control, but excessive doses of mealtime insulins increase the risk of hypoglycemia before the next meal. Sometimes, the best results can be obtained by dividing the meal's carbohydrate intake into two, with the second, smaller intake taken as a between-meal snack. Such regular snacking is not popular with patients but is often necessary in children, especially in the morning, and is probably essential if no prandial insulin is taken with lunch and only morning NPH insulin is used to cover lunch. It is also necessary when daytime background insulinization is suboptimal and dependent on the tail end of the action profile of the mealtime insulin doses. Premeal hypoglycemia may be due to either background or meal-related insulin replacement or a mixture of both. Distinguishing the two can be achieved by omitting a mealtime dose while consuming a carbohydrate-free meal or by sequential post- and premeal glucose testing.

3. With Exercise. Exercise increases glucose uptake and utilization in muscle. Prolonged or vigorous exercise (the terms being relative to the individual's usual activity levels) will deplete muscle and liver glycogen, which can take as long as 24 h to be restored. Thus, hypoglycemia is a risk not only during exercise but also for many hours afterwards. In health, exercise is accompanied by a fall in insulin secretion; in insulin treatment, insulin absorption may be increased as injection sites are mechanically disrupted and blood flow increased. A hot shower afterward may further exacerbate the problem by increasing skin blood flow. In the long term, a further risk for hypoglycemia may be the effect of regular exercise to enhance insulin sensitivity.

Avoidance of exercise-induced hypoglycemia is best achieved by reducing the dose of insulin active at the time of the exercise (and/or taking extra readily available carbohydrate) and, if the exercise is prolonged or vigorous, for the night after the exercise. Decrements of 20–50% may be required. However, insulin should not be entirely withheld during and after exercise, as ketosis may then occur. Different types of exercise will require different strategies, and for major exercise, reducing fast-acting insulin and taking additional carbohydrate is useful.

The current algorithms for reducing background insulin for the night after increased exercise (or alcohol, see below) were worked out for conventional intermediate-acting insulins. The immediate efficacy of reducing doses of long-acting analogs, such as insulin glargine, is not clear, although the rules of pharmacology would suggest that the effect of such reduction may not be immediately apparent. On the other hand, the flatter profile of the long-acting analogs may reduce the drive to nocturnal hypoglycemia. Many patients find reducing analogs as they would with conventional insulins is effective, and others depend more on reducing subsequent doses of morning insulin. It is useful to reduce glargine doses 24–48 h before a major increase in physical activity. There is experimental evidence that exercise can act as a stressor to reduce hormonal responses to later hypoglycemia, and vice versa.

4. With Alcohol. Many alcoholic drinks contain carbohydrate, and the immediate response to such an alcoholic drink is transient hyperglycemia. However, alcohol also inhibits gluconeogenesis, which becomes the main method of endogenous glucose production ~8 h after eating (before which glycogenolysis is the major contributor). Thus, there is enhanced risk for hypoglycemia the morning after significant alcohol intake when followed by normal sleep without food intake. Acutely, alcohol can interfere with the ability to perceive hypoglycemic symptoms, which may also complicate hypoglycemia.

Avoidance of alcohol-induced hypoglycemia is best achieved by either avoidance of alcohol or by reducing overnight background insulin replacement the night of greater-than-usual alcohol intake. This is particularly critical if the increased alcohol intake is associated with exercise, e.g., dancing at a party.

PREVENTION AND TREATMENT OF HYPOGLYCEMIA UNAWARENESS

Epidemiological evidence shows that the most important risk factors for severe hypoglycemia include history of a previous severe hypoglycemic episode, longer duration of diabetes, lower recent A1C, hypoglycemia unawareness, and C-peptide negativity. Anecdotally, autonomic neuropathy is a moderate risk factor for severe hypoglycemia, but classical autonomic neuropathy is not required for the presence of hypoglycemia unawareness. However, even in the presence of these relatively fixed predispositions to hypoglycemia unawareness and severe hypoglycemia risk, there are therapeutic strategies that can restore awareness and protection from severe hypoglycemia, at least to some degree. The underlying principle of these strategies is based on firm evidence that counterregulatory failure and hypoglycemia unawareness can be induced by exposure to quite mild degrees of antecedent hypoglycemia and that avoidance of all exposure to a plasma glucose <54 mg/dl (<3 mmol/l) can produce restoration of symptom responses and to some extent improvement in the catecholamine and sympathetic responses to occasional falls in blood glucose.

Education

The mainstay of hypoglycemia avoidance is patient education by educated health care professionals. In contrast to the data of the DCCT (Diabetes Control and Complications Trial), in which the rate of hypoglycemia appeared inextricably associated with lower A1C, interventions that are based on structured education for patients in the flexible use of insulin in a relatively normal lifestyle have repeatedly shown to achieve reduced A1C in association with reductions (or at the very least no increase) in the rate of episodes of severe hypoglycemia. Such interventions depend on a transfer of skills from the health care professional to the patient, such that the insulin user really understands the pharmacodynamics of his or her insulins and can adjust doses on evidence-based algorithms, which are individualized in response to personal glucose monitoring in structured ways to achieve glycemic targets compatible with minimal risk of diabetes complications. The prototype for such educational courses was the Dusseldorf program, created by Michael Berger et al., using principles of adult education and research into insulin action, and many programs have evolved based on this.

Such patient training is initially time consuming for both patient and health care provider, but the investment of time pays dividends. A recent abstract from the U.K.'s DAFNE (Dose Adjustment for Normal Eating) program has shown that 50% of participants entering the program with hypoglycemia unawareness reported restored awareness 1 year later, which was associated with a significant fall in the severe hypoglycemia rate in the DAFNE graduates as a whole. Such programs teach patients the value of regular home glucose monitoring, focusing especially on premeal and prebedtime values; adjusting meal insulin doses to carbohydrates eaten, corrected for deviation from target; and continuing to reflect on glucose concentrations achieved and adjustment of both meal and background insulins regularly when patterns of failure to achieve targets are observed. Sometimes, participation in such programs leads patients to reduce frequency of home testing, whereas one risk factor for hypoglycemia, especially in children, is failure to monitor, and in some patients with hypoglycemia problems, monitoring may be excessive, leading to anxiety and overcorrection of aberrant values.

Careful education about meal glucose control is especially valuable. Patients checking postmeal blood glucose need to be cautioned against overcorrection. There is some controversial evidence that postprandial hyperglycemia may contribute independently to cardiovascular risk, but it is best tackled prospectively by increasing the relevant mealtime insulin doses on subsequent days. Correcting postmeal hyperglycemia, unless the patient is feeling unwell, often contributes to high hypoglycemia risk as the hyperglycemia may be transient and relate to mismatch between the insulin and the glucose absorption. If the patient finds a high postmeal value, repeating the test in 1 h and only treating if there has been no improvement helps avoid this, but in general the advice should be to change the usual insulin dose for that meal time in the future, if the problem occurs regularly. A similar tendency to hypoglycemia occurs if patients routinely inject insulin after eating, rather than before. Some parents find this necessary because a child's food intake may be unpredictable. When using a rapid-acting analog insulin, this strategy can give acceptable results as long as the injection is immediate, but it is not ideal.

Other educational initiatives such as blood glucose awareness training, which seeks to help patients consider risk factors for hypoglycemia, enhancing their ability to predict and therefore avoid them, have also been shown to reduce hypoglycemia experience. However, it is important to recognize that ~50% of patients with hypoglycemia unawareness do not find resolution as a result of education alone, and many with a history of hypoglycemia find it difficult to avoid hypoglycemia for the long term. Possible explanations for this include the difficulties in maintaining intensive self-monitoring and treatment adjustment indefinitely and perhaps a taught fear of hyperglycemia-related diabetes complications. Some very recent data suggest that a patient with hypoglycemia unawareness may have an altered cortical response to acute hypoglycemia, making him or her unaware not just of the event but also of its danger. This creates a potential barrier to making behavioral change that targets hypoglycemia avoidance, because there is no perception of need.

There is some recent evidence that patients with hypoglycemia-associated autonomic failure may have reduced β-adrenergic sensitivity compared with patients with normal counterregulation. This abnormal sensitivity could be recovered if hypoglycemia is avoided for several months.

Managing hypoglycemia risk is less clear in children, in whom educational strategies are different and parental control is usual. Nevertheless, the same principles of appropriate background and meal-related insulin administration are important, although other factors, such as the willingness of the school to supervise insulin injections and blood testing, may be an issue. Activity levels and food intake may be unpredictable in children, and adjusting food and insulin is often required, as adults adjust regimens after observing the child's actions. Young children have more brisk counterregulatory responses than adults, but, although it has not been tested directly, it is probable that antecedent hypoglycemia has similar ability to reduce defenses against subsequent hypoglycemia. Although insulin-resistant poorly controlled adolescents may experience symptoms of hypoglycemia at quite high blood glucose concentrations, this may not protect them from severe sudden hypoglycemia after erratic insulin administration and/or activity and food intake.

Glucose Sensing

Research continues to examine the molecular mechanisms for glucose sensing and of hypoglycemia awareness and unawareness and seeks pharmacological methods for enhancing the hypoglycemia defenses. In some studies, caffeine has been shown to increase the generation or perception of hypoglycemic symptoms. In contrast, nonselective β-blockers may alter the symptoms of hypoglycemia, and although specific research has shown this not to have major impact on perception of experimental hypoglycemia, it is prudent that people who need to use these medications should be particularly vigilant about routine blood glucose testing.

Continuous glucose monitoring with subcutaneous sensors is now available for detecting hypoglycemia, and devices with sophisticated software can be used to show the patient an estimation of his or her blood glucose (the devices measure interstitial fluid glucose but are calibrated to a plasma glucose measurement) in real time. Early studies with such continuous glucose monitors have shown them to be popular with users, but no major impact has yet been shown on diabetes control or even hypoglycemia rate in unselected patients trained to use conventional self-monitoring well. However, the development of alarms that activate when blood glucose is falling quickly or when hypoglycemia occurs has obvious attraction. Larger studies, perhaps in patients experiencing problems with hypoglycemia as well as having more experience in how to use the real-time data, are eagerly awaited.

Transplantation

The patient presenting with problematic hypoglycemia needs a full review of his or her therapy and lifestyle and optimization of insulin regimen. At the very least this will entail exclusion of comorbidities, improving use of background and mealtime insulins, appropriate use of home glucose monitoring, and increasing use of newer technologies such as insulin pump therapy and continuous glucose monitoring systems. Closing the loop by linking continuous glucose monitors to insulin delivery devices remains a target for research. But replacement of nature's own glucose-dependent insulin delivery device by replacing the destroyed β-cells in pancreatic islets, either as islet transplantation or in whole-organ transplantation, now forms part of the armamentarium. Neither procedure is well enough established, efficient, or safe enough to be considered in all but a very few patients in whom all other strategies have failed. But for those people whose lives are being destroyed by recurrent severe hypoglycemia, despite their best efforts with well-supported conventional therapies, transplantation does prevent hypoglycemia while the transplants continue to function.

COMPLICATIONS OF SEVERE HYPOGLYCEMIA

Hypoglycemia causes physical and psychosocial morbidity and may rarely cause death. Physical morbidity ranges from unpleasant symptoms to errors in judgment, accidents, decreased performance, and behavioral changes leading to episodes that can be mistaken for alcohol intoxication or illegal drug use. More extreme cases may lead to severe neurological manifestations, including focal or generalized seizures or coma. Permanent neurological sequelae are rare, and the evidence for functional or structural change after recurrent hypoglycemia from which a full recovery appears to have been made at the time is very equivocal. Hypoglycemic hemiplegia is a specific condition that follows unsuspected nocturnal hypoglycemia. The patient wakes with a hemiplegia but may no longer be hypoglycemic on discovery of the problem. The hemiplegia resolves after a few hours, and although the literature is not entirely consistent, there is usually no underlying brain or vascular disease, and the condition has no prognostic significance.

Permanent focal neurological damage after severe hypoglycemia is rare and most commonly seen after deliberate or accidental insulin overdosage. There is evidence of harm in the developing brain, however, with children experiencing multiple severe hypoglycemic episodes in childhood performing less well on cognitive function testing (IQ tests, speed in processing information, and reduced motor speed tasks) as adolescents. The data in adults are much less clear, as studies showing impaired cognitive performance are often not controlled for differences in mood state, and comparisons are rarely made with other patient groups with nonhypoglycemic long-term conditions. In animal studies of profound hypoglycemia, structures involved in memory are readily damaged, and anecdotally, patients may complain of memory problems. However, some clinical problems may be more related to the failure to establish a memory during hypoglycemia than permanent damage to the neurological structures responsible for memory.

Some studies suggest impaired cognitive function or faster loss of IQ points is seen in people with multiple episodes of hypoglycemia, but others have found the relationship only in association with other diabetes complications, specifically peripheral neuropathy. Data from the DCCT show no deterioration in cognitive function with intensive insulin therapy, despite much higher rates of hypoglycemia. For an individual patient complaining of cognitive problems, expert assessment of cognitive function should be arranged.

Although rare, death can occur as a result of hypoglycemia, either because of trauma sustained during confusion (e.g., car accidents) or as a direct effect of the hypoglycemia. Hypoglycemia as a cause of car accidents remains controversial. There is clear evidence that driving performance rapidly deteriorates in hypoglycemia but little evidence to suggest that diabetic drivers have more accidents—possibly because they are more cautious. Certainly it is important (and in some countries mandatory) that people using insulin check blood glucose prior to driving and during prolonged drives at ~90-min intervals. Although people with good hypoglycemia awareness may be safe to drive at normoglycemia, those with unawareness of any degree should be advised to use a higher cutoff for driving of 126 mg/dl (7 mmol/l).

It is very difficult to ascertain the mortality rate directly due to hypoglycemia, but one retrospective study estimated deaths due to hypoglycemia at 4% of deaths in diabetes. At least some of these deaths are likely to be cardiac in origin. Hypoglycemia prolongs the QTc interval of the electrocardiogram, and this is associated with increased risk of arrhythmia. Although a neurological hypoglycemic death would be expected to be associated with evidence of seizure, cardiac arrythmias are the suspected cause of the so-called "dead in bed" syndrome, in which the patient is found in an apparently undisturbed state.

TREATMENT OF ACUTE HYPOGLYCEMIA

Everyone taking insulin should be taught how to recognize warning symptoms of hypoglycemia and how to treat it promptly, even if symptoms are subtle, to prevent progression to neuroglycopenia. Similarly, everyone living with someone with diabetes should be taught to recognize the signs of developing hypoglycemia and instructed in what action to take. Ideally, patients should check blood glucose before treating to avoid unnecessary treatment. Even verification of blood glucose level immediately after treatment of suspected hypoglycemia is useful, helping the patient recognize unusual or unexpected symptoms in subsequent episodes. In case of doubt, it is always safe to treat confusion in someone with diabetes as hypoglycemia, although proper diagnosis and treatment of other conditions should follow immediately. The goal of treatment of hypoglycemia is to increase the blood glucose to a safe level to prevent sequelae, using an intervention that works quickly and relieves symptoms quickly while avoiding rebound hyperglycemia.

The ideal treatment of hypoglycemia is self-administered oral glucose: 15–20 g carbohydrate in an adult or 3–5 g/10 kg body wt for a child. Parenteral treatment should not be used if the patient is able to swallow.

Oral glucose should be taken in readily absorbed form, i.e., glucose tablets or sugary drinks that provide 15–20 g glucose. A greater volume of fresh fruit juice will be needed (5–6.75 oz [150–200 ml]), because fruit juice contains sucrose, as well as similar volumes of sugary drinks, such as regular carbonated drinks and colas, to treat hypoglycemia. Diet drinks are not useful. Honey is sometimes convenient (and may be safer than a liquid if it is administered to a confused child) but contains only 5 g glucose in 1 teaspoon (5 ml), being 50–60% fructose. Commercially available glucose gel can be a convenient way to carry emergency hypoglycemia treatment. Glucose is absorbed through the buccal cavity, but if a patient is too confused to swallow, formal parenteral therapy (see below) is preferable to filling the mouth with gel or honey. Sugared milky drinks and chocolate bars and drinks are not a good treatment as the fat content delays absorption of the glucose.

Oral treatment should never be deferred. Patients should be discouraged from waiting because a meal is due shortly. Absorption of carbohydrate in the meal will be delayed by any fat or protein component, and the time delay may easily be enough to allow the hypoglycemia to progress to being profound enough to cause confusion. After the initial treatment is taken, the patient should wait 15 min before rechecking or retreating to minimize the risk of posthypoglycemic hyperglycemia.

If a meal is not due to be eaten within the next hour, the immediate treatment should be followed by 10–20 g of slowly absorbed carbohydrate in the form of fruit, a cookie or two, a slice of bread, or breakfast cereal. This is not necessary if the patient is about to eat, although reducing the usual mealtime insulin dose (by

~1 unit for every 54 mg/dl [3 mmol/l] the patient wishes the glucose to rise) is helpful. Maintaining the mealtime dose but changing the dose-to-meal interval is not useful because it simply increases the mismatch of meal to insulin absorption. Glucose requirements for treating hypoglycemia may be much higher if there has been an error with the insulin dose or a missed meal.

Parenteral therapy is required if there is loss of consciousness or confusion to a degree that might inhibit the normal automatic protection of the airway. Patients' friends and relatives should be taught to administer glucagon: 1 mg (for children aged <5 years, 0.5 mg), intramuscularly or subcutaneously, which will raise blood glucose over 10 min, with a peak effect that lasts ~1 h. Nevertheless, the patient should receive additional oral carbohydrate on recovery because the degree of glucose deficit will have been greater than in a mild episode. Twenty grams of rapidly absorbed carbohydrate, followed by 40 g of slowly absorbed carbohydrate, is recommended. Glucagon works by stimulating immediate release of glucose from liver glycogen and will be less effective in situations where glycogen stores may be depleted, e.g., after very strenuous or prolonged exercise, prolonged fasting and malnutrition, hypoglycemia associated with chronic alcoholism, very high doses of insulin, or recurrent hypoglycemia. Nausea and sometimes vomiting may occur after glucagon administration, so monitoring of blood glucose levels should be continued until the patient is able to eat normally.

Health care professionals use intravenous glucose for the most rapid response to severe hypoglycemia, and it is very effective. The common practice of using 50% glucose solutions is dangerous. The solution is extremely hyperosmolar, and extravasation will cause tissue damage. Larger volumes of more dilute glucose will work equally efficiently and with less risk: 75 ml of 20% or 150 ml 10% glucose will provide sufficient glucose and can be given rapidly. In hospitalized sick patients in whom volume overload may be a problem (renal failure, cardiac failure), 25 ml 50% glucose may be given through a central venous line, but even in cardiac failure, 75 ml 20% glucose solution—or even 150 ml—is preferable if a central line is not in place.

If severe hypoglycemia is thought to be due to excessive amounts of long-acting insulin, such as insulin glargine, or very large insulin overdosage, hospital admission should be considered, as the hypoglycemia is likely to recur. Patients should be warned that, despite the common occurrence of posthypoglycemic hyperglycemia (a combination of overzealous treatment and the insulin resistance engendered by the stress response), a further severe hypoglycemia is statistically more likely to happen in the ensuing 24–48 h. This may be in part because of continuation of the cause of the original hypoglycemia (e.g., effect of exercise or alcohol) and in part because of the ability of hypoglycemia to downregulate the stress response to a subsequent hypoglycemic stimulus and make the next episode even less symptomatic. Scrupulous self-monitoring of blood glucose, while resisting the natural tendency to take extra insulin to correct the posthypoglycemic high glucose concentrations that will be seen, should be carried out during this time.

Whenever hypoglycemia occurs, the patient (with or without professional help) should consider why it might have happened. This will enable adjustments to insulin regimens in specific situations or avoidance of particular behaviors that increase risk of hypoglycemia in the future.

BIBLIOGRAPHY

Amiel SA, Evans ML: Iatrogenic hypoglycaemia. In *Joslin's Diabetes Mellitus.* 14th ed. Kahn CR, Weir GC, King GL, Moses AC, Smith RJ, Jacobson AM, Eds. Baltimore, MD, Lippincott Williams & Wilkins, 2004, p. 671–686

Bartley PC, Bogoev M, Larsen J, Philotheou A: Long-term efficacy and safety of insulin detemir compared to neutral protamine hagedorn insulin in patients with type 1 diabetes using a treat-to-target basal-bolus regimen with insulin aspart at meals: a 2-year, randomized, controlled trial. *Diabet Med* 25:442–449, 2008

Bingham EM, Dunn J, Smith D, Sutcliffe-Goulden J, Reed LJ, Marsden PK, Amiel SA: Differential changes in brain glucose metabolism in hypoglycaemia accompany loss of hypoglycaemia awareness in men with type 1 diabetes mellitus: an [^{11}C]-3-O-methyl-D-glucose PET study. *Diabetologia* 48:2080–2089, 2005

Chase HP, Lockspeiser T, Peery B, Shepherd M, MacKenzie T, Anderson J, et al.: The impact of the Diabetes Control and Complications Trial and Humalog insulin on glycohemoglobin and severe hypoglycemia in type 1 diabetes. *Diabetes Care* 24:430–434, 2001

Clarke WL, Cox DJ, Gonder-Frederick LA, Julian D, Schlundt D, Polonsky W: Reduced awareness of hypoglycemia in adults with IDDM: a prospective study of hypoglycemic frequency and associated symptoms. *Diabetes Care* 18:517–522, 1995

Cox DJ, Kovatchev B, Koev D, Koeva L, Dachev S, Tcharaktchiev D, Protopopova A, Gonder-Frederick L, Clarke W: Hypoglycemia anticipation, awareness and treatment training (HAATT) reduces occurrence of severe hypoglycemia among adults with type 1 diabetes mellitus. *Int J Behav Med* 11:212–218, 2004

Cranston I, Lomas J, Maran A, Macdonald I, Amiel SA: Restoration of hypoglycaemia awareness in patients with long-duration insulin-dependent diabetes. *Lancet* 344:283–287, 1994

DAFNE Study Group: A randomised, controlled trial of training in flexible, intensive insulin management to enable dietary freedom in people with type 1 diabetes: the DAFNE (Dose Adjustment For Normal Eating) trial. *BMJ* 13:197–204, 2002

DCCT Research Group: Hypoglycemia in the Diabetes Control and Complications Trial. *Diabetes* 46:271–286, 1997

Diabetes Control and Complications Trial/Epidemiology of Diabetes Interventions and Complications Study Research Group, Jacobson AM, Musen G, Ryan CM, Silvers N, Cleary P, Waberski B, Burwood A, Weinger K, Bayless M, Dahms W, Harth J: Long-term effect of diabetes and its treatment on cognitive function. *N Engl J Med* 356:1842–1852, 2007

Dunn J, Cranston IC, Marsden PK, Amiel SA, Reed LJ: Attenuation of amydgala and frontal cortical responses to low blood glucose concentration in asymptomatic hypoglycemia in type 1 diabetes: a new player in hypoglycemia unawareness? *Diabetes* 56:2766–2773, 2007

Fanelli C, Pampanelli S, Lalli C, Del Sindaco P, Ciofetta M, Lepore M, et al.: Long-term intensive therapy of IDDM patients with clinically overt autonomic neuropathy: effects on hypoglycemia unawareness and counterregulation. *Diabetes* 46:1172–1181, 1997

Fritsche A, Stefan N, Haring H, Gerich J, Stumvoll M: Avoidance of hypoglycemia restores hypoglycemia unawareness by increasing beta-adrenergic sensitivity in patients with type 1 diabetes. *Ann Intern Med* 134:729–736, 2001

Gold AE, MacLeod KM, Frier BM: Frequency of severe hypoglycemia in patients with type 1 diabetes with impaired awareness of hypoglycemia. *Diabetes Care* 17:697–703, 1994

Hamman A, Matthaei S, Rosak C, Sivestre L: A randomized clinical trial comparing breakfast, dinner or bedtime administration of insulin glargine in patients with type 1 diabetes. *Diabetes Care* 26:1738–1744, 2003

Heller SR, Cryer PE: Reduced neuroendocrine and symptomatic responses to subsequent hypoglycemia after 1 episode of hypoglycemia in nondiabetic humans. *Diabetes* 40:223–226, 1991

Jeitler K, Horvath K, Berghold A, Gratzer TW, Neeser K, Pieber TR, Siebenhofer A: Continuous subcutaneous insulin infusion versus multiple daily insulin injections in patients with diabetes mellitus: systematic review and meta-analysis. *Diabetologia* 51:941–951, 2008

Jones TW, Porter P, Sherwin RS, Davis EA, O'Leary P, Frazer F, et al.: Decreased epinephrine responses to hypoglycemia during sleep. *N Engl J Med* 338:1657–1662, 1998

Ludvigsson J, Samuelsson U: Continuous insulin infusion (CSII) or modern type of multiple daily injections (MDI) in diabetic children and adolescents a critical review on a controversial issue. *Pediatr Endocrinol Rev* 5:666–678, 2007

Murphy NP, Ford-Adams ME, Ong KK, Harris ND, Keane SM, Davies C, Ireland RH, MacDonald IA, Knight EJ, Edge JA, Heller SR, Dunger DB: Prolonged cardiac repolarisation during spontaneous nocturnal hypoglycaemia in children and adolescents with type 1 diabetes. *Diabetologia* 47:1940–1947, 2004

Northam EA, Rankins D, Cameron FJ: Therapy insight: the impact of type 1 diabetes on brain development and function. *Nat Clin Pract Neurol* 2:78–86, 2006

Pedersen-Bjergaard U, Pramming S, Heller SR, Wallace TM, Rasmussen AK, Jørgensen HV, Matthews DR, Hougaard P, Thorsteinsson B: Severe hypoglycaemia in 1076 adult patients with type 1 diabetes: influence of risk markers and selection. *Diabetes Metab Res Rev* 20:479–486, 2004

Robinson RT, Harris ND, Ireland RH, Macdonald IA, Heller SR: Changes in cardiac repolarization during clinical episodes of nocturnal hypoglycaemia in adults with type 1 diabetes. *Diabetologia* 47:312–315, 2004

Sämann A, Mühlhauser I, Bender R, Kloos Ch, Müller UA: Glycaemic control and severe hypoglycaemia following training in flexible, intensive insulin therapy to enable dietary freedom in people with type 1 diabetes: a prospective implementation study. *Diabetologia* 48:1965–1970, 2005

Siebenhofer A, Plank J, Berghold A, Jeitler K, Horvath K, Narath M, Gfrerer R, Pieber TR: Short acting insulin analogues versus regular human insulin in patients with diabetes mellitus. *Cochrane Database Syst Rev* no. CD003287, 2006

Siebenhofer A, Plank J, Berghold A, Horvath K, Sawicki PT, Beck P, Pieber TR: Meta-analysis of short-acting insulin analogues in adult patients with type 1 diabetes: continuous subcutaneous insulin infusion versus injection therapy. *Diabetologia* 47:1895–1905, 2004

Slama G, Traynard PY, Desplanque N, Pudar H, Dhunputh I, Letanoux M, et al.: The search for an optimized treatment of hypoglycemia: carbohydrates in tablets, solution, or gel for the correction of insulin reactions. *Arch Intern Med* 150:589–593, 1990

Truong W, Lakey JR, Ryan EA, Shapiro AM: Clinical islet transplantation at the University of Alberta—the Edmonton experience. *Clin Transpl* 153–172, 2005

Workgroup on Hypoglycemia, American Diabetes Association: Defining and reporting hypoglycemia in diabetes: a report from the American Diabetes Association Workgroup on Hypoglycemia. *Diabetes Care* 28:1245–1249, 2005

Dr. Amiel is the RD Lawrence Professor of Diabetic Medicine at King's College London School of Medicine, London, U.K.

33. Insulin Allergy and Immunological Insulin Resistance

S. Edwin Fineberg, MD, and John H. Holcombe, MD

As stringent purification methods and recombinant DNA technology were applied to insulin production, the incidence of immunological complications of insulin therapy dramatically decreased. However, reports of insulin allergy and resistance continue with all formulations of insulins, including highly purified animal-sourced insulin, unmodified human insulin, and analogs of human insulin. Anti-insulin antibodies occur de novo in individuals prone to type 1 diabetes, in patients treated with certain drugs, and in certain viral and neoplastic disorders. The development of anti-insulin antibodies in response to insulin therapy is affected by the patient's age, immune response genes, and site of insulin delivery and by the formulation, structure, and degradation products of the insulin molecules themselves. Despite the relatively higher incidence of antibody formation in patients with type 1 diabetes, the overall incidence of immunological complications of therapy is roughly equal in type 1 and type 2 diabetes. All classes of immunoglobulin antibodies have been seen in response to insulin therapy, but IgG antibodies predominate, with increased levels of anti-insulin IgE in many individuals with insulin allergy. Immunological insulin resistance and the insulin autoimmune syndrome are associated with anti-insulin IgG.

It is likely that animal insulins will continue to be available in the less-developed world. These insulins are inherently more immunogenic than human insulins, and it would be expected that a higher incidence of adverse immune sequelae might be seen in animal insulin–treated patients. The incidence of dermal reactions to insulin has been reported to be 12.9% with mixed bovine-porcine, 3.4% with porcine, and 2.4% with human insulins. It is controversial whether the presence of high levels of insulin antibodies per se leads to increased insulin dosage requirements, alteration in insulin absorption profiles, antibody-mediated insulin resistance, diabetic ketoacidosis, or increases in hypoglycemic episodes.

Long-acting and rapidly acting human insulin analogs do not differ in their inherent immunogenicity from unmodified human insulins since their structural modifications do not affect the most antigenic portions of the insulin molecule. The currently available short-acting human insulin analogs are insulins lispro, aspart, and glulisine. Structural modifications lead to decreases in the insulin's tendency to self-associate and their rapid onset of action after subcutaneous injection. The long-acting insulin analog insulin glargine precipitates in the subcutaneous space and is slowly absorbed. Insulin detemir, another basal insulin, is coupled with myristic acid. When injected, determir forms hexamers and is eventually absorbed as monomers bind to serum albumin.

Circulating antibodies to protamine have been detected in ~40% of individuals treated with NPH insulins. These antibodies are rarely the cause of insulin-associated allergic phenomena but have been associated with anaphylaxis during the reversal of intraoperative heparin anticoagulation. However, the presence of antibodies to protamine does not predict protamine-related anaphylaxis. In patients previously treated with NPH insulins, heparin anticoagulation should be allowed to reverse spontaneously; if protamine reversal is necessary, it should be carried out with precautions against anaphylaxis.

Insulin aggregates and oxidative products form during the storage of pharmaceutical insulins, especially at high temperatures; only the former incite specific antibodies. There are few cases of zinc-related insulin allergy, despite the common demonstration of skin test reactions to zinc acetate or zinc sulfate. Rarely, patients may react to plasticizers, preservatives, or latex contaminants. Human insulin of recombinant DNA origin is made by inserting insulin genes into the DNA of bacteria (*Escherichia coli*) or yeast, yet no patients who have developed antibodies to yeast or bacterial peptides have been reported.

Local insulin allergic phenomena are encountered in 2–3% of patients treated with human insulins. Systemic allergy has rarely been reported to be associated with human insulins when individuals have only taken that type of insulin. In cases of systemic allergy, a desensitization procedure using human insulin or an insulin analog is often successful. Desensitization is the process of introducing low but increasing doses of an allergen, insulin in this case, to decrease the allergic response to that allergen. Insulin antibody–mediated insulin resistance resulting in insulin requirements of >1.5 units/kg/day (>10 nmol/l per kg/day) in adults or >2.5 units/kg/day (>16.7 nmol/l per kg/day) in children is an extremely rare complication of therapy and has been seen in few individuals begun on human insulin therapy. All three human insulin analogs (insulins lispro, aspart, and glargine) have proven useful in treating insulin allergic reactions.

Table 33.1 Allergic Reactions to Insulin

Type	Description
Local	
Isolated wheal-and-flare reaction	Occurs within 30 min, resolves within 1 h; wheal-and-flare reaction followed by a late-biphasic phase reaction peaking in 4–6 h and persisting for 24 h
Arthus reaction	Develops over 4–6 h, peaks at 12 h
Delayed (tuberculin-like)	Develops nodule or "deep hive" over 8–12 h, peaks in 24 h
Systemic	
Urticaria to anaphylaxis	Immediate reaction

Modified from DeShazo (1987).

PATHOPHYSIOLOGY OF INSULIN ALLERGY

Local and systemic allergy may be associated with anti-insulin IgE (type 1 immediate hypersensitivity reactions) or IgG (type 3 intermediate immune complex–mediated reactions) antibodies. Type 4, delayed hypersensitivity, cell-mediated reactions, have also been reported. Immediate hypersensitivity reactions occur in <1% of patients.

1. Insulin allergy is usually local and occurs within the first 2 weeks of therapy (Table 33.1). About 90% of individuals with local allergy have spontaneous remissions within 2 months while on the same therapy, and an additional 5% will improve within 6–12 months.
2. Isolated wheal-and-flare and biphasic reactions are mediated by reaginic antibodies (IgE). The late phase of a biphasic reaction is characterized by pain and erythema and peaks in 12–24 h. Such reactions may very rarely presage anaphylaxis.
3. Arthus reactions (inflammatory response to the deposition of antigen-antibody complexes) are uncommon and are characterized by localized small-vessel injury and neutrophilic infiltrates.

Table 33.2 Therapy for Persistent Severe Local Allergy to Human Insulin (Present for 14–30 Days)

Rule out improper injection technique (also infection and contaminated alcohol).

↓

Skin test to select least-reactive insulin, 0.02-ml intradermal injections of 1:1 dilution of U-100 human regular insulin, insulin lispro, or insulin aspart diluted in phenol-saline; 700 µg/ml (4.3 mmol/l) zinc sulfate, ~0.1 mg/ml (0.48 mmol/l) histamine phosphate (positive control); and phenol-saline (negative control). Observe for reactions at 20 min, 6 h, and ~24 h. A positive wheal-and-flare reaction is 5 mm > phenol-saline 20 min after injection, surrounded by erythema. Significant induration is >1 cm.

↓

Treat with least-reactive insulin.

↓

If the severe local allergy persists:

↓

Divide dosage and deliver into multiple sites; use soluble insulin delivered by continuous subcutaneous insulin infusion; add dexamethasone to each unit of insulin delivered (1 or 2 mg dexamethasone/1,000-unit vial); systemic antihistamines; two relatively untested approaches have been suggested: cimetidine 300 mg t.i.d. or oral insulin plus aspirin in individuals unresponsive to dermal desensitization.

If reactive to zinc sulfate, consider using low-zinc insulin, such as NPH. If reactive to NPH insulins, avoid protamine. Protamine insulins are typically low in zinc. Modified from DeShazo (1987) and Galloway (1990).

Table 33.3 Therapy for Systemic Insulin Allergy

Is insulin necessary? —No→ Diet and exercise, with or without oral antidiabetic agents

Yes ↓

Skin test for least-reactive insulin: at 20-min intervals, 0.02 ml by intradermal injections of 0.001, 0.01, and 0.1 units (0.007, 0.07, and 0.7 nmol/l, respectively) of human insulin diluted in sterile phenol-saline or neutral insulin-dilution fluid. If wheal-and-flare reaction is 5 mm > phenol-saline control 20 min after injection of any dilution, proceed to insulin lispro or insulin aspart. A positive test results in a wheal-and-flare reaction 5 mm greater than negative control. If initial testing is negative, then proceed to test with 1 unit of insulin and, if negative, proceed to treat the patient with this insulin. If skin testing is positive, proceed to formal desensitization. Use saline and/or insulin-diluting fluid as negative-control solutions. If negative (<5 mm larger than control), test with 1 unit (6.7 nmol/l).

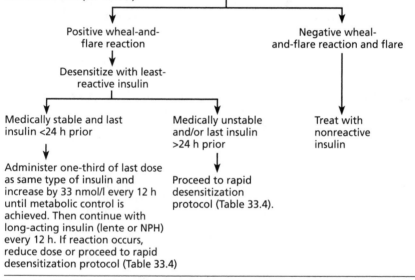

Positive wheal-and-flare reaction ↓
Desensitize with least-reactive insulin

Negative wheal-and-flare reaction and flare

Medically stable and last insulin <24 h prior ↓

Medically unstable and/or last insulin >24 h prior ↓

Treat with nonreactive insulin

Administer one-third of last dose as same type of insulin and increase by 33 nmol/l every 12 h until metabolic control is achieved. Then continue with long-acting insulin (lente or NPH) every 12 h. If reaction occurs, reduce dose or proceed to rapid desensitization protocol (Table 33.4)

Proceed to rapid desensitization protocol (Table 33.4).

Neutral insulin-diluting fluid and empty insulin mixing vials are available from Lilly. Modified from Galloway (1990).

4. Delayed reactions are indurated and often pruritic and painful, with well-defined borders. Histologically, these lesions are associated with perivascular "cuffing" with mononuclear cells.
5. Systemic allergic reactions are seen most commonly in individuals with histories of atopy and/or intermittent insulin therapy. Anti-insulin IgG and IgE levels are not predictive of types of local reactions but are significantly elevated in individuals with systemic insulin allergy.

Table 33.4 Rapid Desensitization Protocol

Prepare serial 1:10 dilutions of least-reactive insulin (after an initial 1:1 dilution of U-100 insulin, then serial 1:10 dilutions of the least-reactive insulin in neutral insulin-diluting fluid of 50, 5, 0.5, 0.05, and 0.005 units/ml).

| | Step (every 20–30 min) | | | | | | | | | | | |
| | Intradermal | | | | | | | | | Subcutaneous | | |
	1	2	3	4	5	6	7	8	9	10	11	12
Volume (ml)	0.02	0.04	0.08	0.02	0.04	0.08	0.02	0.04	0.08	0.02	0.04	0.08
Units/ml	0.05	0.05	0.05	0.5	0.5	0.5	5	5	5	50	50	50
Units	0.001	0.002	0.004	0.004	0.02	0.04	0.1	0.2	0.4	1	2	4

Instructions
1. Precede with skin testing as described in Table 31.3.
2. Carry out in the hospital under medical supervision. If reactions have been severe, carry out procedure in intensive care unit.
3. Avoid concomitant use of antihistamines or steroids. Have a syringe filled with 1 ml of 1:1,000 epinephrine, life-support equipment, and an allergy consultant available.
4. If patient reacts to initial dosage, begin with 0.005 units/ml.
5. If patient has more than a wheal-and-flare reaction or induration >1 cm, reduce by two dilution steps and then proceed again.
6. After step 12, double dose subcutaneously every 4 h until metabolic stability is established. Then, long-acting insulin may be administered (lente or NPH as described in Table 31.3).

Insulin: 1 pmol/l = 0.139 mU/ml.

THERAPY FOR INSULIN ALLERGY

1. In individuals with severe persistent local allergy and individuals with systemic allergy, further therapy is indicated and is summarized in Tables 33.2–33.4.
2. Therapy of systemic allergy is based on intradermal testing to ascertain the least-reactive insulin (i.e., insulin evoking the least hypersensitivity in the patient), desensitization, and, less frequently, the use of glucocorticoids and/or antihistamines.
3. With systemic or severe insulin allergy, insulin therapy must be continued to avoid future anamnestic reactions. Both human and insulin analogs have been used successfully for desensitization. More than 94% of individuals with systemic allergy can be desensitized as described above. Glucocorti-

Table 33.5 Identification and Treatment of Antibody-Mediated Insulin Resistance

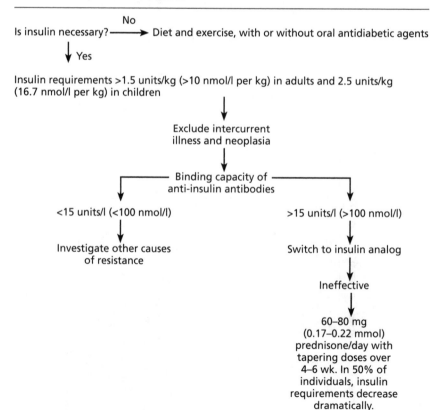

coids and/or antihistamines may rarely be required to modify persisting insulin allergic symptoms.

ANTI-INSULIN ANTIBODY–MEDIATED INSULIN RESISTANCE

1. Individuals with this complication of therapy commonly have histories of intermittent insulin therapy or atopy. Historically, therapy with beef-containing insulin often preceded the antibody-mediated insulin resistance. However, patients treated only with human insulin are now being reported.
2. Because many patients with high levels of insulin antibodies have been shown not to have insulin resistance, one must exclude other causes of insulin resistance, including intercurrent illness, neoplasia, and factitious resistance (e.g., resistance absent when insulin is administered by an MD or RN).
3. Insulin antibody–mediated insulin resistance may be an early manifestation of the insulin autoimmune syndrome or the manifestation of a lymphoma. Identification and treatment of such insulin resistance is described in Table 33.5.
4. The use of a human insulin analog may be advantageous. The use of U-500 regular human insulin may also be of benefit, in lieu of a course of steroid therapy, or if such therapy fails to decrease insulin volume requirements. U-500 insulin, because of its concentration, promotes insulin self-association and acts as a repository insulin.
5. In general, immunological resistance spontaneously remits in <1 year, but durations of up to 5 years have been reported.
6. Approximately 50% of patients will benefit from a course of high-dose glucocorticoid (initially 40–80 mg prednisone daily) that is tapered over 2–4 weeks. Hospitalization is recommended because dramatic decreases in insulin dosage requirements are often seen within days after the institution of such therapy.

BIBLIOGRAPHY

Castera V, Dutour-Meyer A, Koeppel M, Petitjean C, Darmon P: Systemic allergy to human insulin and its rapid and long acting analogs: successful treatment by continuous subcutaneous insulin lispro infusion. *Diabetes Metab* 31:391–400, 2005

Davidson JK, DeBra DW: Immunologic insulin resistance. *Diabetes* 27:307–318, 1978

DeShazo RD, Mather P, Grant W, Carrington D, Frentz JM, Lueg M, et al.: Evaluation of patients with local reactions to insulin with skin tests and in vitro techniques. *Diabetes Care* 10:330–336, 1987

Fineberg SE, Kawabata TT, Finco-Kent D, Fountaine RJ, Finch GL, Krasner AS: Immunologic responses to exogenous insulin. *Endocrine Rev* 28:625–652, 2007

Galloway J, DeShazo R: Insulin chemistry and pharmacology: insulin allergy, resistance, and lipodystrophy. In *Ellenberg and Rifkin's Diabetes Mellitus: Theory and Practice*. 4th ed. Rifkin H, Porte D, Eds. New York, Elsevier, 1990, p. 504–508

Lassmann-Vague V, Belicar P, Alessis C, Raccah D, Vialettes B, Vague P: Insulin kinetics in type I diabetic patients treated by continuous intraperitoneal insulin infusion: influence of anti-insulin antibodies. *Diabet Med* 13:1051–1055, 1996

Lahtela JT, Knip M, Paul R, Antonen J, Salmi J: Severe antibody-mediated human insulin resistance: successful treatment with the insulin analog lispro. *Diabetes Care* 20:71–73, 1997

Lindholm A, Jensen LB, Home P, Raskin P, Boehn BO, Rastam J: Immune responses to insulin aspart and biphasic insulin aspart in people with type 1 and type 2 diabetes. *Diabetes Care* 25:876–882, 2002

Moriyama H, Nagata M, Fujihira K, Yamada K, Chowdhury SA, Chakrabarty S, et al.: Treatment with human analog (GlyA21, ArgB31, ArgB32) insulin glargine (HOE901) resolves a generalized allergy to human insulin in type 1 diabetes. *Diabetes Care* 24:411–412, 2001

Ottesen JL, Nilsson P, Jami J, Weilguny D, Duhrkop M, Bucchini D, et al.: The potential immunogenicity of human insulin and insulin analogues evaluated in a transgenic mouse model. *Diabetologia* 37:1178–1185, 1994

Peters A, Klose O, Hefty R, Keck F, Kerner W: The influence of insulin antibodies on the pharmacokinetics of NPH insulin in patients with type 1 diabetes treated with human insulin. *Diabet Med* 12:925–930, 1995

Van Haeften TW, Gerich JE: Complications of insulin therapy. In *Principles and Practices of Endocrinology and Metabolism*. Becker KL, Ed. Philadelphia, PA, J.B. Lippincott, 1990, p. 1112–1118

Weiler JM, Gellhaus MA, Carter JG, Meng RL, Benson PM, Hottel RA, et al.: A prospective study of the risk of an immediate adverse reaction to protamine sulfate during cardiopulmonary bypass surgery. *J Allergy Clin Immunol* 85:713–719, 1990

Dr. Fineberg is Emeritus Professor of Medicine at the Indiana University School of Medicine, Indianapolis, Indiana, and Clinical Professor of Medicine at the University of Alabama at Birmingham School of Medicine, Birmingham, Alabama. Dr. Holcombe is a Medical Fellow at Eli Lilly and Company, Indianapolis, Indiana.

34. Drugs and Hormones That Increase Blood Glucose Levels

HIMANI CHANDRA, MD, AND DEREK LEROITH, MD, PHD

In an era characterized by rapid medical advancement and powerful pharmaceutical companies, it is important to realize that the majority of the world's population regularly ingests one or more substances for either symptomatic relief or disease remedy. These substances, whether prescription, over-the-counter, hormonal, or herbal, often have untoward side effects, such as hyperglycemia, that must be acknowledged, identified, and treated to prevent subsequent morbidity and mortality.

MEDICATIONS

Many prescription and nonprescription medications have been associated with hyperglycemia (Table 34.1). The following paragraphs will highlight some of these drugs and briefly discuss the molecular mechanisms by which they have been shown to elevate blood glucose levels.

Antihypertensive Agents

At high doses, thiazide diuretics are associated with an increased risk of diabetes. The main mechanism of action is thought to be through their resultant depletion of total body potassium stores. This hypokalemia results in a net decrease in pancreatic β-cell insulin secretion and ensuing hyperglycemia. In fact, several studies have shown that thiazide-induced hyperglycemia is often reversed by potassium replacement or drug discontinuation. Similarly, loop diuretics, such as furosemide, can cause glucose intolerance (but less commonly so than thiazides for reasons that remain unclear), whereas potassium-sparing diuretics, such as spirinolactone, have virtually no effect on glucose metabolism.

β-Adrenergic stimulation promotes insulin secretion from the pancreatic β-cell in response to glucagon or glucose; therefore, blockade of this signal may result in insulinopenia and hyperglycemia. This effect is seen more commonly with the nonselective β-blocker propranolol, but hyperglycemia has also been observed in patients treated with metoprolol and atenolol. Interestingly, the mixed α- and β-adrenergic antagonist, carvedilol, actually improves insulin sensitivity through its anti–β-adrenergic effects.

Calcium channel blockers cause decreased insulin secretion from the β-cell. Several case reports link these medications to the induction of hyperglycemia. Inda-

Table 34.1 Medications Associated with Development of Hyperglycemia

Antihypertensive agents

Diuretics
Acetazolamide
Chlorthalidone
Ethacrynic acid
Furosemide
Indapamide
Thiazide
Triamterene

β-Adrenergic blockers
Atenolol
Metoprolol
Propranolol
Calcium channel blockers
Diltiazem
Nicardipine
Nifedipine
Verapamil
α-**Adrenergic agonists**
Clonidine
Methyldopa

Others
Alcohol
Alloxan
Amiodarone
Calcitonin
Cimetidine
Droperidol
Levodopa
Lithium
Mannitol/sorbitol
Morphine
Minoxidil
Nicotinic acid
Octreotide
Oral contraceptives
Phenytoin/diphenylhydantoin (pesticide)
Quinine
Theophylline
TPN

Psychiatric medications
Chlorpromazine
Clozapine
Haloperidol
Mianserin
Olanzapine
Quetiapine
Risperidone
Tricyclic antidepressants

Antibiotics
Gatifloxacin
Isoniazid, rifampicin
Pentamidine, dapsone
Streptozocin

Immunomodulatory agents
Asparaginase
Cyclophosphamide
Cyclosporine
Cytokines (TNF-α, IL-1 and -6)
Mycophenolate mofetil

Nucleoside analogs
Protease inhibitors
Tacrolimus

Anti-inflammatory agents
Glucocorticoids
Glucosamine sulfate
Indomethacin
Megestrol

Neuromodulatory agents
Amphetamines
β-Adrenergic agonists
α-Adrenergic agonists
Caffeine
Catecholamines, dopamine
Endosulfan
Nicotine
Organophosphates
Vacor (rodenticide)

pamide, acetazolamide, and minoxidil have all been associated with hyperglycemia in a few patients. The central β-adrenergic agonist clonidine has been shown to cause hyperglycemia in animals, but there have been no known human cases.

In general, hyperglycemia may be more commonly seen in hypertensive patients because of an increased prevalence of the metabolic syndrome in this population. Clinical judgment should therefore be exercised in evaluating patients with hyperglycemia who are also on antihypertensive medication, so that a more serious disease process is not overlooked.

ANTI-INFLAMMATORY AGENTS

Glucocorticoids (GCs) cause hyperglycemia by increasing hepatic glucose output, by increasing the synthesis and release of catecholamines, and by creating insulin resistance. Their effects are dose related, and a rise in blood glucose levels is seen within 24 h of dose administration. Even topical GCs can result in hyperglycemia, especially the more potent preparations applied over prolonged periods of time, large surface areas, or in conjunction with occlusive dressings. The hyperglycemia that GCs cause may be reversible in normal patients or may progress to frank diabetes in those patients who have underlying glucose intolerance. Glucosamine therapy for arthritis and indomethacin therapy for psoriatic arthritis have also both been observationally associated with hyperglycemia.

Sympathomimetic and Neuromodulatory Agents

One of the functions of the sympathetic nervous system is to protect against hypoglycemia. Drugs that mimic this sympathetic response result in hyperglycemia via increased glycogenolysis and gluconeogenesis. These drugs also cause decreased tissue insulin sensitivity and inhibit insulin secretion. A concomitant increase in growth hormone (GH) after the use of a sympathomimetic agent further contributes to insulin resistance. These effects are seen after treatment with β-adrenergic agonists such as catecholamines, caffeine, and nicotine.

β-Adrenergic stimulation can also result in hyperglycemia by impairing insulin secretion and increasing both glycogenolysis and lipolysis. Agents such as terbutaline, used in the treatment of premature labor, are associated with an increased risk of gestational diabetes, especially when combined with corticosteroid therapy. Hyperglycemia has not been associated with inhaled β-adrenergic agonists.

The rodenticide vacor acts as a nicotinamide antagonist and causes severe, potentially irreversible β-cell toxicity that can result in diabetes and ketoacidosis. Organophosphate insecticides that cause anticholinesterase poisoning result in hyperglycemia in some cases, although hypoglycemia has also been observed. Endosulfan, a chlorinated hydrocarbon insecticide similar to DDT, acts as a central nervous system stimulant and can lead to hyperglycemia after acute ingestion.

Antipsychotics

The second-generation or atypical antipsychotics, most notably olanzapine and clozapine, can increase the risk of impaired glucose tolerance and type 2 diabetes by up to fourfold. They all cause varying degrees of weight gain and subsequent insulin resistance, but studies have shown that the changes in glucose metabolism that occur from this class of drugs are often independent of adiposity. Atypical antipsychotics also cause insulin resistance by increasing counterregulatory hormones, stimulating free fatty acid release from adipose tissue, and interfering with the insulin action cascade. In addition, they directly inhibit the pancreatic β-cell via the 5-HT_{1A} (5-hydroxytryptamine [serotonin] 1A) receptor, leading to a net decrease in insulin secretion.

The older, more typical antipsychotics, such as haloperidol and chlorpromazine, have been observed to cause elevations in blood glucose levels in humans, whereas tricyclic antidepressants have been shown to do so only in mice and rabbit models. Although selective serotonin reuptake inhibitors, through an increase in serotonergic activity and subsequent increase in insulin secretion, are often beneficial in people with diabetes, there have been isolated case reports of sertraline-, fluvoxamine-, and paroxetine-induced hyperglycemia.

Antibiotics

Infection creates an insulin-resistant state, so there is an expected incidence of concurrent hyperglycemia. Most antibiotics do not raise blood glucose levels on their own. One exception, however, is gatifloxacin, a broad-spectrum fluoroquinolone that has been closely linked to hyperglycemia and diabetes in multiple studies. As a result, it was removed from the U.S. market in 2006 and is now only available as an ophthalmic solution. Pentamidine is β-cell toxic and causes direct injury to the pancreas in a dose- and time-dependent manner. Streptozocin is also β-cell toxic and has been used extensively to produce experimental mice models of type 1 diabetes.

Immunomodulatory Agents

A reversible hyperglycemia, with decreased insulin and elevated glucagon levels, has been seen with asparaginase treatment. Cyclosporine, mycophenolate mofetil, and tacrolimus therapy in transplant patients has been associated with the development of diabetes. The effects of these drugs are usually dose dependent, and they act by directly inhibiting islet cell function and/or contributing to insulin resistance. These immunosuppressants are often used in conjunction with steroids, which adds to the risk of hyperglycemia.

Circulating levels of tumor necrosis factor (TNF)-α and interleukins (IL)-1 and -6 have been shown to be elevated in cases of impaired glucose tolerance. Similarly, infusions of these molecules have been observed to cause an increase in plasma catecholamines, and subcutaneous injections of IL-6 are associated with an increase in glucagon in normal subjects. Cases of hyperglycemia have not yet been documented but are thus a theoretical and plausible result of cytokine therapy. As more and more patients are treated with these immunomodulatory agents, it is only a matter of time before frank hyperglycemia will present itself.

Antiretrovirals, most notably the protease inhibitors, are notorious inducers of hyperglycemia. In addition to conferring insulin resistance via the development of hypertriglyceridemia and centripetal obesity, they also inhibit cytoplasmic retinoid acid–binding protein type 1 (CRABP-1). Inhibition of CRABP-1 results in increased apoptosis of peripheral adipocytes, leading to elevated serum levels of free fatty acids and, hence, further insulin resistance. The nucleoside analogs didanosine and stavudine are also linked to hyperglycemia via two mechanisms: direct injury to β-cells and suppression of insulin release by associated hypokalemia.

Others

Multiple studies have demonstrated a U-shaped relationship between alcohol consumption and risk for diabetes, with moderate alcohol ingestion (one to three drinks per day) resulting in a reduced incidence, and heavy ingestion, as defined by more than three drinks per day, resulting in up to 43% higher incidence of diabetes. The hyperglycemia induced by alcohol is usually seen in the setting of chronic ingestion. It may be caused by an increased insulin resistance that occurs at the cellular level, leading to decreased insulin-mediated glucose disposal in muscle and a dysregulation of hepatic glucose metabolism in the liver, as seen in patients with alcoholic steatohepatitis. In addition, chronic alcohol use often leads to deterioration in self-care behavior, and the ensuing poor medication, dietary, and exercise compliance worsens the hyperglycemia.

Nicotinic acid used in the treatment of hypertriglyceridemia may contribute to an insulin-resistant state, especially in people with existing diabetes, by increasing gluconeogenesis and reducing the body's capacity to respond to hyperglycemic stimuli. Cimetidine, diphenylhydantoin, and phenytoin all result in hyperglycemia by decreasing insulin secretion, and this hyperglycemia is often reversible upon discontinuation of the culprit medication. Quinine acts as a glycogenolytic agent, whereas morphine increases glucagon secretion. Alloxan kills pancreatic β-cells and is used to induce diabetes in laboratory animals. Elevated blood glucose levels can occur in certain cases of drug overdose, such as acute intoxication with aspirin, acetaminophen, theophylline, and isoniazid.

Total parenteral nutrition (TPN) and hyperglycemia frequently occur simultaneously. Most patients receiving TPN in the hospital setting are critically ill and are therefore in a stressed state marked by an excess of catecholamines and cytokines. This milieu of insulin resistance prevents the adequate clearance of the TPN's glucose load, and, consequently, hyperglycemia ensues.

HORMONES

Because blood glucose levels are hormonally mediated, treatment with exogenous hormones, along with certain disease states of endogenous hormonal excess, are both associated with hyperglycemia (Table 34.2).

GH

GH, when acutely administered, causes an increase in insulin-like effects, but this effect only lasts a short time. Chronic administration or pathological states of GH excess, like acromegaly, are characterized by insulin resistance with elevated hepatic glucose output and increased lipid breakdown. This enhanced lipolysis results in the release of free fatty acids, which in turn inhibit insulin action at the target tissues, e.g. liver and muscle.

Glucagon

Glucagon promotes both hepatic gluconeogenesis and glycogenolysis, thereby contributing to hyperglycemia. In addition, this hormone enhances the release of epinephrine, which serves to inhibit pancreatic insulin secretion. Hyperglucagonemia may be caused by a glucagon-secreting tumor, but it is more commonly seen in conditions of ketoacidosis, hyperosmolar syndrome, renal failure, and acute pancreatitis. The most common clinical situation of elevated glucagon levels is after the administration of intramuscular or intravenous glucagon as a treatment

Table 34.2 Hormones Associated with the Development of Hyperglycemia

Hormone	Associated Condition
Growth hormone	Acromegaly
Glucagon	Glucagonoma
Thyroid hormone	Thyrotoxicosis
Cortisol	Cushing's syndrome
Catecholamines	Pheochromocytoma, acute stress response
Somatostatin	Somatostatinoma
Human somatomammotropin	Pregnancy
Testosterone	Androgen excess, polycystic ovarian syndrome
Estrogen/progesterone	Pregnancy, oral contraceptives, hormone replacement medicines

for profound hypoglycemia. In this setting, the glucagon injection temporarily raises the blood glucose level, but blood glucose will rapidly fall again unless the underlying etiology of the hypoglycemia is treated.

Thyroid Hormone

Thyroid hormone, when in excess, augments glucose-6-phosphatase activity and thus causes increased hepatic glucose production. Hyperthyroidism also results in a depletion of pancreatic insulin reserves, thereby decreasing the insulin secretory capacity of β-cells. Thyrotoxicosis is a hypermetabolic stressed state that affects glucose metabolism in a fashion similar to catecholamine excess. Hyperglycemia does not occur in conjunction with exogenous administration of thyroid hormone as long as serum levels are maintained within a normal physiological range.

Cortisol

Excess GCs, such as cortisol and exogenous steroids, promote hyperglycemia and impaired glucose tolerance. In addition to causing the release of amino acids and free fatty acids, they upregulate phosphoenolpyruvate carboxykinase, the key enzyme in gluconeogenesis. GCs also serve to decrease both the β-cell secretion of insulin and the subsequent cellular uptake of glucose. GC-induced hyperglycemia is common and has been well documented because these hormones are widely used in the treatment of inflammatory conditions.

Catecholamines

Norepinephrine and epinephrine, through β- and α-adrenergic stimulation, antagonize the actions of insulin and augment the release of glucagon. Consequently, this process results in an increase in blood glucose by the stimulation of gluconeogenesis, glycogenolysis, and lipolysis. Whereas glucagon secretion is mediated through both α- and β-adrenergic stimulation, insulin secretion from the pancreatic β-cell is promoted solely by α-adrenergic stimulation. In states of catecholamine excess, however, the α-adrenergic system often exerts the dominant action, thus resulting in an inhibition of insulin release.

Somatostatin

Somatostatin inhibits the secretion of neuropeptides such as insulin and glucagon. Hyperglycemia and diabetes may occur in patients with somatostatin-producing tumors, yet pharmacological use of somatostatin analogs for the treatment of neuroendocrine tumors has not been associated with diabetes. These synthetic compounds, however, can result in impaired glucose tolerance, most notably postprandial hyperglycemia. The difference in effect on carbohydrate metabolism between endogenous and synthetic somatostatin may be due to variable stimulation of the somatostatin receptor subtypes.

Human Somatomammotropin (Human Placental Lactogen)

Human somatomammotropin, a hormone that increases throughout the first 3 months of pregnancy and then plateaus at an elevated level, antagonizes the action of insulin and promotes free fatty acid release, thereby stimulating gluconeogenesis. Excess of this hormone serves to create an abundance of nutrients available to the developing fetus and may contribute to the development of gestational diabetes in predisposed mothers.

Testosterone/Estrogen/Progesterone

Elevated androgens, whether administered exogenously in male patients or occurring in conjunction with polycystic ovarian syndrome in female patients, have been associated with insulin resistance and hyperglycemia. Both estrogen and progesterone decrease peripheral tissue insulin sensitivity. Estrogen acts mainly by increasing GH and cortisol levels, and progesterone decreases both the number and affinity of insulin receptors on cell surface membranes. Higher-dose formulations of oral contraceptives were shown to cause hyperglycemia, but this relationship has not been supported by studies using modern low-dose or triphasic preparations.

TREATMENT OF DRUG-INDUCED HYPERGLYCEMIA

When a medication or hormonal substance is suspected of causing hyperglycemia, the agent should be discontinued if possible, and the patient should be reevaluated. In many cases, this cessation of the culprit agent will return the patient to a euglycemic state. On the other hand, if the hyperglycemia-inducing medication cannot be stopped, an additional antihyperglycemic agent should be initiated to optimize blood glucose levels.

Before starting therapy with either a drug or hormone that may elevate blood glucose, patients should be carefully evaluated for their risk of developing hyperglycemia. The coexistence of or family history of obesity, hypertension, diabetes, and dyslipidemia confers a greater risk for the development of drug-induced hyperglycemia. In high-risk patients, a fasting blood glucose and/or oral glucose tolerance test is helpful to establish the diagnosis of either pre-diabetes or frank diabetes before initiating drug therapy. Throughout the course of the drug treatment, physicians should monitor patients closely for the development of hyperglycemia by asking about the presence of any hyperglycemic symptoms (e.g., polyuria or polydipsia) and by obtaining periodic laboratory data. Patients with preexisting diabetes, as well as those at high risk for developing hyperglycemia, should periodically monitor their own fingerstick glucose levels with home glucose meters and then be treated accordingly by their physicians.

Traditionally, short-term treatment of drug or hormone-induced hyperglycemia has been achieved by using insulin therapy. In type 1 diabetic patients, the patient's existing insulin regimen may be increased or adjusted to treat an exacerbated hyperglycemia. In type 2 diabetic patients, however, as well as in patients who develop new hyperglycemia, the choice of agent to use to treat the hyperglycemia is less apparent. A trial of diet and exercise may improve insulin sensitivity, yet this intervention may not be adequate alone. Because of its rapid action and effect, insulin may be the drug of choice for even a type 2 diabetic or newly diagnosed diabetic patient who only requires short-term therapy with the hyperglycemia-inducing medication.

Insulin's mode of administration often makes its initiation quite cumbersome, so oral antihyperglycemic agents may indeed be more effective in some patients. Given their risk of hypoglycemia and drug-drug interactions, sulfonylureas should be used with caution. Shorter-acting insulin secretagogues, such as repaglinide and nateglinide, are often better agents to use, especially when dealing with postprandial hyperglycemia. In contrast, patients who are characterized mainly by insulin resistance rather than deficiency may not respond to therapy that causes an increase in circulating insulin levels. In such cases, insulin sensitizers, such as metformin or thiazolidinediones, may be more appropriate; however, the effects of thiazolidinediones can take 1–2 months to appear, so they are not the best "acute" therapy. One must bear in mind that there have been only a handful of clinical trials studying the safety and efficacy of oral agents in the setting of drug-induced hyperglycemia.

CONCLUSION

In summary, there are a number of pharmaceutical agents and hormones that have been demonstrated to cause hyperglycemia in humans. Patients being treated with such agents should be vigilantly monitored for any signs or symptoms of elevated blood glucose levels. If hyperglycemia does develop, appropriate therapy should be initiated in a timely manner, and its efficacy should be ascertained. Long-term, poorly controlled hyperglycemia is associated with the development of diabetic micro- and macrovascular complications. Because some patients may require treatment with these hyperglycemia-inducing agents for several years, an aggressive approach toward elevated blood glucose levels is both indicated and warranted; only then can further morbidity and mortality be adequately prevented.

BIBLIOGRAPHY

Becker KL, Bilezikian JP, Bremner WJ, Hung W, Kahn CR, Loriaux DL, NylTn ES, Rebar RW, Robertson GL, Snider RH Jr, Wartofsky L: *Principles and Practice of Endocrinology and Metabolism*. 3rd ed. Philadelphia, PA, Lippincott, 2001

Chan NN, Osaki R, Chow CC, Chan JC, Cockram CS: Drug-related hyperglycemia. *JAMA* 287:714–715, 2002

Haupt DW: Differential metabolic effects of antipsychotic treatments. *Eur Neuropsychopharmacol* 16:S149–S155, 2006

Howard AA, Arnsten JH, Gourevitch MN: Effect of alcohol consumption on diabetes mellitus: a systematic review. *Ann Intern Med* 140:211–219, 2004

Knowler WC, Barrett-Connor E, Fowler SE, Hamman RF, Lachin JM, Walker EA, Nathan DM, Diabetes Prevention Program Research Group: Reduction in the incidence of type 2 diabetes with lifestyle intervention or metformin. *N Engl J Med* 346:393–403, 2002

LeRoith D, Taylor SI, Olefsky JM: *Diabetes Mellitus: A Fundamental and Clinical Text*. 2nd ed. Philadelphia, PA, Lippincott, 2000

Luna B, Feinglos MN: Drug-induced hyperglycemia. *JAMA* 286:1945–1948, 2001

Padwal R, Laupacis A: Antihypertensive therapy and incidence of type 2 diabetes: a systematic review. *Diabetes Care* 27:247–255, 2004

Pandit MK, Burke J, Gustafson AB, Minocha A, Peiris AN: Drug-induced disorders of glucose intolerance. *Ann Intern Med* 118:529–539, 1993

Yip C, Lee AJ: Gatifloxacin-induced hyperglycemia: a case report and summary of the current literature. *Clinic Therapeut* 28:1857–1866, 2006

Zillich AJ, Garg J, Basu S, Bakris GL, Carter BL: Thiazide diuretics, potassium, and the development of diabetes: a quantitative review. *Hypertension* 48:219–224, 2006

Thomson Micromedex website. Available from http://www.micromedex.com. Accessed 4 March 2009

Dr. Chandra is Staff Physician and Instructor of Medicine in the James J. Peters VA Medical Center, Division of Endocrinology, Bronx, New York. Dr. LeRoith is Director of the Metabolism Institute, Chief of the Division of Endocrinology, Diabetes, & Bone Diseases, Mt. Sinai School of Medicine, New York, New York.

35. Diabetic Dyslipidemia

SALILA KURRA, MD, AND HENRY N. GINSBERG, MD

Numerous prospective cohort studies have indicated that diabetes is associated with a three- to fourfold increase in risk for coronary heart disease (CHD). The increase in risk is particularly evident in younger age-groups and in women: female patients with type 2 diabetes appear to lose a great deal of the protection that characterizes nondiabetic women. Furthermore, patients with diabetes have 50% greater in-hospital mortality and a twofold increased rate of death within 2 years of surviving a myocardial infarction. Overall, CHD is the leading cause of death in individuals with diabetes who are over the age of 35 years.

Although a significant portion of this increased risk is associated with the presence of well-characterized risk factors for CHD, a significant proportion remains unexplained. Patients with diabetes, particularly those with type 2 diabetes, have abnormalities of plasma lipids and lipoprotein concentrations that are less commonly present in nondiabetic individuals. Patients with poorly controlled type 1 diabetes can also have a dyslipidemic pattern, although this is much less common and probably occurs on a background of insulin resistance or the metabolic syndrome.

In recent years, several large clinical trials have shown that reducing levels of LDL cholesterol and plasma triglycerides and/or raising levels of HDL cholesterol is associated with reduced rates of CHD events. There is now strong evidence that health care professionals caring for patients with diabetes should treat lipid abnormalities aggressively. This review will provide a brief pathophysiological basis for the dyslipidemia commonly present in patients with diabetes and then review treatment approaches. Because of the much greater prevalence of lipid abnormalities in type 2 diabetes, most of the emphasis in this review will focus on that group of patients.

LIPOPROTEIN METABOLISM IN DIABETES

Lipoproteins are spherical, macromolecular complexes carrying various lipids and proteins in plasma. The hydrophobic triglyceride and cholesteryl ester molecules comprise the core of the lipoproteins, and this core is covered by amphipathic (both hydrophobic and hydrophilic) phospholipids and proteins. Hundreds to thousands of triglyceride and cholesteryl ester molecules are carried in the core of different lipoproteins. Apolipoproteins are the proteins on the surface of the lipoproteins. They not only help to solubilize the core lipids but also play a critical role in the regulation of plasma lipid and lipoprotein transport. Apolipoprotein (apo) B100 is required for the secretion of hepatic-derived VLDLs, intermediate-density lipoproteins (IDLs), and LDLs. ApoB48 is a truncated form of apoB100 that is required for secretion of chylomicrons from the small intestine. ApoA-I is the major structural protein in HDLs. Other apolipoproteins will be discussed in the context of their roles in lipoprotein metabolism.

ABNORMAL CHYLOMICRON METABOLISM IN DIABETES

After ingestion of a meal, dietary fat (triglyceride) and cholesterol are absorbed into the cells of the small intestine and are incorporated into the core of nascent chylomicrons, which traverse the lymphatic system and enter the circulation via the superior vena cava. In the capillary beds of adipose tissue and muscle, chylomicrons interact with the enzyme lipoprotein lipase (LpL), the chylomicron core triglyceride is hydrolyzed, and the generated free fatty acids are taken up by fat cells and made back into triglyceride or by muscle cells, where they can be used for energy. Chylomicron remnants, products of this lipolytic process that have lost >75% of their triglyceride, interact with several receptor pathways on hepatocytes and are removed rapidly from the circulation by the liver. Hepatic triglyceride lipase (HL), which hydrolyzes chylomicron remnant triglycerides, also plays a role in remnant removal. Defective metabolism of chylomicrons and chylomicron remnants has been observed commonly in type 2 diabetes, where LpL may be modestly reduced. Recent studies in animal models and in humans suggest that chylomicron formation in intestinal cells may also be increased in insulin-resistant states such as type 2 diabetes. Patients with well-controlled type 1 diabetes usually have normal fasting and postprandial triglyceride levels. The role of HL in the defective chylomicron metabolism in diabetes is unclear. In uncontrolled type 1 diabetes, however, LpL can be significantly reduced, and marked postprandial lipemia has been observed. In most of those cases, however, a partial genetic defect in LpL production or function probably plays a key role along with insulin deficiency.

ABNORMAL VLDL METABOLISM IN DIABETES

VLDLs are assembled in the liver. The core of the VLDL comprises triglycerides and cholesteryl esters. ApoB100 and phospholipids form its surface. Recent studies indicate that an increased flow of fatty acids to the liver from adipose tissue (Fig. 35.1), along with the possibility for increased insulin-mediated fatty acid synthesis in the liver, can drive the increased assembly and secretion of VLDL that is central to the dyslipidemia present in patients with type 2 diabetes (Fig. 35.2). Hepatic insulin resistance can affect insulin's normal role to target apoB for degradation prior to secretion; thus, hepatic insulin resistance can play a role in increased secretion of apoB and VLDL from the liver. Abnormalities of cholesterol metabolism, with excess hepatic cholesterol, may also contribute to the overproduction of VLDL. Such abnormalities have not been well defined in patients with diabetes.

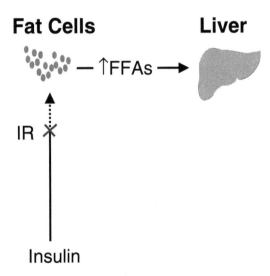

Figure 35.1 Insulin resistance (IR) at the level of the fat cells leads to increased release of free fatty acids (FFAs) into the circulation. The fatty acids are mainly cleared from the circulation by the liver.

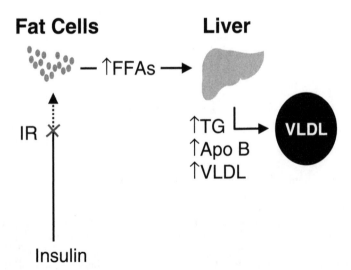

Figure 35.2 Increased fatty acids entering the liver will stimulate triglyceride (TG) synthesis, and this will stimulate the assembly and secretion of increased numbers of VLDL particles. FFA, free fatty acid; IR, insulin resistance.

Once in the plasma, VLDL triglyceride is hydrolyzed by LpL, generating smaller and more dense VLDL and then IDL. IDLs are similar to chylomicron remnants, except that IDLs, in addition to removal by the liver, can undergo further plasma catabolism to become LDLs. Some LpL activity appears necessary for normal functioning of the metabolic cascade from VLDL to IDL to LDL. It also appears that HL, apoE (another surface apolipoprotein), and LDL receptors also play important roles in this process. ApoB100, the sole protein on the surface of LDL, is a ligand for the LDL receptor, and the concentration of LDL in plasma is determined by both the production of LDL and the availability of LDL receptors.

Plasma levels of VLDL triglyceride are commonly elevated in patients with type 2 diabetes. In population studies, levels of triglyceride >90th percentile for nondiabetic individuals are two to three times more common in individuals with diabetes. Overproduction of VLDL, with increased secretion of both triglyceride and apoB100, seems to be the common etiology of the increased plasma VLDL levels. Individuals with type 1 diabetes who have good glycemic control usually have average or better-than-average plasma triglyceride levels. This may be due in part to the ability of insulin to inhibit apoB100 secretion from the liver. As noted above, decreased LpL-mediated hydrolysis of VLDL triglycerides may contribute significantly to elevated triglyceride levels, particularly in patients with either type 1 or type 2 diabetes who have poor glycemic control. Obesity and insulin resistance are important contributors to the hypertriglyceridemia of type 2 diabetes. Regulation of plasma levels of LDL cholesterol in type 2 diabetes is complex. In the presence of hypertriglyceridemia, small, dense, cholesterol-depleted, triglyceride-enriched LDLs are present (Fig. 35.3). This means that there will be more LDL particles for any LDL cholesterol level compared with people without diabetes who have LDLs of normal size and composition (it is important to remember that lipoprotein particles enter the artery wall). Removal of LDL, mainly via LDL receptor pathways, can be increased, normal, or reduced in type 2 diabetes. Glycosylated and/or oxidatively modified lipoproteins, which can be present in increased amounts in the blood of patients with either type 1 or type 2 diabetes, interact less efficiently with the LDL receptor and have the potential to increase plasma LDL levels. On the other hand, modified LDLs can be removed from plasma by alternative metabolic pathways, including retention in the arterial wall. Insulin also plays a role in stimulating the expression of the gene for LDL receptors. Severe insulin deficiency in poorly controlled type 1 or type 2 diabetes may be associated with reduced LDL receptor function and increased LDL cholesterol levels.

ABNORMAL HDL METABOLISM IN DIABETES

HDL may be the most complex of all the lipoprotein classes. The majority of HDLs are formed by the coalescence of individual apolipoproteins, including apoA-I, apoA-II, and apoA-VI, with phospholipids. The resulting nascent disc-like HDLs, also called pre-β HDLs, function as acceptors of cellular-free cholesterol and are the initial HDL particles involved in reverse cholesterol transport (the movement of cholesterol from peripheral tissues to the liver for excretion from the body). The movement of cellular free cholesterol to apoA-I is mediated via a recently discovered protein, ATP-binding cassette transporter A1. Conver-

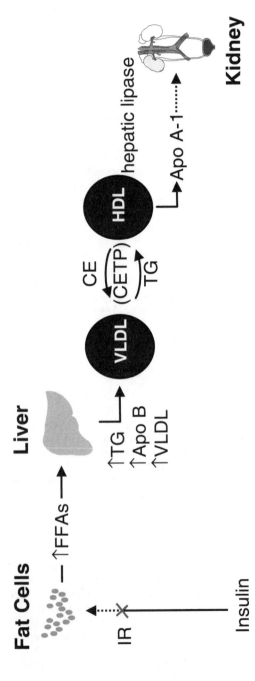

Figure 35.3 Increased VLDL in the circulation, in the presence of CETP, will stimulate increased exchange of HDL cholesterol for VLDL triglycerides (TG). This will deplete HDL of cholesterol. Additionally, hepatic lipase in the capillary bed of the liver will hydrolyze the TG in HDL, the HDL will become smaller, and apoA-I will dissociate. Free apoA-I will be cleared much faster than normal from the circulation, leading to fewer HDLs in the blood. FFAS, free fatty acids; IR, insulin resistance.

sion of cholesterol to cholesteryl ester, by the addition of a fatty acid in a reaction catalyzed by the plasma enzyme, LCAT (lecithin cholesterol acyl transferase), produces HDL_3. HDL_3 can accept more cellular free cholesterol via a second recently characterized protein, ABCG1 (ATP-binding cassette, sub-family G1). The latter process allows HDL_3 to continue to accumulate cholesteryl ester and become HDL_2, which can deliver cholesteryl ester to the liver via a process called selective uptake. The selective uptake of cholesteryl esters from HDL to several organs, including the liver (without entry of the entire HDL particle), was demonstrated to be the result of the HDL interaction with a receptor called SRB-1 (scavenger receptor B-1). Whole–HDL particle uptake into cells can occur by undefined pathways. Finally, plasma HDL cholesteryl esters can move from the HDL particle into VLDL and chylomicron particles in the presence of the cholesteryl ester transfer protein (CETP). LpL activity can modulate HDL levels by influencing plasma levels of triglyceride in VLDL or chylomicrons. HL can affect HDL levels by breaking down phospholipids on the surface of the particles; this leads to dissolution of the HDL and loss of apoA-I from the circulation.

Low levels of plasma HDL cholesterol are almost universally present in patients with type 2 diabetes. An important underlying mechanism for this is the CETP-mediated transfer of cholesteryl ester from HDL into VLDL and chylomicrons, both of which are increased in most patients with type 2 diabetes (Fig. 35.4). Low HDL cholesterol levels in type 2 diabetes can also be present in the absence of fasting hypertriglyceridemia. Although the mechanism for this is undefined, it may reflect high postprandial triglyceride levels or some direct effect of insulin resistance. HDL cholesterol levels are normal or even increased in patients with well-controlled type 1 diabetes, and this seems to be related to effects of insulin treatment, possibly through suppression of HL.

THERAPEUTIC APPROACHES TO DIABETIC DYSLIPIDEMIA

Dietary Therapy

The centerpiece of therapy for the treatment of diabetes is always diet, irrespective of the absence or presence of dyslipidemia. However, the presence of dyslipidemia increases the rationale for intensive diet intervention. It is important to remember that improvements in plasma triglyceride and total cholesterol levels during dietary intervention can be observed even in the absence of weight loss. Thus, reductions in dietary simple carbohydrates, saturated fat intake, and cholesterol consumption can improve the lipid profile even if caloric intake is unchanged.

There is, however, a long-standing and continuing controversy concerning the composition of the "optimal diet" for patients with diabetes. Clearly, reducing dietary saturated fat and cholesterol intake is central to lipid lowering. Such changes will lower LDL ~10%; this may not seem like much, but this degree of reduction is equivalent to almost two doublings of the dose of a hydroxymethylglutaryl (HMG)-CoA reductase inhibitor once the starting dose has been initiated. The optimal replacement for saturated fat is the focus of the controversy. Certainly, high-fiber (not just "complex") carbohydrates should be consumed, and even then,

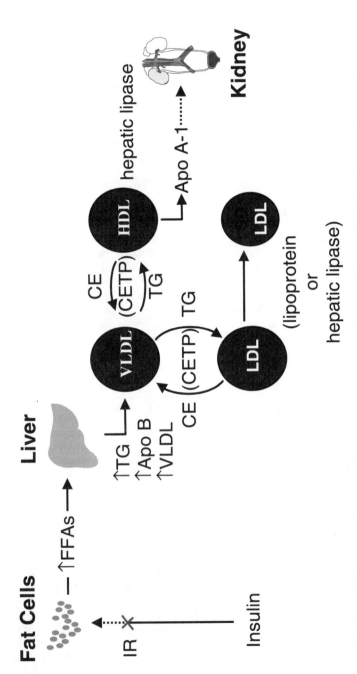

Figure 35.4 Increased VLDL in the circulation, in the presence of CETP, will stimulate an increased exchange of LDL cholesterol for VLDL triglycerides (TG). This will deplete LDL of cholesterol. Additionally, hepatic lipase and/or lipoprotein lipase will hydrolyze the TG in LDL, producing small, dense LDL. FFAs, free fatty acids; IR, insulin resistance.

high-fiber carbohydrates are not a panacea. The recently published DELTA (Diet Effects on Lipids and Thrombogenic Activity) study demonstrated that a diet in which monounsaturated fatty acids replaced saturated fat was associated with a modest but significant decrease in plasma triglycerides and a small but significant increase in HDL cholesterol levels compared with carbohydrate replacement. A diet that is varied in poultry and fish, with many vegetables and legumes and with skim or 1% dairy products, should be recommended for patients with diabetes who need plasma lipid modification. Most importantly, because almost all individuals with type 2 diabetes would benefit from weight loss, removing saturated fat from the diet without replacing it is the optimal approach, at least initially.

Weight Loss

Weight reduction is an essential part of dietary therapy in individuals with type 2 diabetes; it may not be an issue in patients with type 1 diabetes. Weight loss has been shown not only to improve glycemic control and reduce insulin resistance, but also to positively affect lipoprotein patterns as well. Several groups have shown that when weight reduction is achieved and maintained in type 2 diabetic patients, there is a sustained decrease in triglyceride levels. Most, but not all, studies show an increase in HDL cholesterol with weight loss. The optimal weight-loss diet in individuals with diabetes is controversial. Most physicians would agree that a lower-fat diet, with high-fiber foods replacing high-fat foods, is a reasonable approach. In the recently published results of Look AHEAD (Action for Health in Diabetes), which is a large multicenter randomized control trial in overweight and obese individuals with type 2 diabetes, intensive lifestyle intervention resulted in clinically significant weight loss. Obesity-associated factors improved as well. For example, triglyceride levels fell 18% and HDL cholesterol increased 8% in the intensive-therapy group—changes that were twice as great as in the control group.

Glycemic Control

Therapy of type 2 diabetes with either insulin or oral agents only partly corrects lipid abnormalities in the majority of patients. This is almost certainly because dyslipidemia is closely related to insulin resistance. Therapeutic approaches to type 2 diabetes that affect insulin sensitivity, such as metformin and thiazolidinediones, should theoretically lower VLDL secretion from the liver by improving body-wide insulin sensitivity. This would lead to reduced fatty acid flux to the liver, lower plasma insulin levels with less stimulation of hepatic lipogenesis, and possibly decreased apoB secretion. Improved LpL function may also result from such therapies. However, clinical trials indicate that metformin only lowers plasma triglyceride concentrations ~10%, whereas pioglitazone treatment is associated with ~15–20% reductions in plasma triglyceride levels. Unexpectedly, rosiglitazone does not affect triglyceride concentrations in plasma. The effects of the two thiazolidinediones on plasma LDL cholesterol have been variable, although rosiglitazone seems to increase LDL cholesterol 5–15%, whereas pioglitazone is either neutral or associated with ~5% increases in LDL cholesterol. Metformin has been observed to reduce LDL 5–10%. Insulin treatment tends to lower LDL, whereas sulfonylurea therapy has little or no effect. Intensive insulin treatment in patients with type 1 diabetes lowers triglyceride and LDL cholesterol levels significantly.

Control of hyperglycemia does not correlate well with HDL cholesterol levels in patients with type 2 diabetes. Therapy with sulfonylureas does not seem to increase HDL cholesterol concentrations. However, modest increases in HDL levels, concomitant with modest decreases in triglyceride concentrations, have been observed with metformin therapy. More recently, the thiazolidinediones have been shown to raise HDL cholesterol levels in patients with type 2 diabetes. Of interest, although rosiglitazone and pioglitazone appear to differ in their effects on plasma triglyceride levels, they raise HDL cholesterol concentrations similarly. Recently, the U.S. Food and Drug Administration (FDA) has issued "black box" warnings for both thiazolidinediones regarding an increased risk for the development of congestive heart failure. In addition, the FDA has added a warning that rosiglitazone (but not pioglitazone) may be associated with increased risk for cardiovascular disease.

Overall, with better glycemic control, some improvement should be expected in plasma lipid levels. In individuals with type 2 diabetes, however, lipid-altering therapy will almost always be necessary. In patients with type 1 diabetes, tight glycemic control with intensive insulin treatment may be adequate, depending on the individual's CHD risk profile.

Lipid-Lowering Drugs

If therapeutic goals have not been achieved after an adequate trial of diabetes control, diet, weight loss, and exercise, then drug therapy should be initiated for the treatment of dyslipidemia. The length of time devoted to lifestyle changes should depend on the initial presentation of the patient, the severity of the dyslipidemia, and the presence of other risk factors for CHD or CHD itself. Patients with many correctable lifestyle habits and/or poorly controlled glycemia require more time devoted to those problems before initiation of specific hypolipidemic drug treatment. It is clear that lipid-lowering agents will be less efficacious, or actually ineffective, if these related factors are not approached first. In contrast, when patients are severely dyslipidemic, and/or have very high risk for development of CHD, earlier progression to pharmacotherapy may be prudent. If the patient already has clinically significant CHD or other vascular disease, then drug treatment should be initiated concomitant with lifestyle interventions. The severity of the dyslipidemia, independent of glycemic control, is an indicator of the presence of other genetic causes of lipid abnormalities, and this can also be taken into account when considering initiation of specific lipid-lowering therapy. Clearly, physicians cannot "wait forever" to control plasma glucose or achieve significant weight loss before moving on to specific lipid-altering treatment.

The American Diabetes Association (ADA) in its 2009 Standards of Care recommends that diabetic patients aged >40 years should receive statin therapy to achieve LDL cholesterol reduction of 30–40% irrespective of baseline LDL cholesterol levels. The ADA goals suggest that individuals with overt cardiovascular disease can be targeted to an LDL cholesterol level <70 mg/dl. The National Cholesterol Education Program (NCEP) has also taken an aggressive approach, issuing a "white paper" that suggests that an LDL cholesterol level <70 mg/dl is a viable therapeutic option in patients with both cardiovascular disease and diabetes. In both guidelines, however, the goal of treatment for patients without overt cardiovascular disease, once initiated, is an LDL cholesterol level <100 mg/dl. Goals for triglycerides and HDL cholesterol are less well defined, but it is reasonable to try to reach a triglyceride level <150 mg/dl and an HDL cholesterol concentration >45 mg/dl. Women should attempt to get an HDL cholesterol level >50 mg/dl.

HMG-CoA Reductase Inhibitors

During the past two decades, the treatment of hypercholesterolemia has undergone a revolution with the availability of potent, safe HMG-CoA reductase inhibitors, also known as statins. Lovastatin, pravastatin, fluvastatin, simvastatin, atorvastatin, and rosuvastatin are available drugs in this category in the U.S. These drugs work to competitively inhibit HMG-CoA reductase, the rate-limiting enzyme in cholesterol synthesis, and this results in both decreased hepatic production of apoB100-containing lipoproteins and upregulation of LDL receptors. The overall effect is a dramatic lowering of plasma levels of LDL cholesterol. VLDL triglyceride concentrations are also reduced in many subjects with moderate hypertriglyceridemia, including patients with type 2 diabetes. The reduction of triglycerides is directly related to the reduction of LDL cholesterol achieved. At their starting doses, which now range between 10 and 40 mg/day, statins lower LDL cholesterol by 25–40%. The most potent statins (simvastatin, atorvastatin, and rosuvastatin), at the highest doses, can lower LDL cholesterol by up to 45–60% and decrease triglycerides 20–45%. The reduction in triglycerides achieved at these high levels of LDL cholesterol reduction will also depend on the starting triglyceride level; higher baseline triglycerides can be lowered more. Reductase inhibitors can raise HDL cholesterol by up to 5–10% but should not be considered as first-line HDL-raising drugs.

The most worrisome side effect associated with statin therapy is a myositis, characterized by diffuse, moderate to severe muscle tenderness and weakness and elevated levels of creatine phosphokinase (usually >1,000 units). In severe cases, rhabdomyolysis and concomitant myoglobinemia can place patients at risk for renal failure due to myoglobinuria. This is a risk particularly in patients with diabetes who have preexisting proteinuria. However, the incidence of this severe type of myositis when statins are used as monotherapy is ~1 in 2,000 patients, and careful patient instruction about the signs and symptoms, with advice to stop the medication and consume large volumes of liquids if symptoms occur, should obviate more serious outcomes. Less severe myalgias, with normal creatine phosphokinase levels, occurs in 3–5% of patients on statins. Although there is no risk for rhabdomyolysis or renal failure if the creatine phosphokinase levels are normal, patients often refuse to continue on therapy because of symptoms. The basis for their symptoms is unclear. Statins can also cause non–clinically significant elevations in liver function tests in 1–2% of patients, but only at the higher doses of each agent. It is important for physicians and patients to realize that, despite the package insert warnings and the need for liver function tests at initiation of treatment, the statins are not hepatotoxic drugs; clinically significant hepatotoxicity is extremely rare. The statins do not appear to affect diabetic control.

Importantly, we now have results from several very large clinical trials, including the Heart Protection Study (HPS) and the Treat to New Targets (TNT) trial, demonstrating reductions in CHD events and deaths in subgroups of patients with type 2 diabetes receiving statins. In HPS, benefit was observed regardless of the baseline LDL cholesterol level of the participants: even those with baseline

LDL levels <100 mg/dl benefited from statin treatment. In TNT, greater LDL reductions with 80 mg/day of atorvastatin were associated with greater benefit than lesser reductions with 10 mg/day atorvastatin. In addition, the Collaborative Atorvastatin Diabetes Study (CARDS) demonstrated that treatment with atorvastatin reduced the risk for a first cardiovascular event in patients with type 2 diabetes regardless of baseline LDL cholesterol levels. It should be noted that the ASPEN (Atorvastatin Study for Prevention of Coronary Heart Disease Endpoints in non–insulin-dependent diabetes) trial showed no significant benefit in a similar population. Overall, however, these studies support the use of statins for the first-line approach to diabetic patients with isolated high levels of LDL cholesterol, with combined hyperlipidemia, or with moderate hypertriglyceridemia and an LDL cholesterol level above the NCEP goal. Thus, even though the most common lipid abnormality in diabetes is a dyslipidemia characterized by high triglycerides and low HDL cholesterol levels, with average or slightly elevated LDL cholesterol concentrations, statins should be considered as the first agents to be used.

Bile Acid–Binding Resins

Cholestyramine, colestipol, and colesevelam are resins that bind bile acids in the intestine, thus interrupting the enterohepatic recirculation of those molecules. A fall in bile acids returning to the liver results in increased conversion of hepatic cholesterol to bile acids, which results in a diminution of a regulatory pool of hepatic cholesterol and upregulation of the gene for hepatic LDL receptors. All of these changes lead to decreased plasma LDL concentrations. Usual doses are 8–24 g/day for cholestyramine, 10–30 g/day for colestipol (both as granular powders), and 6.5 g/day for colesevelam (as tablets). Cholestyramine is mixed with sucrose, but there is a "light" form that is made with aspartame. Colestipol is also available in 1-g tablets. Colesevelam is available in tablets—six tablets per day is the standard dose. At full doses, cholestyramine and colestipol can reduce LDL levels ~25%; however, compliance is usually low, and, in most patients, only mid-level doses are achieved. At six tablets per day, colesevelam lowers LDL cholesterol by 15–20%, and compliance is significantly better. Bile acid–binding resins are not absorbed and therefore have no systemic toxicities. A drawback to the use of bile acid–binding resin in patients with diabetes is an increase in hepatic VLDL triglyceride production and plasma triglyceride levels commonly associated with their use. This may be less of a problem with colesevelam. The bile acid–binding resins should be used with caution in patients with both hypercholesterolemia and significant hypertriglyceridemia. An additional major side effect of these agents is bloating and constipation, which may pose a significant problem in the diabetic patient with gastroparesis. The resins can also interfere with the absorption of other oral medications, although this problem is significantly less common with colesevelam. With the availability of HMG-CoA reductase inhibitors, however, the need for resins has been markedly reduced. However, they can add greatly to LDL lowering when added to statins. Of interest, recent studies with cholestyramine and colesevelam indicate that they also modestly reduce A1C levels (~0.4%) in patients with type 2 diabetes. The mechanism underlying this action is undefined.

Fibric Acid Derivatives

Fibric acid derivatives are peroxisome proliferator–activated receptor-α agonists that have potent lipid-altering effects and are very useful in patients with diabetes. In general, fibrate use in patients with type 2 diabetes results in lowering of triglycerides from 35 to 50% and increases in HDL cholesterol from 10 to 20%. Fenofibrate and gemfibrozil are the agents currently available in the U.S. (clofibrate is still available, but its use has been restricted by the FDA). Several other agents are available in Europe and Canada. Several mechanisms have been suggested for the triglyceride-lowering effects of fibrates, including increased fatty acid oxidation, decreased synthesis of apoC-III (an inhibitor of LpL), increased synthesis of apoA-5 (an activator of LpL), and possibly increased synthesis of LpL. These agents appear to work by both decreasing hepatic VLDL production and increasing the fractional removal of VLDL triglyceride from plasma. Unfortunately, fibrates have modest and variable effects on LDL cholesterol in most patients with diabetes. That is because fibrates can have some LDL cholesterol–lowering effect, no effect, or even an LDL cholesterol–raising effect in patients with hypertriglyceridemia. The basis for these variable outcomes is complex and has to do with the efficiency with which VLDL is converted to LDL, how efficiently LDL is removed from plasma, and the cholesterol content of LDL. In the latter instance, fibrate treatment, with concomitant triglyceride lowering, usually converts small, dense, cholesterol-depleted LDL into more normal cholesterol-enriched LDL. The usual dose is 600 mg gemfibrozil twice daily and 145 mg once daily for micronized fenofibrate. These agents are contraindicated in patients with gallstones, and because they are tightly bound to plasma proteins, levels of other drugs (e.g., Coumadin) should be carefully monitored. Fibrates do not significantly affect glycemic control.

The rise in LDL cholesterol concentration that can accompany reduced triglyceride levels during fibrate therapy must be viewed in the context of clinical trials of fibrate therapy that included patients with diabetes. In the Helsinki Heart Study, the two groups with hypertriglyceridemia (with and without concomitant elevations in LDL cholesterol) had increases or no changes in LDL cholesterol levels during gemfibrozil therapy and yet achieved the same reduction in CHD events as the group with isolated LDL elevations, in which LDL cholesterol levels fell 10–12% with treatment. The two groups in which LDL changed little or not at all included the majority of participants with diabetes (a small number overall). A more recent study, the Veterans Administration HDL Intervention Trial, showed that gemfibrozil was efficacious in a group of men who had CHD and a mean LDL cholesterol that was low (111 mg/dl) at baseline and did not change during the trial. The treated group did show a 7% increase in HDL cholesterol and a 25% reduction in triglycerides; these changes were associated with a 22% reduction in CHD events. In the 25% of the subjects in this trial who had diabetes (most almost certainly type 2 diabetes), relative benefit was equal to that seen in the nondiabetic cohort. The subjects with diabetes had, as expected, higher absolute rates of events in both the placebo and the treatment group. However, a recent large trial of fenofibrate to prevent cardiovascular disease in patients with diabetes (Fenofibrate Intervention and Event Lowering in Diabetes [FIELD]) was negative for the primary end point of coronary heart disease, death, or nonfatal myocardial infarction (11% reduction, P = NS). Fenofibrate did have a benefit on the secondary end point, which was the composite of cardiovascular disease death, myocardial infarction, stroke, and coronary and carotid revascularization (11%, $P = 0.35$). Why the FIELD trial was negative may never be known for certain. It is possible that fenofibrate, which reversibly raises serum creatinine and homocysteine levels much more than gemfibrozil, is not as effective in preventing cardiovascular events as gemfibrozil. Unfortunately, in the FIELD trial, there was a significant imbalance in the use of nonprotocol statins; twice as many participants on placebo were prescribed statins by their own physicians than were participants receiving fenofibrate. This imbalanced use of statins severely compromises the interpretation of the results.

When statins have been compared with fibrates in patients with type 2 diabetes, the expected results were observed. The statins produced much greater LDL lowering, whereas the fibrates lowered triglycerides and raised HDL cholesterol more than the statins. Importantly, several recent studies of combination treatment of patients with type 2 diabetes have shown the powerful, positive effects on the entire dyslipidemic pattern with this approach. Of note, however, is that the risk of significant myositis increases from ~1 per 2,000 to ~1 per 300 patients when statins are combined with gemfibrozil. However, there does not seem to be increased risk of significant myositis when fenofibrate is used with a statin. In any event, myositis (a creatine phosphokinase level >10 times the upper limit of normal and muscle pain) should never progress to rhabdomyolysis if the patient and the doctor pay attention to the symptoms and if the patient stops the drugs and drinks large volumes of fluids if symptoms occur. More importantly, the question remains: when one considers adding a fibrate to a statin, should the fibrate be gemfibrozil, which has been proven to prevent cardiovascular events but also to increase the risk of myositis, or should the fibrate be fenofibrate, which is safer but possibly ineffective? It is important to note that there are no cardiovascular end point trials showing that the addition of a fibrate to a statin will further reduce cardiovascular events. The results of the ACCORD trial, in which fenofibrate plus simvastatin is compared with simvastatin alone in people with diabetes, will be reported next year.

Cholesterol Absorption Inhibitors

In October 2002, ezetimibe became the first available agent in a new class of molecules that interferes with cholesterol absorption by selectively inhibiting the uptake of cholesterol from the intestinal lumen. Ezetimibe is given as a 10-mg daily dose and has been shown to decrease LDL cholesterol ~17–20%. Studies in patients with type 2 diabetes have demonstrated that ezetimibe combined with statin causes greater reduction in LDL cholesterol and triglyceride levels than either therapy alone. To date, however, there are no completed and published clinical trials demonstrating a cardiovascular benefit of ezetimibe when added to a statin.

Nicotinic Acid (Niacin)

As noted above, the most common lipid abnormalities present in patients with diabetes are elevated triglycerides and low HDL cholesterol levels. Niacin, when used in pharmacological doses (1–3 g/day), has the ability to potently lower triglycerides (20–35%) and raise HDL cholesterol (15–30%). Niacin also lowers

LDL cholesterol (10–20%), and this adds to its potential efficacy in a high-risk population. Of note, niacin can also reduce levels of lipoprotein(a) between 15 and 25%. The mechanism of action of niacin is generally thought to be through lowering hepatic VLDL apoB100 production and increasing the synthesis of apoA-I. Unfortunately, niacin has several side effects that often limit its utility in nondiabetic individuals: regular niacin produces a prostaglandin-mediated flush that occurs ~30 min after ingestion and can last as long as 1 h; patients turn red and feel hot. Pruritus can accompany the flush. An intermediate-release niacin (Niaspan), which is taken once daily at night, may cause slightly less flushing per dose and can be better tolerated by most patients. Both forms of niacin can also cause gastric irritation and can exacerbate peptic ulcer disease, have been associated with dry skin, cause hyperuricemia, can precipitate gouty attacks, and are associated with elevations of hepatic transaminases in ~3–5% of patients. Rarely, niacin can also cause clinically significant hepatitis. All of these side effects can occur in anyone using niacin, but in patients with type 2 diabetes, hyperuricemia is already more common. Most importantly, some studies have demonstrated that niacin therapy worsens diabetic control, likely by inducing insulin resistance. This finding is interesting at a theoretical level because niacin's ability to inhibit lipolysis and lower plasma free fatty acid levels after a single dose might be expected to improve insulin sensitivity. Two recent studies in patients with diabetes, one using regular short-acting niacin and the other using Niaspan, demonstrated that niacin was efficacious in terms of lipid-altering activity with modest but manageable effects on glycemic control. If a physician is faced with persistent low HDL and/or significant hypertriglyceridemia after statin treatment, or even statin plus fibrate therapy, addition of niacin in either of the available forms can be considered. Of note, "long-acting, no flush" niacin preparations can cause severe hepatotoxicity and should not be used. Niaspan appears to have the same safety profile as short-acting niacin. There are some "no-flush" short-acting niacin preparations available (i.e., niacin inositol), but neither their efficacy nor their safety have been well documented.

n-3 Fatty Acid Supplements

Fatty fish from the northern oceans are enriched in n-3 fatty acids, docosahexanoic acid (DHA), and eicosapentanoic acid (EPA). Consumption of fish has, in epidemiological studies, been associated with lower rates of cardiovascular disease. Diets rich in plant sources of the n-3 fatty acid α-linolenic acid have also been associated with reduced cardiovascular events. n-3 fatty acids provided as supplements, in doses of 3–6 g/day, are potent triglyceride-lowering agents and can be very useful in rare diabetic patients who have triglyceride levels >600 mg/dl, especially those who are not responsive to other drug therapies. The question of whether low doses of n-3 fatty acids, as supplements, should be given to patients with type 2 diabetes remains incompletely answered. In the GISSI (Gruppo Italiano per lo Studio della Sopravvivenza nell'Infarto) Prevention trial, 1 g of an n-3 fatty acid supplement significantly reduced fatal and nonfatal myocardial infarction and stroke in both nondiabetic individuals and subjects with diabetes. A prevailing theory is that these fatty acids reduce arrhythmic sudden death. The use of 1 g/day of n-3 fatty acids is not associated with alterations of glycemic control, but their use with aspirin therapy could increase the risk of bleeding. In the recent

JELIS (Japan EPA Lipid Intervention Study), investigators found that patients with hypercholesterolemia who received 1.8 g/day of EPA with a statin, as opposed to statin alone, had fewer major coronary events. Unfortunately, this was not a double-blind study.

Hormone Replacement Therapy

In prospective observational studies of mostly nondiabetic women, estrogen replacement therapy was associated with a significant decrease in risk for CHD. About one-third of the beneficial effects of hormones in these studies has been estimated to be caused by changes in lipid levels, specifically reductions in LDL cholesterol and increases in HDL cholesterol. Oral estrogen given alone raises HDL levels by 10–20% by increasing apoA-I synthesis and decreasing hepatic lipase activity. Estrogen alone also lowers LDL cholesterol ~20% by increasing LDL receptor number on cells, particularly in the liver. Another benefit relates to the ability of estrogen to lower lipoprotein(a) levels ~20%. A potentially negative effect of estrogen administration on diabetic dyslipidemia is the increase in plasma triglycerides that occurs via increased hepatic secretion of VLDL. Severe hyperlipidemia and pancreatitis have been observed in women with preexisting hypertriglyceridemia who were receiving oral estrogen treatment. Addition of a progestational agent has been associated with much less HDL raising, but also less triglyceride raising, compared with estrogen therapy alone.

Early studies with high-dose estrogen-containing oral contraceptives indicated that glucose intolerance could occur, probably in women with the metabolic syndrome. There was a fear that estrogen treatment could "induce" diabetes in predisposed women. However, three intervention trials have assessed hormone therapy in women with type 2 diabetes for treatment periods of 6–12 weeks. All three showed that isolated estrogen treatment lowered blood glucose levels and A1C levels without raising plasma insulin concentrations or causing insulin resistance. Lipid profiles were also improved, with lower LDL and higher HDL cholesterol levels, and with no significant rise in plasma triglycerides in two of the three studies. Interestingly, estrogen replacement therapy appears to improve postprandial lipemia in normal subjects, despite its effect to raise fasting triglyceride levels. It appears that, overall, hormone replacement therapy in women with type 2 diabetes can induce favorable lipid changes (particularly if micronized progesterone is used as the progestational agent) and has no detrimental effect on glycemic control.

With that said, the results from HERS (Heart and Estrogen/Progestin Replacement Study), the WAVE (Women's Angiographic Vitamins and Estrogen) study, and the Womens' Health Initiative showed no benefit in women with or without prior myocardial infarction who received combined therapy with equine conjugated estrogens (Premarin) plus low-dose medroxyprogesterone (Provera). Furthermore, there was no effect on incidence of cardiovascular disease, even in the estrogen-only arm of the Womens' Health Initiative. Thus, it does not seem appropriate at this time to use hormone replacement therapy as a way to reduce cardiovascular risk. Diabetic women receiving postmenopausal hormone replacement therapy for severe symptoms of systemic estrogen deficiency (osteoporosis should be treated with drugs specific for that problem) should understand that there may be an increased risk for cardiovascular disease and breast cancer.

SUMMARY

When rationally approached, the patient with diabetes and hyperlipidemia can be well managed through both lifestyle interventions and pharmacotherapy. Close guidance and monitoring is needed, however, in choosing the proper approach. A variety of options are available to improve plasma lipids and thus reduce risk of CHD. The key, however, based on many clinical trials, is that significant benefit can be obtained by aggressively lowering LDL cholesterol; it is also likely that raising HDL cholesterol/lowering triglycerides will add further benefit.

When specific lipid-altering therapy is indicated, the physician has effective and safe agents from which to choose. Even though the characteristic diabetic dyslipidemia is one of higher triglycerides, lower HDL cholesterol, and average or slightly higher-than-average LDL cholesterol levels, the evidence from clinical trials indicates that lowering LDL cholesterol should be a central priority. Treatment with statins, regardless of initial LDL cholesterol levels, will, based on the HPS, CARDS, and TNT study, reduce event rates significantly. Whether statin therapy should always be first is a question that cannot be answered with full confidence, but it seems prudent to say that at least 90% (arguably 100%) of patients with diabetes should get a statin as part of their overall cardioprotective therapy.

For the diabetic patient without a prior cardiovascular event but with isolated hypertriglyceridemia and low HDL cholesterol (LDL cholesterol <100 mg/dl), fibric acid derivatives could be an alternative as the first choice for drug therapy. In some cases, fibric acid derivatives will be all that is necessary. If the LDL cholesterol increases during fibrate treatment and goes >100 mg/dl, the physician has several choices. First, a bile acid–binding resin could be added to the fibrate; this would lower LDL cholesterol without, in the presence of the fibrate, significantly affecting triglyceride levels. Bile acid–binding resins have been shown to reduce cardiovascular events. The second alternative would be to add ezetimibe. Although more efficacious than bile acid–binding resins, ezetimibe has not yet been shown to reduce events. The third would be to switch to an HMG-CoA reductase inhibitor. This would be the logical choice if the triglyceride elevation (before or during fibrate treatment) was only moderate (<250 mg/dl).

The physician could add the reductase inhibitor to the fibrate. The latter combination is effective in correcting severe combined hyperlipidemia but carries an increased risk of myositis. The risk for increased severe myositis with fenofibrate appears to be minimal, whereas it increases significantly (but is still <1%) with gemfibrozil in combination with statin. As noted above, gemfibrozil has reduced events in prior studies, whereas fenofibrate has not convincingly done so. We believe that this combination can be used successfully, particularly if the patient knows clearly that he or she must stop the medications, drink large quantities of liquids, and call a physician if diffuse, symmetric muscle pain occurs. The patient should have liver function tests obtained regularly with the use of fibrates or reductase inhibitors alone or in combination. Importantly, there is no evidence that the combination of statin and fibrate will reduce events more than statins alone. The ACCORD trial, which is expected to report in 2010, will answer this question.

The final choice, nicotinic acid, could be used in patients with severe, combined hyperlipidemia or extremely low levels of HDL cholesterol. Both short-acting and intermediate-release niacin preparations are efficacious when used with a statin, and the risk of myositis is extremely low with this combination. As noted earlier, close attention must be paid to the potential adverse effects of nicotinic acid on glycemic control; modification of the diabetes treatment regimen may be required. Two large trials of niacin in combination with statin versus statin alone (AIM HIGH [Atherothrombosis Intervention in Metabolic Syndrome with Low HDL/High Triglycerides and Impact on Global Health Outcomes] and HPS2-THRIVE [Heart Protection Study 2—Treatment of HDL to Reduce the Incidence of Vascular Events]) are testing the hypothesis that the combination is better than statin monotherapy for the prevention of cardiovascular events in people with type 2 diabetes.

Therapy for the diabetic patient with an isolated reduction in HDL cholesterol is not clearly defined. Fibrates have not been demonstrated to be very effective in raising HDL cholesterol levels in nondiabetic individuals with isolated reductions in HDL, although no similar studies have been carried out in patients with diabetes. Niacin may be more effective in elevating HDL cholesterol concentrations when they are low in the absence of hypertriglyceridemia, but all of the caveats of niacin use in diabetes would apply here as well. An alternative to raising HDL in these subjects would be to more aggressively treat LDL cholesterol levels, with the goal of reducing them to much less than 100 mg/dl. It must be clear, however, that there are no end point trials supporting any approach to isolated reductions in HDL cholesterol, either in nondiabetic individuals or patients with diabetes.

Finally, in those patients with diabetes who have isolated high levels of LDL cholesterol, an HMG-CoA reductase inhibitor should be the first approach to treatment. The combination of statin with either bile acid–binding resin or ezetimibe has been shown to be effective in those individuals with extremely high levels of LDL cholesterol resistant to monotherapy. Triglyceride levels need to be observed closely in those patients placed on resins.

BIBLIOGRAPHY

American Diabetes Association: Dyslipidemia management in adults with diabetes (Position Statement). *Diabetes Care* 27 (Suppl. 1):S68–S71, 2004

American Diabetes Association: Standards of medical care in diabetes—2009 (Position Statement). *Diabetes Care* 32 (Suppl. 1):S13–S61, 2009

Anderson GL, Limacher M, Assaf AR, Bassford T, Bereford SA, Black H, et al.: Effects of conjugated equine estrogen in postmenopausal women with hysterectomy: the Women's Health Initiative randomized controlled trial. *JAMA* 291:1701–1712, 2004

Bays HE, Moore PB, Drehobl MA, Rosenblatt S, Toth PD, Dujovne CA, et al.: Effectiveness and tolerability of ezetimibe in patients with primary hypercholesterolemia: pooled analysis of two phase II studies. *Clin Ther* 23:1209–1230, 2001

Ballantyne CM, Houri J, Notarbartolo A, Melani L, Lipka LJ, Suresh R, et al.: Effect of ezetimibe coadministered with atorvastatin in 628 patients with primary hypercholesterolemia: a prospective, randomized, double-blind trial. *Circulation* 107:2409–2415, 2003

Berglund L, Lefevre M, Ginsberg HN, Kris-Etherton PM, Elmer PJ, Stewart PW, et al.: Comparison of monounsaturated fat with carbohydrates as a replacement for saturated fat in subjects with a high metabolic risk profile: studies in the fasting and postprandial states. *Am J Clin Nutr* 86:1611–1620, 2007

Chahil T, Ginsberg HN: Diabetic dyslipidemia. *Endo Metab Clin North Am* 35:491–510, 2006

Chesney CM, Elam MB, Herd JA, Davis KB, Garg R, Hunninghake D, et al.: Effect of niacin, warfarin, and antioxidant therapy on coagulation parameters in patients with peripheral arterial disease in the Arterial Disease Multiple Intervention Trial (ADMIT). *Am Heart J* 140:631–636, 2000

Colhoun HM, Betteridge DJ, Durrington PN, Hitman GA, Neil HA,Livingston SJ et al.: Primary prevention of cardiovascular disease with atorvastatin in type 2 diabetes in the Collaborative Atorvastatin Diabetes Study (CARDS): multicentre randomised placebo-controlled trial. *Lancet* 364:685-696, 2004

Ellen RLB, McPherson R: Long-term efficacy and safety of fenofibrate and a statin in the treatment of combined hyperlipidemia. *Am J Cardiol* 81:60B–65B, 1998

Expert Panel on Detection, Evaluation, and Treatment of High Blood Cholesterol in Adults: Executive summary of the third report of the National Cholesterol Education Program (NCEP) Expert Panel on Detection, Evaluation, and Treatment of High Blood Cholesterol in Adults (Adult Treatment Panel III). *JAMA* 285:2486–2497, 2001

Garg A, Grundy SM: Cholestyramine therapy for dyslipidemia in non-insulin dependent diabetes mellitus: a short-term, double-blind, crossover trial. *Ann Intern Med* 121:416–422, 1994

Ginsberg HN, Bonds D, Lovato LC, Crouse JR, Elam MB, Linz PE, et al.: Evolution of the lipid trial protocol of the Action to Control Cardiovascular Risk in Diabetes (ACCORD) Trial. *Am J Cardiol* 99 (Suppl.):56i–67i, 2007

Ginsberg HN, Illingworth DR: Postprandial dyslipidemia: an atherogenic disorder common in patients with diabetes mellitus. *Am J Cardiol* 88:9H–15H, 2001

Goldberg RB, Mellies MJ, Sacks FM, Moye LA, Howard BV, Howard WJ, et al.: Cardiovascular events and their reduction with pravastatin in diabetic and glucose-intolerant myocardial infarction survivors with average cholesterol levels: subgroup analysis in the Cholesterol and Recurrent Events (CARE) trial. *Circulation* 98:2513–2519, 1998

Grundy SM, Cleeman JI, Merz CN, Brewer HB Jr, Clark LT, Hunninghake DB, et al.: Implications of recent clinical trials for the National Cholesterol Education Program Adult Treatment Panel III Guidelines. *Circulation* 110:227–239, 2004

Grundy SM, Vega GL, McGovern ME, Tulloch BR, Kendall DM, Fitz-Patrick D, et al.: Diabetes Multicenter Research Group: efficacy, safety, and tolerability of once-daily niacin for the treatment of dyslipidemia associated with type 2 diabetes: results of the assessment of diabetes control and evaluation of the efficacy of niaspan trial. *Arch Intern Med* 22:1568–1576, 2002

Haffner SM: Management of dyslipidemia in adults with diabetes (Technical Review). *Diabetes Care* 21:160–178, 1998

Heart Protection Study Collaborative Group: MRC/BHF Heart Protection Study of cholesterol lowering with simvastatin in 20,536 high-risk individuals: a randomised placebo-controlled trial. *Lancet* 360:7–22, 2002

Hulley S, Grady D, Bush T, Furberg C, Herrington D, Riggs B, et al.: Randomized trial of estrogen plus progestin for secondary prevention of coronary heart disease in postmenopausal women: Heart and Estrogen/progestin Replacement Study Research Group. *JAMA* 280:605–613, 1998

Kannel WB, D'Agostino RB, Wilson PWF, Bleanger AJ, Gagnon DR: Diabetes, fibrinogen, and risk of cardiovascular disease: the Framingham experience. *Am Heart J* 120:672–676, 1990

Keech A, Simes RJ, Barter P, Best J, Scott R, Taskinen MR, et al.: Effects of long-term fenofibrate therapy on cardiovascular events in 9795 people with type 2 diabetes mellitus (the FIELD study): randomised controlled trial. *Lancet* 366:1849–1861, 2005

Knopp RH, d'Emden M, Smilde JG, Pocock SJ: Efficacy and safety of atorvastatin in the prevention of cardiovascular end points in subjects with type 2 diabetes: the Atorvastatin Study for Prevention of Coronary Heart Disease Endpoints in Non-insulin-dependent diabetes mellitus (ASPEN). *Diabetes Care* 29:1478–1485, 2006

Look AHEAD Research Group: Reduction in weight and cardiovascular disease risk factors in individuals with type 2 diabetes. *Diabetes Care* 30:1374–1383, 2007

Pyorala K, Pedersen TR, Kjekshus J, Faegerman O, Olsson AG, Thorgeirsson G: Cholesterol lowering with simvastatin improves prognosis of diabetic patients with coronary artery disease: a subgroup analysis of the Scandinavian Simvastatin Survival Study. *Diabetes Care* 20:614–620, 1997

Rubins HB, Robins SJ, Collins D, Fye CL, Anderson JW, Elam MB, et al.: Gemfibrozil for the secondary prevention of coronary heart disease in men with low levels of high-density lipoprotein cholesterol: Veterans Affairs High-Density Lipoprotein Cholesterol Intervention Trial Study Group. *N Engl J Med* 341:410–418, 1999

Shepherd J, Barter P, Carmena R, Deedwania P, Fruchart JC, Haffner S, et al.: Effect of lowering LDL cholesterol substantially below currently recommended levels in patients with coronary heart disease and diabetes: the Treating to New Targets (TNT) study. *Diabetes Care* 29:1220–1226, 2006

Tikkanen MJ, Laakso M, Ilmonen M, Helve E, Kaarsalo E, Kilkki E, et al.: Treatment of hypercholesterolemia and combined hyperlipidemia with simvastatin and gemfibrozil in patients with NIDDM: a multicenter comparison study. *Diabetes Care* 21:477–481, 1998

Writing Group for the Women's Health Initiative: Risks and benefits of estrogen plus progestin in healthy postmenopausal women: principal results from the Women's Health Initiative randomized controlled trial. *JAMA* 288:321–333, 2002

Yokoyama M, Origasa H, Matsuzaki M, Matsuzawa Y, Saito Y, Ishikawa Y, et al.: Effects of eicosapentaenoic acid on major coronary events in hypercholesterolaemic patients (JELIS): a randomised open-label, blinded endpoint analysis. *Lancet* 369:1090–1098: 2007

Zieve FJ, Kalin MF, Schwartz SI, Jones MR, Bailey WL: Results of the glucose lowering effect of WelChol Study (GLOWS): a randomized, double-blind, placebo controlled pilot study evaluating the effect of colesevelam hydrochloride on glycemic control in subjects with type 2 diabetes. *Clin Ther* 29:74–83, 2007

Dr. Kurra is a postdoctoral fellow in the Division of Endocrinology, Department of Medicine, Columbia University College of Physicians and Surgeons, New York, New York. Dr. Ginsberg is the Irving Professor of Medicine and Director of the Irving Institute for Clinical and Translational Research, Columbia University College of Physicians and Surgeons, New York, New York.

36. Treatment-Associated Renal Dysfunction in Patients with Diabetes

Irena Duka, MD, and George Bakris, MD

There is a similar risk in the development of nephropathy between type 1 and type 2 diabetes, i.e., about one in three people will develop nephropathy. Factors known to slow nephropathy include glycemic control at levels <7%, blood pressure reduction to <130/80 mmHg using renin-angiotensin system blockade, and, lastly, lipid control (1–3).

BLOOD PRESSURE APPROACH TO OPTIMALLY SLOW NEPHROPATHY

The incidence of hypertension in people with type 2 diabetes is >80% (4). The goal of blood pressure reduction is lower in patients with diabetes than in the general population. Epidemiological studies demonstrate that people whose blood pressure is >130/80 mmHg have a greater likelihood of progressing to end-stage renal disease (5).

From all available data from clinical trials, it is clear the blockade of the renin-angiotensin-aldosterone system (RAAS) is the foundation for slowing progression of proteinuric diabetic kidney disease (Table 36.1). Adequately dosed RAAS blockade alone, however, fails to provide optimal protection in the absence of complementary antihypertensive agents that help achieve blood pressure targets, as indicated by the results of clinical trials (6,7).

Although RAAS blockade is the cornerstone of slowing nephropathy progression, many physicians avoid the use of these classes due to perceived worsening of kidney function. Note that in clinical trials that show benefits of these agents, the patients recruited, i.e., those with glomerular filtration rates (GFRs) of <50 ml/min with proteinuria >500 mg/day, are exactly the ones not getting RAAS blockade due to this perceived worsening of kidney function by RAAS blockers. In a captopril trial, 409 patients with overt proteinuria and a plasma creatinine concentration ≤2.5 mg/dl were randomly assigned to therapy with either captopril or placebo. This trial showed that patients who had a serum creatinine level >2 mg/dl showed a 74% risk reduction in doubling of the serum creatinine in response to ACE inhibitor therapy, whereas patients with baseline creatinine of 1 mg/dl and a similar degree of blood-pressure reduction experienced only a 4% risk reduction in doubling of serum creatinine (8).

Table 36.1 Long-term Outcome of Renal Function in Clinical Trials in Persons With Renal Disease: Impact of ACEI Therapy*

Study	n†	Duration of Follow-up (years)	Achieved MAP (mm Hg)	Renal Function‡ 6 months	Renal Function‡ Trial End
Diabetic subjects					
Captopril Trial	207	3	105	?	−0.15 (Cr clear)
Bakris et al.	18	5	98	−9.47 (GFR)§	−0.02 (Cr clear)
Lebovitz et al.	28	3	104	?	−6.3 (GFR)
Nielsen et al.	21	3	112	−3.97(GFR)§	−7.1 (GFR)
Bjorck et al.	40	2.2	102	−3.8 (GFR)	−2.0 (GFR)
Nondiabetic subjects					
AIPRI Trial	300	3	100	+26 (Cr)	+31 (Cr)
REIN Trial	78	3.5	106	?	−6.3 (GFR)
Zucchelli et al.	32	3	100	?	−0.04 (Cr clear)
Hannedouche et al.	52	3	105	?	−4.8 (GFR)
MDRD Trial	255	3	105	−5.7 (GFR)	−3.8 (GFR)
			94	−14.4 (GFR)	−2.9 (GFR)
Ihle et al.	36	2	101	−0.42 (GFR)	−0.7 (GFR)
Kamper et al.	35	2.2	99	−3 (GFR)	−2.4 (GFR)

*ACEI, ACE inhibitor; MAP, mean arterial pressure; AIPRI, Angiotensin-Converting Enzyme Inhibitionin Progressive Renal Insufficiency; REIN, Ramipril Efficacy in Nephropathy; MDRD, Modification of Dietary Protein in Renal Disease.

†Number of patients randomized to an ACEI in a given trial. Note that for the last 3 trials listed in the table, although many of these patients with a GFR of 13 to 24 mL/min received an ACEI, they were not randomized to this class. They were randomized to a MAP level of either 102 to 107 mm Hg or less than 92 mm Hg.

‡GFR is expressed as milliliters per minute; creatinine clearance (Cr Clear), milliliters per second; and serum creatinine (Cr), micromoles per liter. To convert creatinine clearance values to milliliters per minute, divide by 0.01667; to convert serum creatinine to milligrams per deciliter, divide by 88.4.

§These values were converted to the annual decline rates by converting the GFRs obtained at or before 4 months. Note also that with the exception of 1 study, all rates of GFR decline are slower at study end, especially in those with average blood pressures <130/85 mmHg.

The beneficial response on slowing kidney disease progression by captopril, which was seen in both hypertensive and normotensive subjects, is consistent with smaller studies, which suggested that antihypertensive therapy, particularly with RAAS blockers, slowed the rate of progression in diabetic nephropathy (9,10).

Thus, among patients with diabetic nephropathy, including some with advanced disease, remission or regression may occur with aggressive control of systemic blood pressure utilizing a RAAS blocker.

Another type of RAAS blocker is the angiotensin receptor blocker (ARB). Two major randomized trials demonstrate a clear benefit on slowing kidney disease progression when ARBs are used as part of the initial "antihypertensive cocktail" in patients with proteinuric nephropathy due to type 2 diabetes (11,12).

In the Irbesartan Diabetic Nephropathy Trial (IDNT), 1,715 hypertensive patients with nephropathy due to type 2 diabetes were randomly assigned to irbesartan (300 mg/day), amlodipine (10 mg/day), or placebo (12). At 2.6 years, irbesartan was associated with a risk of the combined end point (doubling of the plasma creatinine, development of end-stage kidney disease, or death from any cause) that was 23 and 20% lower than with amlodipine and placebo, respectively; the values were 37 and 30% lower for doubling of the plasma creatinine. These benefits were independent of the differences in the magnitude of blood pressure reduction among the groups.

In the RENAAL (Reduction of Endpoints in NIDDM with the Angiotensin II Antagonist Losartan) trial, 1,513 patients with type 2 diabetes and nephropathy were randomly assigned to losartan (50 mg, titrating up to 100 mg once daily) or placebo, both in addition to conventional antihypertensive therapy (but not ACE inhibitors) (13). Compared to placebo, losartan reduced the incidence of a doubling of the plasma creatinine by 25% and end-stage renal disease by 28%; the mean follow-up was 3.4 years. These benefits were again not associated with differences in blood pressure levels between the groups.

Although there are no randomized comparative outcome trials on progression of diabetic nephropathy with ACE inhibitors and ARBs, there are the results of the Diabetics Exposed to Telmisartan and Enalapril (DETAIL) trial, which compared an ARB, telmisartan, to an ACE inhibitor, enalapril, on change in GFR in 250 patients with stage 2 nephropathy and hypertension with microalbuminuria (14). In the DETAIL trial, early nephropathy was defined by albuminuria (82% microalbuminuria and 18% macroalbuminuria to a maximum of 1.4 g/day) and a baseline GFR (measured isotopically) of ~93 ml/min per 1.73 m^2 (14). At 5 years, there was a smaller decline in GFR in the enalapril group that was not significant (14.9 vs. 17.9 ml/min per 1.73 m^2 with telmisartan). Both groups had similar rates or findings for the secondary end points, which included annual changes in GFR, blood pressure, serum creatinine, urinary albumin excretion, end-stage kidney disease, cardiovascular events, and mortality.

The results of the DETAIL trial, while underpowered, are similar to what was recently observed when an ARB, telmisartan, was compared to the ACE inhibitor ramipril on cardiovascular outcomes in ONTARGET (Ongoing Telmisartan Alone and in Combination with Ramipril Global Endpoint Trial), i.e., there was no difference between agents (15). Thus, it appears that if blood pressure is at or close to recommended guideline levels, either of these classes of RAAS blocker may be used with a benefit on slowing diabetic kidney disease progression.

Use of RAAS blockers in people with preexisting kidney disease often results in an acute rise in serum creatinine, a fall in GFR, or a rise in serum creatinine (16). This rise in serum creatinine has lead to physician reluctance in continuing

RAAS-blocking therapy in exactly the people who would most benefit from this therapy. As a result, many patients with advanced-stage nephropathy are deprived of strategies that are known to delay the progression of renal disease.

To properly use RAAS blockers in those with advanced kidney disease, one must understand the changes that occur within the kidney circulation. The most common cause of an acute elevation in serum creatinine associated with RAAS blockers is their use in people who have preexisting volume depletion. These agents should not be used in this setting, or volume depletion should be first corrected and then the patient treated. Another major reason for the limited rise in serum creatinine is a renal hemodynamic effect, i.e., loss of the kidney's ability to autoregulate pressure throughout the nephron (17,18). Specifically, as kidney function declines, the kidney loses its ability to vasoconstrict the afferent arteriole and, hence, can't reduce elevated systemic pressure if it is elevated. Moreover, the "remnant nephrons," i.e., those filtering units still functioning in the presence of renal insufficiency, filter at a relatively higher baseline pressure to maintain stable renal function (19,20). Hence, these nephrons see the actual systemic blood pressure. Couple this with RAAS inhibition with either an ARB or ACE inhibitor, which will dilate the efferent arteriole, which is already constricted by increased effects of angiotensin II, and this is a setup for dramatic, but reversible, reductions in intraglomerular pressure of most nephrons if blood pressure is substantially lowered (21,21a) (Fig. 36.1). Thus, the fewer functional nephrons seen in patients with higher serum creatinine level, the greater the likelihood that GFR will

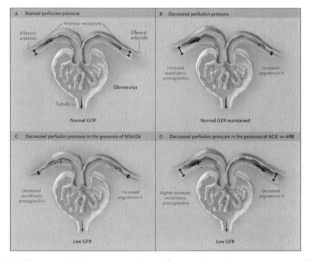

Figure 36.1 Changes in intrarenal perfusion in the presence of different clinical situations. Note that when there is loss of autoregulation and efferent dilation, the intraglomerular pressure markedly falls as a function of the systemic pressure. Reprinted with permission from Abuelo (21a). ©2007 Massachusetts Medical Society. All rights reserved.

decrease when RAAS activity is reduced. This reduction in renal function may not be reflected as a fall in GFR unless blood pressure falls substantially, i.e., at least to levels well below 140/90 mmHg (22,23).

Inhibition of the RAAS blunts the maximal capacitance of organs, such as the heart and kidney, to respond to increased metabolic and physical demands. This is a similar effect to giving β-blockers to the heart; maximal heart rate is reduced with exercise. This is also known to reduce cardiovascular risk. Likewise, in the kidney, clinical trial data support the observation that a small reduction in GFR or rise in serum creatinine level markedly slows renal disease progression (Fig. 36.2). Data from the Modification of Dietary Protein in Kidney Disease (MDRD) study demonstrate that the significant reductions seen in kidney function early in the study translated to long-term slowed decline in kidney function (24). This was also true in two smaller long-term follow-up studies.

A strong association exists between acute increases in serum creatinine of up to 30% that stabilize within the first 2 months of RAAS-blocking therapy and long-term preservation of kidney function (16). This relationship holds for individuals with creatinine values >1.4 mg/dl. Thus, withdrawal of RAAS blockade in such patients should occur only when the rise in creatinine exceeds 30% above baseline within the first 2 months of RAAS initiation or hyperkalemia develops, i.e., serum potassium level ≥5.6 mmol/l (16). A suggested paradigm for RAAS blocker use in patients with renal insufficiency is outlined in Fig. 36.3.

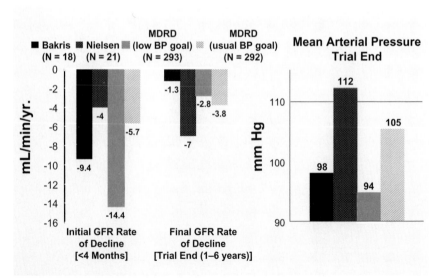

Figure 36.2 Changes in early and late kidney function from clinical trials in the context of blood pressure change. Note those who had better blood pressure control had greater initial reductions in kidney function but better outcomes.

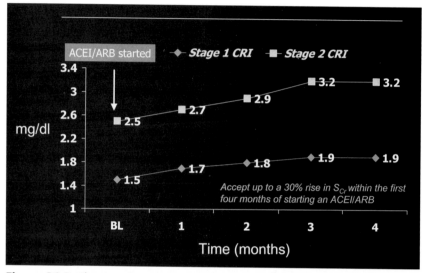

Figure 36.3 Changes in serum creatinine and eGFR in two different patient types, illustrating what is accepted based on guidelines and studies. ACEI, ACE inhibitor.

Note that there are little data about this relationship in people with stage 4 nephropathy, i.e., estimated GFR (eGFR) <30 ml/min. Once marked elevations in serum creatinine are present and renal reserve is lost (serum creatinine >3.0 to 3.5 mg/dl in individuals aged >50 years and normal body habitus), the unique benefits of ACE inhibitors may not exceed that of achieving the recommended level of blood-pressure reduction alone. The hemodynamic changes will be similar to those described previously, and a rise in creatinine may be inevitable once blood pressure comes to the recommended goal. Thus, in a person with preexisting renal insufficiency, aggressive blood pressure control itself, in the absence of ACE inhibition, may lead to a rise in serum creatinine.

A pilot study examined the long-term effect of RAAS blockade on changes in GFR in patients with type 2 diabetes (16). In this study, patients were followed for >5 years on an ACE inhibitor, and then the drug was stopped and clonidine substituted to maintain blood pressure control. It was observed that GFR returned to the earlier baseline where it was 5 years earlier (Fig 36.4).

NON–RAAS-BLOCKING THERAPY IN DIABETIC NEPHROPATHY

There are limited data on use of calcium antagonists in the absence of RAAS blockade in diabetic nephropathy. The best clinical trial that illustrates a lack of protection against declines in kidney function compared to RAAS blockers is the

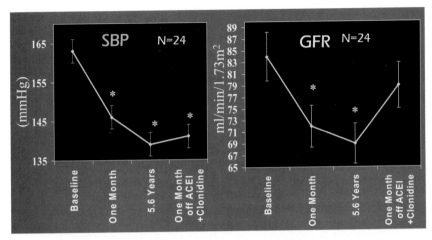

Figure 36.4 Systolic blood pressure and GFR changes over 6 years in patients with type 2 diabetes on an ACE inhibitor who were converted to a centrally acting sympathetic α_2 agonist. *$P<0.05$ from baseline.

IDNT (12). In this trial, the amlodipine arm was no different than placebo on progression of nephropathy.

One predictor of benefit in all outcome trials of kidney disease progression is the magnitude of proteinuria reduction (25). In all outcome studies, those who had >30% reduction in proteinuria within the first 6 months of treatment had slower kidney disease progression. Dihydropyridine calcium antagonists, unlike nondihydropyridine calcium channel blockers, do not have significant antiproteinuric action, despite effective blood pressure reduction (26–28). Only diltiazem and verapamil appear to be as consistently effective as an ACE inhibitor or ARB in lowering protein excretion in diabetic patients (29); furthermore, the antiproteinuric effects of verapamil and an ACE inhibitor may be additive. In one study of patients with type 2 diabetes, lisinopril or verapamil alone lowered protein excretion from 5.8 to 2.7 g/day (22). In comparison, using roughly one-half the dose of both drugs (mean of 16 mg of lisinopril and 187 mg of sustained-release verapamil) had a much greater antiproteinuric effect—from 6.8 down to 1.7 g/day. The low-dose combination regimen was also associated with fewer drug-induced side effects (such as constipation with verapamil and dizziness with lisinopril). A similar antiproteinuric advantage has been demonstrated with combination therapy with verapamil and trandolapril (30). In addition to a small reduction in intraglomerular pressure, nondihydropyridine calcium channel blockers may have other protective actions (31). Some studies in animals suggest that calcium channel blockers may minimize progressive glomerular injury by reducing the associated glomerular hypertrophy (32).

In humans, antiproteinuric effects with diltiazem may also be due to improved glomerular size permselectivity (33). To further solidify this observation, a recent study examined the changes in glomerular permselectivity between amlodipine and verapamil on background ACE inhibitor therapy in patients with proteinuric nephropathy. It was noted that the verapamil combination resulted in an additional 500-mg reduction in proteinuria compared to amlodipine, with a significant improvement in glomerular permeability at similar blood pressure levels (34). Thus, in advanced proteinuric kidney disease, use of either diltiazem or verapamil will yield greater proteinuria reductions compared with amlodipine.

Diuretics can also lead to worsening kidney function that is directly related to development of volume depletion. This worsening of kidney function would be even more exaggerated in the presence of RAAS blockade. Among diuretics, aldosterone antagonists appear to reduce proteinuria when used alone (35) and to have an additive effect on proteinuria when used in combination with an ACE inhibitor or an ARB in both type 1 and type 2 diabetes (36,37). These effects of spironolactone were illustrated in a double-blind trial of 59 patients with type 2 diabetes already on an ACE inhibitor or ARB who were randomly assigned to spironolactone or placebo (37). In this study, the urine albumin-to-creatinine ratio decreased by 40% in the spironolactone group, with no change in the control group. Further blood pressure reduction may partially explain the beneficial effect, although an anti-inflammatory mechanism has also been proposed (38).

The efficacy and safety of eplerenone, a selective aldosterone blocker, has also been examined in a randomized trial of 268 patients with type 2 diabetes already treated with an ACE inhibitor (39). Compared with placebo, eplerenone therapy at a dose of 50 or 100 mg/day was associated with a significant reduction in urinary albumin excretion (40–50 vs. <10%). The authors concluded that eplerenone in combination with an ACE inhibitor provides an additive antiproteinuric effect, with the rate of hyperkalemia being similar to placebo. In clinical practice, the use of this combination should be used with caution in patients with GFR levels <40 ml/min. Patients should be instructed to reduce dietary potassium and avoid nonsteroidal anti-inflammatory drugs (NSAIDs) and cyclooxygenase (COX)-2 inhibitors, and they probably should be prescribed a concomitant kaliuretic diuretic therapy. The risk of hyperkalemia may possibly be lower with an ARB (16).

APPROACH TO PATIENT RAAS-ASSOCIATED RENAL DYSFUNCTION

A schema is presented in Fig. 36.5 to illustrate management plans for possible scenarios that may occur after initiation of RAAS-blocking treatment. A key point before making any change in medication dose or type is to ensure that patients avoid nephrotoxic medications, such as NSAIDs and aminoglycosides.

It is recommended that therapy should not be altered if the change in serum creatinine is small, i.e., <30% increase in serum creatinine concentration. The fall in GFR in this setting does not reflect structural injury and, to the degree that it is mediated by a reduction in intraglomerular pressure, may be associated with a long-term slowing in the rate of nephropathy progression (16,40). The initial decrease in filtration is reversible (16) (Fig. 36.3). Additionally, this was illustrated

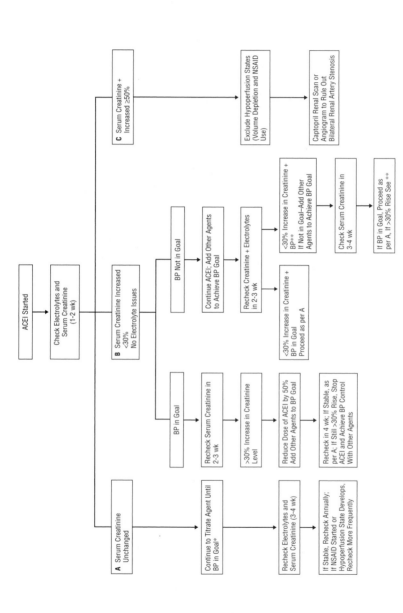

Figure 36.5 A suggested approach to deal with changes in kidney function in the presence of RAAS-blocking therapy. ACEI, ACE inhibitor; BP, blood pressure. Reprinted with permission from Bakris and Weir (16). Copyright ©2000 American Medical Association. All rights reserved.

in a report of 42 patients with type 1 diabetes and hypertension; cessation of anti-hypertensive therapy led to a rise in both blood pressure and glomerular filtration rate (from 76 to 81 ml/min) (40).

BIBLIOGRAPHY

1. Gaede P, Vedel P, Larsen N, Jensen GV, Parving HH, Pedersen O: Multifactorial intervention and cardiovascular disease in patients with type 2 diabetes. *N Engl J Med* 348:383–393, 2003

2. Manley S: Haemoglobin A1c--a marker for complications of type 2 diabetes: the experience from the UK Prospective Diabetes Study (UKPDS). *Clin Chem Lab Med* 41:1182–1190, 2003

3. Strippoli GF, Navaneethan SD, Johnson DW, Perkovic V, Pellegrini F, Nicolucci A, et al.: Effects of statins in patients with chronic kidney disease: meta-analysis and meta-regression of randomised controlled trials. *BMJ* 336:645–651, 2008

4. KDOQI: KDOQI Clinical Practice Guidelines and Clinical Practice Recommendations for Diabetes and Chronic Kidney Disease. *Am J Kidney Dis* 49 (2 Suppl. 2):S12–S154, 2007

5. Bakris GL: Progression of diabetic nephropathy: a focus on arterial pressure level and methods of reduction. *Diabetes Res Clin Pract* 39 (Suppl.):S35–S42, 1998

6. Lewis EJ, Hunsicker LG, Bain RP, Rohde RD: The effect of angiotensin-converting-enzyme inhibition on diabetic nephropathy: the Collaborative Study Group. *N Engl J Med* 329:1456–1462, 1993

7. Bakris GL, Weir MR, Shanifar S, Zhang Z, Douglas J, van Dijk DJ, et al.: Effects of blood pressure level on progression of diabetic nephropathy: results from the RENAAL study. *Arch Intern Med* 163:1555–1565, 2003

8. Rodby RA, Firth LM, Lewis EJ: An economic analysis of captopril in the treatment of diabetic nephropathy: the Collaborative Study Group. *Diabetes Care* 19:1051–1061, 1996

9. Fried LF, Orchard TJ, Kasiske BL: Effect of lipid reduction on the progression of renal disease: a meta-analysis. *Kidney Int* 59:260–269, 2001

10. Parving HH, Lehnert H, Brochner-Mortensen J, Gomis R, Andersen S, Arner P: The effect of irbesartan on the development of diabetic nephropathy in patients with type 2 diabetes. *N Engl J Med* 345:870–878, 2001

11. Brenner BM, Cooper ME, de Zeeuw D, Keane WF, Mitch WE, Parving HH, et al.: Effects of losartan on renal and cardiovascular outcomes in patients with type 2 diabetes and nephropathy. *N Engl J Med* 345:861–869, 2001

12. Lewis EJ, Hunsicker LG, Clarke WR, Berl T, Pohl MA, Lewis JB, et al.: Renoprotective effect of the angiotensin-receptor antagonist irbesartan in patients with nephropathy due to type 2 diabetes. *N Engl J Med* 345:851–860, 2001

13. Zhang Z, Shahinfar S, Keane WF, Ramjit D, Dickson TZ, Gleim GW, et al.: Importance of baseline distribution of proteinuria in renal outcomes trials: lessons from the reduction of endpoints in NIDDM with the angiotensin II antagonist losartan (RENAAL) study. *J Am Soc Nephrol* 16:1775–1780, 2005

14. Barnett AH, Bain SC, Bouter P, Karlberg B, Madsbad S, Jervell J, et al.: Angiotensin-receptor blockade versus converting-enzyme inhibition in type 2 diabetes and nephropathy. *N Engl J Med* 351:1952–1961, 2004

15. ONTARGET Investigators, Yusuf S, Teo KK, Pogue J, Dyal L, Copland I, Schumacher H, Dagenais G, Sleight P, Anderson C: Telmisartan, ramipril, or both in patients at high risk for vascular events. *N Engl J Med* 358:1547–1559, 2008

16. Bakris GL, Weir MR: Angiotensin-converting enzyme inhibitor-associated elevations in serum creatinine: is this a cause for concern? *Arch Intern Med* 160:685–693, 2000

17. Anderson S, Rennke HG, Brenner BM: Nifedipine versus fosinopril in uninephrectomized diabetic rats. *Kidney Int* 41:891–897, 1992

18. Griffin KA, Hacioglu R, bu-Amarah I, Loutzenhiser R, Williamson GA, Bidani AK: Effects of calcium channel blockers on "dynamic" and "steady-state step" renal autoregulation. *Am J Physiol Renal Physiol* 286:F1136–F1143, 2004

19. Brown SA, Brown CA: Single-nephron adaptations to partial renal ablation in cats. *Am J Physiol* 269:R1002–R1008, 1995

20. Yoshioka T, Shiraga H, Yoshida Y, Fogo A, Glick AD, Deen WM, et al.: "Intact nephrons" as the primary origin of proteinuria in chronic renal disease: study in the rat model of subtotal nephrectomy. *J Clin Invest* 82:1614–1623, 1988

21. Tarif N, Bakris GL: Preservation of renal function: the spectrum of effects by calcium-channel blockers. *Nephrol Dial Transplant* 12:2244–2250, 1997

21a. Abuelo JG: Normotensive ischemic acute renal failure. *N Engl J Med* 357:797–805, 2007

22. Bakris GL, Barnhill BW, Sadler R: Treatment of arterial hypertension in diabetic humans: importance of therapeutic selection. *Kidney Int* 41:912–919, 1992

23. Griffin KA, Picken MM, Bakris GL, Bidani AK: Class differences in the effects of calcium channel blockers in the rat remnant kidney model. *Kidney Int* 55:1849–1860, 1999

24. Sarnak MJ, Greene T, Wang X, Beck G, Kusek JW, Collins AJ, et al.: The effect of a lower target blood pressure on the progression of kidney disease: long-term follow-up of the modification of diet in renal disease study. *Ann Intern Med* 142:342–351, 2005

25. Nathan S, Pepine CJ, Bakris GL: Calcium antagonists: effects on cardio-renal risk in hypertensive patients. *Hypertension* 46:637–642, 2005

26. Abbott K, Smith A, Bakris GL: Effects of dihydropyridine calcium antagonists on albuminuria in patients with diabetes. *J Clin Pharmacol* 36:274–279, 1996

27. Bohlen L, de Courten M, Weidmann P: Comparative study of the effect of ACE-inhibitors and other antihypertensive agents on proteinuria in diabetic patients. *Am J Hypertens* 7:84S–92S, 1994

28. Remuzzi G, Chiurchiu C, Ruggenenti P: Proteinuria predicting outcome in renal disease: nondiabetic nephropathies (REIN). *Kidney Int Suppl* 92:S90–S96, 2004

29. Bakris GL, Weir MR, Secic M, Campbell B, Weis-McNulty A: Differential effects of calcium antagonist subclasses on markers of nephropathy progression. *Kidney Int* 65:1991–2002, 2004

30. Bakris GL, Weir MR, DeQuattro V, McMahon FG: Effects of an ACE inhibitor/calcium antagonist combination on proteinuria in diabetic nephropathy. *Kidney Int* 54:1283–1289, 1998

31. Brown SA, Walton CL, Crawford P, Bakris GL: Long-term effects of antihypertensive regimens on renal hemodynamics and proteinuria. *Kidney Int* 43:1210–1218, 1993

32. Dworkin LD, Tolbert E, Recht PA, Hersch JC, Feiner H, Levin RI: Effects of amlodipine on glomerular filtration, growth, and injury in experimental hypertension. *Hypertension* 27:245–250, 1996

33. Smith AC, Toto R, Bakris GL: Differential effects of calcium channel blockers on size selectivity of proteinuria in diabetic glomerulopathy. *Kidney Int* 54:889–896, 1998

34. Boero R, Rollino C, Massara C, Berto IM, Perosa P, Vagelli G, et al.: The verapamil versus amlodipine in nondiabetic nephropathies treated with trandolapril (VVANNTT) study. *Am J Kidney Dis* 42:67–75, 2003

35. Rachmani R, Slavachevsky I, Amit M, Levi Z, Kedar Y, Berla M, et al.: The effect of spironolactone, cilazapril and their combination on albuminuria in patients with hypertension and diabetic nephropathy is independent of blood pressure reduction: a randomized controlled study. *Diabet Med* 21:471–475, 2004

36. Sato A, Hayashi K, Naruse M, Saruta T: Effectiveness of aldosterone blockade in patients with diabetic nephropathy. *Hypertension* 41:64–68, 2003

37. van den Meiracker AH, Baggen RG, Pauli S, Lindemans A, Vulto AG, Poldermans D, et al.: Spironolactone in type 2 diabetic nephropathy: effects on proteinuria, blood pressure and renal function. *J Hypertens* 24:2285–2292, 2006

38. Han SY, Kim CH, Kim HS, Jee YH, Song HK, Lee MH, et al.: Spironolactone prevents diabetic nephropathy through an anti-inflammatory mechanism in type 2 diabetic rats. *J Am Soc Nephrol* 17:1362–1372, 2006

39. Epstein M, Williams GH, Weinberger M, Lewin A, Krause S, Mukherjee R, et al.: Selective aldosterone blockade with eplerenone reduces albuminuria in patients with type 2 diabetes. *Clin J Am Soc Nephrol* 1:940–951, 2006

40. Hansen PM, Goddijn PP, Kofoed-Enevoldsen A, van Tol KM, Bilo HJ, Deckert T: Diurnal variation in glomerular charge selectivity, urinary albumin excretion and blood pressure in insulin-dependent diabetic patients. *Kidney Int* 48:1559–1562, 1995

Drs. Duka and Bakris are from the Department of Medicine, Hypertensive Diseases Unit, Section of Endocrinology, Diabetes and Metabolism, University of Chicago Pritzker School of Medicine, Chicago, Illinois.

37. Skin and Subcutaneous Tissues

JEAN L. BOLOGNIA, MD, AND IRWIN M. BRAVERMAN, MD

The cutaneous disorders discussed in this chapter are waxy skin and stiff joints, scleredema, diabetic dermopathy, necrobiosis lipoidica (NL; diabeticorum), disseminated granuloma annulare, eruptive xanthomas, lipodystrophy, acanthosis nigricans, diabetic bullae, necrolytic migratory erythema (NME; glucagonoma syndrome), and reactions to oral hypoglycemic drugs and insulin. Cutaneous infections (e.g., candidiasis and mucormycosis) and lower-extremity ulcerations are covered in other chapters in this book.

PATHOPHYSIOLOGY

The underlying pathophysiology is theoretical in most of the cutaneous disorders associated with diabetes. In the skin lesions of NL and diabetic dermopathy, there is histological evidence of microangiopathy, and this presumably plays a role in the formation of lesions. In waxy skin associated with stiff joints, the thickened dermis may be the result of an increase in glycosylated insoluble collagen. The epidermal hyperplasia seen in lesions of acanthosis nigricans is thought to result from the action of circulating insulin on insulin-like growth factor receptors on keratinocytes and fibroblasts, whereas the epidermal necrosis seen in NME may be a reflection of glucagon-induced hypoaminoacidemia. Hypertriglyceridemia and eruptive xanthomas in the setting of diabetes are presumably due to the effects of hypoinsulinemia on lipid metabolism in that they quickly resolve after insulin administration.

WAXY SKIN AND STIFF JOINTS (CHEIROARTHROPATHY)

Up to 30% of young patients (aged 1–28 years) with type 1 diabetes have painless limited mobility of the small and large joints, and in individuals with diabetes for >5 years, the severity of joint disease is correlated with microvascular complications. Although involvement of the small joints of the hands can be demonstrated by the failure of the palmar surfaces of the interphalangeal joints to approximate ("prayer sign") (Fig. 37.1) or the inability to place the palms flat on a tabletop ("tabletop sign"), clinical detection may require passive extension of the digits. Approximately 30% of patients with limited joint mobility have tight, thick, waxy

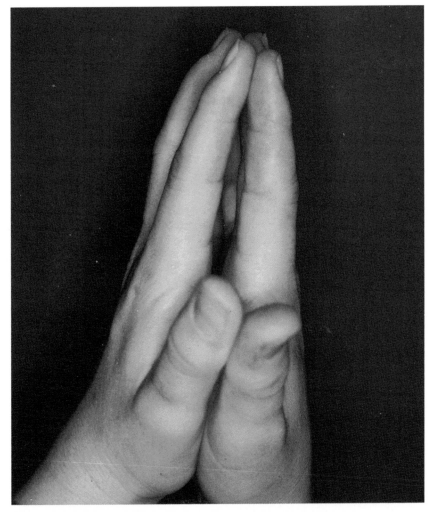

Figure 37.1 Failure of the palmar surfaces of interphalangeal joints to approximate in a patient with stiff joints and waxy skin.

skin of the dorsal aspect of the hands that is difficult to tent, i.e., is less extensible. This increased thickness can be confirmed by high-resolution ultrasonography, whereas thickening and enhancement of the flexor tendon sheaths may be seen by magnetic resonance imaging. Of note, thickened skin has been observed primarily in individuals with moderate to severe joint disease. These skin findings may reverse with improved control of diabetes, including pancreatic transplant; otherwise, there is no well-established treatment.

SCLEREDEMA

In scleredema, there is a thickening of the skin due to the deposition of glycosaminoglycans (in particular, hyaluronic acid) within the dermis. Areas of involvement may not be visually apparent, although they can develop a peau d'orange appearance as a result of prominent and depressed follicular openings (Fig. 37.2). The extent of involvement is best appreciated by palpation of the induration. Because scleredema is found most commonly on the upper back and posterior neck, the patient may be unaware of its presence. However, on physical examination, there is often decreased range of motion of the neck, especially dorsal extension. Less common sites of involvement include the face, upper arms, chest, lower back, and tongue. Rarely, there is cardiac, muscular, or esophageal involvement.

Scleredema has been associated with a monoclonal gammopathy or preceding streptococcal and viral infections as well as type 1 and type 2 diabetes (usually type 2 and long-standing). In the form seen in patients with diabetes, the induration may be accompanied by erythema (Fig. 37.2), which might be misdiagnosed as treatment-resistant cellulitis.

There is no consistently effective treatment for scleredema, although sometimes, especially in nondiabetic patients, spontaneous resolution may occur. In symptomatic patients, a 12-week course of PUVA [psoralens (8-methoxypsoralen,

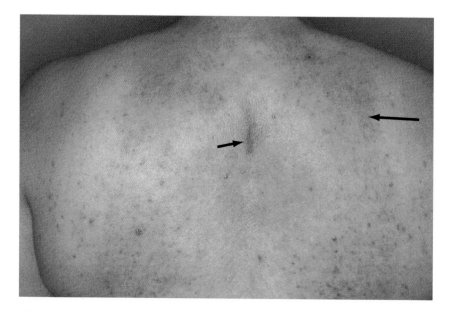

Figure 37.2 Scleredema of the upper back with overlying erythema (*large arrow*) and development of peau d'orange appearance centrally (*small arrow*).

0.4–0.6 mg/kg) plus ultraviolet A (UVA)] or UVA1 (340–400 nm) can be considered.

DIABETIC DERMOPATHY

Diabetic dermopathy is characterized by multiple hyperpigmented macules on the extensor surface of the distal lower extremities (Fig. 37.3). The individual lesions range in size from 0.5 to 2 cm, are oval or circular, and may have associated atrophy and scale. These skin changes have also been referred to as "shin spots" or "pigmented pretibial patches" and are thought to represent an abnormal response to trauma. In one series of 393 patients with type 2 diabetes, 12.5% had evidence of diabetic dermopathy, whereas in a second series of 173 patients (with both type 1 and type 2 diabetes), 40% had such lesions, in particular, individuals >50 years of age. These skin lesions may also be seen in individuals without evidence of glucose intolerance, albeit less often. In general, the dermopathy is asymptomatic except for its appearance, and no effective treatment has been described. However, a higher prevalence of neuropathy, retinopathy, nephropathy, and large-vessel disease has been reported in patients with diabetic dermopathy as compared with individuals without such skin lesions.

NL (DIABETICORUM)

Skin lesions of NL (diabeticorum) are so named because of: *1)* the presence of necrobiosis or degeneration of collagen in the dermis, *2)* the yellow color of most well-developed lesions due to carotene and lipid, and *3)* the association with diabetes. The disorder is characterized by red-brown to violet plaques that enlarge and frequently become yellow centrally. In addition, there is atrophy of the epidermis, which leads to shiny transparent skin and visualization of underlying dermal and subcutaneous vessels (Fig. 37.4). The most common location for NL is the shin (seen in 90% of patients), but lesions can also occur on the scalp, face, and arms. Plaques may ulcerate, especially those on the distal lower extremities.

NL is uncommon, occurring in 0.1–0.3% of the diabetic population, usually in the third or fourth decade of life. However, there is some disagreement as to the proportion of patients with NL who actually have frank diabetes. The range that is usually cited is 40–65%, based primarily on clinical series from the 1950s and 1960s. In a more recent retrospective study of consecutive patients seen over a period of 25 years, only 7 (11%) of 65 patients with classic biopsy-proven NL had diabetes at presentation.

There is no well-established treatment for NL, but in small series, some success has been reported with topical corticosteroids (with or without occlusion), pentoxifylline (400 mg three times per day), nicotinamide (500 mg three times per day), clofazimine (200 mg/day), and dipyridamole (50–75 mg three to four times per day) plus low-dose aspirin (325 mg/day). However, a double-blind, placebo-controlled trial of a combination of the latter two medications showed no significant benefit. Intralesional injections of corticosteroids (5 mg/ml triamcinolone

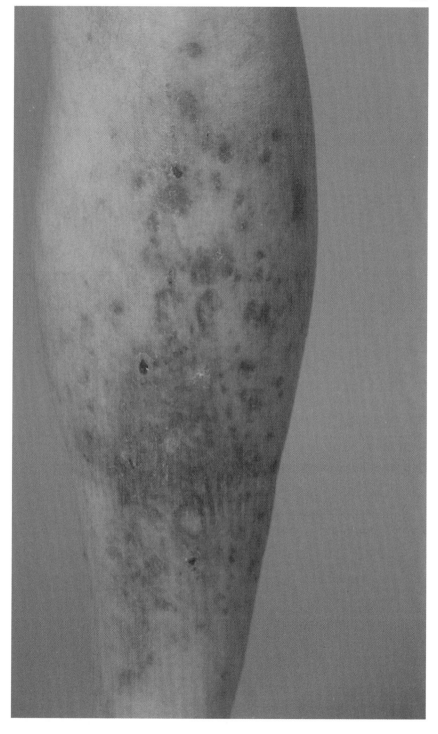

Figure 37.3 Hyperpigmented macules on the shin of a patient with diabetic dermopathy.

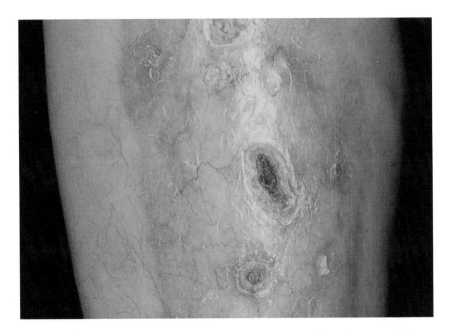

Figure 37.4 NL of the anterior lower extremity with its characteristic yellow color and atrophy leading to visualization of the underlying vessels. There are also multiple sites of ulceration.

acetonide) can be used to treat the active borders of the lesions. If ulceration occurs, the injections should be discontinued.

DISSEMINATED GRANULOMA ANNULARE

Granuloma annulare is characterized by annular or arciform plaques that form from the coalescence of skin-colored, pink, or red-brown papules (Fig. 37.5). The skin in the center of the lesion may be normal or slightly erythematous in appearance. Most commonly, granuloma annulare has an acral distribution, but the lesions can be more numerous, papular, and located on the trunk as well as the extremities. The term generalized or disseminated granuloma annulare is used to describe the latter patients. The clinical diagnosis can be confirmed by performing a skin biopsy. A patient with generalized granuloma annulare should be screened for glucose intolerance because in one series of 100 patients with generalized granuloma annulare, 21% were shown to have diabetes. The etiology of granuloma annulare is unknown, and the treatment is empiric and includes topical and intralesional corticosteroids (5 mg/ml triamcinolone acetonide), topical calcineurin inhibitors (twice daily), oral niacinamide (500 mg three times per day), and, in

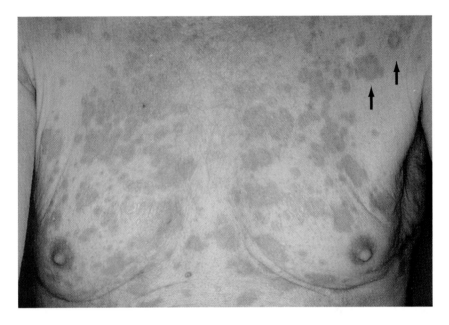

Figure 37.5 Generalized granuloma annulare. The annular shape of the lesions is best seen on the left shoulder.

severe cases, PUVA two to three times per week or oral hydroxychloroquine (200–400 mg/day).

XANTHOMAS

There are several types of cutaneous xanthomas, including eruptive, tendinous, tuberous, and planar, which are reflections of hypercholesterolemia and/or hypertriglyceridemia. Eruptive xanthomas can appear suddenly, and the lesions are usually 4–6 mm in diameter, firm, and yellow with a red base; the elbows, knees, buttocks, and sites of trauma are favored sites (Fig. 37.6). Biopsy findings are diagnostic and demonstrate collections of lipids within the dermis. The most common scenario for the appearance of eruptive xanthomas is hypertriglyceridemia in the setting of poorly controlled diabetes. Administration of insulin results in a decrease in the circulating levels of triglycerides, and the xanthomas quickly resolve. Xanthelasma (plane xanthoma of the eyelids) is the least specific marker of hyperlipidemia because 50% of the patients have normal lipid levels. In addition, there is no clear-cut association between diabetes and xanthelasma.

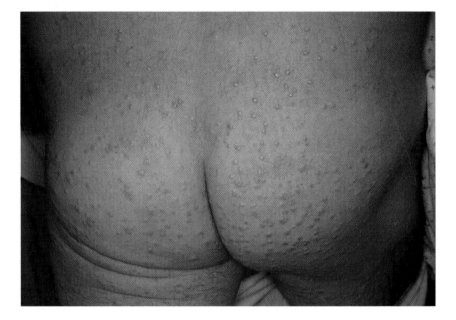

Figure 37.6 Eruptive xanthomas on the buttocks of a patient with poorly controlled diabetes.

LIPODYSTROPHY

Although the diseases outlined in this section are referred to as lipodystrophies, the patients have primarily lipoatrophy, and the lipoatrophy is divided into two major forms: total (generalized) and partial. In the generalized form, the entire body is involved. The onset is congenital (at birth or during infancy) in the inherited (autosomal recessive) form of the disease and during the first to third decades of life in the sporadic form. In contrast, partial lipoatrophy usually involves the extremities or the upper portion of the body (face to hips), is sporadic or less often familial, and has its onset during childhood or at puberty. Occasionally, there is also increased fat (lipohypertrophy) of the hips and legs. In biopsy specimens of areas of subcutaneous fat loss, the fat cells are present, but the cytoplasmic fat is absent.

Both forms of lipoatrophy, total and partial, are associated with insulin-resistant diabetes. Patients with total lipoatrophy also have increased muscle mass, hypertriglyceridemia, and fatty infiltration of the liver. In addition, those with congenital total lipoatrophy have hyperpigmentation, acanthosis nigricans, and generalized hirsutism. In contrast, ~40–50% of those with acquired partial lipoatrophy have evidence of membranoproliferative glomerulonephritis, often in association with hypocomplementemia.

ACANTHOSIS NIGRICANS

In acanthosis nigricans, velvety tan to dark-brown plaques are seen on the sides of the neck, axillae, and groin (Fig. 37.7). Additional sites of involvement include the extensor surface of the small joints of the hand, the elbows, and the knees. Acanthosis nigricans can be a reflection of an underlying malignancy, usually adenocarcinoma of the gastrointestinal tract, but is more commonly associated with insulin resistance and obesity.

The clinical spectrum in obese patients can range from euglycemia with mild hyperinsulinemia and tissue resistance to insulin-requiring diabetes. Acanthosis nigricans is also a cutaneous manifestation of the insulin-resistant syndromes (types A and B) and lipodystrophy (generalized and partial), as well as women with the HAIR-AN (hyperandrogenism, insulin resistance, acanthosis nigricans) syndrome. In obese patients, weight loss and improvement of tissue resistance to insulin has improved their acanthosis nigricans. Otherwise, treatment is limited to topical agents such as tretinoin (0.05–0.1%), urea (10–25%), and α-hydroxy acids (lactic and glycolic), which can improve the cosmetic appearance.

BULLOSIS DIABETICORUM (DIABETIC BULLAE)

The spontaneous formation of bullae in a primarily acral location (feet and distal lower extremities more than forearms and hands) is an uncommon manifestation

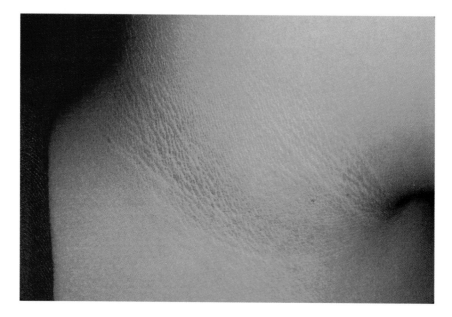

Figure 37.7 Velvety dark-brown plaques on the lateral neck of a patient with acanthosis nigricans.

of diabetes. The lesions arise from normal noninflamed skin and range in size from a few millimeters to several centimeters (Fig. 37.8). The blisters are usually tense and contain clear viscous fluid that is sterile. There is no history of antecedent trauma, and the lesions may recur. Two major forms exist and are distinguished by the site of blister formation: *1*) the blister is intraepidermal and heals without scarring or *2*) it is subepidermal and may heal with atrophy and mild scarring. Both types are found predominantly in middle-aged to elderly patients with long-standing diabetes who often have evidence of peripheral neuropathy. Other than local care (e.g., drainage and topical antibiotics to prevent secondary infection), there is no specific recommended treatment.

NME

Patients with NME have bright erythematous patches that are most frequently seen in the girdle area (lower abdomen, groin, buttocks, and thighs), perioral region, and extremities (Fig. 37.9). The cutaneous finding that distinguishes NME from other migratory eruptions is the presence of superficial bullae at the active borders. Because the bullae rapidly break, only denuded areas and crusts may be observed clinically. These areas then heal with superficial desquamation as the erythema advances.

Histologically, swollen and necrotic keratinocytes are seen in the superficial layers of the epidermis, findings similar to those seen in acrodermatitis enteropathica. In addition to the cutaneous eruption, the patients frequently have glossitis, anemia, weight loss, and diarrhea, as well as diabetes.

Most patients with classic NME have an α-cell tumor of the pancreas and markedly elevated serum glucagon levels (a variant termed "necrolytic acral erythema" is a cutaneous marker of liver disease, usually due to hepatitis C virus). Removal of the pancreatic tumor can result in prompt resolution of the cutaneous eruption. In inoperable cases, intermittent peripheral infusions of amino acids, zinc, and fatty acids; subcutaneous injections of the long-acting somatostatin analog octreotide acetate; or transcatheter arterial embolization of hepatic metastases can lead to improvement.

DRUG REACTIONS TO ORAL HYPOGLYCEMIC AGENTS AND INSULIN

Administration of oral hypoglycemic agents can lead to commonly recognized drug reactions such as pruritus, urticaria, morbilliform eruptions, and Stevens-Johnson syndrome. Phototoxic (dose-related exaggerated sunburn) and photoallergic (idiosyncratic eczematous dermatitis in a photodistribution) eruptions are additional potential cutaneous side effects and are related to the sulfur moiety found in sulfonylureas. A unique reaction is the chlorpropamide alcohol flush, which is similar to the disulfiram alcohol flush.

The cutaneous reactions to insulin can be divided into localized reactions, generalized reactions, and lipoatrophy/lipohypertrophy. The localized reactions

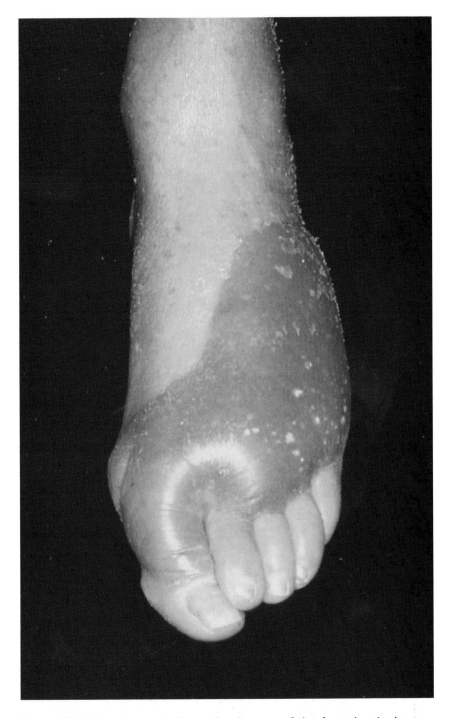

Figure 37.8 Tense large bulla on the dorsum of the foot that is characteristic of bullosis diabeticorum. From Braverman (1998).

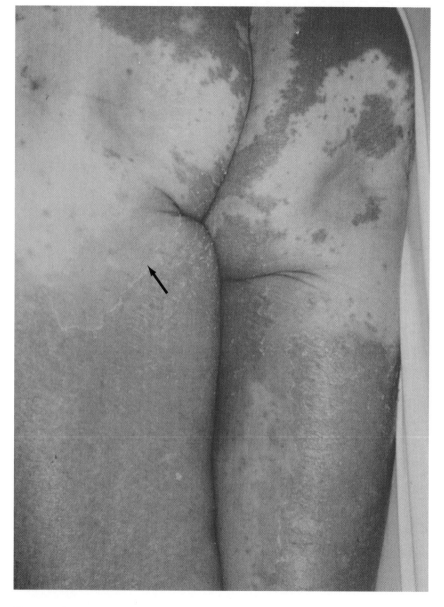

Figure 37.9 Angular erythematous patches on the buttocks and thighs of a patient with a glucagonoma of the pancreas; arrow, peripheral desquamation. From Braverman (1998).

include pruritus, burning, erythema, induration, and, occasionally, ulceration at the insulin injection site. Allergic local reactions vary from the immediate formation of an urticarial lesion at the injection site to the appearance of a pruritic papule or nodule 24–48 h after the injection. The latter lesions represent a delayed hypersensitivity reaction and, as such, heal slowly over a week or more and often leave residual hyperpigmentation. They frequently cease to form after several weeks or months. The primary treatment for persistent localized reactions is a switch to purer forms of insulin; if this is unsuccessful, the possibility of an allergy to the zinc, protamine, or preservative, such as paraben or meta-cresol, in the preparation should be considered as well as small quantities of natural latex rubber antigens from the insulin injection materials.

Generalized systemic reactions are uncommon and are characterized by pruritus, urticaria/angioedema, and serum sickness–like illnesses. The risk of a systemic reaction to insulin is related to the source and purification of the insulin, with bovine insulin having the highest incidence and human insulin the lowest. Diagnosis of IgE-mediated insulin allergy is based on measurement of specific IgE antibodies against insulin and protamine in addition to skin-prick/intracutaneous tests to insulin preparations and insulin additives. Treatment options for individuals already receiving human insulin include induction of tolerance via continuous subcutaneous insulin infusion, induction of tolerance via desensitization, and use of insulin analogs, e.g., lispro. Lipoatrophy at injection sites is seen with subcutaneous administration and is much less common with monocomponent or recombinant human insulin. Improvement in the areas of subcutaneous fat loss has been reported after injection of human insulin into the edge of the lipoatrophy. In patients already receiving human insulin, the use of a jet injector may prove beneficial. Lipohypertrophy (i.e., an increase in the amount of subcutaneous fat) can also be seen at the site of insulin injection. Treatment consists of rotation of injection sites and perhaps liposuction and the use of lispro.

BIBLIOGRAPHY

Bolognia JL, Braverman IM: Cutaneous complications of type 1 diabetes. In *Type 1 Diabetes: Etiology and Treatment.* Sperling MA, Ed. Totowa, NJ, Humana Press, 2003, p. 485–499

Braverman IM: *Skin Signs of Systemic Disease.* 3rd ed. Philadelphia, PA, Saunders, 1998

Heinzerling L, Raile K, Rochlitz H, Zuberbier T, Worm M: Insulin allergy: clinical manifestations and management strategies. *Allergy* 63:148–155, 2008

Jabbour SA: Cutaneous manifestations of endocrine disorders: a guide for dermatologists. *Am J Clin Dermatol* 4:315–331, 2003

Jelenick JE: *The Skin in Diabetes.* Philadelphia, PA, Lea & Febiger, 1986

Perez MI, Kohn SR: Cutaneous manifestations of diabetes mellitus. *J Am Acad Dermatol* 30:519–531, 1994

Radermecker RP, Scheen AJ: Allergic reactions to insulin: effects of continuous subcutaneous insulin infusion and insulin analogues. *Diabetes Metab Res Rev* 23:348–355, 2007

Rosenbloom AL, Silverstein JH, Lezotte DC, Richardson K, McCallum M: Limited joint mobility in childhood diabetes mellitus indicates increased risk for microvascular disease. *N Engl J Med* 305:191–194, 1981

Shemer A, Bergman R, Linn S, Kantor Y, Friedman-Birnbaum R: Diabetic dermopathy and internal complications in diabetes mellitus. *Int J Dermatol* 37:113–115, 1998

Drs. Bolognia and Braverman are Professors of Dermatology at the Yale University School of Medicine, New Haven, Connecticut.

38. Infections

Martin Kramer, MD, and Mary Ann Banerji, MD, FACP

Host immune defenses are altered in patients with diabetes. Hyperglycemia and acidosis alter the functions of phagocytic cells and result in changing their movement toward the site of an infection and impairing their microbiocidal activity. Subtle alterations in cell-mediated immunity predispose the patient to tuberculosis, coccidioidomycosis, and cryptococcosis. The host's metabolic state in diabetes also favors the specific nutritional requirements of some microbes. High glucose concentrations in blood and body fluids promote the overgrowth of certain fungal pathogens—particularly *Candida* species and *Zygomycetes*. *Zygomycetes* also grow more rapidly in an acidotic environment. Finally, mechanical factors largely contribute to the increased susceptibility of patients with diabetes to infections (Table 38.1). Treatment of infection in a patient with diabetes involves both antibiotic therapy and aggressive maintenance of good glycemic control. Table 38.2 provides an empiric antimicrobial treatment scheme for the management of the more common infections affecting diabetic patients. More specific details are described in subsequent sections.

There are now ample clinical data suggesting that hyperglycemia increases the risk for potentially serious infections. A study involving patients in an intensive care unit demonstrated that intensive insulin treatment that maintained blood glucose levels between 80 and 110 mg/dl (4.4 and 6.1 mmol/l) resulted in a significant decrease in mortality when these patients were compared with a control group with hyperglycemia. The largest decrease involved (autopsy-proven) deaths due to multiple end-organ failure with a septic focus. Thus, it is likely that good glycemic control will decrease the incidence and possibly the severity of infections.

SUPERFICIAL TISSUE INFECTIONS

Minor trauma to tissues affected by vascular insufficiency often initiates superficial tissue infection. In addition, peripheral sensory neuropathy leads to the occurrence of an insensibility to minor injuries, which delays care. Infection may take the form of a cellulitis, soft tissue necrosis, draining sinus, or osteomyelitis. Although the feet are most commonly involved in these infections, a similar process can occur in the skin beneath pressure points. In both situations, tissue undermining can be extensive.

Table 38.1 Mechanical Factors Contributing to Infections in Patients with Diabetes

Physiological Change	Disease Process	Result
Ischemic changes	Chronic diabetic vascular disease	Mixed bacterial foot infections
Depressed cough reflex	Cerebrovascular insults	Pneumonia
Impaired bladder emptying	Autonomic neuropathy	UTIs
Fecal incontinence	Autonomic neuropathy	Cutaneous maceration
Impaired mobility	Various abnormalities	Pressure sores

Diabetic Foot Infections

Diabetic foot infections with ulcers can be broadly divided into two categories: non–limb threatening and limb threatening.

Non–limb-threatening infections. Non–limb-threatening infections are associated with shallow ulcers, minimal cellulitis, minimal or no tissue necrosis, and no systemic symptoms. Treatment involves wound care and oral antibiotics. Gram-positive bacteria such as group A streptococci, *Staphylococcus aureus,* and possibly coagulase-negative staphylococci are usually involved. Oral antibiotics that are reasonable to use include dicloxacillin, cephalexin, amoxicillin/clavulanate, or clindamycin. A culture of the exudate would be useful if methicillin-resistant *S. aureus* (MRSA) is prevalent locally. Oral agents for MRSA include clindamycin, trimethoprim/sulfamethoxazole, and doxycycline. The latter two antibiotics generally have poor activity against β-hemolytic streptococci. Local susceptibility patterns should be checked. Maintaining good control of glucose levels is very important. Frequent observation is necessary to ensure that healing occurs.

Limb-threatening infections. Limb-threatening infections are associated with ulcers that are usually deep; the infection extends to the subcutaneous tissue or deeper with significant tissue necrosis and systemic symptoms. Patients must be hospitalized, and surgical evaluation (and often intervention) is essential. The bacteriology of these infections includes the Gram-positive bacteria mentioned above, Gram-negative bacteria (e.g., *Escherichia coli* and *Pseudomonas aeruginosa*), and anaerobic bacteria (e.g., *Bacteroides fragilis* and *Peptostreptococcus* species). Deep-wound cultures and Gram stains (preferably scrapings or curettage of tissue) should be done to determine therapy. In addition to determining the bacteriology, antimicrobial susceptibility must be determined in view of the increasing antimicrobial resistance of Gram-negative and Gram-positive bacteria (i.e., MRSA). Empiric intravenous antibiotic therapy is directed at the presumed organisms mentioned above. Examples of such regimens include piperacillin/tazobactam, ticarcillin/clavulanate, imipenem/cilastatin, or meropenem. There are many other potentially effective regimens (see Stevens, 2005). Any regimen used should take into account

Table 38.2 Empiric Antimicrobial Treatment

Organ System	Usual Organism	Primary	Alternate
Urinary Tract			
Bacteruria			
Asymptomatic male or female		No treatment	
Acute uncomplicated cystitis/urethritis	*E. coli, S. saphrophyticus*	Fluoroquinolone	Trimethoprim/sulfamethoxazole
			Ampicillin/clavulanate
			Vancomycin
	Enterococci	Ampicillin	
Acute pyelonephritis	*E. coli*	Fluoroquinolones	Ticarcillin/clavulanate 3
Hospitalized		Third-generation	or piperacillin/
		cephalosporin	tazobactam
	Enterococci	Ampicillin	Vancomycin
Perinephric abscess (drainage as required)			
With pyelonephritis	*E. coli*	Treat as for	
		pyelonephritis	
With *S. aureus* bacteremia	*S. aureus*	Nafcillin *or* oxacillin	Cephazolin
			Vancomycin
Gall Bladder			
Cholecystitis	Enterobacteriaceae	Piperacillin/tazobactam	Ceftazidime *plus* metronidazole
	Enterococci, Bacteroides	Ampicillin/sulbactam	Aztreonam *plus* clindamycin
		Ticarcillin/clavulanate	Ampicillin *plus* gentamicin with
			or without metronidazole
If life-threatening		Imipenem/cilastatin *or*	
		meropenem	
Emphysematous	Polymicrobial, including	Imipenem/cilastatin	
	Clostridium species	*or* meropenem	

(Continued)

Table 38.2 Empiric Antimicrobial Treatment (Continued)

Organ System	Usual Organism	Primary	Alternate
Ear, Nose, and Throat			
Rhinocerebral mucormycosis	*Mucor* and *Rhizopus* species	Amphotericin B	
Invasive otitis externa	*P. aeruginosa*	Ciprofloxacin Ceftazidime	Imipenem/cilastatin Meropenem Piperacillin
Foot			
Non-limb/life threatening Mild, previously untreated*	*S. aureus, streptococci*	Clindamycin, cephalosporin Amoxicillin/ clavulanate	
Chronic	Polymicrobial: *S. aureus, streptococci,* *E. coli, Proteus, Klebsiela/* Anaerobes (e.g., *B. fragilis*)	Ampicillin/sulbactam Piperacillin/tazobactam Ticarcillin/clavulanate Clindamycin *plus* ceftriaxone or cefotaxime	
Limb/life threatening	Polymicrobial: as above	Imipenem/cilastatin *or* meropenem *plus* vancomycin	
Soft Tissue			
Necrotizing fasciitis	Group A *streptococcus,* *Clostridia* species Polymicrobial	Penicillin G *plus* clindamycin Imipenem/cilastatin Meropenem	

*Shallow and no ischemia, abscess, or osteomyelitis. All antibiotic use and dosing should take into account renal and hepatic function, clinical circumstance, contraindications, and drug toxicity. These are examples of regimens likely to be effective. Other regimens may also be effective in specific circumstances. Examples of fluoroquinolones with enhanced activity are levofloxacin, ciprofloxacin, and moxifloxacin; examples of third-generation cephalosporins are ceftriaxone and cefotaxime.

features such as local antimicrobial susceptibility data (i.e., the prevalence of MRSA), drug toxicity, and contraindications.

Patients with diabetes are more susceptible to developing severe necrotizing/gangrenous infections. These may be monomicrobial (i.e., caused by *Streptococcus* species, primarily β-hemolytic streptococcus such as group A) or polymicrobial. Immediate surgical intervention is warranted. Broad-spectrum antibiotic therapy (see above) is indicated for polymicrobial infection. In group A streptococcal necrotizing fasciitis (which may result in streptococcal toxic shock syndrome [TSS]), both high-dose penicillin and clindamycin should be used. There are anecdotal data that intravenous immune globulin may be beneficial in treating streptococcal TSS.

MALIGNANT OTITIS EXTERNA

Malignant otitis externa is an infection usually caused by *Pseudomonas aeruginosa* that occurs almost exclusively in patients with diabetes. It is a chronic erosive process that initially involves the soft tissue and cartilage around the external auditory canal. There is pain and drainage of purulent material and progressive destruction as the process progresses into the temporal and petrous bones and mastoids. The infection progresses regardless of tissue planes and ultimately reaches cranial nerves, the meninges, and/or the sigmoid sinus. Paralysis of nerves 7, 9, 10, 11, and possibly 12 may occur. Treatment consists of local debridement of necrotic tissue and prolonged therapy with anti-pseudomonal antibiotics. Because osteomyelitis is usually present, the course of therapy should be at least 4–6 weeks. Useful antimicrobial agents are listed in Table 38.2.

URINARY TRACT INFECTIONS

Women with diabetes have a two- to fourfold higher incidence of bacteriuria than nondiabetic women and diabetic men. *E. coli* and other Gram-negative bacteria cause most urinary tract infections (UTIs). Hematogenous infection is most commonly caused by *S. aureus*. In contrast to nondiabetic women, women with diabetes have frequent involvement of the upper urinary tract (43–80% of cases). Acute pyelonephritis has a similar presentation in diabetic patients, and the response to therapy is likewise similar. A failure to respond to appropriate therapy raises the possibility of complications, including perinephric abscess, renal papillary necrosis, emphysematous cystitis, or emphysematous pyelonephritis. These complications need to be rapidly diagnosed and aggressively treated.

When upper UTI is suspected, patients should be hospitalized and treated with intravenous antibiotics and hydration. If there is poor response after 3–4 days of therapy, the above-mentioned complications should be sought using radiological investigations. The usual duration of therapy in uncomplicated infection with intravenous and subsequent oral antibiotics is 14 days.

Asymptomatic bacteriuria is common in women with diabetes. There is no evidence that therapy of asymptomatic bacteriuria is beneficial because relapse rates are high and therapy does not prevent the development of symptomatic

UTIs. Screening for asymptomatic bacteruria in diabetic women is therefore not recommended. *Candida* UTIs are usually associated with indwelling bladder catheters or anatomic abnormalities. Less commonly, hematogenous spread occurs. *Candida* UTIs rarely occur otherwise. The presentation of *Candida* UTIs is similar to that of bacterial cystitis. Paranchymal involvement may result in pyelonephritis, abscess formation, or the development of fungus balls (which may also cause obstruction). Treatment consists of removal of the urinary catheters and/or the correction of anatomic abnormality. Symptomatic infection can be treated with fluconazole. There is no clear benefit to treating asymptomatic infection.

ABDOMINAL INFECTIONS

Emphysematous cholecystitis occurs with an increased frequency in patients with diabetes. Approximately 35% of the cases occur in patients with diabetes, and emphysematous cholecystitis is associated with increased mortality in 15% of patients with diabetes compared with <4% of individuals without diabetes. The presentation is similar to that of uncomplicated cholecystitis. The presence of crepitations, clinical deterioration, or failure to improve with conservative therapy should lead to radiological evaluation. Surgical intervention, in addition to broad-spectrum antimicrobial therapy, may be lifesaving.

FUNGAL INFECTIONS

Mucormycosis (Zygomycosis)

Much less common but much more devastating is infection caused by the agents of mucormycosis (primarily the *Zygomycetes*). The syndrome most often seen in patients with diabetes is rhinocerebral mucormycosis. This is an invasive process caused by the mycelia of the genera *Mucor, Absidia, Rhizopus, Cunninghamella,* and others. The conidia of the organisms are unable to regenerate if ingested by normal macrophages, and the organisms are essentially nonpathogenic in the normal host. The growth of *Rhizopus* is inhibited by normal human serum. However, these fungi can grow rapidly in the presence of high concentrations of glucose and in an acid environment. Both conditions prevail in the patient with ketoacidosis. In such patients, these organisms are able to germinate at the site of infections (usually the nares and the sinuses) and to begin a rapid necrotizing process that characterizes rhinocerebral mucormycosis. Within a few days, the process may extend from a small eschar on the nasal septum to involve the paranasal sinuses and orbit. The infection proceeds without regard for tissue planes. It can track into the brain within a few days, and the result is often lethal if not diagnosed and treated at an early stage.

Diagnosis is by prompt aggressive surgical biopsy, including tissues deep to the area of necrosis. *Zygomycetes* are different from other fungi in that they stain better with hematoxylin and eosin than with methenamine silver. Identification of irregular pleomorphic nonseptate branching hyphae is pathognomonic. *Zygomycetes* must be differentiated from *Aspergillus,* which is the most similar in appearance.

The hyphae of *Aspergillus* do not stain well with hematoxylin and eosin. Treatment of zygomycosis infection includes correction of ketoacidosis, vigorous and repeated surgical debridement, and antifungal therapy with amphotericin B. Azole antifungal drugs are not effective against *Zygomycetes*, although pocaconazole, a recently approved orally administered triazole, has shown promise as salvage therapy. Pocaconazole is not U.S. Food and Drug Administration (FDA)-approved for the treatment of zygomycosis.

PULMONARY INFECTIONS

It is not clear whether diabetes is associated with an increased incidence of pneumonia. However, the spectrum of pneumonia is different in patients with diabetes. There is an increased frequency of infections with Gram-negative bacteria (e.g., *Klebsiella* and *E. coli*), *S. aureus*, *Mycobacterium tuberculosis*, and certain fungi such as *Aspergillus*, *Mucor*, *Cryptococcus*, and *Coccidiodes*. Other infections caused by *Streptococcus pneumoniae* (especially bacteremia), the influenza virus, and *Legionella* may be associated with increased morbidity and mortality. This spectrum of pulmonary infections needs to be considered with regard to diagnosis, (empiric) treatment, and clinical follow-up to ensure that the infection is resolving appropriately. Table 38.3 outlines an empiric approach to antimicrobial treatment for pulmonary infections.

Prevention of pneumonia should be addressed in all patients with diabetes. The Advisory Committee on Immunization Practices recommends that all patients with diabetes be vaccinated once with the pneumococcal vaccine and annually with the influenza vaccine. All patients with diabetes should undergo tuberculin skin testing to diagnose latent tuberculosis infection. The risk of a diabetic patient with a positive skin test developing active tuberculosis is two- to fourfold greater than that for a patient without diabetes with the same positive test. Patients with diabetes with a positive tuberculin skin test >10 mm should be strongly considered for preventive chemotherapy once active tuberculosis is excluded.

BIBLIOGRAPHY

Blumberg HM, Burman WJ, Chaisson RE, Daley CL, Etkind SC, Friedman LN, Fujiwara P, Grzemska M, Hopewell PC, Iseman MD, Jasmer RM, Koppaka V, Menzies RI, O'Brien RJ, Reves RR, Reichman LB, Simone PM, Starke JR, Vernon AA: American Thoracic Society/Centers for Disease Control and Prevention/Infectious Disease Society of America: treatment of tuberculosis. *Am J Respir Crit Care Med* 167:603–663, 2003

Calvert HM, Yoshikawa T: Infections in diabetes. *Infect Dis Clin North Am* 15:407–421, 2001

Harding GKM, Zhanel GG, Nicolle LE, Cheang M, Manitoba Diabetes Urinary Tract Infection Study Group: Antimicrobial treatment in diabetic women with asymptomatic bacteriuria. *N Engl J Med* 347:1576–1583, 2002

Table 38.3 Recommended Empirical Antibiotics for Community-Acquired Pneumonia

Outpatients

1. Previously healthy and no use of antimicrobials within the previous 3 months.
 ■ Macrolide (strong recommendation; level I evidence)
 ■ Doxycycline (weak recommendation; level III evidence)
2. Presence of comorbidities, such as chronic heart, lung, liver or renal disease; diabetes; alcoholism; malignancies; asplenia; immunosuppressing conditions or use of immunosuppressant drugs; or use of antimicrobials within the previous 3 months (in which case an alternative from a different class should be selected)
 ■ Respiratory fluoroquinolone: moxifloxacin, gemifloxacin, or levofloxacin (750 mg) (strong recommendation; level I evidence)
 ■ β-Lactam **plus** a macrolide (strong recommendation; level I evidence)
3. In regions with a high rate (>25%) of infection with high-level (MIC ≥16 µg/ml) macrolide-resistant *Streptococcus pneumoniae*, consider use of alternative agents listed in 2. for patients without comorbidities (moderate recommendation; level III evidence)

Inpatients: non-ICU treatment

■ Respiratory fluoroquinolone (strong recommendation; level I evidence)
■ β-Lactam **plus** a macrolide (strong recommendation; level I evidence)

Inpatients: ICU treatment

■ β-Lactam (cefotaxime, ceftriaxone, or ampicillin/sulbactam) **plus** either azithromycin (strong recommendation; level II evidence) or a respiratory fluoroquinolone (strong recommendation; level I evidence)
 For penicillin-allergic patients, a respiratory fluoroquinolone and aztreonam are recommended.

Special concerns

*If **Pseudomonas** is a consideration*
 ■ An antipneumococcal, antipseudomonal β-lactam (piperacillin/tazobactam, cefepime, imipenem, or meropenem) **plus** either ciprofloxacin or levofloxacin (750 mg)
 or
 ■ The above β-lactam **plus** an aminoglycoside and azithromycin
 or
 ■ The above β-lactam **plus** an aminoglycoside and an antipneumococcal fluoroquinolone (for penicillin-allergic patients, substitute aztreonam for above β-lactam) (moderate recommendation; level III evidence)

*If **CA-MRSA** is a consideration*
 ■ Add vancomycin or linezolid (moderate recommendation; level III evidence).

CA-MRSA, community-acquired methicillin-resistant *Staphylococus aureus*; ICU, intensive care unit. From Mandell et al. (2007). Reprinted with permission by The University of Chicago Press. ©2007 by The University of Chicago Press.

Joshi N, Caputo GM, Weitekamp MR, Karchmer AW: Infections in patients with diabetes mellitus. *N Engl J Med* 341:1906–1912, 1999

Karchmer AW, Gibbons G: Foot infections in diabetes: evaluation and management. *Curr Clin Top Infect Dis* 14:1–22, 1994

Mandell LA, Wunderink RG, Anzueto A, Bartlett JG, Campbell GD, Dean NC, Dowell SF, File TM Jr, Musher DM, Niederman MS, Torres A, Whitney CG, Infectious Diseases Society of America; American Thoracic Society: Infectious Diseases Society of America/American Thoracic Society consensus guidelines on the management of community-acquired pneumonia in adults. *Clin Infect Dis* 44 (Suppl. 2):S27–S72, 2007

Nicolle LE, Bradley S, Colgan R, Rice JC, Schaeffer A, Hooton TM, Infectious Diseases Society of America, American Society of Nephrology, American Geriatric Society: Infectious Diseases Society of America guidelines for the diagnosis and treatment of asymptomatic bacteriuria in adults. *Clin Infect Dis* 40:643–654, 2005 [erratum *Clin Infect Dis* 40:1556, 2005]

Stevens DL, Bisno AL, Chambers HF, Everett ED, Dellinger P, Goldstein EJ, Gorbach SL, Hirschmann JV, Kaplan EL, Montoya JG, Wade JC, Infectious Diseases Society of America: Practice guidelines for the diagnosis and management of skin and soft-tissue infections. *Clin Infect Dis* 41:1373–1406, 2005 [errata *Clin Infect Dis* 41:1830, 2005; *Clin Infect Dis* 42:1219, 2006]

Van den Berghe G, Wouters P, Weekers F, Verwaest C, Bruyninckx F, Schetz M, Vlasselaers D, Ferdinande P, Lauwers P, Bouillon R: Intensive insulin therapy in critically ill patients. *N Engl J Med* 345:1359–1367, 2001

Dr. Kramer is Associate Professor of Clinical Medicine from the Division of Infectious Diseases State University of New York (SUNY) Downstate Medcial Center and Chief of Infection Control at Kings County Hospital, Brooklyn, New York. Dr. Banerji is Professor of Medicine from the Division of Endocrinology, SUNY Downstate Medical Center, Brooklyn, New York.

39. Ocular Complications

Paolo S. Silva, MD, Jerry D. Cavallerano, OD, PhD, Lloyd M. Aiello, MD, and Lloyd Paul Aiello, MD, PhD

D iabetes will affect >350 million people worldwide by the year 2030. Diabetic retinopathy is the most prevalent of the diabetes complications, affecting nearly half of all individuals with diabetes at any point in time. Almost all people with diabetes will eventually develop some degree of diabetic retinopathy. According to the International Diabetes Federation (2003), diabetic retinopathy is the leading cause of new-onset blindness, severe visual loss, and moderate visual loss in individuals of working age in most developed countries.

Diabetic retinopathy and diabetic macular edema (DME) affect individuals with both type 1 and type 2 diabetes. Type 1 diabetic patients, because of the earlier onset and longer duration of diabetes, experience more frequent and severe ocular complications. After 5 years of diabetes, 23% of type 1 diabetic patients have diabetic retinopathy. After 10 and 15 years, this prevalence increases to almost 60 and 80%, respectively. Proliferative diabetic retinopathy (PDR), the most sight-threatening stage of the disease, is present in 25 and 56% of patients with type 1 diabetes after 15 and 20 years, respectively, and often remains asymptomatic until it has progressed substantially beyond the optimal stage for initiating treatment.

In type 2 diabetes, diabetic retinopathy was present in 20% of cases at diagnosis, increasing to 60–85% after 15 years, as assessed by the Wisconsin Epidemiologic Study of Diabetic Retinopathy. PDR was present in 3–4% of patients within 4 years, 5–20% of patients after 15 years, and >50% after ≥20 years. Thus, patients with type 2 diabetes are more likely to have diabetic retinopathy at diagnosis and are more likely to develop diabetic retinopathy sooner after diagnosis than patients with type 1 diabetes.

Of the nearly 24 million Americans estimated to have diabetes by the Centers for Disease Control and Prevention (CDC), 700,000 have PDR and 500,000 have DME, resulting in 12,000–24,000 new cases of blindness each year and making diabetic retinopathy the leading cause of new-onset blindness in the U.S. Fortunately, there are interventions that have significant benefit in preserving vision. Adherence to intensive blood glucose control regimens, as demonstrated by the Diabetes Control and Complications Trial (DCCT) and the U.K. Prospective Diabetes Study (UKPDS), can reduce the rates of onset and progression of diabetic retinopathy. Laser surgery can ameliorate the devastating effects of diabetic retinal disease, particularly when laser surgery is initiated promptly once indicated. Timely laser photocoagulation can reduce the risk of severe visual loss (best vision of 5/200 or worse) from high-risk PDR to <4%. Timely laser surgery of DME can reduce the risk of moderate visual loss (a doubling of the visual angle, e.g., 20/20 reduced to 20/40) by ≥50%. Vitrectomy surgery can restore useful vision by removing vitreous hemorrhage or by relieving retinal traction threatening the macula. Novel therapies, such as intravitreal injection of steroids or anti–vascular endothelial growth factor (VEGF) factors, frequently in conjunction with laser photocoagulation, may further reduce the risk of vision loss and preserve vision; however, results of studies definitively detailing their efficacy and risks are not yet available.

Early detection and treatment of diabetic retinopathy are critical, but it is estimated that only 55% of the diabetic population receives adequate ophthalmic care. Emphasis must therefore be placed on early detection of retinal disorders, with appropriate referral for management and treatment. In addition, careful control of blood glucose levels and concurrent systemic conditions such as hypertension, renal disease, and dyslipidemia is critical.

DIABETIC RETINOPATHY

Pathophysiology

Elevated blood glucose levels result in structural, physiological, and biochemical changes that alter cellular metabolism, retinal blood flow, and retinal capillary competency. Classic pathophysiological processes characterize diabetic retinopathy and include biochemical changes affecting cellular metabolism, decreased retinal blood flow, impaired vascular autoregulation, loss of retinal pericytes, outpouchings of the capillary walls to form microaneurysms, closure of retinal capillaries and arterioles (resulting in retinal ischemia), increased vascular permeability of retinal capillaries (sometimes leading to retinal edema), proliferation of new vessels (with or without vitreous hemorrhage), development of fibrous tissue, and contraction of vitreous and fibrous proliferation with subsequent retinal traction and detachment.

Clinically, these processes are manifested as either PDR, nonproliferative diabetic retinopathy (NPDR), or DME (Table 39.1). These and other processes of diabetic retinopathy may affect the macula, significantly altering function and reading vision. Loss of vision from diabetes usually results from vitreous hemorrhage, PDR leading to fibrous tissue formation and subsequent traction retinal detachment, or DME.

Clinical Care

Current management strategies for diabetic retinopathy are guided by results of large well-designed clinical trials. There have been five landmark studies that have been particularly instrumental in establishing the minimum standard of eye care for diabetic patients to optimally preserve vision and reduce the threat of visual loss.

Table 39.1 Clinical Manifestations of Retinopathy

NPDR

■ Mild—one or both of the following:
  – Few scattered retinal microaneurysms and hemorrhages
  – Hard exudate
■ Moderate—one or more of the following:
  – More extensive retinal hemorrhages and/or microaneurysms
  – Mild IRMAs
  – Early venous beading
■ Severe to very severe—one or more of the following:
  – Severe hemorrhages and/or microaneurysms in all four quadrants
  – Venous beading in at least two quadrants
  – More extensive IRMAs in at least one quadrant

PDR

■ Early
  – Minimal NVD <1/4 disc area without preretinal or vitreous hemorrhage
                              or
  – NVE without preretinal or vitreous hemorrhage
■ High-risk
  – NVD ≥1/4 disc area with or without preretinal or vitreous hemorrhage
                              or
  – NVD <1/4 disc area in extent accompanied by fresh hemorrhage
                              or
  – NVE ≥1/2 disc area with preretinal or vitreous hemorrhage

IRMA, intraretinal microvascular abnormalities; NVD, new vessels on the optic disc; NVE, new vessels elsewhere on the retina. DME may occur at any level of diabetic retinopathy, although it is more common with more advanced retinopathy.

The Diabetic Retinopathy Study (1971–1975) definitively established the beneficial effects of scatter (panretinal) laser photocoagulation for PDR. The Early Treatment Diabetic Retinopathy Study (ETDRS) (1979–1990) demonstrated the benefit of focal laser treatment for DME and provided insight into the most appropriate timing for retinal laser surgery for diabetic retinopathy and DME. The ETDRS also demonstrated that the use of 650 mg aspirin/day is unlikely to have any effect on the progression of diabetic retinopathy or the risk of vitreous hemorrhage in the presence of diabetic retinopathy. The Diabetic Retinopathy Vitrectomy Study (1977–1987) established early guidelines for the timing of surgical intervention after visual loss from vitreous hemorrhage. The Diabetes Control and Complications Trial (1983–1993) demonstrated that intensive control of blood glucose levels in patients with type 1 diabetes, resulting in at least a 1% drop in A1C levels, reduces the risk of onset of any diabetic retinopathy, the progression of retinopathy, and the need for laser surgery. The UKPDS (1977–1999) found similar results of intensive blood glucose control for patients with type 2 diabetes. Additionally, the UKPDS found that more intensive control of blood pressure, with either a β-blocking agent or an ACE inhibitor, reduced the risk of progression of retinopathy.

Diagnosis: Clinical Levels of Diabetic Retinopathy and DME

Diabetic retinopathy can be broadly classified into nonproliferative diabetic retinopathy and proliferative diabetic retinopathy. Based on the presence and degree of retinal lesions, NPDR is clinically classified as mild, moderate, severe, or very severe. PDR is marked by proliferation of new vessels on the optic disc (NVD), new vessels elsewhere on the retina (NVE), preretinal hemorrhage, vitreous hemorrhage, or fibrous tissue proliferation. DME can be present with any level of diabetic retinopathy. Accurate diagnosis of the severity of diabetic retinopathy is essential, since the risk of progression to PDR and high-risk PDR is closely correlated with specific NPDR level. Proper diagnosis of diabetic retinopathy severity establishes the risk of progression to sight-threatening retinopathy and appropriate clinical management both in terms of follow-up schedule and therapeutic options.

NPDR

Mild NPDR, characterized by microaneurysms with or without occasional blot hemorrhages, is virtually ubiquitous after 15–17 years of diabetes. Microaneurysms may resolve slowly with time or show little or no change. Dot hemorrhages and microaneurysms can be considered together clinically as one type of lesion. They are frequently indistinguishable from one another by ophthalmoscopic examination without fluorescein angiography, and identifying them separately does not add any benefit in terms of predicting progression risk. The invasive fluorescein angiography testing is not warranted at this stage of diabetic retinopathy unless macular edema threatening central vision is present. The microaneurysms represent outpouchings of blood vessel walls, possibly secondary to weakness of the capillary wall from loss of pericytes or from increased intraluminal pressure or due to endothelial proliferation.

Rare flecks of hard exudates, representing small white or yellowish white deposits, generally with sharp borders, may be present in the intermediate layers of the retina. Hard exudates are lipid deposits leaked from microaneurysms or compromised capillary beds and may be present at any stage of NPDR and PDR. Patients with mild NPDR can safely be followed every 9–12 months unless macular edema is present (Table 39.1).

Moderate NPDR is characterized by more severe retinal lesions. These lesions represent not only changes in vascular and perivascular tissue, but also changes within the retina associated with the effects of relative retinal hypoxia and circulatory changes. More abundant retinal hemorrhages and microaneurysms are present (Fig. 39.1). Early venous caliber abnormalities may also be present, reflected clinically as tortuous vasculature with varying lumen size. Venous caliber abnormalities may be caused by either sluggish blood flow, blood vessel wall weakening, or hypoxia.

Another vascular change observed in moderate NPDR is intraretinal microvascular abnormalities (Fig. 39.2). Intraretinal microvascular abnormalities are a type of intraretinal neovascularization. Cotton-wool spots may also be present at this stage and represent micro-infarct–induced stasis of axoplasmic flow in the nerve fiber layer of the retina. Cotton-wool spots tend to disappear as NPDR becomes more severe.

Patients with moderate NPDR have more significant retinal disease. These patients are at greater risk for progression to vision-threatening diabetic retinopathy and are best monitored every 4–6 months.

Severe or very severe NPDR is characterized by an abundance of nonproliferative lesions that include venous beading (Fig. 39.3), intraretinal microvascular abnormalities (Fig. 39.2), and/or extensive hemorrhages and microaneurysms (Fig. 39.1). There is a high risk for progression to PDR due to the widespread retinal ischemia, but frank new-vessel growth on the retina is not present. Consultation with an ophthalmologist experienced in the management of diabetic eye disease for possible early laser surgery is urgent, particularly if exacerbating conditions exist (e.g., hypertension, renal disease, or pregnancy) or if the patient seems to be nonadherent or late with follow-up examination. Rates of progression to high-risk PDR approach 45–50% in 2 years and 75% in 5 years if untreated. Patients with type 2 diabetes may be candidates for scatter laser photocoagulation at this time (i.e., before developing high-risk PDR).

PDR

PDR represents a severe form of retinopathy. It is characterized by the growth of new vessels on or within 1 disc diameter of the optic disc (NVD), the growth of NVE, vitreous or preretinal hemorrhage, or preretinal fibrous tissue proliferation.

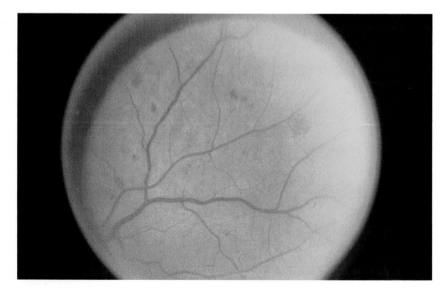

Figure 39.1 This severity and extent of hemorrhages or micro-aneurysms in all four quadrants constitutes severe NPDR. Standard photograph 2A.

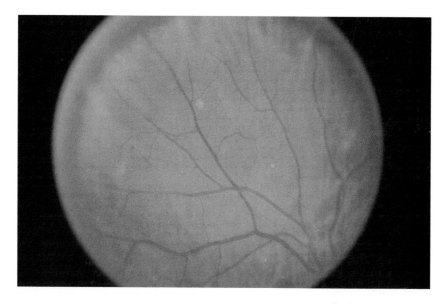

Figure 39.2 This extent of IRMAs in one or more quadrant constitutes severe NPDR. Standard photograph 8A.

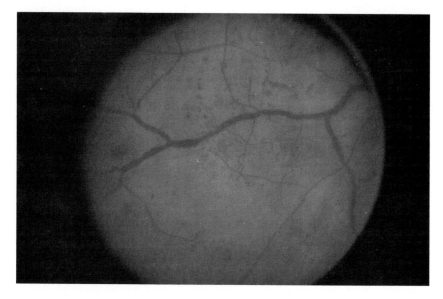

Figure 39.3 Venous beading in two or more quadrants constitutes severe NPDR. Standard photograph 6B.

These vessels grow over the retinal surface and on the posterior surface of the vitreous. They are fragile and rupture easily, causing preretinal and vitreous hemorrhage. The vessels can rupture spontaneously while the person is engaged in vigorous exercise, straining, coughing, or sneezing, or even while the person is asleep.

High-risk PDR puts a person at significant risk for visual loss (Table 39.1). The Diabetic Retinopathy Study revealed a 25–40% risk of severe visual loss (≤5/200, worse than legal blindness) over a 2-year period if high-risk PDR is present. Scatter laser treatment can reduce this risk by ~60%. High-risk PDR is characterized by any one of the following lesions:

- NVD greater than standard photo 10A of the modified Airlie House classification of diabetic retinopathy (i.e., NVD that covers more than one-fourth to one-third of the disc area) (Fig. 39.4)
- NVD less than standard photo 10A if preretinal or vitreous hemorrhage is present
- NVE greater than or equal to one-half of the disc area if preretinal or vitreous hemorrhage is present

Patients with high-risk PDR are candidates for immediate scatter laser photocoagulation. These patients should be referred immediately for laser treatment by an ophthalmologist skilled in the treatment of diabetic retinopathy. These patients generally should not wait more than a few days for laser surgery.

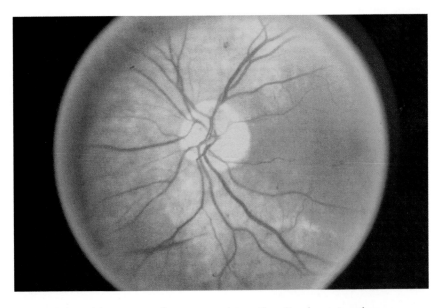

Figure 39.4 This extent of new vessels on the disc (greater than or equal to one-fourth of the disc area) with or without preretinal or vitreous hemorrhage constitutes high-risk diabetic retinopathy. Standard photograph 10A.

The ETDRS demonstrated that scatter laser treatment applied when a person approaches or reaches high-risk PDR can reduce the 5-year risk of severe visual loss to <4% per eye and <2% per individual. In full scatter treatment, 1,200–2,000 lesions are applied to the posterior pole. Two or more sessions are normally required to complete the treatment. The treating ophthalmologist applies the 500-µm laser burns 500 µm apart. Major retinal vessels, the optic nerve, and the central macula are avoided.

The response to full scatter photocoagulation varies depending on the retinal and medical status of the patient. There may be *1*) regression of active neovascularization, *2*) persistent neovascularization without further progression, *3*) continued growth of the neovascularization, and/or *4*) recurrent vitreous hemorrhage. Careful follow-up evaluation by the treating ophthalmologist with additional scatter or local laser photocoagulation and/or vitrectomy may be indicated, especially if continued new-vessel growth or recurrent vitreous hemorrhage occurs.

Fibrous tissue proliferation may lead to traction, which may cause a retinal detachment. If a view of the posterior pole is obscured by vitreous hemorrhage, ultrasound examination may be necessary. Nonresolving vitreous hemorrhage and traction retinal detachments, particularly those threatening detachment of the macula, may be indications for vitrectomy surgery.

Following the natural history of diabetic retinopathy, PDR usually progresses through an active phase, followed by remission. In the remission phase, fibrous tissue usually forms along abnormal vessels but may also form between the retina and posterior vitreous surface. A goal of scatter laser surgery is to shorten the active phase of diabetic retinopathy, leading to remission before major vitreous hemorrhage or fibrous tissue proliferation compromises vision. Patients who undergo scatter laser surgery for PDR may have reactivation of diabetic retinopathy in the future and may require further laser treatments and/or vitrectomy.

Laser photocoagulation is not without potential side effects and complications. The Diabetic Retinopathy Study documented occasional minor decreases in visual acuity levels and peripheral visual fields, particularly in eyes treated with the xenon-arc photocoagulator, a system no longer in use. Today, scatter photocoagulation is performed with newer, more efficient laser systems that may minimize adverse effects, but as with any surgical procedure, the risks need to be weighed against the potential benefits of laser surgery.

Poor diabetes control, hypertension, kidney disease, high cholesterol, and anemia are documented risk factors for the progression of diabetic retinopathy. Many factors affect the progression of diabetic retinopathy in type 1 diabetic patients, including duration of diabetes, diabetic retinopathy status, pregnancy, the use of diuretics, and A1C levels. In type 2 diabetic patients, the age of the patient, severity of diabetic retinopathy, A1C levels, diuretic usage, lower intraocular pressure, smoking, and lower diastolic blood pressure may be risk factors.

DME

DME can be present at any stage of diabetic retinopathy and is a leading cause of moderate visual loss from diabetes. Proper evaluation requires stereoscopic examination of the macula with a slit-lamp biomicroscope, fundus photography, and/or ocular coherence tomography. DME is a collection of fluid or thickening in the macula. Hard exudates within the macula area, nonperfusion of the retina inside the temporal vessel arcades, or any combination of these lesions may also be present. Patients with or suspected of having DME should be referred to an ophthalmologist for evaluation for clinically significant DME (CSME), since laser photocoagulation is frequently indicated at this stage. CSME is macular edema that involves or threatens the center of the macula and is characterized by any of the following retinal lesions:

- Retinal thickening at or within 500 µm from the center of the macula
- Hard exudates at or within 500 µm from the center of the macula if accompanied by thickening of the adjacent retina
- A zone or zones of thickening greater than or equal to one disc area in size, any portion of which is less than or equal to one disc diameter from the center of the macula

Patients with CSME should be referred to an ophthalmologist experienced in the care of diabetic eye disease. The urgency for treatment of DME is not as acute as for high-risk PDR, but consultation and referral should preferably occur within 1 month.

DME can only be adequately evaluated through dilated pupils and with stereoscopic examination of the macula. Stereo fundus photography and ocular coherence tomography are important adjunct examinations for patients who have or are suspected to have DME.

Patients with CSME are candidates for focal laser photocoagulation. The goal of this laser treatment is to maintain acuity at approximately the same level as before treatment by preventing or limiting further leakage in the retina and allowing the leakage already present to reabsorb. Fluorescein angiography is often used to determine whether treatable lesions are present and to guide the application of focal or grid laser surgery. Focal treatment is applied to focal leaks contributing to DME. Grid treatment is applied to areas of diffuse leakage or areas of nonperfusion in the macula area.

The ETDRS demonstrated that in eyes with CSME, the risk of moderate visual loss was 50–60% less for eyes treated with focal laser compared with eyes assigned to deferral of treatment, being reduced from 32 to 15% after 3 years of follow-up. Focal photocoagulation reduced the risk of moderate visual loss, increased the chance of visual improvement, decreased retinal thickening, and was not associated with any major adverse effects.

Emerging Treatment Modalities

Numerous novel therapies for diabetic retinopathy are in various stages of development and testing. Many of these focus on inhibiting growth factors such as VEGF, thought to underlie the development of macular edema and retinal neovascularization. These compounds are injected into the eye on a repetitive basis. Preliminary clinical data suggest beneficial activity, but definitive proof of efficacy and side effects awaits the results of rigorous multicenter randomized clinical trials currently underway. Other compounds attempt to correct the biochemical alterations induced by diabetes. These approaches include use of protein kinase C inhibitors, Celebrex, IGF-I inhibitors (somatostatin), and vitamin E. To date in later-stage trials, Celebrex, somatostatin, and vitamin E have not shown the efficacy suggested in the initial studies. The protein kinase C inhibitor ruboxistaurin showed modest benefit in initial phase III clinical trials, receiving an approvable letter from the U.S. Food and Drug Administration, but still requiring an additional phase III study before registration of the drug can be considered. Numerous other treatments, including integrin antagonists, vitreolysis, metalloproteinases, etc., are in various stages of early clinical evaluation.

NONRETINAL OCULAR COMPLICATIONS

The ocular manifestations of diabetes that receive the most attention are those related to diabetic retinopathy and macular edema because these changes are usually responsible for the most devastating visual threat from diabetes. Diabetic eye disease, however, represents an end-organ response to a systemic medical condition. Consequently, all structures of the eye are susceptible to the deleterious effects of diabetes. Following are some of the ocular problems in addition to diabetic retinopathy that are associated with diabetes:

- Mononeuropathies of cranial nerves III, IV, or VI
- Higher incidence of glaucoma
- Earlier and more rapidly progressing cataracts
- Susceptibility to corneal abrasions and recurrent corneal erosions
- Early presbyopia
- Blurred or fluctuating vision

Lenticular Opacities

Cataracts may occur at a younger age and progress more rapidly in the presence of diabetes. Cataracts are 60% more common in people with diabetes. This increased risk of cataract development occurs in both type 1 and type 2 diabetic populations.

Reversible lenticular opacities related to diabetes can occur in different layers of the lens and are most frequently related to poor glycemic control. The so-called true diabetic cataracts are usually bilateral and are characterized by dense bands of white subcapsular spots that look like snowflakes or fine needle-shaped opacities. Because diabetic cataracts are related to prolonged periods of severe hyperglycemia and untreated diabetes, they are now seldom seen in the U.S. and other industrialized countries.

Management of diabetic cataracts involves the same treatment strategies as management of age-related cataracts. For visual impairment not requiring surgery, optimum refraction for maximum visual acuity is recommended. Glare-control lenses and the use of sunglasses may relieve cataract-induced visual symptoms. Fortunately, cataract extraction with intraocular lens implantation is 90–95% successful in restoring useful vision, but the surgery has potential complications unique to diabetes. Intraocular lens implants provide the most natural postsurgical refractive correction. Careful patient education and consultation with the cataract surgeon is indicated.

A further consideration for the diabetic patient requiring cataract surgery involves the status of diabetic retinopathy. Diabetes is associated with an increased incidence of postoperative neovascularization on the iris and neovascular glaucoma (NVG) after cataract extractions, regardless of the degree of retinopathy before surgery. If active PDR is present before cataract surgery, the risk of subsequently developing neovascularization on the iris, NVG, and vitreous hemorrhage is greater.

To provide appropriate preoperative care, physicians must determine diabetic retinopathy status before cataract extraction. Scatter laser photocoagulation is indicated for patients with high-risk PDR. With cataracts developing in the presence of severe NPDR or PDR without high-risk PDR, early laser treatment may be indicated. Laser treatment may be required a few days after surgery if active PDR is present. Preoperative evaluation may require optical coherence tomography to evaluate the vitreoretinal interface to assess subtle vitreoretinal traction. Presurgical evaluation may influence the decision to perform cataract surgery in conjunction with vitrectomy or intravitreal injection to optimize postsurgical visual outcomes.

Glaucoma

Open-angle glaucoma is 1.2–2.7 times more common in the diabetic population than in the nondiabetic population. The prevalence of glaucoma increases with age and duration of diabetes, but medical therapy for open-angle glaucoma is generally effective. Argon-laser trabeculoplasty may normalize intraocular pressures in some patients if medical therapy proves ineffective. Treatment of open-angle glaucoma for the diabetic patient is essentially the same as for the nondiabetic patient.

NVG is a severe problem and sometimes occurs in eyes with severe diabetic retinopathy or retinal detachments or occasionally after cataract surgery. NVG results from a proliferation of new vessels on the surface of the iris. These vessels are usually first observed at the pupillary border. As these new vessels progress, a fine network of vessels and fibrous tissue grows over the iris tissue and into the filtration angle of the eye. This fibrovascular growth results in peripheral anterior synechie and closure of the filtration angle, resulting in NVG. In some cases, intraocular pressure may be elevated before angle involvement because of protein and cellular leakage from the proliferative vessels. Occasionally, iris neovascularization may be present in the filtration angle while not observed at the pupillary border.

NVG may be difficult to manage and generally requires aggressive treatment. Treatment modalities for neovascularization on the iris and NVG include scatter laser photocoagulation, intraocular anti-VEGF agents, topical antiglaucoma drugs, topical steroids, topical atropine, systemic antiglaucoma drugs, goniophotocoagulation, cyclodestructive procedures, filtration surgery, or a combination of these therapies. Early recognition and prompt retinal photocoagulation with or without pretreatment with an intravitreal anti-VEGF agent may help ameliorate this otherwise frequently devastating condition.

EXAMINATION CRITERIA AND FREQUENCY

Patients with diabetes should be examined *1*) within at least 5 years of diagnosis or during puberty for type 1 diabetic patients and at least yearly thereafter, *2*) at the time of diagnosis for type 2 diabetic patients and at least yearly thereafter, and *3*) before pregnancy for diabetic patients planning to conceive and early in the first trimester and then each trimester during pregnancy and 6 weeks after delivery. The American Diabetes Association recognizes the value of retinal imaging in assessing diabetic retinopathy and states that examinations can be done with retinal photographs with or without pupil dilation read by experienced experts. However, in-person examinations are still necessary when photos are unacceptable and for follow-up of detected abnormalities.

Pregnancy, nephropathy, hypertension, hypercholesterolemia, anemia, and other medical conditions may dictate more frequent examination. The presence of DME or diabetic retinopathy more advanced than mild NPDR indicates a need for more frequent examination. Tables 39.2 and 39.3 outline the examination schedule and guidelines for the care of patients with diabetes.

VISUAL AND PSYCHOSOCIAL REHABILITATION

All patients with diabetes should be informed that proven methods are in place to preserve vision. These methods include regular comprehensive eye and retinal examination; intensive control of blood glucose (as evaluated by A1C levels); control of coexisting medical complications, such as hypertension, kidney disease, and/or dyslipidemia; and appropriate and timely laser surgery or other interventions when indicated for DME or diabetic retinopathy. As a routine part of the health history, all patients with diabetes should be asked whether they have any visual symptoms (Table 39.1), such as any reduction in vision (either at a distance or near), fluctuation of vision, floating spots in field of view, flashing lights in field of view, any metamorphopsia (distortion or waviness) or apparent warping of straight lines, eye redness or pain, or diplopia (double vision).

Table 39.2 Eye Examination Schedule

Diabetes Type	Recommended Time of First Examination	Recommended Follow-Up*
Type 1 diabetes	3–5 years after diagnosis or during puberty	Yearly
Type 2 diabetes	At time of diagnosis	Yearly
Prior to pregnancy	Prior to conception and early in the first trimester	Each trimester or more frequently, as indicated, and 6–8 weeks postpartum

*Abnormal findings dictate more frequent follow-up examinations (Table 39.3). Adapted from the American Academy of Ophthalmology *Preferred Practice Patterns for Diabetic Retinopathy,* San Francisco, CA, 2008.

Table 39.3 Management Recommendations

Status of Retina	Follow-Up (mo)	Color Fundus Photography	Fluorescein Angiography	Laser
Normal or minimal NPDR	12	No	No	No
Mild to moderate NPDR without DME	6–12	Rarely	No	No
Mild to moderate NPDR with clinically insignificant DME	4–6	Occasionally	Rarely	No
Mild to moderate NPDR with CSME	2–4	Yes	Yes	Yes
Severe to very severe NPDR	2–4	Yes	Yes, if CSME	Consider
Non–high-risk PDR	2–4	Yes	Yes, if CSME	Consider
High-risk PDR	2–4	Yes	Yes, if CSME	Yes
High-risk PDR not amenable to photocoagulation	1–6	If possible	No	In connection with vitrectomy if indicated

Adapted from the American Academy of Ophthalmology: *Preferred Practice Patterns for Diabetic Retinopathy.* San Francisco, CA, American Academy of Ophthalmology, 2008.

There are numerous etiologies for reduced vision—some benign and some requiring immediate treatment. In general, patients who report floating spots in their view, flashing lights, or the sensation of a curtain or veil crossing their vision should be referred for immediate ophthalmological attention because they may be experiencing symptoms of a vitreous hemorrhage, retinal detachment, or retinal hole. Patients with metamorphopsia may have significant macular edema or traction in the macular area and should be referred for prompt ophthalmological evaluation, preferably within 1 week.

Fluctuating vision is frequently the result of poor blood glucose control. Elevated blood glucose levels may lead to a myopic shift, enabling presbyopic individuals to read without their glasses, while their distance vision becomes blurred. For some who never wore glasses, distance vision may become blurred, and for those with hyperopia, glasses may no longer be needed for clear distance vision. Blurred vision may be the presenting symptom for a wide range of ocular conditions, such as macular edema and cataracts. In general, if the vision clears with a pinhole, the condition is most likely refractive, and referral is less urgent.

Patients complaining of pain in or above the eye should be evaluated for possible neovascular or angle-closure glaucoma, especially if there is a loss of corneal reflex, irregularity in shape and response of the pupil, or acute redness of the eye. Also, a painful or red eye may reflect a corneal abrasion or corneal erosion. In most cases, patients with anterior-segment complaints should be promptly examined with a slit-lamp biomicroscope to rule out any form of glaucoma, foreign body, corneal abrasion, or iritis. Tonometry to measure intraocular pressure is also advisable. An emergency referral to an ophthalmologist may be critical in these cases.

Patients with new-onset double vision require neuro-ophthalmic and often neurological evaluation. Any patient who shows neovascularization of the optic nerve head or elsewhere in the retina or hard exudates or microaneurysms in the macula area should be promptly referred for complete ophthalmological evaluation. If proliferative retinopathy is present, immediate referral is warranted (Table 39.2).

For those patients who experience significant vision loss, referral for visual rehabilitation (low vision) is beneficial to help maximize visual function. A variety of handheld, stand, spectacle-borne, and electronic magnifiers is useful to assist distance and near vision. Non-optical aids, such as large-print books, "talking books," specially designed computer software, closed-circuit television, and other electronic aids allow a person to perform tasks otherwise hindered by reduced vision. Counseling and support groups may be beneficial for both patients and their families.

Currently, diabetic eye disease cannot be prevented. Therapeutic strategies focus on addressing avenues to delay the onset and slow the progression of eye disease and ensure proper management of proliferative retinopathy and DME when these conditions are present. All patients should be informed of the potential ocular complications of diabetes and should be advised to have a regular comprehensive eye examination with pupil dilation and appropriate referral for management and treatment as indicated to preserve vision.

Patients with significant retinal disease or those who have lost vision from diabetic retinopathy should be encouraged to continue with regular eye care. Vitrectomy surgery can restore useful vision for some individuals who have lost sight from vitreous hemorrhages or fibrous tissue proliferation with traction retinal detachment. Proper refraction, visual rehabilitation (low-vision evaluation), optical aids, and other techniques and devices are available to enable a person to use even severely limited vision. Referral to visual rehabilitation specialists may be appropriate. Support groups for the visually impaired and organizations providing vocational rehabilitation exist in most areas. All practitioners should be familiar with appropriate referral sources for their patients with visual impairment.

Unlike many other eye conditions, diabetic retinopathy is not solely an eye problem but an end-organ response to a chronic systemic condition also affecting other organs (e.g., heart and kidney). Multiple psychological and social issues may also be present. Health care providers should be aware of these problems and be prepared to assist in their appropriate management. Close communication among all members of a patient's health care team is of paramount importance in dealing with the physical and psychological stresses of visual loss from diabetes.

SUMMARY

Diabetes remains the leading cause of new-onset blindness in developed countries. In its earliest stages, diabetic retinopathy causes no symptoms. Visual acuity may be excellent and, on evaluation and diagnosis, a patient may deny the presence or significance of retinopathy. At this stage, the physician should initiate a careful program of education and follow-up. Early institution of routine lifelong follow-up; intensive systemic control of blood glucose, hypertension, and dyslipidemia; and timely therapeutic intervention when required are the hallmarks of appropriate diabetic eye care—and can prevent the majority of visual loss from diabetes.

BIBLIOGRAPHY

Aiello LM: Perspectives on diabetic retinopathy. *Am J Ophthalmol* 136:122–135, 2003

Aiello LP, Cahill MT, Wong JS: Systemic considerations in the management of diabetic retinopathy. *Am J Ophthalmol* 132:760–776, 2001

Aiello LP, Cavallerano J, Prakash M, Aiello LM: Diagnosis, management and treatment of nonproliferative diabetic retinopathy and macular edema. In *The Principles and Practices of Ophthalmology: The Harvard System.* Philadelphia, PA, Saunders, 2008, p. 1775–1791

Aiello LP, Gardner TW, King GL, Blankenship G, Cavallerano JD, Ferris FL III, Klein R: Diabetic retinopathy (Technical Review). *Diabetes Care* 21:143–156, 1998

American Diabetes Association: Retinopathy in diabetes (Position Statement). *Diabetes Care* 27 (Suppl. 1):S84–S87, 2004

Early Treatment Diabetic Retinopathy Study Research Group: Early photocoagulation for diabetic retinopathy: ETDRS report no. 9. *Ophthalmology* 98:766–785, 1991

Early Treatment Diabetic Retinopathy Study Research Group: Effects of aspirin treatment on diabetic retinopathy: ETDRS report no. 8. *Ophthalmology* 98:757–765, 1991

Early Treatment Diabetic Retinopathy Study Research Group: Fundus photographic risk factors for progression of diabetic retinopathy: ETDRS report no. 12. *Ophthalmology* 98:823–833, 1991

Early Treatment Diabetic Retinopathy Study Research Group: Photocoagulation for diabetic macular edema: ETDRS report no. 1. *Arch Ophthalmol* 103:1796–1806, 1985

Ferris FL III: Early photocoagulation in patients with either type I or type II diabetes. *Trans Am Ophthalmol Soc* 94:505–537, 1996

Javitt JC, Aiello LP, Bassi LJ, Canner JK: Detecting and treating diabetic retinopathy: financial and visual savings associated with improved implementation of current guidelines. *Ophthalmology* 98:1565–1574, 1990

Klein R, Klein BEK, Moss SE, Davis MD, DeMets DL: The Wisconsin Epidemiologic Study of Diabetic Retinopathy. II. Prevalence and risk of diabetic retinopathy when age at diagnosis is less than 30 years. *Arch Ophthalmol* 102:520–526, 1984

Klein R, Klein BEK, Moss SE, Davis MD, DeMets DL: The Wisconsin Epidemiologic Study of Diabetic Retinopathy. III. Prevalence and risk of diabetic retinopathy when age at diagnosis is 30 or more years. *Arch Ophthalmol* 102:527–532, 1984

U.K. Prospective Diabetes Study (UKPDS) Group: Intensive blood-glucose control with sulphonylureas or insulin compared with conventional treatment and risk of complications in patients with type 2 diabetes (UKPDS 33). *Lancet* 352:837–853, 1998

Dr. L.P. Aiello is Director of the Beetham Eye Institute, Joslin Diabetes Center, Boston, Massachusetts; Head of the Section of Eye Research, Joslin Diabetes Center, Boston, Massachusetts; and Associate Professor of Ophthalmology at Harvard Medical School, Boston, Massachusetts. Dr. L.M. Aiello is Founding Director at the Beetham Eye Institute, Joslin Diabetes Center, Boston, Massachusetts, and Clinical Professor of Ophthalmology at Harvard Medical School, Boston, Massachusetts. Dr. Cavallerano is Staff Optometrist and Assistant to the Director at Beetham Eye Institute, Joslin Diabetes Center, Boston, Massachusetts, and Assistant Professor of Ophthalmology at Harvard Medical School, Boston, Massachusetts. Dr. Silva is Senior Fellow in Ophthalmology at Beetham Eye Institute, Joslin Diabetes Center, Boston, Massachusetts.

40. Diabetic Nephropathy

Andrew Davis, MD, Irena Duka, MD, and George Bakris, MD

Chronic kidney disease (CKD) affects >50 million people worldwide, and >1 million of them are receiving kidney replacement therapy. Diabetes is the leading cause of CKD in developed countries and is rapidly becoming the leading cause in developing countries as a result of an increase in type 2 diabetes and obesity (1). Data from the 2005 U.S. Renal Data System (USRDS) document that diabetes accounts for 45% of kidney failure, an increase from 18% in 1980 (2).

Studies demonstrate that the risk of diabetic nephropathy is similar in both type 1 and type 2 diabetes. The epidemiology of diabetic nephropathy is best characterized in patients with type 1 because the time of clinical onset is usually known. Twenty to 30% of these patients will have microalbuminuria after a mean duration of diabetes of 15 years. The onset of overt nephropathy in type 1 diabetes is between 10 and 15 years after the onset of the disease. Patients who have no proteinuria after 20–25 years have a risk of developing overt renal disease of only ~1% per year.

In type 2 diabetic patients, the progression to diabetic nephropathy has been studied in the U.K. Prospective Diabetes Study (UKPDS) (3). This study showed that 10 years after diagnosis, the prevalence of microalbuminuria (>30 but <300 mg/day) was 25% and macroalbuminuria (≥300 mg/day) was 5%.

The contribution of diabetic kidney disease (DKD) to patient suffering and disability, cardiovascular disease risk, and all-cause mortality make prevention and mitigation of this condition a pressing clinical concern. The increasing prevalence of diabetes worldwide and the enormous expenses associated with DKD make it a major societal issue as well.

DEFINITION, SCREENING, AND DIAGNOSIS OF DIABETIC NEPHROPATHY

CKD is currently classified in five stages, ranging from stage 1 kidney damage with normal glomerular filtration rate (GFR) to stage 5 kidney failure (Table 40.1). The recent 2007 guidelines from the National Kidney Foundation Kidney Disease Outcomes Quality Initiative (KDOQI) suggest that the term "diabetic nephropathy" be reserved for renal biopsy–confirmed disease (4). Patients with CKD due to diabetes should be referred to as having DKD.

Table 40.1. Classification of Chronic Kidney Disease

KDOQI Classification of CKD

Stage	Description	GFR (ml/min/1.73 m²)
1	Kidney damage with normal GFR	>90
2	Kidney damage with mildly decreased GFR	60–89
3	Moderately decreased GFR	30–59
4	Severely decreased GFR	15–20
5	Kidney failure	<15 (or dialysis)

Diabetic nephropathy is a clinical diagnosis that has been based on the finding of proteinuria in diabetic patients. The latest recommendations suggest that a diagnosis of diabetic nephropathy could be established in most diabetic patients by the presence of macroalbuminuria or estimated GFR (eGFR) <60 ml/min/1.73 m². Progression of microalbuminuria into the macroalbuminuria range is an independent risk marker for the development of CKD and GFR loss; microalbuminuria itself is associated with significantly higher cardiovascular morbidity and mortality (5,6). The prevalence of microalbuminuria varies (depending on the population) from 7 to 22% in type 1 diabetes (7) and from 6.5 to 42% in type 2 diabetes (8). Annual incidence rates of microalbuminuria of 1–2% are reported consistently for both type 1 and type 2 diabetes. In the U.S., microalbuminuria is found in 43% and macroalbuminuria in 8% of those with a history of diabetes.

The lower limit of microalbuminuria is set arbitrarily at an albumin-to-creatinine ratio (ACR) of 30 mg/g or albumin excretion rate (AER) of 20 mg/min. Microalbuminuria is defined as an ACR between 30 and 300 mg/g, whereas macroalbuminuria is defined as an ACR >300 mg/g. The definitions of abnormalities in urinary albumin excretion in spot, 24-h collection, and timed collection are described in Table 40.2. Although macroalbuminuria had historically had a relationship with a progressive decrease in GFR associated with an increase in systemic blood pressure (BP), microalbuminuria is associated with more stable kidney function that does not exclude the risk of development to macroalbuminuria and kidney failure (9).

Although microalbuminuria satisfies nearly all criteria for a screening test, its detection has not be proven to have any effect on clinical end points, such as CKD stage 5, GFR loss, or cardiovascular disease morbidity/mortality. Nevertheless, the American Diabetes Association (ADA) and other diabetes professional societies recommend annual screening for microalbuminuria in patients with diabetes (10). The suggested screening plan, adapted from the ADA guidelines, is shown in Fig. 40.1.

Both assessment of urinary albumin excretion and estimation of GFR are required to screen for and diagnose DKD, as many patients with diabetes with CKD may have normal GFRs in the early years after diagnosis. Screening for CKD should begin 5 years after the diagnosis of type 1 diabetes and at the time of diagnosis in type 2 diabetes. To assess urine albumin excretion, a spot morning-

Table 40.2. Definitions of Abnormalities in Albumin Excretion

Category	Spot collection (mg/g creatinine)	24-h Collection (mg/24 h)	Timed collection (mg/min)
Normoalbuminuria	<30	<30	<20
Microalbuminuria	30–300	30–300	20–200
Macroalbuminuria	>300	>300	>200
Nephrotic Range	>3,500	>3,500	>2,500

urine ACR is preferred, with the measurement of two additional first-void additional samples over the next 3–6 months recommended.

A diagnosis of DKD is considered justified under the KDOQI guidelines if a patient with diabetes has *1*) macroalbuminuria (ACR >300 mg/g on two of three samples) or *2*) microalbuminuria (30–300 mg/g on two of three samples) in the presence of diabetic retinopathy.

False-positive elevations of urine albumin may occur after exercise, and ideally spot urines should not be obtained within 24 h of vigorous activity; however, transient postexercise elevations may predict subsequent persistent microalbuminuria (11).

Sex, racial, and ethnic variations in ACR have been described (12). Macroalbuminuria appears to be more prevalent in non-Hispanic blacks than whites, even adjusting for BP and health care access (13). In the same study, Hispanics with hypertension had higher rates of microalbuminuria relative to hypertensive whites, and among normotensive individuals with diabetes, Asian-Americans appeared to have higher rates of microalbuminuria. Nationally representative prevalence rates of albuminuria and CKD have recently been published and appear to be increasing across racial and ethnic groups (14).

OTHER CAUSES OF NEPHROPATHY IN DIABETIC PATIENTS

The variability in the severity of underlying pathology in type 1 diabetes and the heterogeneous nature of pathology in type 2 diabetes suggest that microalbuminuria may or may not reflect underlying DKD. For example, the presence of elevated albuminuria in diabetes of short duration should raise concern about nondiabetic kidney disease because there is a strong relationship between duration of diabetes and DKD, particularly in type 1 diabetes.

Type 1 diabetic patients with nephropathy nearly always have other manifestations of diabetic microvascular disease, such as retinopathy and neuropathy (15). The absence of retinopathy, especially in the presence of macroalbuminuria, should raise strong suspicion for an alternate diagnosis. In type 2 diabetes, the association with retinopathy is less certain, with perhaps 40% of patients with

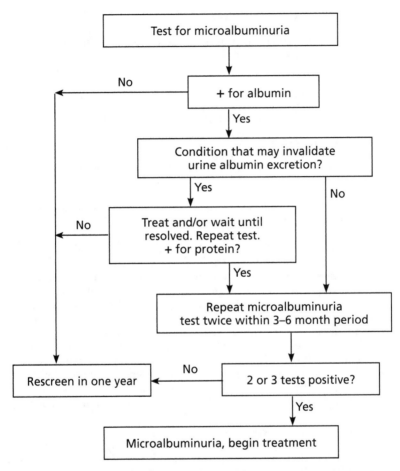

Figure 40.1 Screening for microalbuminuria. Reprinted from Molitch et al. (10).

biopsy-proven diabetic nephropathy lacking retinopathy in one study (16). As described above, the absence of proteinuria, particularly prior to the institution of renin-angiotensin-aldosterone system (RAS) therapy, is an important clue for the cause of kidney disease, other than diabetes (4). This clue and others are listed in Table 40.3 and may help target patients for whom renal biopsy is most informative (17). A recent review has examined the pathological features that help distinguish diabetic nephropathy from other causes of diffuse and nodular glomerulosclerosis (17).

Table 40.3. Clinical Features Suggesting Causes of CKD Other Than Diabetes (KDOQI 2007)

• Absence of diabetic retinopathy
• Low or rapidly declining GFR
• Rapidly increasing proteinuria or nephrotic syndrome
• Onset of proteinuria <5 years from diabetes onset (more reliable type 1 diabetes)
• Refractory hypertension
• Presence of active urinary sediment (such as casts) or RBC alone
• Signs or symptoms of other systemic disease
• >30% reduction in GFR within 2–3 months after initiation of an ACE inhibitor or ARB

PATHOGENESIS OF DIABETIC NEPHROPATHY

Diabetic nephropathy affects up to 35% of those with type 1 and 30–40% of those with type 2 diabetes; the reason why only a fraction of patients with diabetes develop this complication is unknown. One main reason for this heterogeneity of nephropathy development is probably genetic, as the number of Pima Indians who develop nephropathy exceeds that of the general population. Nevertheless, in general, it is clear that the pathogenesis of diabetic nephropathy is not well understood and continues to evolve, with new data emerging annually.

Diabetic nephropathy, characterized best in type 1 diabetes, develops through several distinct phases (Fig. 40.2). It should be noted that all people with diabetes have high GFRs early in their disease course (hyperfiltration) and that almost all develop microalbuminuria. Microalbuminuria development relates more to vascular injury than renal parenchymal injury. Data from follow-up studies in people with diabetes, however, suggest that those with BP increases into the hypertensive range are destined to develop nephropathy (19–21).

There appear to be different pathogenetic processes leading to the pathological mechanisms in diabetic nephropathy. An interaction of hyperglycemia-induced metabolic and hemodynamic factors are postulated to be the mediators of injury to the kidney (22). The hemodynamic factors involve activation of various vasoactive systems, such as RAS and endothelin, in addition to increased systemic and intraglomerular pressure in the individual genetically predisposed to nephropathy.

Metabolic pathways involve nonenzymatic glycosylation, increased protein kinase C (PKC) activity, and abnormal polyol metabolism. Recent studies have supported the fact that inflammatory cells such as cytokines, growth factors, and metalloproteinases are associated with development of diabetic nephropathy (22,23). Studies with the inhibitors of the pathways involved in genesis of diabetic nephropathy have shed a light on the pathogenesis of this condition (24–26).

Glomerular Hyperfiltration

Although glomerular hypertension and hyperfiltration occur in all people with diabetes, not all develop nephropathy. It is clear, however, that lowering intra-glomerular pressure in those with albuminuria by use of RAS blockade is benefi-

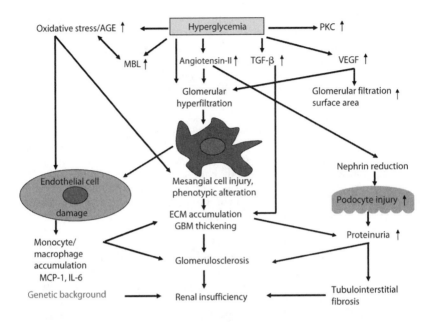

Figure 40.2 Molecular mechanisms of diabetic nephropathy. ECM, extracellular matrix; GBM, glomerular basement membrane; IL, interleukin; MCP-1, monocyte chemoattractant protein-1. Reprinted with permission from Ichinose et al. (23).

cial. Antagonizing the profibrotic effects of angiotensin II may also be a significant factor in benefits observed with these agents (27,28). Transient RAS blockade (for 7 weeks) in pre-diabetic rats reduced proteinuria and improved glomerular structure (29).

Hyperglycemia and Advanced Glycosylation End Products

Hyperglycemia may directly induce mesangial expansion and injury, in part via increased matrix production or glycosylation of matrix proteins. In vitro studies have demonstrated that hyperglycemia stimulates mesangial cell matrix production (30,31) and mesangial cell apoptosis (32,33). Mesangial cell expansion appears to be mediated in part by an increase in the mesangial cell glucose concentration because similar changes in mesangial function can be induced in a normal glucose concentration by overexpression of glucose transporters, thereby enhancing glucose entry into the cells (31).

Glycosylation of tissue proteins may also contribute to the development of diabetic nephropathy and other microvascular complications. In chronic hyperglycemia, some of the excess glucose combines with free amino acids on circulating or tissue proteins, leading to formation of reversible early glycosylation products and later irreversible advanced glycosylation end products (AGEs). The net effect is tissue accumulation of AGEs, in part by cross-linking with collagen, which can contribute to the associated renal and microvascular complications (34).

Other proposed mechanisms by which hyperglycemia might promote the development of diabetic nephropathy include activation of PKC (35) and upregulation of heparanase expression, which may contribute to increased glomerular basement membrane permeability to albumin (36).

Prorenin

Initial clinical studies in children and adolescents suggested that increased plasma prorenin activity was a risk factor for the development of diabetic nephropathy (37,38). The prorenin receptor in the kidney is located in the mesangium and podocytes, and its blockade had beneficial effect on the kidneys of diabetic animal models. This effect is mediated both by RAS-dependent and -independent intracellular signals. Prorenin binds to a specific tissue receptor, which promotes activation of the mitogen-activated protein kinases (MAPKs) p44/p42A (39).

A possible pathogenic role for prorenin in the development of diabetic nephropathy was suggested by an experimental model (streptozotocin diabetes in mice), in which prolonged prorenin receptor blockade abolished MAPK activation and prevented the development of nephropathy, despite an unaltered increase in angiotensin II activity (40).

If prorenin was a key player in the pathogenesis of this disease, data with renin inhibitors that increase prorenin should have a detrimental effect, and to date, no such adverse effect has been seen in animal studies.

Cytokines

Activation of cytokines, profibrotic elements, inflammation, and vascular growth factors (e.g., vascular endothelial growth factor [VEGF]) may be involved in the matrix accumulation in diabetic nephropathy (41). Hyperglycemia stimulates increased VEGF expression (a mediator of endothelial injury in human diabetes) (26,42). Hyperglycemia also increases the expression both of transforming growth factor-β (TGF-β) in the glomeruli and of matrix proteins specifically stimulated by this cytokine (43). TGF-β may contribute to both the cellular hypertrophy and enhanced collagen synthesis that are seen in diabetic nephropathy. Studies have shown that the combination of an anti–TGF-β antibody along with ACE inhibitor completely normalized proteinuria in rats with diabetic nephropathy; proteinuria was only partially lessened with an ACE inhibitor alone. Glomerulosclerosis and tubulointerstitial injury were also improved. Another study demonstrated that the administration of hepatocyte growth factor, which specifically blocks the profibrotic actions of TGF-β, ameliorates diabetic nephropathy in mice (44).

Nephrin Expression

The renal expression of nephrin may be impaired in diabetic nephropathy. When compared with nondiabetic patients with minimal change nephropathy and control subjects, patients with diabetic nephropathy had markedly lower renal nephrin expression and fewer electron-dense slit diaphragms. By comparison, the expression of two other important podocyte/slit diaphragm proteins, podocin and

CD2AP, was similar among the three groups. Similar decreases in renal nephrin expression have been reported in other studies of diabetic nephropathy (45).

RISK FACTORS FOR DIABETIC NEPHROPATHY

Genetic Susceptibility

There is growing evidence that genetic background may be an important determinant of both the incidence and severity of diabetic nephropathy (23,35,46). The increase in risk cannot be explained by the duration of diabetes, hypertension, or the degree of glycemic control, so it is concluded that both environmental and genetic factors play a role in the pathogenesis of diabetic nephropathy. The likelihood of developing diabetic nephropathy is markedly increased in patients with a sibling or parent with diabetes who has diabetic nephropathy; these observations have been made in both type 1 and type 2 diabetes (47,48). One study evaluated Pima Indian families in which two successive generations had type 2 diabetes (48). The likelihood of the offspring developing overt proteinuria was 14% if neither parent had proteinuria, 23% if one parent had proteinuria, and 46% if both parents had proteinuria.

Recent advances in molecular genetics have developed a system for genotyping single-nucleotide polymorphisms and have led to genome-wide association studies to explore loci involved in diabetic nephropathy. In the genome-wide scans for microvascular complications of diabetes in Pima Indians, four loci on chromosomes 3, 7, 9, and 20 were identified (49). Additional loci as diabetic nephropathy susceptibility gene areas were identified on chromosomes 7q21.3, 10p15.3, 14q23.1, and 18q22.3 (50,51).

Candidate gene–based association studies have been the most common approach to identify genes susceptible for diabetic nephropathy. Some of the genes that have been considered a potential genetic risk factor are the genes encoding for ACE, angiotensin II receptor, glucose metabolism, lipids, extracellular matrix, and cytokines.

The ACE gene polymorphism has been studied in several studies as a candidate gene in developing diabetic nephropathy. The ACE insertion/deletion gene polymorphism is responsible for the difference in ACE plasma levels among individuals. In type 2 diabetic patients, the DD polymorphism has been associated with an increased risk for the development of diabetic nephropathy, more severe proteinuria, greater likelihood of progressive renal failure, and mortality on dialysis (52–54).

Other studies have produced controversial data. A critical review of 19 studies examining a possible link between the ACE gene genotype and diabetic nephropathy failed to confirm an association among whites with either type 1 or type 2 diabetes, but it could not exclude a possible association in Asians. An analysis of >1,000 white type 1 diabetic patients found a strong correlation between genetic variation in the ACE gene and the development of nephropathy (55).

Another implicated genetic factor is the angiotensin II type 2 receptor (AT2) gene on the X chromosome. Male type 1 diabetic patients and the AA haplotype of the AT2 gene had a lower GFR than those with the GT haplotype (56).

Recent advances in technology have led to new evidence in the pathogenesis of diabetic nephropathy, especially in the genetics. Many pathways were discovered to be involved in the pathogenesis, making it a complex interaction between different pathways that needs further clarification.

BP

Prospective studies demonstrate higher rates of diabetic nephropathy with a prior diagnosis of hypertension and with poorer control, but it is not clear whether the development of hypertension hastens the development of kidney disease or is simply a marker for more severe renal involvement (57).

Glycemic Control

The value of tight glycemic control in addressing diabetic nephropathy is best demonstrated in type 1 diabetes, where intensive insulin therapy has been demonstrated to reverse glomerular hypertrophy and hyperfiltration, delay the development of microalbuminuria, and stabilize and even decrease protein excretion, particularly after 2 years of improved glycemic control. In a landmark trial of patients in their early 30s with type 1 diabetes, an initial period of near-normal glycemia for a median of 6.5 years resulted in a 60–80% reduction in rates of micro- and macroalbuminuria when assessed 7–8 years later (58). Further support for the importance of treating hyperglycemia comes from studies of patients who have had pancreatic islet cell transplantation. Clear histological regression in their diabetic nephropathy occurs after euglycemia has been maintained for 10 years (59).

Obesity

Higher BMI is associated with higher rates of CKD, and weight loss may reduce proteinuria and improve renal function in diabetic patients (57). It remains unclear whether these effects are independent of the association of obesity with glycemia and BP.

Race

The incidence and severity of diabetic nephropathy are increased in genetically disparate populations, such as African Americans, Mexican Americans, and Pima Indians, suggesting a primary role for sociocultural factors, such as diet, obesity, and poor control of hypertension and glycemia (60). Some of these differences narrow when access to medical care and medication is considered.

EPIDEMIOLOGY AND NATURAL HISTORY OF DKD

Although many diabetic patients develop microalbuminuria and have hypertension, only about one-third of people with either type 1 or type 2 diabetes develop nephropathy. This relates to many factors discussed earlier but also the degree and duration with which known risk factors for nephropathy have been controlled. The time needed to progress between the stages may vary considerably depending on the intensity of glycemic, lipid, and BP control; the use of ACE inhibitors and angiotensin II receptor blockers (ARBs); genetic factors; and perhaps the type of diabetes. The renal prognosis of type 1 diabetes has dramatically improved over the past 20 years in optimally managed patient populations, but there is increasing awareness of the importance of translating this good news from clinical trials into everyday clinical practice (61,62).

Type 1 Diabetes

About 25% of type 1 diabetic patients will develop microalbumin after 15 years, but <50% of these will develop more advanced renal disease. A large trial from Finland followed 20,005 patients over a median period of 17 years and demonstrated a cumulative incidence of end-stage renal disease of 2.2 and 7.8% at 20 and 30 years, respectively (63).

Type 2 Diabetes

Perhaps the best data on the development of diabetic nephropathy comes from a population of 5,000 predominantly white patients studied in the UKPDS (3). The prevalence of microalbuminuria, macroalbuminuria, and a creatinine of ≥2.0 was 25, 5, and 0.8%, respectively, at 10 years after diagnosis. A statistical estimation of the median time spent at each stage before progressing to another nephropathy stage was 19, 11, and 10 years for those with no nephropathy, microalbuminuria, and macroalbuminuria, respectively.

TREATMENT OF DIABETIC NEPHROPATHY

The four keys to reducing the incidence and progression of DKD are strict glycemic control; rigorous BP control, with emphasis on the use of ACE inhibitors or ARBs; and close attention to each patient's urinary excretion of albumin. Reductions of at least 30% below the starting levels correlated with slowed kidney disease progression (64–66). Combinations of RAS blockers are known to further reduce proteinuria by an additional 20% beyond either class of ACE inhibitors or ARBs alone (67). However, they should be used with caution due to the risk of hyperkalemia (67a).

Management of Hyperglycemia

Hyperglycemia is responsible for vascular target-organ complications, including kidney disease. Intensive treatment of hyperglycemia prevents DKD and may slow the progression of established kidney disease. Patients with DKD may be at higher risk for hypoglycemia with attempts at achieving very tight targets. Although some questions remain regarding the accuracy of A1C in patients receiving dialysis, it remains the preferred monitoring test, with lower A1C levels associated with lower mortality in dialysis populations (68,69). Target A1C for patients with diabetes should be <7%, irrespective of the presence or absence of CKD.

Studies in type 1 diabetes have shown that poor glycemic control predicts the development of microalbuminuria (70–72). The Diabetes Complications and Control Trial (DCCT) was a multicenter randomized clinical trial of 1,441 people with type 1 diabetes that compared the effects of intensive glucose control with conventional treatment on the development and progression of the long-term complications of type 1 diabetes (73). After a mean of 6.5 years, intensive therapy reduced the occurrence of microalbuminuria by 34% (95% CI 2–56%) in the primary-prevention group (no retinopathy and urinary AER <28 µg/min at base-line) and by 43% (21–58%) in the secondary-intervention group, who had early complications at baseline (background retinopathy with or without microalbu-minuria) but normal GFR.

Intensive insulin therapy has the following benefits with respect to the kidney: *1)* it can partially reverse the glomerular hypertrophy and hyperfiltration that are thought to be important risk factors for glomerular injury; *2)* it can delay the development of microalbuminuria; and *3)* it can stabilize or decrease protein excretion in patients with microalbuminuria, although this effect may not be apparent until relative normoglycemia has been maintained for 2 years.

Results that were observed in type 1 diabetes were true for type 2 diabetes also, showing an association of glycemic control with development of microalbu-minuria (74,75). Studies have shown that people with diabetes assigned to inten-sive glycemic control developed less albuminuria than those assigned to conventional glycemic control (76,77). In the UKPDS, type 2 diabetic patients were assigned to intensive glucose control with either an insulin or sulfonylurea or to management of hyperglycemia with diet alone. After 9 years of intensive therapy, relative risk reduction for development of microalbuminuria was 24%, with no differences in the way glycemic control was achieved (76).

Of the eight classes of oral hypoglycemic drugs, some agents should be avoided in patients with impaired kidney function (eGFR <50 ml/min) or end-stage renal disease. The sulfonylurea agent glyburide, biguanides (metformin), meglitinides (nateglinide), and α-glucosidase inhibitors are among these. Thiazolidinediones, agonists of the peroxisome proliferator–activated receptor (PPAR)-γ receptors, have beneficial effects in animal models of diabetic nephropathy and reduce uri-nary albumin excretion and BP, as discussed above. Although both pioglitazone and rosiglitazone have been associated with renoprotective effects, pioglitazone is probably preferred over rosiglitazone, given the association of the latter with higher rates of myocardial infarction (78).

The KDOQI guideline is consistent with the ADA guidelines, which recom-mend that diabetic adults achieve an A1C level <7%, or as close to normal as possible without excessive episodes of hypoglycemia, with the goal of reducing all complications of diabetes. Although the ADA does not have a separate guideline for patients with DKD, it is important to tailor the needs of glycemic control to each patient according to their hypoglycemic episode history. The American Association of Clinical Endocrinologists, the International Diabetes Federation Global Guidelines, and the European NIDDM Working Group proposed that the A1C goal be <6.5%. This level is recommended with the goal of reducing all complications of diabetes. None of these organizations has a separate guideline specific to DKD.

BP APPROACH TO TREAT NEPHROPATHY

The majority of people with diabetes who develop nephropathy also have hyper-tension. The incidence of hypertension in type 2 diabetic patients is >80%. The goal of BP reduction is lower in diabetic patients than those in the general population. Studies have shown that people with BP >130/80 mmHg have a greater likelihood of progressing to end-stage renal disease (79).

ACE Inhibitors

Many clinical trials demonstrate slowing of diabetes nephropathy when ACE inhibitors are used as part of antihypertensive therapy (Table 40.4). The benefit of antihypertensive therapy with an ACE inhibitor in type 1 diabetes is demonstrated early in the course of the disease when microalbuminuria is the only clinical manifestation. In one study, for example, the administration of an ACE inhibitor to normotensive type 1 diabetic patients with microalbuminuria decreased both albumin excretion and, at 2 years, progression to overt diabetic nephropathy compared with patients treated with placebo (80,81). Moreover, these studies demonstrate that patients with the greatest degree of proteinuria and renal insufficiency also benefit the greatest from BP reduction by ACE inhibitors (Fig. 40.3). In the Captopril trial, 409 patients with overt proteinuria and a plasma creatinine concentration ≤2.5 mg/dl were randomly assigned to therapy with either captopril or placebo. This trial showed that patients who had a serum creatinine level >2 mg/dl showed a 74% risk reduction in doubling of the serum creatinine in response to ACE inhibitor therapy, whereas patients with a baseline creatinine of 1 mg/dl and a similar degree of BP reduction experienced only a 4% risk reduction in doubling of serum creatinine (81).

The beneficial response to captopril, which was seen in both hypertensive and normotensive subjects, is consistent with smaller studies, which suggested that antihypertensive therapy, particularly with an ACE inhibitor, slowed the rate of progression in diabetic nephropathy (82,83). Among patients with diabetic nephropathy, including some with advanced disease, remission or regression may occur with aggressive control of systemic BP, particularly with ACE inhibitors.

ARBs

More data are currently available on the efficacy of ARBs in patients with nephropathy due to type 2 diabetes. Two major trials have demonstrated a clear

Table 40.4 Long-Term Outcome of Renal Function in Clinical Trials in Patients with Diabetes and Renal Disease on ACE Inhibitor Therapy

Study	*n*	Duration (years)	Achieved BP (mmHg)	GFR-estimated (ml/min)	
				<6 months	Trial end
Captopril Trial	207	3	105	?	–0.15 (Cr clearance)
Bakris et al.	18	5	98	–9.47 (GFR)	–0.02 (Cr clearance)
Lebovitz et al.	28	3	104	?	–6.3 (GFR)
Nielsen et al.	21	3	112	–3.97 (GFR)	–7.1 GFR
Bjork et al.	40	2.2	102	–3.8 (GFR)	–2 (GFR)

benefit in terms of renoprotection with ARBs in patients with nephropathy due to type 2 diabetes. None of these trials compared ARBs to ACE inhibitors in people with diabetes.

In the Irbesartan Diabetic Nephropathy Trial (IDNT), 1,715 hypertensive patients with nephropathy due to type 2 diabetes were randomly assigned to irbesartan (300 mg/day), amlodipine (10 mg/day), or placebo (84). At 2.6 years, irbesartan was associated with a risk of the combined end point (doubling of the plasma creatinine, development of end-stage renal disease, or death from any cause) that was 23 and 20% lower than with amlodipine and placebo, respectively; the values were 37 and 30% lower for doubling of the plasma creatinine, respectively. These benefits were independent of the differences in the magnitude of BP reduction among the groups.

In the RENAAL trial, 1,513 type 2 diabetic patients with nephropathy were randomly assigned to losartan (50 mg titrating up to 100 mg once daily) or placebo, both in addition to conventional antihypertensive therapy (but not ACE

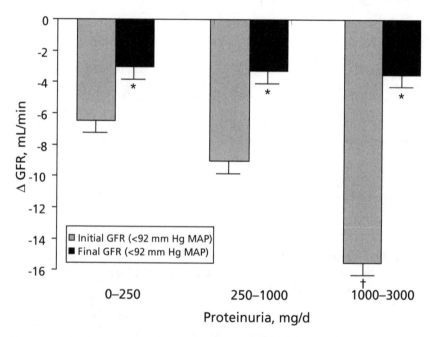

Figure 40.3 Changes in GFR among patients with GFR between 13 and 24 ml/min from the Modification of Dietary Protein in Renal Disease trial as a function of the different levels of proteinuria. *$P < 0.05$ compared with initial fall in GFR; †$P < 0.05$ compared with initial GFR from less proteinic groups; bars, SD; MAP, mean arterial pressure. Reprinted with permission from from Bakris and Weir (126).

inhibitors) (85). Compared to placebo, losartan reduced the incidence of a doubling of the plasma creatinine by 25% and end-stage renal disease by 28%; the mean follow-up was 3.4 years. These benefits were again not associated with differences in BP levels between the groups.

The only randomized controlled trial of ACE inhibitors in people with type 2 diabetes with microalbuminuria or overt proteinuria compared enalapril to the ARB telmisartan in the DETAIL trial of 250 patients with early nephropathy as defined by albuminuria (82% microalbuminuria and 18% macroalbuminuria to a maximum of 1.4 g/day) and a baseline GFR (measured isotopically) of ~93 ml/min per 1.73 m^2 (86). At 5 years, there was a smaller decline in GFR in the enalapril that was not significant (14.9 vs. 17.9 ml/min per 1.73 m^2 with telmisartan). Both groups had similar rates or findings for the secondary end points, which included annual changes in GFR, BP, serum creatinine, urinary albumin excretion, end-stage kidney disease, cardiovascular events, and mortality.

The CALM study randomized patients to candesartan 16 mg or lisinopril 20 mg once daily. The reduction in urinary microalbumin was greater with combination treatment (50%) than candesartan or lisinopril (24 and 39%, respectively) alone and was more effective in reducing BP (87). This additional BP-lowering effect was responsible for the additional antiproteinuric effects.

In contrast, the IMPROVE trial assigned 405 hypertensive patients with albuminuria and increased cardiovascular risk (87% with diabetes) to a 20-week treatment with ramipril plus irbesartan or to ramipril plus placebo. Although there was better BP control in patients receiving combined therapy, there was great variation in AER, and the reduction in albumin excretion was not significantly greater in the combined therapy group (88). Given the available evidence, ACE inhibitors and ARBs appear to provide preferential renoprotection in patients with diabetic nephropathy.

Calcium Channel Blockers

Dihydropyridine calcium channel blockers, unlike nondihydropyridine calcium channel blockers, do not have significant antiproteinuric action, despite effective BP reduction (89,92). Only diltiazem and verapamil appear to be as consistently effective as an ACE inhibitor or ARB in lowering protein excretion in diabetic patients (91); furthermore, the antiproteinuric effects of verapamil and an ACE inhibitor may be additive. In one study of type 2 diabetic patients, lisinopril or verapamil alone lowered protein excretion from 5.8 to 2.7 g/day (93). In comparison, using ~50% the dose of both drugs (mean of 16 mg of lisinopril and 187 mg of sustained-release verapamil) had a much greater antiproteinuric effect—6.8 down to 1.7 g/day. The low-dose combination regimen was also associated with fewer drug-induced side effects (such as constipation with verapamil and dizziness with lisinopril). A similar antiproteinuric advantage has been demonstrated with combination therapy with verapamil and trandolapril (94).

In addition to a possible reduction in intraglomerular pressure, nondihydropyridine calcium channel blockers may have other protective actions. Some studies in animals suggest that calcium channel blockers may minimize progressive glomerular injury by reducing the associated glomerular hypertrophy (95).

In humans, antiproteinuric effects with diltiazem may also be due to improved glomerular size permselectivity (96). These drugs were excluded in the captopril-diabetes trial noted above; as a result, their efficacy in the preservation of renal function in relation to ACE inhibitors has not yet been evaluated in humans.

β-Blockers

β-Blockers have shown a variable response: the fall in protein excretion is generally less than that induced by an ACE inhibitor or ARB (91,97). The cardioselective β-blockers such as metoprolol and atenolol are known to delay the progression of renal disease to a lesser degree than RAS blockers (98). But the newer vasodilating β-blockers such as carvedilol and nebivolol have a different effect on renal hemodynamics and function because of their greater adjunctive β_1-blocking activity (99).

A recent large-scale randomized clinical trial compared carvedilol and metoprolol added to a treatment regimen containing a RAS antagonist in 1,235 diabetic patients with established hypertension. After 5 months of maintenance therapy, BP was decreased to the same extent in both groups, but the mean urinary ACR of the carvedilol group was decreased by 1%, whereas that of the metoprolol group increased by 2.5%. Of those patients with trace protein loss (<30 mg/g at baseline), 47% fewer carvedilol-treated patients progressed to microalbuminuria than those receiving metoprolol (100,101).

Diuretics

Although diuretics have shown a reduction in BP, they generally have not been shown to have an antiproteinuric effect (91,93). Combination of thiazide diuretics with agents that block the RAS are used in 60 and 90% of patients in studies of hypertension treatment in DKD and are more effective than either type of treatment alone for lowering BP and achieving the target BP of <130/80 mmHg (102,103).

Among diuretics, aldosterone antagonists appear to reduce proteinuria when used alone (104) and to have an additive effect on proteinuria when used in combination with an ACE inhibitor or an ARB in both type 1 and type 2 diabetes (105,106). These effects of spironolactone were illustrated in a double-blind trial of 59 type 2 diabetic patients already on an ACE inhibitor or ARB who were randomly assigned to spironolactone or placebo (106). In this study, the urine ACR decreased by 40% in the spironolactone group, with no change in the control group. Further BP reduction may partially explain the beneficial effect, although an anti-inflammatory mechanism has also been proposed (107).

The efficacy and safety of eplerenone, a selective aldosterone blocker, has also been examined in a randomized trial of 268 type 2 diabetic patients already treated with an ACE inhibitor (108). Compared with placebo, eplerenone therapy at a dose of 50 or 100 mg/day was associated with a significant reduction in urinary albumin excretion (40–50 vs. <10%). This study concluded that eplerenone in combination with an ACE inhibitor provides an additive antiproteinuric effect, with the rate of hyperkalemia being similar to placebo. In clinical practice, the use of this combination should be used with caution in patients with reduced GFR. Patients should be instructed for dietary potassium restriction and avoidance of nonsteroidal anti-inflammatory drugs and cyclooxygenase-2 inhibitors, and they probably should be prescribed concomitant kaliuretic diuretic therapy. The risk of hyperkalemia may possibly be lower with an ARB (109).

NONHYPERTENSIVE AGENTS

Pentoxifylline

Small randomized controlled trials in nonhypertensive type 2 diabetic subjects have shown a beneficial effect of pentoxifylline 400 mg t.i.d. (110). Effects on progression to more advanced CKD and on cardiovascular outcomes have yet to be demonstrated.

PPAR Agonists

Preliminary data suggests the value of PPAR-γ agonists such as pioglitazone and rosiglitazone in reducing urinary albumin excretion in diabetic nephropathy (111,112). Animal studies have also suggested the value of PPAR-α/-γ agonists in improving protein loss and renal fibrosis (113). Intriguingly, the PPAR-α agonist fenofibrate reduces progression to microalbuminuria and has also shown benefit in reducing laser requirements in retinopathy (114,115). However, careful analysis of overall risks and benefits of this class of agents will be required before they can be recommended for routine management.

DIETARY APPROACHES

Protein Restriction

It is uncertain whether a low-protein diet influences the preservation of renal function to a similar extent as blockade of the RAS and aggressive control of BP and blood glucose (116,117). That diabetic patients are already on fat and carbohydrate restriction make compliance with diet difficult; however, it is reasonable to avoid a high-protein diet by limiting protein intake to a level at which compliance is not difficult for the patient to reach levels of 0.7–0.8 g/kg/day.

Weight Reduction

In a small randomized controlled trial of overweight patients with chronic proteinuric nephropathy (nearly half with diabetes), proteinuria was significantly decreased at 5 months among dieters who lost on average 4% of body weight (118).

Sodium Restriction

High salt intake blunts the antiproteinuric effects of angiotensin inhibitors as well as calcium channel blockers, even when BP control is adequate (32,119). Moderate restriction to 100–110 mEq/day of sodium (~2.3–2.6 g of sodium) is a reasonable goal.

MANAGEMENT OF DYSLIPIDEMIA AND CARDIOVASCULAR RISK IN CKD

Both diabetes and CKD of any etiology significantly increase cardiovascular risk in a graded independent manner (120). Cardiovascular complications are the leading cause of death in patients with diabetes and renal disease (121,122). The target LDL cholesterol in people with diabetes and CKD stages 1–4 should be <100 mg/dl, with levels <70 mg/dl as a therapeutic option.

Diabetes, CKD stages 1–4, and LDL cholesterol >100 mg/dl should be treated with a statin. Although some observational studies have suggested a mortality benefit to statin therapy in end-stage renal disease (123), based on the only randomized controlled trial in this population, the 2007 KDOQI guidelines do not suggest initiation of a statin in type 2 diabetic patients on maintenance hemodialysis therapy who do not have a specific cardiovascular indication for treatment (124). Ongoing trials (SHARP and AURORA) should shed additional light on the benefits of statin therapy in the dialysis population. Additional benefits of statin therapy in end-stage renal disease may include reduction of hospitalizations for sepsis (125).

SUMMARY AND APPROACH TO PATIENT

In diabetic patients with CKD, aggressive goals are recommended for hyperglycemia, proteinuria, and BP. Antihypertensive therapy is given for both renal protection and cardiovascular protection because CKD and diabetes are independently associated with a marked increase in cardiovascular risk (4). The goals should be an A1C <7%, a reduction in protein excretion of at least 30% of baseline values, and a reduction in BP to <130/80 mmHg. However, evidence among those with nondiabetic proteinuric renal disease suggest that an even lower systolic pressure (125/75 mmHg) may be more effective in slowing progressive renal disease in patients with a spot urine total protein-to-creatinine ratio ≥1,000 mg/g.

These aggressive goals will, in most patients, require therapy with multiple drugs. It seems likely that ACE inhibitors and ARBs are equally effective in the treatment of diabetic nephropathy in patients with type 1 or 2 diabetic nephropathy. KDOQI 2007 clinical practice guidelines for diabetes and CKD prefer initiating therapy with an ACE inhibitor in type 1 diabetic nephropathy and either an ACE inhibitor or an ARB in type 2 diabetic nephropathy. If the BP goal is not reached, a diuretic should be added and, if necessary, followed by diltiazem, verapamil, or a β-blocker (Fig. 40.4).

BIBLIOGRAPHY

1. Zimmet P, Alberti KG, Shaw J: Global and societal implications of the diabetes epidemic. *Nature* 414:782–787, 2001

2. U.S. Renal Data System [website]. Available from www.usrds.org. Accessed 5 March 2008

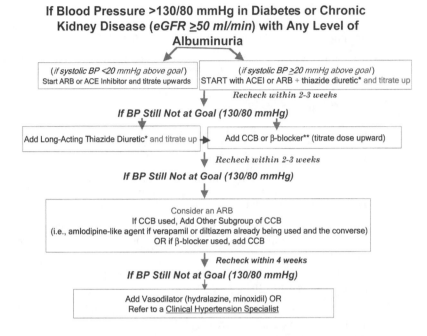

Figure 40.4 An approach to achieving recommended blood pressure goals in diabetic patients. CCB, calcium channel blocker.

3. Adler AI, Stevens RJ, Manley SE, Bilous RW, Cull CA, Holman RR: Development and progression of nephropathy in type 2 diabetes: the U.K. Prospective Diabetes Study (UKPDS 64). *Kidney Int* 63:225–232, 2003

4. KDOQI: KDOQI Clinical Practice Guidelines and Clinical Practice Recommendations for Diabetes and Chronic Kidney Disease. *Am J Kidney Dis* 49 (Suppl. 2):S12–S154, 2007

5. Jones CA, Agodoa L: Kidney disease and hypertension in blacks: scope of the problem. *Am J Kidney Dis* 21 (Suppl. 1):S6–S9, 1993

6. Nielsen FS, Rossing P, Gall MA, Skott P, Smidt UM, Parving HH: Long-term effect of lisinopril and atenolol on kidney function in hypertensive NIDDM subjects with diabetic nephropathy. *Diabetes* 46:1182–1188, 1997

7. U.K. Prospective Diabetes Study. XII. Differences between Asian, Afro-Caribbean, and white Caucasian type 2 diabetic patients at diagnosis of diabetes: U.K. Prospective Diabetes Study Group. *Diabet Med* 11:670–677, 1994

8. Collins VR, Dowse GK, Finch CF, Zimmet PZ, Linnane AW: Prevalence and risk factors for micro- and macroalbuminuria in diabetic subjects and entire population of Nauru. *Diabetes* 38:1602–1610, 1989

9. MacLeod JM, Lutale J, Marshall SM: Albumin excretion and vascular deaths in NIDDM. *Diabetologia* 38:610–616, 1995

10. Molitch ME, DeFronzo RA, Franz MJ: Nephropathy in diabetes. *Diabetes Care* 27 (Suppl. 1):S79–S83, 2004

11. O'Brien SF, Watts GF, Powrie JK, Shaw KM: Exercise testing as a long-term predictor of the development of microalbuminuria in normoalbuminuric IDDM patients. *Diabetes Care* 18:1602–1605, 1995

12. Mattix HJ, Hsu CY, Shaykevich S, Curhan G: Use of the albumin/creatinine ratio to detect microalbuminuria: implications of sex and race. *J Am Soc Nephrol* 13:1034–1039, 2002

13. Young BA, Katon WJ, Von KM: Racial and ethnic differences in microalbuminuria prevalence in a diabetes population: the pathways study. *J Am Soc Nephrol* 16:219–228, 2005

14. Coresh J, Selvin E, Stevens LA, et al.: Prevalence of chronic kidney disease in the U.S. *JAMA* 298:2038–2047, 2007

15. Orchard TJ, Dorman JS, Maser RE, et al.: Prevalence of complications in IDDM by sex and duration: Pittsburgh Epidemiology of Diabetes Complications Study II. *Diabetes* 39:1116–1124, 1990

16. Parving HH, Gall MA, Skott P, et al.: Prevalence and causes of albuminuria in noninsulin-dependent diabetic patients. *Kidney Int* 41:758–762, 1992

17. Mazzucco G, Bertani T, Fortunato M, et al.: Different patterns of renal damage in type 2 diabetes mellitus: a multicentric study on 393 biopsies. *Am J Kidney Dis* 39:713–720, 2002

18. Alsaad KO, Herzenberg AM: Distinguishing diabetic nephropathy from other causes of glomerulosclerosis: an update. *J Clin Pathol* 60:18–26, 2007

19. Mogensen CE: Systemic blood pressure and glomerular leakage with particular reference to diabetes and hypertension. *J Intern Med* 235:297–316, 1994

20. Nielsen S, Schmitz A, Rehling M, Mogensen CE: Systolic blood pressure relates to the rate of decline of glomerular filtration rate in type II diabetes. *Diabetes Care* 16:1427–1432, 1993

21. Mogensen CE: Prediction of clinical diabetic nephropathy in IDDM patients: alternatives to microalbuminuria? *Diabetes* 39:761–767, 1990

22. Raptis AE, Viberti G: Pathogenesis of diabetic nephropathy. *Exp Clin Endocrinol Diabetes* 109 (Suppl. 2):S424–S437, 2001

23. Ichinose K, Kawasaki E, Eguchi K: Recent advancement of understanding pathogenesis of type 1 diabetes and potential relevance to diabetic nephropathy. *Am J Nephrol* 27:554–564, 2007

24. Tilton RG, Chang K, Pugliese G, et al.: Prevention of hemodynamic and vascular albumin filtration changes in diabetic rats by aldose reductase inhibitors. *Diabetes* 38:1258–1270, 1989

25. Flyvbjerg A, Dgnaes-Hansen F, De Vriese AS, Schrijvers BF, Tilton RG, Rasch R: Amelioration of long-term renal changes in obese type 2 diabetic mice by a neutralizing vascular endothelial growth factor antibody. *Diabetes* 51:3090–3094, 2002

26. De Vriese AS, Stoenoiu MS, Elger M, et al.: Diabetes-induced microvascular dysfunction in the hydronephrotic kidney: role of nitric oxide. *Kidney Int* 60:202–210, 2001

27. Sharma K, Eltayeb BO, McGowan TA, et al.: Captopril-induced reduction of serum levels of transforming growth factor-beta1 correlates with long-term renoprotection in insulin-dependent diabetic patients. *Am J Kidney Dis* 34:818–823, 1999

28. Sharma K, Cook A, Smith M, Valancius C, Inscho EW: TGF-β impairs renal autoregulation via generation of ROS. *Am J Physiol Renal Physiol* 288:F1069-F1077, 2005

29. Nagai K, Matsubara T, Mima A, et al.: Gas6 induces Akt/mTOR-mediated mesangial hypertrophy in diabetic nephropathy. *Kidney Int* 68:552–561, 2005

30. Harris RD, Steffes MW, Bilous RW, Sutherland DE, Mauer SM: Global glomerular sclerosis and glomerular arteriolar hyalinosis in insulin-dependent diabetes. *Kidney Int* 40:107–114, 1991

31. Heilig CW, Concepcion LA, Riser BL, Freytag SO, Zhu M, Cortes P: Overexpression of glucose transporters in rat mesangial cells cultured in a normal glucose milieu mimics the diabetic phenotype. *J Clin Invest* 96:1802–1814, 1995

32. Mishra SI, Jones-Burton C, Fink JC, Brown J, Bakris GL, Weir MR: Does dietary salt increase the risk for progression of kidney disease? *Curr Hypertens Rep* 7:385–391, 2005

33. Bakris G, Molitch M, Hewkin A, et al.: Differences in glucose tolerance between fixed-dose antihypertensive drug combinations in people with metabolic syndrome. *Diabetes Care* 29:2592–2597, 2006

34. Singh AK, Mo W, Dunea G, Arruda JA: Effect of glycated proteins on the matrix of glomerular epithelial cells. *J Am Soc Nephrol* 9:802–810, 1998

35. Cooper ME: Pathogenesis, prevention, and treatment of diabetic nephropathy. *Lancet* 352:213–219, 1998

36. Maxhimer JB, Somenek M, Rao G, et al.: Heparanase-1 gene expression and regulation by high glucose in renal epithelial cells: a potential role in the pathogenesis of proteinuria in diabetic patients. *Diabetes* 54:2172–2178, 2005

37. Wilson DM, Luetscher JA: Plasma prorenin activity and complications in children with insulin-dependent diabetes mellitus. *N Engl J Med* 323:1101–1106, 1990

38. Daneman D, Crompton CH, Balfe JW, et al.: Plasma prorenin as an early marker of nephropathy in diabetic (IDDM) adolescents. *Kidney Int* 46:1154–1159, 1994

39. Nguyen G: Renin/prorenin receptors. *Kidney Int* 69:1503–1506, 2006

40. Ichihara A, Suzuki F, Nakagawa T, et al.: Prorenin receptor blockade inhibits development of glomerulosclerosis in diabetic angiotensin II type 1a receptor-deficient mice. *J Am Soc Nephrol* 17:1950–1961, 2006

41. Wolf G: Vasoactive factors and tubulointerstitial injury. *Kidney Blood Press Res* 22:62–70, 1999

42. Hohenstein B, Hausknecht B, Boehmer K, Riess R, Brekken RA, Hugo CP: Local VEGF activity but not VEGF expression is tightly regulated during diabetic nephropathy in man. *Kidney Int* 69:1654–1661, 2006

43. Sharma K, Ziyadeh FN: Hyperglycemia and diabetic kidney disease: the case for transforming growth factor-beta as a key mediator. *Diabetes* 44:1139–1146, 1995

44. Dai C, Liu Y: Hepatocyte growth factor antagonizes the profibrotic action of TGF-β1 in mesangial cells by stabilizing Smad transcriptional corepressor TGIF. *J Am Soc Nephrol* 15:1402–1412, 2004

45. Langham RG, Kelly DJ, Cox AJ, et al.: Proteinuria and the expression of the podocyte slit diaphragm protein, nephrin, in diabetic nephropathy: effects of angiotensin converting enzyme inhibition. *Diabetologia* 45:1572–1576, 2002

46. Adler S: Diabetic nephropathy: linking histology, cell biology, and genetics. *Kidney Int* 66:2095–2106, 2004

47. Trevisan R, Viberti G: Genetic factors in the development of diabetic nephropathy. *J Lab Clin Med* 126:342–349, 1995

48. Pettitt DJ, Saad MF, Bennett PH, Nelson RG, Knowler WC: Familial predisposition to renal disease in two generations of Pima Indians with type 2 (noninsulin-dependent) diabetes mellitus. *Diabetologia* 33:438–443, 1990

49. Imperatore G, Hanson RL, Pettitt DJ, Kobes S, Bennett PH, Knowler WC: Sib-pair linkage analysis for susceptibility genes for microvascular complications among Pima Indians with type 2 diabetes: Pima Diabetes Genes Group. *Diabetes* 47:821–830, 1998

50. Vardarli I, Baier LJ, Hanson RL, et al.: Gene for susceptibility to diabetic nephropathy in type 2 diabetes maps to 18q22.3-23. *Kidney Int* 62:2176–2183, 2002

51. Iyengar SK, Abboud HE, Goddard KA, et al.: Genome-wide scans for diabetic nephropathy and albuminuria in multiethnic populations: the Family

Investigation of Nephropathy and Diabetes (FIND). *Diabetes* 56:1577–1585, 2007

52. Movva S, Alluri RV, Komandur S, et al.: Relationship of angiotensin-converting enzyme gene polymorphism with nephropathy associated with type 2 diabetes mellitus in Asian Indians. *J Diabetes Complications* 21:237–241, 2007

53. Jeffers BW, Estacio RO, Reynolds MV, Schrier RW: Angiotensin-converting enzyme gene polymorphism in noninsulin-dependent diabetes mellitus and its relationship with diabetic nephropathy. *Kidney Int* 52:473–477, 1997

54. Kunz R, Bork JP, Fritsche L, Ringel J, Sharma AM: Association between the angiotensin-converting enzyme-insertion/deletion polymorphism and diabetic nephropathy: a methodologic appraisal and systematic review. *J Am Soc Nephrol* 9:1653–1663, 1998

55. Boright AP, Paterson AD, Mirea L, et al.: Genetic variation at the ACE gene is associated with persistent microalbuminuria and severe nephropathy in type 1 diabetes: the DCCT/EDIC Genetics Study. *Diabetes* 54:1238–1244, 2005

56. Pettersson-Fernholm K, Frojdo S, Fagerudd J, et al.: The AT2 gene may have a gender-specific effect on kidney function and pulse pressure in type I diabetic patients. *Kidney Int* 69:1880–1884, 2006

57. Tapp RJ, Shaw JE, Zimmet PZ, et al.: Albuminuria is evident in the early stages of diabetes onset: results from the Australian Diabetes, Obesity, and Lifestyle Study (AusDiab). *Am J Kidney Dis* 44:792–798, 2004

58. Writing team for the Diabetes Control and Complications Trial/Epidemiology of Diabetes Interventions and Complications Research Group: Sustained effect of intensive treatment of type 1 diabetes mellitus on development and progression of diabetic nephropathy: the Epidemiology of Diabetes Interventions and Complications (EDIC) study. *JAMA* 290:2159–2167, 2003

59. Fioretto P, Stehouwer CD, Mauer M, et al.: Heterogeneous nature of microalbuminuria in NIDDM: studies of endothelial function and renal structure. *Diabetologia* 41:233–236, 1998

60. Kohler KA, McClellan WM, Ziemer DC, Kleinbaum DG, Boring JR: Risk factors for microalbuminuria in black Americans with newly diagnosed type 2 diabetes. *Am J Kidney Dis* 36:903–913, 2000

61. Gaede P, Vedel P, Larsen N, Jensen GV, Parving HH, Pedersen O: Multifactorial intervention and cardiovascular disease in patients with type 2 diabetes. *N Engl J Med* 348:383–393, 2003

62. Joss N, Ferguson C, Brown C, Deighan CJ, Paterson KR, Boulton-Jones JM: Intensified treatment of patients with type 2 diabetes mellitus and overt nephropathy *QJM* 97:219–227, 2004

63. Finne P, Reunanen A, Stenman S, Groop PH, Gronhagen-Riska C: Incidence of end-stage renal disease in patients with type 1 diabetes. *JAMA* 294:1782–1787, 2005

64. Atkins RC, Briganti EM, Lewis JB, et al.: Proteinuria reduction and progression to renal failure in patients with type 2 diabetes mellitus and overt nephropathy. *Am J Kidney Dis* 45:281–287, 2005

65. De Zeeuw D, Remuzzi G, Parving HH, et al.: Albuminuria, a therapeutic target for cardiovascular protection in type 2 diabetic patients with nephropathy. *Circulation* 110:921–927, 2004

66. Chua DC, Bakris GL: Is proteinuria a plausible target of therapy? *Curr Hypertens Rep* 6:177–181, 2004

67. Kunz R, Friedrich C, Wolbers M, Mann JF: Meta-analysis: effect of monotherapy and combination therapy with inhibitors of the renin angiotensin system on proteinuria in renal disease. *Ann Intern Med* 148:30–48, 2008

67a. Sarafidis PA, Bakris GL: Renin-angiotensin blockade and kidney disease. *Lancet* 372:511–512, 2008

68. Morioka T, Emoto M, Tabata T, et al.: Glycemic control is a predictor of survival for diabetic patients on hemodialysis. *Diabetes Care* 24:909–913, 2001

69. Stadler M, Auinger M, Anderwald C, et al.: Long-term mortality and incidence of renal dialysis and transplantation in type 1 diabetes mellitus *J Clin Endocrinol Metab* 91:3814–3820, 2006

70. Bojestig M, Arnqvist HJ, Karlberg BE, Ludvigsson J: Glycemic control and prognosis in type I diabetic patients with microalbuminuria. *Diabetes Care* 19:313–317, 1996

71. Chantelau E: Decay of hemoglobin A1C upon return to normoglycemia. *Diabetologia* 35:191, 1992

72. Chase HP, Jackson WE, Hoops SL, Cockerham RS, Archer PG, O'Brien D: Glucose control and the renal and retinal complications of insulin-dependent diabetes. *JAMA* 261:1155–1160, 1989

73. Keen H: Insulin resistance and the prevention of diabetes mellitus. *N Engl J Med* 331:1226–1227, 1994

74. Gilbert RE, Tsalamandris C, Bach LA, et al.: Long-term glycemic control and the rate of progression of early diabetic kidney disease. *Kidney Int* 44:855–859, 1993

75. Kawazu S, Tomono S, Shimizu M, et al.: The relationship between early diabetic nephropathy and control of plasma glucose in noninsulin-dependent diabetes mellitus: the effect of glycemic control on the development and progression of diabetic nephropathy in an 8-year follow-up study. *J Diabetes Complications* 8:13–17, 1994

76. U.K. Prospective Diabetes Study Group: Efficacy of atenolol and captopril in reducing risk of macrovascular and microvascular complications in type 2 diabetes: UKPDS 39. *BMJ* 317:713–720, 1998

77. Levin A: Consequences of late referral on patient outcomes. *Nephrol Dial Transplant* 15 (Suppl. 3):S8–S13, 2000

78. Singh S, Loke YK, Furberg CD: Long-term risk of cardiovascular events with rosiglitazone: a meta-analysis. *JAMA* 298:1189–1195, 2007

79. Bakris GL: Progression of diabetic nephropathy: a focus on arterial pressure level and methods of reduction. *Diabetes Res Clin Pract* 39 (Suppl. 1):S35–S42, 1998

80. Viberti G: Prognostic significance of microalbuminuria. *Am J Hypertens* 7:69S–72S, 1994

81. Microalbuminuria Captopril Study Group: Captopril reduces the risk of nephropathy in IDDM patients with microalbuminuria. *Diabetologia* 39:587–593, 1996

82. Kasiske BL, Kalil RS, Ma JZ, Liao M, Keane WF: Effect of antihypertensive therapy on the kidney in patients with diabetes: a meta-regression analysis. *Ann Intern Med* 118:129–138, 1993

83. Parving HH, Lehnert H, Brochner-Mortensen J, Gomis R, Andersen S, Arner P: The effect of irbesartan on the development of diabetic nephropathy in patients with type 2 diabetes. *N Engl J Med* 345:870–878, 2001

84. Lewis EJ, Hunsicker LG, Clarke WR, et al.: Renoprotective effect of the angiotensin-receptor antagonist irbesartan in patients with nephropathy due to type 2 diabetes. *N Engl J Med* 345:851–860, 2001

85. Zhang Z, Shahinfar S, Keane WF, et al.: Importance of baseline distribution of proteinuria in renal outcomes trials: lessons from the Reduction of Endpoints in NIDDM with the Angiotensin II Antagonist Losartan (RENAAL) study. *J Am Soc Nephrol* 16:1775–1780, 2005

86. Barnett AH, Bain SC, Bouter P, et al.: Angiotensin-receptor blockade versus converting-enzyme inhibition in type 2 diabetes and nephropathy. *N Engl J Med* 351:1952–1961, 2004

87. Mogensen CE, Neldam S, Tikkanen I, et al.: Randomized controlled trial of dual blockade of renin-angiotensin system in patients with hypertension, microalbuminuria, and noninsulin-dependent diabetes: the Candesartan and Lisinopril Microalbuminuria (CALM) study. *BMJ* 321:1440–1444, 2000

88. Bakris GL, Ruilope L, Locatelli F, et al.: Treatment of microalbuminuria in hypertensive subjects with elevated cardiovascular risk: results of the IMPROVE trial. *Kidney Int* 72:879–885, 2007

89. Bakris GL, Weir MR, Secic M, Campbell B, Weis-McNulty A: Differential effects of calcium antagonist subclasses on markers of nephropathy progression. *Kidney Int* 65:1991–2002, 2004

90. Bakris GL, Copley JB, Vicknair N, Sadler R, Leurgans S: Calcium channel blockers versus other antihypertensive therapies on progression of NIDDM associated nephropathy. *Kidney Int* 50:1641–1650, 1996

91. Bohlen L, de Courten M, Weidmann P: Comparative study of the effect of ACE-inhibitors and other antihypertensive agents on proteinuria in diabetic patients. *Am J Hypertens* 7:84S–92S, 1994

92. Ruggenenti P, Fassi A, Ilieva AP, et al.: Preventing microalbuminuria in type 2 diabetes. *N Engl J Med* 351:1941–1951, 2004

93. Bakris GL, Barnhill BW, Sadler R: Treatment of arterial hypertension in diabetic humans: importance of therapeutic selection. *Kidney Int* 41:912–919, 1992

94. Bakris GL, Weir MR, DeQuattro V, McMahon FG: Effects of an ACE inhibitor/calcium antagonist combination on proteinuria in diabetic nephropathy. *Kidney Int* 54:1283–1289, 1998

95. Dworkin LD, Tolbert E, Recht PA, Hersch JC, Feiner H, Levin RI: Effects of amlodipine on glomerular filtration, growth, and injury in experimental hypertension. *Hypertension* 27:245–250, 1996

96. Smith AC, Toto R, Bakris GL: Differential effects of calcium channel blockers on size selectivity of proteinuria in diabetic glomerulopathy. *Kidney Int* 54:889–896, 1998

97. Nielsen FS, Rossing P, Gall MA, Skott P, Smidt UM, Parving HH: Impact of lisinopril and atenolol on kidney function in hypertensive NIDDM subjects with diabetic nephropathy. *Diabetes* 43:1108–1113, 1994

98. Bakris GL, Hart P, Ritz E: Beta blockers in the management of chronic kidney disease. *Kidney Int* 70:1905–1913, 2006

99. Hart PD, Bakris GL: Should β-blockers be used to control hypertension in people with chronic kidney disease? *Semin Nephrol* 27:555–564, 2007

100. Bakris GL, Fonseca V, Katholi RE, et al.: Differential effects of β-blockers on albuminuria in patients with type 2 diabetes. *Hypertension* 46:1309–1315, 2005

101. Bakris GL, Fonseca V, Katholi RE, et al.: Metabolic effects of carvedilol vs. metoprolol in patients with type 2 diabetes mellitus and hypertension: a randomized controlled trial. *JAMA* 292:2227–2236, 2004

102. Brenner BM, Cooper ME, de Zeeuw D, et al.: Effects of losartan on renal and cardiovascular outcomes in patients with type 2 diabetes and nephropathy. *N Engl J Med* 345:861–869, 2001

103. Lewis EJ, Hunsicker LG, Bain RP, Rohde RD: The effect of angiotensin-converting-enzyme inhibition on diabetic nephropathy: the Collaborative Study Group. *N Engl J Med* 329:1456–1462, 1993

104. Rachmani R, Slavachevsky I, Amit, et al.: The effect of spironolactone, cilazapril, and their combination on albuminuria in patients with hypertension and diabetic nephropathy is independent of blood pressure reduction: a randomized controlled study. *Diabet Med* 21:471–475, 2004

105. Sato A, Hayashi K, Naruse M, Saruta T: Effectiveness of aldosterone block-ade in patients with diabetic nephropathy. *Hypertension* 41:64–68, 2003

106. van den Meiracker AH, Baggen RG, Pauli S, et al.: Spironolactone in type 2 diabetic nephropathy: effects on proteinuria, blood pressure, and renal func-tion. *J Hypertens* 24:2285–2292, 2006

107. Han SY, Kim CH, Kim HS, et al.: Spironolactone prevents diabetic neph-ropathy through an anti-inflammatory mechanism in type 2 diabetic rats. *J Am Soc Nephrol* 17:1362–1372, 2006

108. Epstein M, Williams GH, Weinberger M, et al.: Selective aldosterone blockade with eplerenone reduces albuminuria in patients with type 2 dia-betes. *Clin J Am Soc Nephrol* 1:940–951, 2006

109. Bakris GL, Siomos M, Richardson D, et al.: ACE inhibition or angiotensin receptor blockade: impact on potassium in renal failure: VAL-K Study Group. *Kidney Int* 58:2084–2092, 2000

110. Rodriguez-Moran M, Gonzalez-Gonzalez G, Bermudez-Barba MV, et al.: Effects of pentoxifylline on the urinary protein excretion profile of type 2 diabetic patients with microproteinuria: a double-blind, placebo-controlled randomized trial *Clin Nephrol* 66:3–10, 2006

111. Bakris G, Viberti G, Weston WM, Heise M, Porter LE, Freed MI: Rosigli-tazone reduces urinary albumin excretion in type II diabetes. *J Hum Hyper-tens* 17:7–12, 2003

112. Agarwal R: Anti-inflammatory effects of short-term pioglitazone therapy in men with advanced diabetic nephropathy. *Am J Physiol Renal Physiol* 290:F600–F605, 2006

113. Cha DR, Zhang X, Zhang Y, et al.: Peroxisome proliferator–activated recep-tor α/γ dual agonist tesaglitazar attenuates diabetic nephropathy in db/db mice *Diabetes* 56:2036–2045, 2007

114. Ansquer JC, Foucher C, Rattier S, Taskinen MR, Steiner G: Fenofibrate reduces progression to microalbuminuria over 3 years in a placebo-con-trolled study in type 2 diabetes: results from the Diabetes Atherosclerosis Intervention Study (DAIS). *Am J Kidney Dis* 45:485–493, 2005

115. Keech AC, Mitchell P, Summanen PA, et al.: Effect of fenofibrate on the need for laser treatment for diabetic retinopathy (FIELD study): a random-ized controlled trial. *Lancet* 370:1687–1697, 2007

116. Fouque D, Aparicio M: Eleven reasons to control the protein intake of patients with chronic kidney disease. *Nat Clin Pract Nephrol* 3:383–392, 2007

117. Hansen HP, Tauber-Lassen E, Jensen BR, Parving HH: Effect of dietary protein restriction on prognosis in patients with diabetic nephropathy. *Kid-ney Int* 62:220–228, 2002

118. Morales E, Valero MA, Leon M, Hernandez E, Praga M: Beneficial effects of weight loss in overweight patients with chronic proteinuric nephropathies. *Am J Kidney Dis* 41:319–327, 2003

119. Jones-Burton C, Mishra SI, Fink JC, et al.: An in-depth review of the evidence linking dietary salt intake and progression of chronic kidney disease. *Am J Nephrol* 26:268–275, 2006

120. Go AS, Chertow GM, Fan D, McCulloch CE, Hsu CY: Chronic kidney disease and the risks of death, cardiovascular events, and hospitalization. *N Engl J Med* 351:1296–1305, 2004

121. Foley RN, Murray AM, Li S, et al.: Chronic kidney disease and the risk for cardiovascular disease, renal replacement, and death in the United States Medicare population, 1998 to 1999. *J Am Soc Nephrol* 16:489–495, 2005

122. Ruilope L, Kjeldsen SE, de la Sierra A, et al.: The kidney and cardiovascular risk—implications for management: a consensus statement from the European Society of Hypertension. *Blood Press* 16:72–79, 2007

123. Seliger SL, Weiss NS, Gillen DL, et al.: HMG-CoA reductase inhibitors are associated with reduced mortality in ESRD patients. *Kidney Int* 61:297–304, 2002

124. Wanner C, Krane V, Marz W, et al.: Atorvastatin in patients with type 2 diabetes mellitus undergoing hemodialysis. *N Engl J Med* 353:238–248, 2005

125. Gupta R, Plantinga LC, Fink NE, et al.: Statin use and hospitalization for sepsis in patients with chronic kidney disease. *JAMA* 297:1455–1464, 2007

126. Bakris GL, Weir MR: Angiotensin-converting enzyme inhibitor-associated elevations in serum creatinine: is this a cause for concern? *Arch Intern Med* 160:685–693, 2000

Dr. Davis is Associate Professor of Medicine at the University of Chicago, Chicago, Illinois. Dr. Duka is a Fellow in the Department of Medicine at the University of Chicago, Chicago, Illinois. Dr. Bakris is Professor of Medicine and Director of Hypertensive Diseases Unit at the University of Chicago, Chicago, Illinois.

41. Chronic Kidney Disease

ELI A. FRIEDMAN, MD

Individuals with either type 1 or type 2 diabetes risk injury to their kidneys. This injury begins as histological changes to glomeruli and small arterioles that may progress to irreversible renal failure, termed end-stage renal disease (ESRD). Of those individuals who express nephropathy, in about one-third of subjects with diabetes, both diabetes types manifest the same clinical changes culminating in uremia. While differences between the course of progressive kidney disease in type 1 or type 2 diabetes have been noted in some reports, both diabetes types follow similar time-related sequences.

As tabulated in the U.S. Renal Data System (USRDS) Annual Report for 2007, of 106,912 patients begun on therapy for ESRD during 2005, 46,851 (43.8%) had diabetes, an incidence rate of 152 per million population. Reflecting their relatively higher death rate compared to other causes of ESRD, the prevalence of U.S. diabetic ESRD patients on 31 December 2005 was 36.9% (179,157 of 485,012 patients).

Initially held to be the reason for exclusion from ESRD treatment in the 1960s and 1970s, ESRD attributed to diabetic nephropathy emerged as a continuously expanding treatable cause of renal failure to the extent that in the U.S., Japan, and industrialized Europe, diabetes is the leading cause of ESRD, surpassing glomerulonephritis and hypertension. In the U.S., in addition to the above-noted 44% of incident-treated patients in 2005, an additional 6.5% of patients who commenced ESRD therapy had diabetes that was not noted on their Medicare Report Form. A further 10% of incident ESRD patients had diabetes diagnosed during their first year of ESRD treatment, meaning that in the U.S., a minimum of 6 of 10 new ESRD patients had diabetes. ESRD and diabetes were intertwined as drains on health resources.

After years of hyperglycemia (usually accompanied by hypertension) and hyperlipidemia, diabetic nephropathy may reduce renal function to the extent that life is no longer possible without replacement therapy (i.e., hemodialysis, peritoneal dialysis, or kidney transplantation). Kidney malfunction in diabetes typically follows a well-demarcated sequence of microalbuminuria preceding proteinuria that in turn is followed by azotemia over several years to a decade or longer. Chronic kidney disease (CKD), however, may develop suddenly because of a vascular catastrophe (atheroembolic disease), sustained hypotension complicating coronary artery surgery or other major surgery, or treatment with a nephrotoxic drug or antibiotic.

In health, urinary protein excretion for an adult woman or man is <25 mg/day. Microalbuminuria, defined as a 24-h urinary albumin excretion rate of 20–200 µg/min (30–300 mg/24 h), is a laboratory finding predictive of subsequent nephropathy. The upper limit corresponds approximately to a total urinary protein concentration of 0.5 g/l, the hallmark of clinical nephropathy. Increased mortality is observed in both type 1 and type 2 diabetic patients who have microalbuminuria. The usual course of diabetic nephropathy, however, entails months to years of a nephrotic syndrome (proteinuria >3.5 g/day, hypoalbuminuria, hyperlipidemia, and anasarca) followed by azotemia, which signals the onset of CKD. CKD has been defined as a progressive deterioration of glomerular filtration rate (GFR) through five stages (1–5). ESRD is the typical termination of CKD stage 5. Severe CKD induces myriad extrarenal diverse symptoms, physical signs, and abnormal laboratory values that, in the aggregate, constitute the uremic syndrome. Appropriate therapy for the microalbuminuric and/or proteinuric individual with diabetes is remarkably effective in retarding progression of nephropathy, delaying ESRD in some individuals for a decade or longer.

Untreated uremia results in orange-yellow skin discoloration (urochrome pigmentation), easy bruisability, wasting of muscle and fat, and a blunted, dull affect stressed by a reversed diurnal sleep pattern. Anemia, acidosis, and azotemia are the cardinal laboratory findings in CKD stages 4 and 5. Agonal ESRD may present with fibrinous pericarditis and pericardial tamponade, bowel ulceration (colitis, gastritis), and neurological syndromes (grand mal seizures, transient cortical blindness, and motor nerve paralysis). When treated by hemodialysis, peritoneal dialysis, or kidney transplantation, life extension for several years to more than three decades is attainable for many individuals with diabetes who develop ESRD.

THERAPY

Every person with diabetes and a kidney syndrome should understand the overall strategy for care, termed a "life plan." Management approaches to diabetic nephropathy have three main objectives:

1. Detect and eliminate potentially reversible factors that can decrease renal functional reserve.
2. Preserve GFR by modulating blood pressure, metabolic control, and dietary protein intake. The choice of antihypertensive medications should include (unless precluded by drug toxicity such as hyperkalemia and/or an incapacitating dry cough) an ACE inhibitor and/or an angiotensin receptor blocker (ARB) because of their renoprotective effects. Recent trials indicate that the combination of an ACE inhibitor plus an ARB consistently stabilizes diabetic nephropathy and may prevent GFR loss for ≥5 years.
3. Prepare the patient and his or her family for kidney replacement therapy while preserving work, school, or home activities when uremia supervenes. These decisions include:

   - Scheduling treatment of comorbid extrarenal conditions, especially diabetic retinopathy, heart disease, foot infections, and peripheral arterial disease

- Making an intrafamilial kidney transplant feasible
- When a familial donor is absent, registering for a deceased donor kidney at the nearest regional transplant facility
- Selecting a dialysis technique (peritoneal or hemodialysis) when a renal transplant is unlikely
- Gaining familiarity with variations in dialytic therapy, including daily hemodialysis
- Constructing a vascular access for hemodialysis access if that therapy is chosen
- Electing a locale (home or facility) if hemodialysis is chosen
- Identifying markers indicating that ESRD therapy must be initiated

When constructing an individual's life plan, every opportunity should be taken to fortify the patient's emotions for coming stressful arduous components of kidney replacement therapy. An intensive patient educational program under the auspices of a nurse educator should include consideration of normal and abnormal renal function and descriptions of dialysis and kidney transplantation. To minimize stress to patients, provide literature from the American Association of Kidney Patients and suggest that patients visit their website (www.aakp.org). Also, introduce patients to other patients currently undergoing ESRD therapy. Key components of therapy are given in Table 41.1.

Preserving Renal Functional Reserve

Use caution when administering nephrotoxic drugs such as aminoglycoside antibiotics to avoid superimposed iatrogenic injury. Drugs that should not be administered to patients with azotemia include nitrofurantoin, spironolactone, amiloride, triamterene, metformin, and phenformin. Abruptly deteriorating renal function may be the consequence of interstitial nephritis (not directly induced by diabetes) caused by captopril, cimetidine, methicillin sodium, allopurinol, phenylhydantoin, nonsteroidal anti-inflammatory drugs, or furosemide. The ACE inhibitors may reversibly worsen azotemia and/or precipitate hyperkalemia and incapacitating nonproductive cough in up to 20% of individuals with diabetes. ARBs regulate hypertensive blood pressure, reduce proteinuria, and slow the course of nephropathy, but they may also trigger renal functional deterioration and, less often, nonproductive cough. Dosage reductions according to residual GFR of cyclophosphamide, cimetidine, clofibrate, digoxin, and many antibiotics (particularly aminoglycosides) are required for azotemic patients.

Because of the risk of urinary infection, bladder catheterization in a diabetic patient with azotemia should be restricted to the few instances when the information to be gained is unobtainable by other means. Easing the measurement of daily urinary output is insufficient justification for an indwelling bladder catheter.

There is serious risk of worsening renal insufficiency when radiographic contrast medium is administered to diabetic patients with serum creatinine levels >2.5 mg/dl (>227.3 µmol/l) or estimated GFR (eGFR) <40 ml/min. Under circumstances where radiographic contrast medium must be given, e.g., before a limb arterial bypass, prior hydration with half-normal saline and mannitol infusion (25 g in 2 liters 0.45% saline solution) may protect against renal injury. Early trials in small numbers of diabetic patients suggest that pretreatment with *N*-acetylcysteine

Table 41.1 Therapy for Azotemic Diabetic Patients

1. Discontinue nephrotoxic drugs and limit exposure to radiocontrast agents.
2. When radiocontrast agents must be administered, maintain patient hydration.
3. Detect and treat urinary infection, including asymptomatic bacteriuria.
4. Correct electrolyte imbalance with special attention to hyperkalemia.
5. Establish a daily log to record weight, blood pressure, and blood glucose excursions.
6. Decrease excess extracellular volume (anascara) by combining metolazone (10–40 mg) with 40–240 mg furosemide in a twice-daily regimen until a stable "dry weight" is obtained. Record and monitor daily weight as well as self-measured daily blood glucose values. Report unusual weight increases (fluid retention) or decreases (excess diuretic effect) to primary physician.
7. Expand plasma volume if contracted.
8. Control hypertension, striving for continuous blood pressure levels <125/75 mmHg. Include ACE inhibitor and/or ARB, as tolerated.
9. With the assistance of a nutritionist, construct acceptable diet, restricting dietary protein to ≤40–60 g/day.
10. Correct hyperlipidemia by diet or pharmacological means using a standard hypolipidemic regimen plus a statin drug to a target LDL cholesterol <100 mg/dl.
11. Control hyperphosphatemia by diet and calcium-based phosphate binders (calcium carbonate).
12. Reduce hyperuricemia if >12 mg/dl or at lower levels if symptomatic gout occurs.
13. Add 1.2–4.8 g/day oral bicarbonate for severe acidosis, especially if renal tubular acidosis is present.
14. Administer synthetic vitamin D, with careful attention to avoid hypercalcemia.
15. For symptomatic anemia, when hematocrit is at <30%, after excluding blood loss and other extrarenal causes, administer recombinant erythropoietin 50–150 units/kg subcutaneously three times per week, maintaining iron stores as needed. Consider darbepoetin alfa given once every 1–3 weeks subcutaneously in an equivalent or reduced dosage.
16. Avoid volume depletion, radiocontrast media, nephrotoxic drugs, and bladder catheterization.

(600 mg orally twice daily) coupled with hydration with saline solution or infusion of sodium bicarbonate will in several studies preempt contrast medium injury. However, the question of optimal protection against contrast media nephropathy remains open.

Minimizing the Rate of GFR Loss

The rate of renal functional decline in diabetic nephropathy is slowed by normalization of hypertension and dietary protein restriction. In microalbuminuric individuals who are not hypertensive, treatment with an ACE inhibitor and/ or an ARB reduces the rate of increase in albumin excretion. Thus, regardless of blood pressure level, every individual with type 1 or type 2 diabetes should be treated with an ACE inhibitor and/or an ARB when microalbuminuria is discovered. For individuals who cannot tolerate ACE inhibitors because of drug allergy, nonproductive cough, or a rise in serum potassium or creatinine concentration, a trial with an ARB alone will achieve the same objective of retarding the course of nephropathy.

Preservation of bone integrity is the objective of treatment with intestinal phosphate binders. No clear superiority of calcium-based versus calcium-free phosphate binders such as resin polymers or lanthium has been established.

The American Diabetes Association advises that patients with diabetes be maintained at a target blood pressure ≤130/80 mmHg. Hypertension due to diabetic nephropathy is often associated with intravascular volume expansion and anasarca resulting from hypoalbuminemia consequent to nephrotic-range proteinuria. Reduction of the amount of intravascular and extracellular excess fluid is a vital component of blood pressure control. Diuresis can usually be affected in CKD stages 1–3 by graded doses of furosemide (40–120 mg twice a day). Metolazone (5–40 mg once or twice per day) induces diuresis even when the creatinine clearance has fallen in CKD stages 4 and 5 to <10 ml/min.

Close observation of the patient, with recording of daily weight, is mandatory when prescribing a potent diuretic regimen. Once edema is reduced, doses of metolazone and furosemide should be decreased while monitoring daily weight to avoid dehydration, intravascular volume contraction, and vascular collapse. As GFR declines to <15 ml/min (CKD stage 5), patient compensation straddles a narrow range between dehydration and extracellular volume overload—the difference in weight between the two extremes may be as little as 3–6 kg, underscoring the necessity for recording daily weight. GFR stabilization by intensified antihypertensive treatment is possible in patients with overt diabetic nephropathy, even if renal function is markedly impaired. For hypertension resistant to diuretics, ACE inhibitors, and calcium channel blockers, a trial-and-error regimen of vasodilators and β-blockers may be attempted.

When successive trials of ACE inhibitors, ARBs, calcium channel blockers, vasodilators, β-blockers, as well as α-blockers fail to attain satisfactory blood pressure regulation, minoxidil in doses of 2.5–70 mg/day almost always reduces blood pressure to <140/90 mmHg. Careful observation of minoxidil-treated patients for tachycardia and fluid retention is required, and the abnormalities are managed by the addition of diuretics and β-blockers. Single daily doses of long-acting antihypertensive drugs such as nifedipine (a calcium channel blocker) and lisinopril (an ACE inhibitor) facilitate patient adherence over that attained with multidose regimens.

Dietary protein restriction may retard renal injury that ends as glomerulosclerosis. Although convincingly effective in retarding renal functional deterioration in rats, trials in small groups of patients with progressive renal disorders, including diabetic nephropathy, indicate that a diet containing 40–60 g/day protein (with or without addition of essential amino acids or their precursor) slows but does not stop renal functional loss. Appreciating that the benefit of protein restriction on the progress of diabetic nephropathy is unproven, the prudent physician may nevertheless opt to prescribe a diet containing <80 g/day dietary protein while suggesting modest protein restriction (40–60 g/day).

Maintenance of the Metabolic Environment

Perturbed lipid metabolism is characteristic of diabetic patients with nephropathy, especially when accompanied by a nephrotic syndrome. Hypertriglyceridemia and low levels of HDL are typical of azotemic patients with diabetic nephropathy; the risk of coronary artery disease, expressed as the ratio of total cholesterol to

HDL cholesterol, is elevated. Partial correction of these lipid abnormalities may be affected by weight reduction in obese individuals with a low-fat diet, nicotinic acid, a statin, or a fibrate. The American Diabetes Association advises that patients with diabetes be maintained at a target LDL cholesterol level ≤100 mg/dl.

As the GFR falls below ~30 ml/min, hyperphosphatemia and reduced renal synthesis of active vitamin D may cause reciprocal hypocalcemia and hyperparathyroidism. Hyperphosphatemia can be controlled by limiting phosphate intake to 500–800 mg/day; dairy products are high in phosphate content. Premeal ingestion of intestinal phosphate-binding drugs, e.g., aluminum hydroxide and aluminum carbonate or magnesium hydroxide (1–2 g three times per day), and calcium supplementation (calcium carbonate 1–3 g three times per day) will lower the serum phosphate concentration to 5 mmol/l. Unfortunately, when reducing the serum phosphate concentration to normal, treatment with phosphate binders may be complicated by hypermagnesemia, hypercalcemia, aluminum-induced vitamin D–resistant bone disease, and neurological disorders. Aluminum toxicity is also associated with a syndrome of dementia and anemia. For these reasons, a calcium-based phosphate binder became the first choice, and aluminum gels are no longer used. More expensive regimens for reducing hyperphosphatemia, including sevelamer, a polymeric amine, and lanthanum carbonate, have not been shown to afford any clear advantage.

Hypocalcemia in the absence of marked hyperphosphatemia is effectively treated by daily administration of 1,25-dihydroxyvitamin D_3. Treatment with this vitamin early in the course of progressive renal insufficiency prevents renal bone disease and reverses secondary hyperparathyroidism.

In advanced diabetic nephropathy, attention to the amount of dietary sodium and potassium is important as the GFR falls below 15 ml/min (CKD stage 5). A small subset of diabetic patients—those with concurrent interstitial renal disease—may lose large quantities of urinary sodium, similar to salt-wasting individuals with Addison's disease. In contrast, most azotemic individuals with diabetes predominantly have glomerular disease, which causes retention of salt and water. Defining a correct dietary salt prescription for the individual patient requires a process of trial and error termed "salt balancing." Daily weights are the keystone to the regimen, which begins with a diet made up of 40 g protein and 2 g salt. The salt waster's weight will decrease, necessitating supplementation with sodium bicarbonate tablets (600 mg) given up to four times per day. With continued weight loss, the amount of sodium bicarbonate is increased by increments of 1.2 g/day until a stable weight results. At the other extreme, the nephrotic salt retainer may evince pulmonary congestion and peripheral edema with the initial 2-g salt prescription, in which case furosemide (40–80 mg three times per day) is added.

Dietary potassium restriction is rarely required before the daily urine output falls below 1 liter or the patient is under treatment with drugs that impair K^+ excretion (e.g., an ACE inhibitor). Hyperkalemia <6 mEq/l can usually be managed by reducing dietary intake of K^+, especially in citrus juices. More severe K^+ retention requires administration of a cation-exchange resin (e.g., sodium polystyrene sulfonate). A trial discontinuance of ACE inhibitors and other K^+-retaining or -elevating drugs is a key step in managing hyperkalemia.

Anemia in diabetic patients with reduced renal function is mainly the consequence of diminished renal secretion of erythropoietin. In patients with ESRD who are sustained by hemodialysis or peritoneal dialysis, correction of typical anemia (hematocrit of 20–25% raised to 32–38%) is effected by thrice-weekly subcutaneous injections of recombinant erythropoietin (2,000–8,000 units). Indications for erythropoietin administration in predialysis patients include advanced anemia (hematocrit <31%), coronary artery disease, and inordinate fatigue.

Raising erythrocyte mass in the azotemic individual with diabetes is an important component of sustaining daily activities before developing ESRD. Broad use of erythropoietin, a genetically engineered form of human erythropoietin, indicates that correction of anemia in predialysis patients achieves substantive benefit in terms of life quality, ability to continue employment, and subjective assessment of severity of illness. Introduction of darbepoetin alfa, another engineered variant of human erythropoietin (in prefilled syringes containing 40–200 µg) that can be injected subcutaneously as infrequently as once every 2 weeks, simplified the regimen, although high cost continues to be an impediment to universal acceptance of the need for raising hematocrit levels to normal. A recent concern, precipitating a U.S. Food and Drug Administration black box warning for prescribed erythropoietin and darbepoeitin, cautions: "Patients experienced greater risks for death and serious cardiovascular events when administered erythropoiesis-stimulating agents to target higher versus lower hemoglobin levels (13.5 vs. 11.3 g/dl; 14 vs. 10 g/dl) in two clinical studies. Individualize dosing to achieve and maintain hemoglobin levels within the range of 10–12 g/dl is advised." Like so many other aspects of modern medicine, a powerful advance must be used with awareness of potential side effects.

Comprehensive management of declining renal function in a person with diabetes involves:

- Normalization of hypertensive blood pressure ≤130/80 mmHg
- Treatment of blood glucose to an A1C ≤7.0%
- Correction of hyperlipidemia LDL cholesterol ≤100 mg/dl
- Reduction of hyperphosphatemia with phosphate binders
- Administration of synthetic 1,25-dihydroxyvitamin D_3
- Cautiously raising the hematocrit with recombinant erythropoietin

During progressive loss of GFR, periodic (monthly to weekly as GFR falls) measurements of weight, hematocrit, blood urea nitrogen, serum creatinine, serum potassium, and serum calcium should be performed at each visit. Insulin and other small peptide hormones are partially degraded by the kidney. On reduction of GFR to <25 ml/min, insulin catabolism within the kidney lessens to the extent that progressively intensive hypoglycemic episodes may interfere with metabolic control in a previously stable individual. When the serum creatinine level increases to >5 mg/dl (>442 µmol/l), the need for kidney replacement therapy is urgent.

HEMODIALYSIS

Maintenance hemodialysis is the kidney replacement regimen used for >90% of people with diabetes who develop ESRD in the U.S. Of prevalent patients in 2006, 93.4% were sustained by hemodialysis, according to the 2008 report of the U.S. Renal Data System. Performance of maintenance hemodialysis requires vascular access to the circulation. Deciding to undergo hemodialysis or any other renal replacement therapy should be the consequence of a clear presentation of options, including answering questions raised by patient and family. An intrafamilial kidney transplant is the most desired choice, yielding the best survival and overall rehabilitation of any uremia therapy. Should hemodialysis be selected (as the preferred treatment modality), early creation of a radial artery-to-vein internal fistula in the nondominant forearm at the wrist is a federal standard of care. Appreciating that it usually takes ≥2 months for an arteriovenous fistula to mature, meaning to induce easily cannulated forearm veins, and the procedure is usually more difficult in a patient with diabetes than in a nondiabetic person because of systemic atherosclerosis, planning should be initiated as soon as ESRD is projected. For many diabetic patients with peripheral vascular calcification and/or atherosclerosis, establishment of an access for hemodialysis necessitates use of synthetic (Dacron) prosthetic vascular grafts. In both sexes and in all age-groups, survival of individuals with diabetes treated with maintenance hemodialysis has been inferior to that of nondiabetic patients. More recent data indicate that survival in diabetes on dialysis is improving to the extent that the curves for those with and without diabetes coincide for the first 5 years of dialytic therapy. Currently, the added value of daily hemodialysis is under evaluation as a means of enhancing quality of life, reducing the need for erythropoietin and antihypertensive drugs, and improving nutritional status, as judged by a rising serum albumin concentration. The main concerns in delivering maintenance hemodialysis for diabetic patients are listed in Table 41.2.

PERITONEAL DIALYSIS

Peritoneal dialysis has been used effectively to sustain life in 5–10% of individuals with diabetes who develop ESRD. Continuous ambulatory peritoneal dialysis (CAPD), a self-treatment, has grown rapidly in application because of its advantages (compared with home hemodialysis) of rapid training, reduced cardiovascular stress, and avoidance of heparin (Table 41.3); home hemodialysis requires 3–16 weeks of training. As a facilitating procedure for peritoneal dialysis, an intraperitoneal catheter is sewn in place several days before CAPD is begun. Motivated diabetic patients, including those who are blind, are able to learn to perform CAPD at home within 3 weeks. In practice, patients exchange 2–3 liters of commercially prepared sterile dialysate four to five times per day. Insulin, antibiotics, and other drugs are added by the patient to each dialysate exchange.

Simplification of peritoneal dialysate exchanges has been brought about by use of a mechanical cycler in the therapeutic variation called continuous cyclic peritoneal dialysis (CCPD). Both CAPD and CCPD subject the diabetic patient to the constant risk of peritonitis and a gradual decrease in peritoneal surface area. Peritonitis has an incidence rate of about once every 10 months of peritoneal dialysis.

KIDNEY TRANSPLANTATION

Kidney transplantation is the preferred therapeutic option for selected patients with ESRD because of diabetic nephropathy. Both patient survival and degree of

Table 41.2 Concerns or Issues in Conducting Maintenance Hemodialysis in Patients with Diabetes

- Meet with patient, provide instructional literature until the patient is sufficiently informed to permit selection of a specific option in uremia therapy.
- If hemodialysis is preferred, determine type and date for surgical creation of vascular access that may be either:
  1. Internal arteriovenous fistula
  2. Teflon arteriovenous graft
- Metabolic regulation
  1. Take frequent fingerstick glucose measurements (insulin-treated diabetes).
  2. Use fractional insulin doses or insulin pump (type 1 diabetes).
  3. Reeducate patients about diet and exercise.
  4. Instruct patient in American Diabetes Association targets for glucose and A1C.
- Normalize weight and introduce daily activity (exercise).
- When there is a propensity to hypotension:
  1. Establish patient's "dry weight."
  2. Minimize intradialytic weight gain.
  3. Use bicarbonate dialysate.
  4. Perform gradual ultrafiltration for fluid extraction during hemodialysis.
- To preserve vision:
  1. Collaborate with ophthalmologist.
  2. Use lowest effective heparin dosage during hemodialysis.
  3. Use two or more pillows for head elevation during active retinopathy.
- To preserve lower extremities:
  1. Wear heel booties.
  2. Collaborate with podiatrist.
- When obstipation complicates use of phosphate binders:
  1. Prescribe detergent with antacid gel for phosphate sorption.
  2. Metoclopramide stimulates bowel motility and is taken before meals. Also taken is a non–glucose-containing stool softener such as psyllium seed husks (Metamucil), a soluble plant fiber that is often labeled as a laxative, but is not. Fibers become gelatinous and sticky in water, are not absorbed in the small bowel, and are broken down in the large bowel, becoming a food source for bacteria in the colon.
- For depression:
  1. Obtain membership in patient self-help organizations, especially the American Association of Kidney Patients (www.aakp.org).
  2. Enlist patient, patient's family, and individuals who give social support in overall planning.

rehabilitation in diabetic transplant recipients are sharply superior to results attained by dialytic therapy. With cyclosporine or tacrolimus as the main immunosuppressive drugs coupled with induction therapy, including monoclonal anti-lymphocyte antibodies, kidney transplantation has improved progressively to the extent that patient survival at 1 and 2 years is equivalent in recipients with and without diabetes, whereas kidney graft survival is <10% lower in individuals with diabetes than in nondiabetic recipients at 2 years. Newer immunosuppressive drugs in clinical trials, including rapamycin, sirolimus, lefunomide, and mycophenolate mofetil, offer promise of still further reduced allograft rejection with less nephrotoxicity.

Table 41.3 CAPD or CCPD in Patients with Diabetes

By way of direct meeting, provision of literature, and discussion of any questions, enable the patient to make an informed selection of a specific option in uremia therapy. Should peritoneal dialysis be preferred, schedule date for surgical insertion of abdominal catheter.

- Advantages
  1. Rapid establishment as a home therapy
  2. Partner not essential, although required for home hemodialysis
  3. Few profound hypotensive episodes compared with hemodialysis
  4. Insulin regimen simplified by direct addition to dialysate
  5. Enthusiastic patient acceptance of freedom from machine (CAPD)
  6. Survival equivalent to hemodialysis, at least for first 3 years
  7. Minimal stress to cardiovascular system; no extracorporeal circulation
- Disadvantages
  1. Intra-abdominal catheter-related complications
  2. Pain, bleeding, dialysate leak
  3. Obstruction of intraperitoneal catheter
  4. Perforation of abdominal viscus during catheter insertion
- Mechanical
  1. Abdominal hernia
  2. Hydrothorax, ascites
- Peritoneal
  1. Peritonitis as frequent as once every 10 months
  2. Peritoneal thickening (sclerosis) and loss of dialyzing surface
- Neuropsychiatric
  1. Depression over daily necessity for multiple exchanges
  2. Restriction on swimming and some strenuous activities
  3. Boredom with regimen and altered self-image
  4. Time required for multiple daily fluid exchanges

Kidney replacement therapy is more difficult to initiate and sustain, and the course is stressful in diabetic patients because of excessive morbidity and mortality imparted by extrarenal disease. Variables in selecting therapy are presented in Table 41.4. Preparation for a kidney transplant in a patient with diabetes, for example, requires careful cardiac evaluation to detect and treat coronary artery disease, the major cause of death in the azotemic diabetic patient. A dobutamine or exercise stress test with thallium imaging will suffice, if normal, as a prelude to a kidney or kidney-pancreas transplantation. Cardiac catheterization and corrective coronary artery bypass grafting or intracoronary stent placement may preempt unanticipated death from heart disease during the posttransplant period.

Consultations with an ophthalmologist and a podiatrist familiar with abnormalities of the diabetic eye and foot, respectively, are also desirable during transplant evaluation. Assistance from other specialists, including a gastroenterologist and neurologist, is usually required before kidney replacement therapy. Unappreciated gastroparesis may interfere with regimens contingent on relating the timing of food ingestion to insulin injections. Once discovered, metoclopramide given in doses of 5–10 mg before meals usually corrects gastric hypomotility.

Table 41.4 Comparison of Options in Kidney Replacement Therapy in Diabetes

Variable	Peritoneal Dialysis	Hemodialysis	Kidney Transplant
Extensive extrarenal disease	No limitation	No limitation except where hypotension interdicts sufficient extracorporeal blood flow	Excluded in cardiovascular insufficiency, liver failure, active hepatitis, bone marrow depression, active malignancy
Geriatric patients (>65 yr)	No age restriction	No age restriction	Arbitrary exclusion of older patients; age cutoff (65–75 yr) determined by some programs
Complete rehabilitation	Rare, if ever, unless high residual GFR	Very few individuals unless high residual GFR	Common as long as allograft functions at GFR >40 ml/min, contingent on proactive approach to eye, heart, and vascular disease
Death rate	Higher than for nondiabetic peritoneal dialysis patients	Higher than for nondiabetic hemodialysis patients	About the same as nondiabetic transplant recipients for the first 2 yr, then higher death rate
First-year patient survival	<87%	<79%	93–97%
Survival to second decade	Rare; only 5% alive after 10 yr	Unusual <5% living after 10 yr	One in two recipients of either live or deceased donor kidneys survive 10 yr
Progression of complications	Usual and unremitting; hyperglycemia and hyperlipidemia accentuated	Usual and unremitting	Interdicted by functioning pancreas + kidney; regression of neuropathy reported; vasculopathy progresses in recipients of renal allografts
Special advantage	Can be self-performed; rapid training; avoids swings in solute and intravascular volume level	Can be self-performed; extraction of solute and water in hours	Cures uremia; freedom to travel; offers best survival and superior rehabilitation

(continued)

Table 41.4 Comparison of Options in Kidney Replacement Therapy in Diabetes (*Continued*)

Variable	Peritoneal Dialysis	Hemodialysis	Kidney Transplant
Disadvantage	Peritonitis, hyperinsulinemia, hyperglycemia, hyperlipidemia; long hours of treatment; more days hospitalized than either hemodialysis or transplant patients	Blood access a hazard for clotting, hemorrhage, and infection; cyclical hypotension, weakness; aluminum toxicity, amyloidosis	Cosmetic disfigurement from corticosteroids and cyclosporine; hypertension; personal expense for cytotoxic drugs; induced malignancy; HIV transmission; corticosteroids and tacrolimus aggravate glycemic control
Patient acceptance	Variable, after initial enthusiasm, usual compliance with passive tolerance for regimen	Variable, often noncompliant with dietary, metabolic, or antihypertensive component of regimen	Buoyant during periods of good renal allograft function; joyful when pancreas transplant establishes euglycemia
Bias in comparison	Delivered as first choice by enthusiasts, but in U.S., substantially higher mortality than for hemodialysis; in Canada, peritoneal dialysis has lower mortality than hemodialysis	Treatment by default; often complicated by inattention to progressive cardiac and peripheral arterial disease	Kidney transplant programs preselect patients with fewest complications; exclusion of those >45 yr for pancreas + kidney simultaneous grafting obviously favorably biasing outcome
Relative cost	Approximately $70,000 annually for 2003–2005 according to U.S. Renal Data System	Approximately $82,000 annually for 2003–2005 according to U.S. Renal Data System	Pancreas + kidney engraftment most expensive uremia therapy for diabetes (more than $180,000); kidney transplant alone approximately $120,000, then $25,000 annually according to U.S. Renal Data System

REFERRAL TO A RENAL SPECIALIST

First referral to a nephrologist is advisable when urinary protein excretion is constant at >500 mg/day. Initial renal evaluation will be directed toward quantifying renal reserve by measuring GFR and excluding causes of nephropathy other than diabetes. Resorting to percutaneous renal biopsy is indicated when the renal syndrome is atypical for diabetes: absence of retinopathy, associated gross hematuria, or pyuria. Subsequent nephrology consultations at yearly intervals will chart progress of renal functional loss, increase in proteinuria, and regulation of blood pressure. The use of synthetic vitamin D and erythropoietin to manage hyperphosphatemia (hypocalcemia) and anemia should be guided by a kidney specialist. Once azotemia is noted (serum creatinine concentration >1.5 mg/dl in men and >1.2 mg/dl in women), the frequency of contact with a nephrologist should increase to bimonthly, and later, monthly (frequency of follow-up visits is contingent on the rate of loss of GFR). When it is anticipated that dialytic therapy or a kidney transplantation will be needed within 6 months (serum creatinine ≥5 mg/dl [≥442 µmol/l]), the main responsibility for management should shift to the collaborating nephrologist. Provision of comprehensive care in which collaborating specialists are orchestrated by a team-leading nephrologist is a central theme of successful management of advanced diabetic nephropathy.

BIBLIOGRAPHY

Abbott KC, Bakris GL: What have we learned from the current trials? *Med Clin North Am* 88:189–207, 2004

American Diabetes Association: Standards of medical care in diabetes—2009. *Diabetes Care* 32 (Suppl. 1):S13–S62, 2009

Bakris GL: Slowing nephropathy progression: focus on proteinuria reduction. *Clin J Amer Soc Nephrol* 3 (Suppl. 1):S3–S10, 2008

Berman DH, Friedman EA, Lundin AP: Aggressive ophthalmological management in diabetic ESRD: a study of 31 consecutively referred patients. *Am J Nephrol* 12:344–350, 1992

Biesenback G, Janko O, Zazgornik J: Similar rate of progression in the predialysis phase in type I and type II diabetes mellitus. *Nephrol Dial Transplant* 9:1097–1102, 1994

Bode BW, Schwartz S, Stubbs HA, Block JE: Glycemic characteristics in continuously monitored patients with type 1 and type 2 diabetes: normative values. *Diabetes Care* 28:2361–2366, 2005

Coyle D, Rodby RA: Economic evaluation of the use of irbesartan and amlodipine in the treatment of diabetic nephropathy in patients with hypertension in Canada. *Can J Cardiol* 20:71–79, 2004

Diaz-Sandoval LJ, Kosowsky BD, Losordo DW: Acetylcysteine to prevent angiography-related renal tissue injury (the APART trial). *Am J Cardiol* 89:356–358, 2002

Jerums G, Panagiotopoulos S, Premaratne E, Power DA, Macisaac RJ: Lowering of proteinuria in response to antihypertensive therapy predicts improved renal function in late but not in early diabetic nephropathy: a pooled analysis. *Am J Nephrol* 28:614–627, 2008

Johnson DW: Evidence-based guide to slowing the progression of early renal insufficiency. *Intern Med J* 34:50–57, 2004

Kaplan NM: Management of hypertension in patients with type 2 diabetes mellitus: guidelines based on current evidence. *Ann Intern Med* 135:1079–1083, 2001

Kelly AM, Dwamena B, Cronin P, Bernstein SJ, Carlos RC: Meta-analysis: effectiveness of drugs for preventing contrast-induced nephropathy. *Ann Intern Med* 148:284–294, 2008

Klahr S, Morrissey J, Hruska K, Wang S, Chen Q: New approaches to delay the progression of chronic renal failure. *Kidney Int* 61 (Suppl. 80):23–26, 2002

Kong AP, So WY, Szeto CC, Chan NN, Luk A, Ma RC, Ozaki R, Ng VW, Ho CS, Lam CW, Chow CC, Cockram CS, Chan JC, Tong PC: Assessment of glomerular filtration rate in addition to albuminuria is important in managing type II diabetes. *Kidney Int* 69:383–387, 2006

Lane JT: Microalbuminuria as a marker of cardiovascular and renal risk in type 2 diabetes mellitus: a temporal perspective. *Am J Physiol Renal Physiol* 286:F442–F450, 2004

Levey AS, Eckardt KU, Tsukamoto Y, Levin A, Coresh J, Rossert J, Zeeuw D, Hostetter TH, Lameire N, Eknoyan G: Definition and classification of chronic kidney disease: a position statement from Kidney Disease: Improving Global Outcomes (KDIGO). *Kidney Int* 67:2089–2100, 2005

McCarter RJ, Hempe JM, Chalew SA: Mean blood glucose and biological variation have greater influence on HbA$_{1c}$ levels than glucose instability: an analysis of data from the Diabetes Control and Complications Trial. *Diabetes Care* 29:352–355, 2006

Nakai S, Shinzato T, Nagura Y, Masakane I, Kitaoka T, Shinoda T, Yamazaki C, Sakai R, Ohmori H, Morita O, Iseki K, Kikuchi K, Kubo K, Suzuki K, Tabei K, Fushimi K, Miwa N, Wada A, Yanai M, Akiba T; Patient Registration Committee, Japanese Society for Dialysis Therapy, Tokyo: An overview of regular dialysis treatment in Japan (as of 31 December 2001). *Ther Apher Dial* 8:3–32, 2004

Nangaku M: Mechanisms of tubulointerstitial injury in the kidney: final common pathways to end-stage renal failure. *Intern Med* 43:9–17, 2004

Parving HH, Chaturvedi N, Viberti G, Mogensen CE: Does microalbuminuria predict diabetic nephropathy? *Diabetes Care* 25:406–407, 2002

Remuzzi G, Schieppati A, Ruggenenti P: Clinical practice: nephropathy in patients with type 2 diabetes. *N Engl J Med* 346:1145–1151, 2002

Rippin JD, Barnett AH, Bain SC: Cost-effective strategies in the prevention of diabetic nephropathy. *Pharmacoeconomics* 22:9–28, 2004

Ruilope LM, Segura J: Losartan and other angiotensin II antagonists for nephropathy in type 2 diabetes mellitus: a review of the clinical trial evidence. *Clin Ther* 25:3044–3064, 2004

Sferra L, Kelsberg G, Dodson S: Do ACE inhibitors prevent nephropathy in type 2 diabetes without proteinuria? *J Fam Pract* 53:68–69, 2004

Thomas MC, Rosengard-Barlund M, Mills V, Ronnback M, Thomas S, Forsblom C, Cooper ME, Taskinen MR, Viberti G, Groop PH: Serum lipids and the progression of nephropathy in type 1 diabetes. *Diabetes Care* 29:317–322, 2006

U.S. Renal Data System: *USRDS 2007 Annual Data Report Atlas of End-Stage Disease in the United States.* Bethesda, MD, National Institutes of Health, National Institute of Diabetes and Digestive and Kidney Diseases, 2007

Weisbord SD, Palevsky PM: Prevention of contrast-induced nephropathy with volume expansion. *Clin J Am Soc Nephrol* 3:273–280, 2008

Dr. Friedman is a Distinguished Teaching Professor of Medicine at the Downstate Medical Center, Brooklyn, New York.

42. Painful or Insensitive Lower Extremity

ANDREW J. M. BOULTON, MD, FRCP

Peripheral neuropathy and obstructive arterial disease are common causes of leg pain in patients with diabetes. Whereas sensory neuropathy is usually the precipitant of painful symptoms, other neuropathic syndromes may also result in pain (Table 42.1). Reduced sensation to sensory stimuli, including pain, temperature, touch, and vibration in the feet and lower parts of the legs in diabetic patients, is invariably a result of sensory neuropathy and may go unnoticed by patients for years unless specifically tested for and demonstrated. Paradoxically, some patients may experience spontaneous painful or paresthetic symptoms while concurrently having marked loss of sensation on neurological examination—a condition described as the "painful/painless leg." The explanation for this not uncommon finding is that the sensory nerves to the feet are severely diseased and fail to conduct stimuli. Proximally, however, spontaneous electrical activity in diseased peripheral axons is interpreted by the patient as pain and is perceived in the area (i.e., the foot) that the nerve used to innervate.

PATHOPHYSIOLOGY

The true causes of diabetic neuropathy remain enigmatic. However, evidence from large trials such as the Diabetes Control and Complications Trial and the U.K. Prospective Diabetes Study clearly implicate chronic hyperglycemia as the prime abnormality that results in many of the mechanisms summarized in Table 42.2.

EPIDEMIOLOGY

Peripheral sensory neuropathy is common, affecting up to 50% of older type 2 diabetic patients. The average endocrine practice with a mixed age range of patients would expect a neuropathy prevalence of ~33%. Neuropathy is more prevalent with increasing age and duration of diabetes (Table 42.3). Of 100 patients with sensory neuropathy, up to 50 may be asymptomatic, and only 10–20 would be expected to have significant symptoms that require treatment.

Table 42.1 Conditions that Result in Pain in Lower Limbs of Diabetic Patients

- Sensory neuropathy
  - ☐ Acute sensory
  - ☐ Chronic sensorimotor
- Entrapment neuropathy
  - ☐ Meralgia paresthetica
- Proximal motor neuropathy (amyotrophy)
- Peripheral arterial disease
  - ☐ Intermittent claudication
  - ☐ Rest pain

DIAGNOSIS

Because up to half of all patients with diabetic distal sensory neuropathy may experience no symptoms, the diagnosis cannot be made by history alone. Careful clinical examination of the feet is indicated in all patients on at least an annual basis.

HISTORY

Take a careful history, inquiring about pain, discomfort, or numbness in the legs. Patients with no spontaneously volunteered symptoms might, if asked, describe numbness or say that their feet "feel dead." Remember, diabetic neuropathy is a diagnosis of exclusion of other causes. Atypical features that might suggest a nondiabetic cause of neuropathy include rapid progression, foot drop, back or neck pain, marked asymmetry, weight loss, and family history.

EXAMINATION

A careful inspection of the feet is indicated. In longstanding sensorimotor neuropathy, small muscle wasting may be seen. Dry skin suggests coexisting sympa-

Table 42.2 Proposed Pathogenetic Mechanisms for Neuropathy

- Hyperglycemia
- Nonenzymatic glycation
- Oxidative stress
- Ischemic/hypoxic factors
- Nerve growth factor abnormalities
- Polyol pathway activation
- Immunological abnormalities

Table 42.3 Risk Factors for Neuropathy

- Age
- Duration of diabetes
- Glycemic control
- Cholesterol/triglyceride level
- Hypertension
- Other microvascular complications
- Smoking

thetic dysfunction. Look for ulcers, deformities, or Charcot changes. Simple neurological assessment ideally would include:

- Pressure sensation (use a 10-g monofilament)

Plus one of the following

- Pinprick sensation
- Light touch
- Vibration (use a 128-Hz tuning fork at the apex of the hallux)
- Ankle reflexes

All these tests should be performed bilaterally, and the patient should be observed walking after the shoes have been inspected. Patients with severe sensory loss but no symptoms are often unsteady during normal gait because of the loss of proprioception.

The diagnosis of diabetic neuropathy is normally a clinical one. Quantitative assessment of sensory modalities and electrophysiological studies may help to define the severity of the neuropathy but will not distinguish between neuropathy due to diabetes or to other causes (Table 42.4). It is particularly important to exclude malignant disease. For example, an older male diabetic patient who smokes and has typical neuropathic symptoms and signs coupled with weight loss might well have a paraneoplastic syndrome associated with a bronchogenic carcinoma, giving rise to the neurological symptoms and signs.

Table 42.4 Other Causes of Peripheral Neuropathy

- Malignant disease
- Toxins (e.g., alcohol)
- Uremia
- Infections (e.g., HIV)
- Metabolic disorders (e.g., uremia, hypothyroidism)
- Iatrogenic agents (e.g., cytotoxic drugs, isoniazid)
- Inflammatory disease (e.g., chronic inflammatory demyelinating polyneuropathy)

PAINFUL NEUROPATHY

As stated above, the differential diagnosis of pain in the diabetic leg includes a number of conditions (Table 42.1), the most common of which is sensory neuropathy.

Sensory Neuropathy

Distal sensory neuropathy includes the common chronic sensorimotor variety and the relatively rare acute sensory neuropathy. The symptoms are of similar character and commonly comprise burning discomfort, pain of an electrical nature, stabbing, prickling, pricking, and shooting or stabbing pains symmetrically in the feet and lower legs. Pins and needles (Novocain like) and other dysesthetic symptoms are also common. All these symptoms are prone to nocturnal exacerbation with characteristic bed cloth hyperesthesia.

Patients with troublesome nocturnal symptoms may benefit from getting up and walking around, in contrast to enduring ischemic rest pain. They may occasionally immerse their legs in cold water to relieve the burning discomfort.

Acute sensory neuropathy tends to follow periods of metabolic instability (such as ketoacidosis) or a sudden change of metabolic control, such as after rapid improvement of control after starting insulin (insulin neuritis). Symptoms are severe, signs are few, and the prognosis for disappearance of symptoms is good (in a matter of weeks or months).

Chronic sensorimotor neuropathy is the most common variety of diabetic neuropathy and is of insidious onset with symptoms that wax and wane. Although symptoms are sensory, as described above, signs are both sensory and motor, with small muscle wasting and absent reflexes, hence "sensorimotor neuropathy."

The symptoms of this type of neuropathy were well described by Dr. Pavy of London in 1884 as being "of a burning and unremitting character." These symptoms may last intermittently for years but gradually tend to improve; this improvement is often accompanied by progressive sensory loss, leaving the patient at risk of insensitive foot injuries.

Entrapment Neuropathy

Entrapment of the lateral cutaneous nerve of the thigh can give rise to localized neuropathic symptoms in its area of innervation, the lateral area of the midthigh. This pain is localized and usually unilateral, in contrast to symmetrical distal sensory neuropathy. It is known as "meralgia paresthetica."

Amyotrophy (Proximal Motor Neuropathy)

Amyotrophy typically affects older male type 2 diabetic patients with neuropathic pain in the thigh region together with proximal motor weakness.

Peripheral Arterial Disease

Claudication, a classic symptom of peripheral arterial disease, should not be confused with neuropathic pain. It is usually described as a cramping in the calf muscles, induced by exercise and relieved by rest without changing positions.

TREATMENT OF PAINFUL SENSORY NEUROPATHY

Many patients with severely painful conditions believe that they have malignant disease; thus, reassurance that this is not the case and that treatment is available for these symptoms, which may well resolve in due course, is an important part of management. The first step in symptom management is to stabilize glycemic control. There is increasing evidence that blood glucose flux may exacerbate neuropathic pain, so avoiding swings of glycemia from hypoglycemia to hyperglycemia may help. Insulin is not always needed in type 2 diabetic patients if control is satisfactory on oral agents. Most patients will also require some form of pharmacotherapy for the painful symptoms, as summarized in Table 42.5.

Tricyclic drugs remain a useful therapy in some patients because they have proven efficacy in several randomized trials. Their pain-relieving effects are usually apparent in a matter of days, in contrast to their antidepressant actions. The predictable side effects of drowsiness and anticholinergic symptoms (particularly dry mouth) limit their use, and up to one-third of patients cannot tolerate them at all. To avoid these effects, start with a low dose given at bedtime (e.g., 10–25 mg amitriptyline) and build up gradually until symptoms are relieved.

Gabapentin is a useful anticonvulsant, again with efficacy confirmed in randomized trials; however, it has been replaced in many cases by the newer agent pregabalin, which appears to have equivalent efficacy but can usefully be given twice daily.

Duloxetine, the selective serotonin and norepinephrine reuptake inhibitor, has been demonstrated to have useful pain-relieving effects in a number of trials of patients with painful diabetic neuropathy. Additionally, it has antidepressive properties.

Among the other listed drugs, tramadol, an opioid-like centrally acting synthetic nonnarcotic analgesic, has also been shown to be efficacious in the management of neuropathic pains, although only short-term (up to 6 months) use is recommended. More recently, other opioids such as oxycodone-CR (controlled release) have been shown to be useful in patients with severe neuropathic pain

Table 42.5 Drug Treatment of Neuropathic Symptoms

Agent/Group	Drug	Daily Dosage	Side Effects
Tricyclics	Amitriptyline Imipramine	10–150 mg hs 10–150 mg hs	Drowsiness Anticholinergic
Anticonvulsants	Gabapentin Pregabalin Carbamazepine	900–3,000 mg divided 150–600 mg divided Up to 800 mg divided	Central side effects: dizziness, somnolence
Dual reuptake inhibitor	Duloxetine	60–120 mg daily	Drowsiness, nausea
Opioid-like	Tramadol Oxycodone-CR	50–400 mg divided	Nausea, constipation, drowsiness

hs, bedtime.

often unresponsive to any of the above agents. However, these agents are invariably accompanied by typical opioid side effects. Topical agents such as capsaicin may be helpful in cases of localized pain, and acupuncture has been shown to be of use in a long-term open study.

THE INSENSITIVE FOOT

Any patient found on clinical examination to have reduced sensation to modalities such as vibration, touch, or pain must be considered to be at risk of insensitive injury. Methods to avoid further complications such as ulceration or Charcot neuroarthropathy should be actively pursued in such individuals. These typically include education in personal foot care, regular visits to a podiatrist, more frequent visits to the physician, and advice on footwear.

BIBLIOGRAPHY

Boulton AJM, Malik RA, Arezzo JC, Sosenko JM: Diabetic somatic neuropathies. *Diabetes Care* 27:1458–1486, 2004

Boulton AJM, Vinik AI, Arezzo JC, Bril V, Feldman EL, Freeman R, Malik RA, Mase RE, Sosenko JM, Ziegler D: Diabetic neuropathies: a statement by the American Diabetes Association. *Diabetes Care* 28:958–962, 2005

Boulton AJM, Cavanagh PR, Rayman G (Eds.): *The Foot in Diabetes.* 4th ed. New York, Wiley, 2006

Boulton AJ, Armstrong DG, Albert SF, Frykberg RG, Hellman R, Kirkman MS, Lavery LA, LeMaster JW, Mills JL, Mueller MJ, Sheehan P, Wukich DK: Comprehensive foot examination and risk assessment: a report of the task force of the foot care interest group of the American Diabetes Association, with endorsement by the American Association of Clinical Endocrinologists. *Diabetes Care* 31:1679–1685, 2008

Bowker JH, Pfeifer MA (Eds.): *Levin and O'Neil's "The Diabetic Foot."* 7th ed. St. Louis, MO, Mosby, 2008

Casellini CM, Vinik AI: Clinical manifestations and current treatment options for diabetic neuropathies. *Endocrin Pract* 13:550–556, 2007

Veves A (Ed.): *Clinical Management of Diabetic Neuropathy.* 2nd ed. Totowa, NJ, Humana Press, 2007

Ziegler D: Painful diabetic neuropathy: treatment and future aspects. *Diabetes Metab Res Rev* 24 (Suppl. 1):S52–S57, 2008

Dr. Boulton is Visiting Professor of Medicine, University of Miami School of Medicine, Miami, Florida; and Professor of Medicine, University of Manchester, and Consultant Physician, Manchester Royal Infirmary, Manchester, U.K.

43. Diabetic Monoradiculopathy/ Amyoradiculopathy

Aaron Vinik, MD, PHD, FCP, MACP, and Archana Nakave, MD

Peripheral neuropathies in diabetes comprise a variety of peripheral nerve afflictions. Of the various subgroups, length-dependent distal symmetric polyneuropathy (DSPN) is the most common type of peripheral nerve damage. However, all anatomical parts of the peripheral nervous system may be affected by diabetes, and this creates difficulties in proper diagnosis and selection of optimal therapy. The focal and multifocal neuropathies are confined to the distribution of single or multiple peripheral nerves, and their involvement is referred to as mononeuropathy or mononeuritis multiplex. A focal neurological deficit in the nerve distribution at the brachial or lumbosacral plexus is known as diabetic plexopathy or, when at the nerve roots, as radiculopathy. Each neurological abnormality has different pathogenesis, mode of onset, course of disease, signs and symptoms, and associated laboratory and clinical information from that of DSPN, and if this is understood and recognized, then response to treatment can be quite salutary. Table 43.1 distinguishes the features of classic DSPN from those of the asymmetric mono-/polyneuropathies.

FOCAL NEUROPATHIES (MONONEURITIS) AND ENTRAPMENT SYNDROMES

Focal neuropathies are distinguished by their presentation and distribution of clinical symptoms (Table 43.2). They have the following characteristics:

- Focal (asymmetric unilateral or bilateral muscle weakness)
- Painful (pain is one of the most disabling features)
- Acute or subacute (all signs and symptoms develop in a few days to 2 months)
- Self-limited (spontaneous complete recovery or significant improvement of clinical signs is the rule)

Mononeuropathies are due to a vasculitis with subsequent ischemia or infarction of nerves. They heal spontaneously, usually within 6–8 weeks. Mononeuropathies involve the median (5.8% of all diabetic neuropathies), ulnar (2.1%), radial (0.6%), and common peroneal nerves. Cranial neuropathies are extremely rare (0.05%); involve primarily cranial nerves III, IV, VI, and VII (Boulton et al. 2005); and occur in older individuals with a long duration of diabetes (Vinik et al.

Table 43.1 Differentiation of DSPN from Mono-/Amyoradiculopathies

	DSPN	Mono-/Amyoradiculopathies
Onset	Insidious	Acute/subacute
Distribution	Distal, length dependent	Proximal, asymmetric
Leading signs and symptoms	Mild to moderate sensory symptoms (negative or positive) and mild motor symptoms	Severe sensory (positive pain) and motor (weakness and atrophy) symptoms
Course of disease	Slow progression	Monophasic
Glycemic control	Dependent	Independent
Duration of diabetes	Dependent	Independent
Association with retinopathy and nephropathy	Associated	Not associated

2006). Their onset is acute and associated with pain, and their course is self-limiting, resolving over a period of 6 weeks.

Pathogenesis

Mononeuropathies are thought to occur because of a microvascular "infarct," which, in the majority of cases, resolves spontaneously over several months. Electrophysiological studies show a reduction in both nerve conduction and amplitude, suggestive of underlying demyelination and axonal degeneration (Boulton et al. 2005).

Mononeuropathies must, however, be distinguished from entrapment syndromes, which start slowly, progress, and persist without intervention (Table 43.3). Common entrapment syndromes involve the following:

- Median nerve with impaired sensation in the first three fingers and positive Tinel sign over the wrist
- Ulnar nerve with decreased sensory perception in the little and ring fingers and Tinel sign over the ulnar canal at the elbow (ulnar entrapment)
- Lateral cutaneous nerve of the thigh with pain in the upper anterior aspect of the thigh and hyper- or hypoesthesia in the nerve distribution (the condition is known as meralgia paresthetica, and the nerve is trapped under the inguinal ligament)
- Peroneal nerve with pain in the outer anterior aspect of the tibial region and weakness during dorsiflexion of the foot
- Median and lateral plantar nerves with decreased sensation in the inside and outside of the feet, respectively (medial and lateral plantar entrapments)

Electrophysiological studies are most helpful in identifying blocks in conduction at the entrapment sites. Spinal stenosis is also common in people with diabe-

Table 43.2 Common Mononeuropathies

Cranial	3rd, 4th, 6th, 7th
Thoracic	Mononeuritis multiplex
Peripheral	Peroneal
	Sural
	Sciatic
	Femoral
	Ulnar
	Median

tes and needs to be distinguished from the proximal neuropathies and amyotrophy (Boulton et al. 2005). In mononeuropathies, such as peroneal palsy, where weakness is a prominent feature, physical therapy may be necessary to maintain good muscle tone and prevent contractures.

MONONEUROPATHIES

Painful Ophthalmoplegia

Severe retro- and periorbital pain with radiation into the frontal and temporal areas is the first symptom of painful ophthalmoplegia. Diplopia due to ocular mononeuropathy or partial lesion of all oculomotor nerves follows the acute pain syndrome resembling either retro-orbital infection or acute brain pathology. Sparing of the pupillary reaction is a very important sign in differentiating diabetic ophthalmoplegia from structural ophthalmoplegia. Diabetic ophthalmoplegia is self-limited, and spontaneous recovery occurs over a period of 6–8 weeks. The lesion is a vascular occlusion to an interfascicular neuron, and other fascicles take over the function. It is imperative to distinguish diabetic ophthalmoplegia from the other causes of painful ophthalmoplegia because it is a common presentation of orbital, and paraorbital, diseases as well as brainstem catastrophes. Posterior communicating aneurysm rupture can be distinguished because it presents with loss of the pupillary reaction to light and accommodation, and this is spared in diabetic oculomotor palsy. Other causes of painful ophthalmoplegia, such as cavernous sinus thrombosis, orbital infection, cranial arteritis, primary or metastatic tumors, Tolosa-Hunt syndrome, and Gradenigo's syndrome, should be excluded because they require active intervention as opposed to diabetic ophthalmoplegia.

Diabetic Thoracoabdominal Neuropathy

Diabetic thoracoabdominal neuropathy is characterized by manifestations of symptoms and signs along single or multiple intercostal nerves. Pain is the leading complaint and often results in unnecessary surgical treatment, especially in low thoracic root involvement, when acute abdominal pathology can be sug-

Table 43.3 Comparison of Features of Mononeuritis and Entrapment

	Mononeuritis	Entrapment
Onset	Sudden	Gradual
Pain	Acute	Chronic
Multiplex	Occurs	Rare
Course	Resolves	Persists without intervention
Treatment	Physical therapy	Rest, splints, steroid and local anesthetic injections, surgery

gested. Pain in thoracoabdominal neuropathy is mostly burning and tingling in character and associated with hyperesthesia and allodynia. It resembles herpetic pain or sunburn-type pain and is rarely followed by numbness and hypoesthesia in the corresponding dermatomes. Profound anterior or anterior-lateral abdominal and thoracic involvement is characteristic, whereas back pain is atypical. Muscle weakness is also common. It is prominent with lower thoracic root affliction and creates a "false" hernia with bulging of the abdominal muscles because of loss of tone. Superficial pain and hyperesthesia in combination with painless deep palpation can be useful diagnostic criteria to exclude underlying visceral involvement. The course of the disease and prognosis are the same as in the proximal neuropathies.

Treatment of Diabetic Mononeuropathy with α-Lipoic Acid

As indicated above, for the most part, treatment of mononeuropathy is conservative and usually results in spontaneous resolution. However, as in DSPN, it has been suggested that oxidative stress participates in the pathogenesis of mononeuropathies by inducing neurovascular defects that result in endoneural hypoxia and subsequent nerve dysfunction (Rice et al. 2007). α-Lipoic acid is a universal antioxidant, exerting direct (directly scavenges free radicals) and indirect (participates in the process of recycling of other natural antioxidants, e.g., reduced glutathione and vitamins C and E) antioxidant activity (Dawson 1993, Cornblath et al. 2007, Vinik et al. 2008, Barohn et al. 1991). It has been established that α-lipoic acid protects from lipid peroxidation and increases the activity of the antioxidant enzymes—catalase and superoxide dismutase—in peripheral nerves (Leedman et al. 1988). By decreasing oxidative stress, α-lipoic acid normalizes the impaired endoneural blood flow as well as the impaired nerve conduction velocity (Leedman et al. 1988). Several studies have established the neuroregenerative and neuroprotective effects of α-lipoic acid. It appears to be an effective drug in the treatment for not only peripheral and autonomic diabetic neuropathy but also diabetic mononeuropathy of the cranial nerves, leading to recovery of the patients, and it has also been proven to be effective in some cases of mononeuritis multiplex (Tankova et al. 2005). Similarly, the antiepileptic drug topiramate exerts neuroprotective effects and has been shown to reverse phrenic nerve palsy refractory to conventional medical therapy (Rice et al. 2007).

ENTRAPMENT SYNDROMES

Carpal Tunnel Syndrome

Carpal tunnel syndrome (CTS) occurs thrice as frequently in the diabetic population as in the healthy population. Its increased prevalence in diabetes may be related to repeated undetected trauma, metabolic changes, or accumulation of fluid or edema within the confined space of the carpal tunnel. It is more common in female individuals and in obese individuals (BMI >30 kg/m^2) and affects the dominant hand. It occurs in 2% of the general population, 14% of diabetic patients without diabetic proximal neuropathy (DPN), and 30% of diabetic patients with DPN. It peaks at ~40–60 years of age, and an increased wrist index is a risk factor. CTS used to be associated with work-related injury but now seems to be common in people in sedentary positions and is probably related to the use of keyboards and typewriters. Dentists are particularly prone to CTS. Smoking appears to be an important risk factor for entrapments, and systemic disorders such as hypertension, hypothyroidism, rheumatoid arthritis, and acromegaly all contribute to its occurrence.

If recognized, the diagnosis can be confirmed by an electrophysiological study. The unaware physician seldom realizes that symptoms may spread to the whole hand or arm in CTS, and the signs may extend beyond those subserved by the nerve entrapped. Tinel sign for median nerve (percussion at the wrist) is positive in 61% and Phalen's test (wrist flexion) in only 46%. Thus, the very nature of the trouble goes unrecognized, and an opportunity for successful therapeutic intervention is often missed. Electromyogram–nerve conduction velocity can be particularly useful in distinguishing CTS from DSPN and the double crush syndrome of C7-8 radiculopathy. The high sensitivity and specificity of a nerve conduction study makes it the most valuable diagnostic method for diagnosing CTS (80% positive). Moreover, it is the only technique to establish subclinical cases and differentiate CTS from DSPN. Impaired nerve conduction at the wrist over the median nerve with normal ulnar nerve conduction is characteristic of CTS. Combined entrapment of the median and ulnar nerves can mimic DSPN and can only be distinguished by electromyogram–nerve conduction velocity with nerve stimulation in the palm. Treatment of CTS involves rest, splinting the wrist in a neutral position, use of a diuretic to reduce edema, liberal use of nonsteroidal anti-inflammatory agents, and injections of steroids and local anesthetics under the ligament. Surgical release may be required in cases unresponsive to these medical measures.

Ulnar Nerve Entrapment

The second common entrapment syndrome is that of the ulnar nerve (ulnar nerve entrapment). Sensory symptoms and weakness of the fourth and fifth fingers, accompanied by hypothenar atrophy, are the typical signs of ulnar nerve entrapment. Etiology of ulnar nerve entrapment includes trauma, arthritis, and systemic diseases (less often than in CTS). As in CTS, conduction through the elbow is decreased. A C8-T1 radiculopathy must be excluded. Response to local injections is less rewarding than in CTS, and surgical release is only of value if done early, before there is wasting of the interosseous muscles.

Peroneal Nerve Entrapment

Peroneal nerve entrapment at the level of the fibula head is the most common entrapment syndrome in the lower limbs and is due to the ease of external compression of the peroneal nerve under general anesthesia, when crossing the legs (especially in older people while sleeping), and with weight loss. It needs to be distinguished from an L5 radiculopathy with foot drop. Tripping and fractures are a consequence of impaired peroneal nerve function, especially in older people.

Tarsal Tunnel Syndrome

Tarsal tunnel syndrome is a painful lower-limb entrapment. Passing through the tarsal tunnel, the tibial nerve innervates only muscles of the sole, and clinical signs are mostly sensory. Foot pain may be severe, burning, or worse on standing and walking. Tinel sign on the underside of the medial malleolus, with atrophy of the sole muscles, is typical. Weakness is rare because most of the small foot muscles (flexor hallucis longus) are not damaged in tarsal tunnel syndrome. Nerve conduction velocity can be informative in the case of a normal plantar response from one leg and an abnormal response from the symptomatic side in unilateral tarsal tunnel syndrome. Tarsal tunnel syndrome is not difficult to diagnose clinically when DSPN is not severe and nerve conduction velocity is moderately abnormal. Mild symmetric peroneal and tibial nerve conduction velocity abnormality with intact ankle jerks and sensation of the dorsal aspect of the foot with the above-mentioned clinical signs are the most important diagnostic features of tarsal tunnel syndrome. When neuropathy is severe, diagnosis may be impossible.

The mainstays of nonsurgical treatment are avoiding use of the joint, placing a splint in a neutral position for day and night use, and using anti-inflammatory medications and targeted injections of local anesthetics and steroids. Surgical treatment consists of sectioning the offending ligament. The decision to proceed with surgery should be based on several considerations, including severity of symptoms, appearance of motor weakness, and failure of nonsurgical treatment (Dawson 1993).

Surgical Decompression for Diabetic Sensorimotor Polyneuropathy

While it is clear that surgical decompression may be of value when there is bona fide compression demonstrable by a conduction block at known sites of entrapment, "the utility of surgical decompression for symptomatic diabetic neuropathy received a grade IV rating, i.e., based on evidence from uncontrolled studies, case reports, or expert opinion" (Cornblath et al. 2007). Surgical decompression was assigned a U grading, which is defined as "data inadequate or conflicting given current knowledge, treatment is unproven" (Cornblath et al. 2007). "We believe the findings of the American Academy of Neurology's evidence-based review should be strong evidence that the procedures should not be considered care but, rather, subjected to further research until proven beneficial. Only well-controlled, randomized, double-masked, sham-procedure, controlled clinical trials will allow us to know whether these surgeries are safe and effective for this indication—the same standard that any drug for DPN would have to meet" (Cornblath et al. 2007, Vinik et al. 2008).

DPN

DPN is one of the most unpleasant and disabling conditions of diabetes. It was first reported by Bruns and Garland as subacute proximal leg weakness with moderate pain, and the term "diabetic amyotrophy" was coined by Garland in 1961 to emphasize prominent thigh muscle affliction (Barohn et al. 1991). Based on clinical and neurophysiological findings, the same condition was described variably as "diabetic femoral neuropathy," "diabetic polyradiculopathy," "proximal motor neuropathy," and "diabetic lumbosacral plexopathy." Despite this diversity of terminology and some disagreement on the complement and severity of symptoms and signs, DPN is now a well-known and established entity. DPN presents clinically with the following features:

- It primarily affects older adults (>64 years of age) with type 2 diabetes (Boulton et al. 2005) and almost exclusively affects male patients.
- It can be gradual or abrupt in onset.
- It begins with jabbing, knifelike pain with hyperesthesia and allodynia, usually in the anterior thigh region, spreading to the buttocks and down the leg. It usually starts on one side and then spreads to the other.
- Sensory loss is atypical.
- Pain is followed by significant pelvifemoral muscle weakness (quadriceps, iliopsoas, hip adductors, hamstrings, and glutei), with predominantly thigh muscles involved; the inability to rise from a chair or rise from the kneeling position occurs.
- DPN begins unilaterally and spreads bilaterally.
- Knee reflexes are absent.
- It coexists with DSPN.
- Patients include individuals with chronic inflammatory demyelinating polyneuropathy (CIDP), monoclonal gammopathy of unknown significance (MGUS), GM1 antibody syndrome, and inflammatory vasculitis as well as subjects with diabetes.
- It was formerly thought that DPN was often a self-limited condition and resolved spontaneously in 1.5–3.0 years.
- Current thinking is that DPN is an inflammatory condition with vasculitis or immune-mediated nerve damage and can resolve within days on appropriate therapy, and immune-mediated epineurial microvasculitis has been demonstrated in nerve biopsies (Boulton et al. 2005).
- This condition is unrelated to blood glucose control and is not associated with triopathies.
- A more severe diffuse distal-proximal DSPN with strongly pronounced weight loss is known as "diabetic neuropathic cachexia," and weight loss may amount to as much as 10–20 kg.

Proximal motor neuropathy can be clinically identified based on proximal muscle weakness and muscle wasting with fasciculation and/or twitching of muscles. It may be symmetric or asymmetric in distribution. The condition is readily recognizable clinically, with prevailing weakness of the iliopsoas, obturator, and adductor muscles, together with relative preservation of the gluteus maximus and minimus and the hamstrings. Individuals affected have great difficulty rising out of a chair unaided and often climb up their bodies (Gowers' maneuver). Heel or toe standing is surprisingly good (Leedman et al. 1988). In the classic form of diabetic amyotrophy, axonal loss is the predominant process, and the condition coexists with DSPN. However, this accounts for <9% of cases. Electrophysiological evaluation reveals lumbosacral plexopathy. In contrast, 91% of cases are due to a demyelinating condition, and there is an 11-fold greater risk of CIDP in people with diabetes, and 12% of diabetic patients develop some form of MGUS or monosialoganglioside neuropathy (GM1). If demyelination predominates and the motor deficit affects proximal and distal muscle groups, the diagnosis of CIDP, MGUS, vasculitis, and GM1 syndrome should be considered. The clinical differences between these syndromes are given in Table 43.4. It is important to divide proximal syndromes into these two subcategories because the autoimmune and inflammatory variants respond dramatically to intervention, whereas amyotrophy runs its own course over months to years. Until more evidence is available, we will consider them as separate syndromes.

DIAGNOSIS

It has been difficult to establish the exact site of the lesion, but recent studies labeled DPN as "diabetic lumbosacral polyradiculoplexus neuropathy," pointing to the multifocal proximal nerve involvement. Indeed, the most important conditions to exclude are the proximal myopathies (e.g., carcinoid, thyrotoxicosis, Cushing's syndrome or steroid treatment, and carcinoma). Lumbosacral outlet syndrome must also be excluded on an anatomical basis and usually requires magnetic resonance imaging with contrast. Bilateral painless proximal motor weakness is common in the genetically determined myopathies, motor neuron disorders, and neuromuscular junction lesions. The clinical picture usually serves to distinguish them from DPN. Electromyogram findings are typical. A detailed electromyogram examination and blood work, including immunoelectrophoresis, antibodies to nerve structures, and paraneoplastic antibodies, are necessary to establish that the primary demyelination in diabetes is due to MGUS, CIDP, vasculitis, or a paraneoplastic syndrome. If doubt remains as to the diagnosis, then a cerebrospinal fluid tap combined with immunohistochemical evaluation of an obturator nerve biopsy will usually establish the diagnosis (Chia et al. 1996).

An electromyogram is helpful in distinguishing these syndromes because diabetes per se lowers amplitudes. CIDP and MGUS cause severe demyelination and prolong conduction velocities, and specific nerve root entrapments in the lum-

Table 43.4 Distribution (%) of Symptoms and Signs of Proximal Neuropathies in Diabetes

Clinical Presentation	Vasculitis	CIDP	MGUS	Diabetes
DSPN (motor/sensory)	3	91	100	67
Distal (asymmetric)	27	9	0	0
Multifocal	70	0	0	33

bosacral outlet can be identified. These investigations make it possible to direct therapy to the appropriate condition.

THERAPIES FOR PROXIMAL NEUROPATHIES

Treatment of proximal neuropathies can now be rational and based on the nature of the underlying pathogenesis. The following is an outline of what is available, and specific details can be found in the Bibliography.

Vasculitis: Withdraw drugs and treat with steroids or immunosuppressive agents.
CIDP: Give intravenous immunoglobulin (1.0 g/kg) on 2 consecutive days and repeat at 2-week intervals for three treatments. Further treatment depends on the response. Plasmapheresis and immunosuppressive therapy (steroids and azathioprine) are alternative treatments.
MGUS: Undergo plasmapheresis.
Diabetes: Achieve glycemic control.
Sacral outlet syndrome: Undergo physical therapy/surgery (Krendel et al. 1995).

BIBLIOGRAPHY

Barohn RJ, Sahenk Z, Warmolts JR, Mendell JR: The Bruns-Garland syndrome (diabetic amyotrophy): revisited 100 years later. *Arch Neurol* 48:1130–1135, 1991

Boulton AJ, Vinik AI, Arezzo JC, Bril V, Feldman EL, Freeman R, Malik RA, Maser RE, Sosenko JM, Ziegler D: Diabetic neuropathies: a statement by the American Diabetes Association. *Diabetes Care* 28:956–962, 2005

Chia L, Fernandez A, Lacroix C, Adams D, Plante V: Contribution of nerve biopsy findings to the diagnosis of disabling neuropathy in the elderly: a retrospective review of 100 consecutive patients. *Brain* 119:1091–1098, 1996

Cornblath DR, Vinik A, Feldman E, Freeman R, Boulton AJ: Surgical decompression for diabetic sensorimotor polyneuropathy. *Diabetes Care* 30:421–422, 2007

Dawson DM: Entrapment neuropathies of the upper extremities. *N Engl J Med* 329:2013–2018, 1993

Krendel DA, Costigan DA, Hopkins LC: Successful treatment of neuropathies in patients with diabetes mellitus. *Arch Neurol* 52:1053–1061, 1995

Leedman PJ, Davis S, Harrison LS: Diabetic amyotrophy: reassessment of the clinical spectrum. *Aust N Z J Med* 18:768–773, 1988

Rice AL, Ullal J, Vinik AI: Reversal of phrenic nerve palsy with topiramate. *J Diabetes Complications* 21:63–67, 2007

Tankova T, Cherninkova S, Koev D: Treatment for diabetic mononeuropathy with α-lipoic acid. *Int J Clin Pract* 59:645-650, 2005

Vinik A, Casellini C, Nakave A, Patel C: Diabetic neuropathies. In *Diabetes and Carbohydrate Metabolism*. Goldfine ID, Rushakoff RJ, Eds. Available from www. endotext.org. Accessed March 2009

Vinik A, Ullal J, Parson H, Casellini C: Diabetic neuropathies: clinical manifestations and current treatment options. *Nat Clin Pract Endocrinol Metab* 2:269–281, 2006

Dr. Vinik is Professor of Medicine at the Eastern Virginia Medical School (EVMS) and Director of the EVMS Diabetes Research Center in Norfolk, Virginia. Dr. Nakave is a neuroendocrine fellow at the EVMS Diabetes Research Center and Neuroendocrine Unit, Norfolk, Virginia.

44. Gastrointestinal Disturbances

Aaron I. Vinik, MD, PhD, FCP, MACP, Archana Nakave, MD,
Maria del Pilar Silva Chuecos, MD, and David A. Johnson, MD

Gastrointestinal (GI) disturbances caused by autonomic neuropathy are common and often a disabling complication of diabetes. Between 20 and 40% of diabetic patients develop dysfunction of the autonomic nervous system. This may be a functional disturbance, which occurs with severe hyperglycemia or ketoacidosis, or a consequence of autonomic neuropathy. Diabetes can affect every part of the GI tract (i.e., the esophagus, stomach, small intestine, and colon). Thus, the GI manifestations are quite variable and include the following:

- dysphagia
- abdominal pain
- nausea
- vomiting
- malabsorption
- fecal incontinence
- diarrhea
- constipation (1)

The clinical spectrum of these complaints can range from relatively silent to life threatening. This chapter focuses on the clinical features, pathophysiology, diagnosis, and treatment of GI disturbances in diabetic patients (2).

PATHOGENESIS

GI complications of diabetes appear to be more common in patients with long-standing disease and poorly controlled blood glucose levels. The most prevalent GI complication is a motility disturbance of the viscera, which is generally the result of widespread autonomic neuropathy. Clinical symptoms of enteric diabetic neuropathy are more common in patients with long-standing diabetes, poor glucose control, increased age, and symptoms of peripheral or cardiovascular autonomic neuropathy (3).

The clinical features of certain diabetic enteropathies resemble those caused by surgical resection of the nerve plexus supplying that organ. Unfortunately, convincing morphological demonstration of gross neuropathology in human diabetic enteropathy is lacking, and correlation of GI symptoms with other signs of end-organ neuropathic damage is sometimes poor. Further complicating the understanding of this condition is a relatively high incidence of affective anxiety disorders in diabetic patients with GI symptoms that often resemble those of autonomic dysfunction. Microangiopathic changes, as seen in the retina or kidney, do not seem to cause disease in the GI tract.

Disturbed release of gut hormones may play some role in the symptom complex and the pathogenesis of GI complications of diabetes. Whereas autonomic dysfunction is associated with marked abnormalities in hormonal secretions, their role in the cause of symptoms is less clear. Cholinergic neuromuscular transmission in the myenteric plexus of the intestinal tract may be diminished. Additionally, failure of gut muscle to react appropriately on neurostimulation may be the result of relative deficiencies of stimulatory neurotransmitters such as motilin, neuropeptide Y, and methionine-enkephalin. Defective postprandial release of pancreatic polypeptide has also been demonstrated in diabetic patients with autonomic neuropathy but may only reflect loss of vagal integrity (4,5).

Metabolic abnormalities such as hyperglycemia and electrolyte imbalances undoubtedly play at least a contributory role in the disruption of GI motility in patients with diabetes. Clinically, this is most apparent when diabetic ketoacidosis occurs and the typical features of anorexia, nausea, vomiting, or abdominal pain develop. As the metabolic derangements are controlled, the GI symptoms resolve. It is well demonstrated that acute hyperglycemia inhibits GI motility. Some of the motor disturbances described with diabetes may therefore be directly related to glycemic control and are functional, and the integrity of the autonomic nervous system is intact (6).

ESOPHAGEAL DYSFUNCTION

Esophageal motor disorders have been described in 75% of patients with diabetes. Esophageal dysfunction is so common in patients with diabetic autonomic neuropathy that its absence in patients with GI symptoms casts doubt on the diagnosis of diabetic enteropathy. Motor abnormalities include impairment of peristaltic activity with double-peak and tertiary contractions or impaired peristalsis and diminished lower esophageal sphincteric pressures. These factors may further predispose the patient to gastroesophageal reflux disease, particularly in the setting of impaired gastric emptying.

Esophageal disturbances may be asymptomatic, although dysphagia has been described in up to one-third of patients. The presence of esophageal dysfunction in individuals with diabetes in the absence of symptoms suggests an underlying sensory autonomic diabetic neuropathy, similar to that observed with painless myocardial infarction. Interestingly, neuropsychiatric profiles of diabetic patients with abnormalities of esophageal motility have shown that abnormal contractions are more frequent during episodes of anxiety and depression. Esophageal dysfunction is of particular concern with ingestion of drugs such as oral bisphosphonates, which may cause ulceration, perforation, bleeding, and mediastinitis.

Patients with diabetes are prone to *Candida* esophagitis. This should be suspected where pharyngeal thrush is evident or clinical symptoms of odynophagia or dysphagia exist.

GASTRIC DYSFUNCTION

With the advent of electrogastrography, it has now been established that functional disturbances such as arrhythmias, tachygastria, bradygastria, pylorospasm, and hypomotility may occur in patients with diabetes. Organic lesions include gastroparesis, antral dilatation and obstruction, ulceration, inflammation, and bezoar formation.

Gastroparesis diabeticorum can be detected in 25% of diabetic patients. This is usually clinically silent, although severe diabetic gastroparesis is one of the most debilitating of all the GI complications of diabetes. The prevalence of gastric motility abnormalities ranges from 20 to 30%. Physiology of gastric emptying largely depends on vagus nerve function, which may be grossly disturbed in diabetes. Liquid emptying is controlled by the proximal stomach (fundus) and depends on the volume of gastric contents. With impaired vagal function, the proximal stomach is less relaxed, and liquid emptying may actually be increased in diabetic patients. Solid-phase emptying is affected by powerful contractions of the distal stomach (antrum). These contractions, known as phase 3 contractions, grind and mix solid food into particles of <1 mm in size, which then pass through the pylorus into the duodenum. Phase 3 contractions of the interdigestive migratory motor complex are frequently absent in diabetic patients. This results in poor antral grinding and emptying, which may result in gastric retention. Furthermore, there may be disordered integration of gastric and duodenal motor function resulting from disturbances in receptor relaxation of the stomach. Pylorospasm may occur because of disturbed contractility, which causes a functional resistance to gastric outflow. Impaired gastric emptying puts the patient at particular risk for gastric bezoar formation.

The exact pathophysiology of gastric motor disturbances is not certain. It is clear that vagal parasympathetic function disturbances may occur. The release of the peptide motilin, which regulates GI motility, is under vagal control. Motilin stimulates the initiation of phase 3 motor activity of the migrating motor complex of the stomach in patients with gastroparesis. High levels of this peptide have been reported in patients with gastroparesis. High motilin levels may therefore be partly compensatory. Further support is the observation that motilin levels fall in patients who have gastroparesis and receive treatment with prokinetic agents. Hyperglycemia itself may cause delayed gastric emptying in both healthy individuals and individuals with diabetes (7).

Now, with the discovery of the gastric hormone ghrelin, it has been shown that circulating levels of ghrelin rise before and decrease after a meal (8). Secretion rates of ghrelin 30–60 min after a meal in obese patients were significantly lower than those in normal-weight patients. Plasma ghrelin levels are elevated in diabetes. Elevated endogenous ghrelin enhances antropyloric coordination, which accelerates gastric emptying in the early stages of diabetes (9).

The importance of insulin and glucagons to maintain postprandial glycemic excursions within a narrow range is well established (10). However, alterations in gastric emptying, another potentially important factor (13), are not generally considered to be of clinical significance for postprandial hyperglycemia diabetes unless diabetic late complications such as gastroparesis have emerged (11,12).

Rapid gastric emptying can be seen in subgroups of patients in the early stages of type 2 diabetes and neuropathy-free, insulin-dependent diabetes (type 1 diabetes). During the early stages of diabetes, gastric emptying is often accelerated, rather than delayed (9). Solid gastric emptying is accelerated in obese type 2 diabetic patients without patent autonomic neuropathy when compared to obese nondiabetic patients (13). Normally, the rate of postprandial gastric emptying is tightly regulated as a result of neural and hormonal feedback triggered by the interaction of nutrients with the small intestine, known as the ileal break mechanism. This feedback is caloric load dependent, relates to the length of small intestine exposed to nutrient, and regulates the overall rate of emptying from ~2 to 3 kcal/min. The presence of nutrients in the small intestine is associated with relaxation of the gastric fundus, suppression of antral contractions, and stimulation of tonic and phasic pyloric contractions. The main hormones involved include cholecystokinin, glucagon-like peptide-1 (GLP-1), peptide YY, and amylin. The neural feedback involves both intrinsic (the enteric nervous system) and extrinsic (the autonomic and central nervous systems) components (Fig. 44.1). Nitric oxide (NO), an important inhibitory neurotransmitter in the gut, plays a role in the neural feedback pathway. In diabetes, there is impaired meal-induced relaxation of the gastric fundus, increased pyloric motor activity, fewer antral contractions, and impaired antroduodenal coordination. Disturbances of the gastric electrical rhythm, measured by electrogastrography, also occur frequently (14).

The pancreatic β-cell hormone islet amyloid polypeptide (IAPP) is cosecreted with insulin in a fixed molar ratio (15). IAPP has potent inhibitory effects on gastric emptying (16). Thus, type 1 diabetic patients even without concomitant enteric neuropathy should have increased rather than delayed rates of gastric emptying because they are IAPP deficient (17); physiological hyperglycemia delays gastric emptying in patients with type 1 diabetes (18) and this should contribute to postprandial hyperglycemia in patients with type 1 diabetes. In studies suggesting that insulin may be another important regulator of gastric emptying in healthy volunteers (19), the effects of hyperinsulinemia on gastric emptying were found to be marginal (19).

Gastric emptying is modulated by feedback mechanisms arising from the interaction of nutrients with the small intestine (20), known as the extrinsic pathway. Both intestinal vagus nerve activity, as well as intestinal peptides, regulate gastric emptying. GLP-1 inhibits gastric emptying (21). Its secretion, however, is stimulated by the intestinal nutrient content and flow rather than by plasma glucose concentration itself (22).

In the intrinsic pathway, hyperglycemia has been reported to cause profound inhibition of vagal activity accompanied by substantial IAPP secretion (23). In contrast, however, in IAPP-deficient type 1 diabetic patients, hyperglycemia did not affect vagal activity (18). Because the inhibitory effect of IAPP on gastric emptying seems to be mediated via inhibition in vagal nerve activity (23), findings consistent with the concept that hyperglycemia-induced delay in gastric emptying may be at least partially regulated via an IAPP-mediated inhibitory effect on vagal nerve activity.

Teleologically, the slowing of gastric emptying during hyperglycemia can be seen as an important defense mechanism to prevent hyperglycemia. IAPP secretion is linked to insulin release (15). As a response to hyperglycemia, the pancreatic β-cell with its glucose sensor increases insulin and IAPP secretion. Insulin suppresses hepatic glucose output and increases peripheral glucose uptake (24) while IAPP slows gastric emptying.

Taken together, these studies highlight the importance of a delay in gastric emptying response to hyperglycemia to minimize postprandial glucose excursions, a defense mechanism not operative in type 1 diabetic patients, which may be explained at least partially by IAPP deficiency. Perhaps on a more sobering note is the question of what would transpire if pramlintide were to be given to patients with autonomic nerve dysfunction with reduction in vagal activity. Would this lead to obstruction and bezoar formation, or would the loss of vagal function be a failsafe device in which the actions of IAPP to slow gastric emptying would be lost? Clearly, this is a very complex arena, and further studies on the effects of inhibition of IAPP (if and when an antagonist becomes available) and the impact of autonomic dysfunction might serve to resolve some of these issues (15).

Gastroparesis is a relatively rare late-diabetes complication caused by irreversible intestinal nerve damage (25) and has to be distinguished from the physiologi-

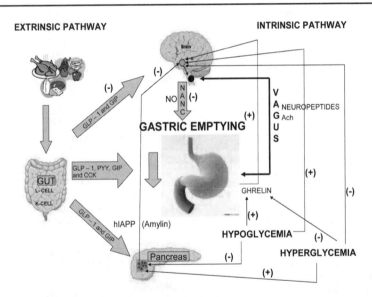

Figure 44.1 Regulation of Gastric Emptying
EXTRINSIC PATHWAY: When food reaches the intestine, L and K cells in the distal small bowel are stimulated to produce GLP-1 and glucose-dependent insulinotropic peptide (GIP), respectively, both of which exert their effects on different targets. In the brain they act on the hypothalamus, reducing appetite, but they also send signals via the vagus nerve (parasympathetic nervous system: cholinergic and peptidergic neu-

cal inhibitory effects of acute hyperglycemia on gastric motility (26,27). The latter has been proposed as a defense mechanism to minimize postprandial hyperglycemia by reducing the rate of efflux of glucose into the circulation from the gut (28). This may be of special importance for people with type 1 diabetes because they have been reported to have a reduced ability to delay gastric emptying in response to hyperglycemia (18).

Symptoms

Typical symptoms of gastroparesis (Table 44.1) include the following:

- nausea
- vomiting
- early satiety
- abdominal bloating
- epigastric pain
- anorexia

---

rotransmission) directly to the stomach, inhibiting antral and stimulating pyloric motility, both of which contribute to inhibition of gastric emptying. GLP-1 and GIP stimulate glucose-dependent insulin release from pancreatic islet β-cells, as well as amylin, and simultaneously inhibit glucagon secretion from pancreatic α-cells. Insulin plays a role in the reduction of food intake through an action in the satiety center in the hypothalamus, and amylin (or human IAPP [hIAPP]), via parasympathetic stimulation, slows the gastric emptying rate. NO also plays a role in slowing the gastric emptying rate mediated by NANC, producing relaxation of the GI smooth muscle. All these effects will have one common final outcome, which is prevention of postprandial hyperglycemia.

INTRINSIC PATHWAY: Involves the action of hyper- or hypoglycemia. In the hyperglycemic state, the pancreas is stimulated to produce insulin and amylin, and the secretion of glucagon is inhibited as is the secretion of ghrelin from the stomach. The increase in amylin and decrease in ghrelin slow the gastric emptying rate by producing a parasympathetic signal. Hypoglycemia exerts the opposite effect, stimulating ghrelin secretion from the stomach. Elevated endogenous ghrelin enhances antropyloric coordination, which accelerates gastric emptying, this signal is also transmitted via the vagus nerve. Glucagon and ghrelin both act on the satiety center in the hypothalamus to enhance food intake. Hypo- and hyperglycemia can act directly in the hypothalamus, increasing or decreasing appetite respectively, but they also activate the parasympathetic system and send signals to increase (hypoglycemia) or decrease (hyperglycemia) the gastric emptying rate.

Table 44.1 GI Disturbances in Diabetes

Condition	Symptom	Treatment
Esophagial dysfunction	Dysphagia	Metoclopramide
Gastroparesis	Nausea, vomiting, early satiety, anorexia, epigastric pain	Blood glucose control, care with hypoglycemia, bethanecol, metoclopramide, domperidone, tegaserod, mosapride ghrelin, Botox, cGMP PDIE inhibitors, gastric pacing
Hemorrhagic gastritis	Repeated vomiting and hematamesis (ketoacidosis and gastroparesis)	Erythromycin, clonidine, levosulpiride, treat cause
Cholelithiasis	Gallstone biliary colic, cholecystitis	Dissolution therapy, lithotripsy, or surgery
Pancreatic insufficiency	None (steatorrhoea)	Enzyme replacement
Diabetic diarrhea	Paroxysamal, nocturnal, painless, explosive diarrhea	Gluten-free diet, pancreatic enzymes, antibiotics, cholestyramine, diphenoxylate, loperamide, sandostatin (octreotide)
Fecal incontinence	Soiling without awareness	Treat diarrhea, biofeedback training
Constipation	Infrequent bowel actions, abdominal pain	Improve toilet habits, increase fluid intake, psyllium, metoclopramide, mistoprostil
Liver dysfunction	Abdominal pain	Test for hepatitis C, control blood glucose, lower lipids, stop hepatotoxic drugs

Classically, patients with gastroparesis have emesis of undigested food consumed many hours or even days previously. Postprandial vomiting is a rule, but more subtle presentation, such as morning nausea or even nonproductive retching may also occur. Even with mild symptoms, gastroparesis interferes with nutrient delivery to the small bowel and therefore disrupts the relationship between glucose absorption and exogenous insulin administration. This may result in wide swings of glucose levels and unexpected episodes of postprandial hypoglycemia. Gastroparesis should therefore always be suspected in patients with erratic glucose control. It may, in its most troublesome form, cause chronic nausea and anorexia, punctuated by bouts of prolonged emesis requiring hospitalization for dehydration and uncontrolled hyperglycemia. Inexplicably, symptoms are variable and may fluctuate markedly over a period of weeks to months (29).

Role in Brittle Diabetes

Delayed gastric emptying is one of the major causes of brittle diabetes. Type 1 diabetes is an intrinsically unstable condition. However, the term "brittle diabetes" is reserved for those cases in which the instability, whatever its cause, results in disruption of life and often recurrent and/or prolonged hospitalization. It affects 3/1,000 type 1 diabetic patients, mainly young women. Its prognosis is poor with lower quality-of-life scores, more microvascular and pregnancy complications, and shortened life expectancy. Three forms have been described: recurrent diabetic ketoacidosis, predominant hypoglycemic forms, and mixed instability. Main causes of brittleness include malabsorption, certain drugs (alcohol, antipsychotics), defective insulin absorption or degradation, defect of hyperglycemic hormones (especially glucocorticoid and glucagon), and above all delayed gastric emptying as a result of autonomic neuropathy (30). Thus, in brittle diabetes one must focus on achieving normal gastric emptying. Gastroparesis is associated with changes in the gastric enteric nervous system. Histological examination in patients with brittle diabetes with severe gastroparesis revealed increased fibrosis in the muscle layers as well as significantly fewer nerve fibers and myenteric neurons as assessed by PGP9.5 (a pan-neuronal antigen) staining. Further, significant reduction was seen in staining for neuronal NO synthase (nNOS), heme oxygenase-2, tyrosine hydroxylase, as well as c-KIT (31), suggesting that nitrergic stimulation was essential for normal gastric emptying.

Chronic gastritis and gastric atrophy have been noted with a high prevalence in diabetic patients. The role of *Helicobacter pylori* is not clear. This organism seems to play a minor role, if any, in disturbances in the upper alimentary tract of diabetic patients (32). Interestingly, there is a significantly lower incidence of *H. pylori* infections in diabetic patients with delayed gastric emptying compared with individuals with normal emptying. Furthermore, gastric atrophy and hypochloridia are not uncommon, especially with type 1 diabetes (33), and there is the potential predisposition for bacterial overgrowth. Chronic gastritis and gastric atrophy are often associated with significant titers of antiparietal antibodies and antithyroid antibodies. This partly explains the high incidence of pernicious anemia and hypothyroidism in diabetic patients. Awareness of these associations is necessary to appropriately direct replacement therapies. Acute hemorrhagic gastritis is common in patients with repeated emesis of gastroparesis or ketoacidosis. Additionally, bleeding may develop from Mallory-Weiss tears, particularly in patients with repetitive emesis.

Diagnosis

Upper GI symptoms should not be attributed to gastroparesis until conditions such as gastric ulcer, duodenal ulcer, severe gastritis, and gastric cancer have been excluded. An upper GI endoscopy or high-quality barium series should be performed. The finding of retained food in the stomach after an 8- to 12-h fast, in the absence of obstruction, is diagnostic of gastroparesis. The lack of this finding, however, does not rule out the diagnosis.

Nuclear medicine scintigraphy is the gold standard for evaluation of gastric emptying. This involves ingestion of a standard radiolabeled meal and provides a useful means to not only diagnose but objectively follow patients' response to therapy. Newer noninvasive imaging tests have also been developed recently.

Magnetic resonance imaging and percutaneous electrogastrography hold promise for future clinical application. Gastroduodenal manometrics may be helpful in select patients (e.g., symptomatic patients with apparently normal emptying to look for pylorospasm or incoordinate gastric and duodenal motility). This test is generally cumbersome, available only in a few research centers interested in motility disorders, and at this point does not dictate therapeutic strategies.

Electrogastrography

Electrogastrography is the recording and measurement of gastric myoelectrical activity from electrodes placed on the surface of the epigastrium. Normal electrogastrograms (EGGs) reflect 3 cycles per min (cpm) gastric myoelectrical activity produced by specialized pacemaker cells, the interstitial cells of Cajal, located in the muscular wall of the gastric corpus and antrum. Gastric dysrhythmias (tachygastrias and bradygastrias) are disturbances of the normal gastric pacesetter potentials and are associated with symptoms of nausea, epigastric fullness, and bloating and with hyperglycemia and delayed gastric emptying. In diabetic gastropathy, the normal 3-cpm electrical rhythm is replaced with bradygastrias, tachygastrias, and mixed or nonspecific dysrhythmias. Diagnosis of gastric dysrhythmias identifies an objective neuromuscular abnormality in diabetic patients with upper GI symptoms. Correction of gastric dysrhythmias decreases upper GI symptoms and may improve gastric emptying, all of which may enhance glucose control. The EGG diagnosis of gastric dysrhythmias provides new insights into gastric neuromuscular abnormalities and guides therapies to improve upper GI symptoms in diabetic patients (34).

The EGG signal is by nature a nonstationary signal in terms of its frequency, amplitude, and wave shape. Unlike the other methods, discrete wavelet analysis (DWT) was designed for nonstationary signals. For automatic assessment of EGG, we used artificial neural networks (ANNs) that have been widely used in pattern recognition due to their great potential of high performance, flexibility, robust fault tolerance, cost-effective functionality, and capability for real-time applications. So we developed a new method for classification of EGG based on DWT and ANN (35).

Gastric myoelectrical rhythm derangement is present in a large proportion of young diabetic patients. Bradygastria is the most prominent EGG abnormality. Weak correlation was found between EGG parameters and diabetes metabolic control (36).

Derangement of the gastric myoelectrical activity is present in 71% of children with early-stage type 1 diabetes. Glucose levels influence gastric myoelectrical activity, whereas long-term glucose control (A1C level) does not correlate with EGG parameters (37).

Treatment

Initial treatment of diabetic gastroparesis should focus on blood glucose control. Hyperglycemia, even acute, may interfere with gastric contractility. Physiological control of blood glucose levels may improve gastric motor dysfunction. Overregulation of blood glucose control should be avoided when gastric emptying is impaired because of the danger of severe hypoglycemia resulting from a variable pattern of gastric emptying. Patients who complain of early satiety and bloating may benefit from a low-fat, low-fiber diet and several small meals throughout the day. Fiber, vegetables, and poorly digestible solids should be avoided because of their predisposition to gastric bezoar formation.

Pharmacological therapy is usually necessary in patients with clinically significant gastroparesis. Evaluation of ancillary medications is critical before treating with prokinetic medications. Any drugs with anticholinergic potential that may further decrease gastric emptying should be withdrawn. Avoidance of medications such as carafate or psyllium may help to decrease gastric bezoar potential.

Metoclopramide

Metoclopramide is a dopamine antagonist that stimulates acetylcholine release in the myenteric plexus. This drug acts centrally on the chemoreceptor triggers in the floor of the fourth ventricle, which provides an important antiemetic activity. Controlled trials documenting the efficacy of metoclopramide have been unable to consistently show an improvement in gastric emptying rate. This drug is given at a dose of 10–30 mg 1 h before meals and at bedtime. For patients with severe impairment of gastric emptying, use of the elixir form seems to be more effective. In addition, metoclopramide can be given subcutaneously, allowing for a more sustained effect in complicated patients. Intravenous administration of this medication may be helpful in hospitalized patients. Administration of a 25-mg rectal suppository dose of metoclopramide has been effective in some patients. The effectiveness of this drug typically wanes because of a tachyphylaxis effect, so its efficacy is short lived (<6 months) in most patients. However, patients may respond after reintroduction of the medication after a period of withdrawal. Side effects of metoclopramide include drowsiness, lethargy, and depression, especially at higher doses. If Parkinson-like tremor occurs, medication should be discontinued immediately. Galactorrhea and breast tenderness may occur because of increased prolactin secretion caused by metoclopramide. Metoclopramide may lower the seizure threshold in patients with epilepsy and should be used with extreme caution in these patients.

Domperidone

Domperidone is similar to metoclopramide in that it is a dopamine antagonist, but it has little action on acetylcholine release in the myenteric plexus. It does not cross the blood-brain barrier and thus has limited side effects. It does reach the hypothalamus, which is outside the barrier. The dose is 20–40 mg taken 1 h before meals and at bedtime. Domperidone stimulates prolactin secretion and may cause breast tenderness and galactorrhea. Intravenous administration of domperidone causes cardiac dysrhythmias. Domperidone appears to be most useful for patients who have responded well to metoclopramide but are unable to take it because of side effects. Domperidone is free of tachyphylaxis with long-term treatment, and improvements in gastric emptying persist for 6 months to 1 year.

Erythromycin

The macrolide erythromycin and its derivatives duplicate the action of motilin, which is responsible for the migrating motor complex activity, by binding to and activating motilin receptors. Intravenous administration of this antibiotic enhances the emptying rate of both liquids and solids. The effects are not as dramatic with oral therapy, although clinical efficacy has been demonstrated with erythromycin in a dose of 250 mg 0.5 h before meals. Substitution of the enteric-coated form may be better tolerated in some patients. Erythromycin has the downside of creating antibiotic-related resistance problems. However, it appears to be an effective therapeutic alternative to more established forms of treatment in patients with diabetic gastroparesis, especially when other drugs have failed (38). A recent focus of pharmaceutical investigation has been the development of motilin receptor agonists exhibiting prokinetic capabilities but without antimicrobial properties. An early motilin agonist, ABT-229, actually worsened symptoms in diabetic patients with nausea and vomiting compared with placebo and showed no benefits in functional dyspepsia (44,45). A newer agent, mitemicinal, exhibits potent prokinetic action in the stomach, and early results in diabetic gastroparesis show good effects (39).

Levosulpiride

Levosulpiride is a new prokinetic drug that is a selective antagonist for D2-dopamine receptors. Recent studies have suggested that this medication, given at a dosage of 25 mg three times a day orally for 6 months, shows maintained improvement in gastric emptying and improved glycemic control in diabetic subjects with gastroparesis. Further studies are forthcoming. The drug is not yet freely available (40).

Clonidine

Clonidine is a specific α_2-adrenergic receptor antagonist used to control diabetic diarrhea. A recent study has demonstrated significant improvement in diabetic patients with chronic refractory symptoms of bloating, nausea, and vomiting. Patients were treated with 0.1 mg clonidine two or three times a day. This preliminary work suggests that improvement of adrenergic influences on GI motility may play a role in diabetic gastroparesis. Therefore, clonidine may be helpful in select cases, but dosing must be cautious because of the danger of orthostatic hypotension (41).

Tegaserod

Tegaserod, a selective 5-HT4 (5-hydroxytryptamine 4) agonist, has been shown to improve gastric emptying in diabetic patients with gastroparesis. Clinical studies have demonstrated stimulation of GI tract motility and improvement of visceral sensitivity in irritable bowel syndrome, which is associated with abdominal pain, bloating, and constipation. Tegaserod (6 mg orally twice daily) increases colonic motility and proximal colonic filling, accelerates orocecal transit, and improves esophageal acid clearance. Preclinical studies have demonstrated the antinociceptive effects of Zelnorm (tegaserod), which are supposedly the result of pain threshold alteration. Unfortunately, the drug has been shown to affect cardiac conductance and has been removed from the market (42). Other 5-HT4 receptor agonists have been developed and show efficacy in gastroparesis. Mosapride accelerates gastric emptying in healthy volunteers and patients with diabetic gastroparesis. Furthermore, the drug may improve glycemic control in diabetic patients with delayed gastric emptying. In contrast to cisapride, mosapride has little effect on potassium channel activity and appears to exhibit a significantly lesser cardiac dysrhythmogenic potential. Renzapride is a combined 5-HT4 receptor agonist and 5-HT3 receptor antagonist. Future studies are needed to determine whether renzapride exhibits efficacy in gastroparesis (39).

Ghrelin

Ghrelin is a natural ligand for the growth hormone secretagogue receptor and is known for its ability to provoke growth hormone secretion. It is produced predominantly in epithelial cells lining the fundus of the stomach. It increases gastric motility. Regulation of ghrelin levels is said to be impaired in diabetic gastroparesis (43). Ghrelin increases gastric emptying in patients with diabetic gastroparesis. This is independent of vagal tone. It has been proposed that analogues of ghrelin may represent a new class of prokinetic agents (44).

Role of NO in Gastric Emptying and Use of cGMP Phosphodiesterase Inhibitors

NO is an important neurotransmitter in the gut and has been demonstrated to be a key physiological mediator of nonadrenergic noncholinergic (NANC) relaxation of GI smooth muscle (45). (Fig. 44.2) It is generated by neuronal NO synthase (nNOS) resident in the NANC neuron.

It acts in the stomach, pylorus, and the duodenum and regulates gastric emptying of solid meals by partially inhibiting pyloric and proximal duodenal contractions (46). NO-cGMP transduction pathway is involved in the inhibitory effect of sildenafil (higher doses) on the GI smooth muscles and in its potential application in patients with diabetic gastroparesis (45). Phosphodiesterase type 5 hydrolyzes and inactivates cyclic guanosine monophosphate produced by the NO-stimulated guanylate cyclase. Sildenafil is a potent, reversible, and highly selective inhibitor of this phosphodiesterase. It causes smooth-muscle relaxation by increasing intracellular concentrations of cyclic guanosine monophosphate. Sildenafil alters the intragastric distribution of food and does not cause gastric stasis (47). It has restored gastric emptying of liquids in an animal model of diabetes. It reduces dysrhythmia of stomach induced by experimental hyperglycemia in humans. It significantly increases postprandial gastric volume and slows liquid emptying rate, though not solid. It inhibits interdigestive motor activity of antrum and duodenum (48).

Effects of Exenatide (GLP-1 Analog) and "Gliptins" (Dipeptidyl Peptidase-4 Inhibitors)

GLP-1 is an enterogastrone that inhibits antral and stimulates pyloric motility, both of which contribute to inhibition of gastric emptying (49). Exenatide, a mimetic of the incretin GLP-1, and sitagliptin, an inhibitor of the enzyme dipeptidyl peptidase-4 (DPP-4), which breaks down GLP-1, are both known to delay gastric emptying and reduce food intake (50).

Exenatide has potent effects on glucose-dependent insulin release and also inhibits glucagon secretion. It has been mainly used for the treatment of type 2 diabetes, resulting in significant improvement in A1C levels. In addition, preliminary studies have shown improved glucose control in a selected cohort of type 1 diabetic patients who had received islet allografts and were treated with exenatide (11).

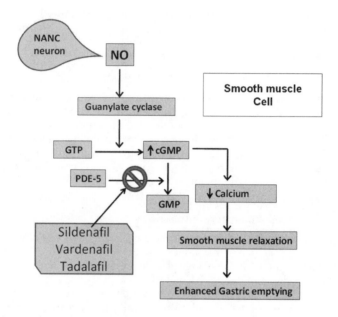

Figure 44.2 Gastric smooth muscle has nitrergic innervation and depends on NO generated by induction of nNOS resident in NANC neurons in gastric mucosa, causing its relaxation and facilitating gastric emptying.

Due to its effect on gastric emptying, GI symptoms are common with exenatide, including nausea 57.1%, vomiting 17.4%, and diarrhea 8.5% in patients (51), and its discontinuation rate is 36% (52).

In patients with gastroparesis, exenatide may cause further delay in gastric emptying, predisposing these patients to bezoars, with the risk of other complications (i.e., obstruction, pancreatitis, and intestinal perforation). According to a case study report, a patient who was a type 1 diabetic with long-term complications (retinopathy, neuropathy, and end-stage renal disease) who had undergone a recent islet after kidney transplant and was put on exenatide for improving glycemic control, was found to develop severe gastroparesis and food content bezoar 11 months later. Exenatide was stopped and restarted after removing the bezoar endoscopically, which only led to recurrence of GI symptoms and another gastric bezoar. So exenatide was discontinued, and the patient's condition remained stable after that with help of intrapyloric botulinum injection. An incidence of pancreatitis has also been observed in patients during exenatide treatment (53).

Management of Complex Gastroparesis

There is a substantial subgroup of patients with troublesome gastroparesis in whom explanation, education, dietary manipulation, and sequential or incremental trials of prokinetic drugs and/or antiemetics fail to provide adequate relief. Those most refractory to treatment are likely to include markedly symptomatic patients with evidence of profound delay in gastric emptying. Additional strategies might be considered in these complex patients (35).

Gastric Neurostimulation

Paced gastric neurostimulation (54) using an implantable stimulator (Enterra Therapy; Medtronic, Minneapolis, MN) has been approved by the U.S. Food and Drug Administration. Electrical stimulation is delivered by two electrodes implanted laparoscopically or at laparotomy onto the serosal surface overlying the pacemaker area on the greater curve of the stomach and ~2 cm apart. Leads from the electrodes connect to a neurostimulator, which resembles a cardiac pacemaker that is implanted in the anterior abdominal wall. Enterra generates a high-frequency (12 cycles/min), low-energy, short-duration pulse. A wireless remote controller allows settings to be adjusted to optimize symptom control. Overall, 79% of patients had a ≥50% decrease in vomiting. The benefits, measured by a symptom score of nausea, vomiting, bloating, fullness, satiety, and pain, were significant, but less so than for vomiting alone. A reduction in medication use with fewer hospital admissions has been reported, and other uncontrolled series have reported benefit. Gastric electrical stimulation is reported to enhance nutritional status, reduce the requirement for supplemental feeds, and improve glycemic control in diabetic patients. There is a special need in diabetes being considered for renal and/or pancreas transplantation, where it is important that the immunosuppressive agents will be absorbed (39).

The effect of Enterra on gastric emptying is controversial with different outcomes reported in the literature. However, there is general agreement that symptom relief is disproportionate to any effect on gastric pump function. Symptom improvement is probably because of another action, and there is speculation that electrical stimulation of vagal afferents might suppress the vomiting center in the brain. Electrostimulation has, however, also been reported in patients with postsurgical gastroparesis who have undergone vagotomy. Infection is the major complication associated with neurostimulator implantation, resulting in removal of the device in 5–20% of patients. Despite its apparent value in refractory gastroparesis, most authorities recommend that neurostimulators should be implanted in the context of long-term controlled trials (55).

Intrapyloric Injection of Botulinum Toxin

Manometric studies of patients with diabetic gastroparesis show prolonged periods of increased pyloric tone and phasic contractions, known as pylorospasm. Botulinum toxin is a potent inhibitor of neuromuscular transmission and has been used to treat spastic somatic muscle disorders as well as achalasia. Intrapyloric injection of botulinum toxin has been reported to be efficacious in several open-label studies. In a preliminary report, saline or Botox 4×25 units was injected into the pylorus of 12 patients with gastroparesis, 2 with diabetes and 10 idiopathic, in a double-blind, placebo-controlled, crossover study. Gastric emptying of solids improved with Botox treatment, but the symptoms were not different at the end of each arm of the study .

In a large, open-label, observational study, 43% had a response to botulinum toxin treatment that lasted a mean of ~5 months. Male sex was associated with a response to this therapy; however, durability of response was unrelated to sex. Vomiting as a major symptom predicted no response. In summary, the available information does not yet support the widespread application of this treatment modality in gastroparesis (48).

Gastrostomy or Jejunostomy Placement

Medical treatment is effective in most people with gastroparesis. However, 2–5% of patients are refractory to drug therapy and require multiple hospitalizations. In refractory patients with severe nausea and vomiting, placement of a gastrostomy tube for intermittent decompression by venting or suctioning may provide symptom relief, especially of interdigestive fullness and bloating secondary to retained intragastric gas and liquids. Venting gastrostomy may be needed to relieve severe gastric stasis. Venting jejunostomy in patients with chronic intestinal pseudo-obstruction needing total parenteral nutrition was shown to reduce the need for repeat hospitalizations by a factor of five compared with a historical control period. Venting gastrostomies or jejunostomies may be placed endoscopically, surgically, or by interventional radiology. The results of endoscopically placed venting (percutaneous endoscopic gastrostomy or jejunostomy) for gastroparesis are still unclear. For patients with gastroparesis who are unable to maintain nutrition with oral intake, placement of a feeding jejunostomy may decrease symptoms and reduce hospitalizations. The therapeutic response to jejunostomy infusion may be predicted by a trial of nasojejunal feedings. Jejunostomy tubes are effective for providing nutrition, fluids, and medications if there is normal small intestinal motor function. Except in cases of profound malnutrition or electrolyte disturbance, enteral feedings are preferable to chronic parenteral nutrition because of the significant risks of infection and liver disease with the latter treatment, especially in diabetic patients (48,56,57).

Other Surgical Options

Gastrectomy has been reported in a final attempt to manage severe, intractable, and refractory gastroparesis. The procedure carries a substantial morbidity and mortality, and there is little experience to guide practice. Highly selected small case series suggest that the procedure is likely to succeed in diabetic gastroparesis. There have also been reports of symptom improvement in diabetic patients after pancreatic transplantation. As there are no prospective controlled trials of gastrectomy, this treatment should only be considered in rare instances in expert tertiary referral centers (48).

BILIARY DISEASE

Earlier data suggesting that diabetic patients have a higher incidence of cholelithiasis (reported incidence 1.5 times that of the normal population) are controversial. The high incidence of type 2 diabetes in populations at risk for cholelithiasis (e.g., women, obese people, and patients with hyperlipoproteinemia) makes it difficult to identify diabetes as an independent risk factor. Most recent studies have suggested gallstone disease is multifactorial, and it is an independent risk factor only in type 2 diabetic female patients (58).

Theoretically, diabetic autonomic neuropathy predisposes patients to gallstone formation because diminished gallbladder contractility leads to stasis. This stasis causes the bile to become supersaturated with cholesterol, which predisposes to stone formation. The role of prophylactic cholecystectomy in diabetic patients with asymptomatic gallstones is controversial. More recent studies have assessed the outcome of acute cholecystitis in diabetic patients and suggest there is no incremental risk of morbidity or mortality (59). Accordingly, there seems to be no role for routine prophylactic cholecystectomy in diabetic patients with cholelithiasis.

Medical treatment for cholesterol gallstones with dissolution therapy may be an alternative to surgery in patients with symptomatic gallstones. Laparoscopic cholecystectomy, however, will probably have fewer and fewer applications in symptomatic cholelithiasis. Medical therapy is being investigated to attempt to augment abnormal gallbladder motility with the intent to decrease bile stasis. Levosulpiride D2, a dopamine antagonist, has shown preliminary effectiveness in augmenting gallbladder emptying in patients with diabetic cholecystoparesis.

PANCREAS

Exocrine pancreatic function is reduced in >50% of type 1 diabetic patients. The degree of impairment progresses with greater duration of the disease. This may be the consequence of chronic insulin deficiency and resultant autonomic neuropathy. Clinically significant pancreatic insufficiency is rare, however, because 90% of exocrine function must be lost before steatorrhea occurs.

Diabetes and pancreatic cancer are known to be associated, but the cause of the association and whether diabetes is a risk factor for pancreatic cancer remain controversial. Pancreatic cancer may occur with increased frequency among patients with long-standing diabetes (>5 years). It is important to recognize that new-onset diabetes in older patients without a family history of diabetes may develop as the "form fruste" of pancreatic cancer or a neuroendocrine tumor (i.e., somatostatinoma) and is presumably caused by the tumor itself.

LIVER DISEASE

Certain types of liver disease are usually associated with glucose intolerance or diabetes. The liver is the principal organ responsible for insulin metabolism. Approximately 50% of the insulin secreted by the pancreas is removed by the first passage through the liver. In the presence of cirrhosis, there is decreased extraction by the liver, and the peripheral circulating insulin is increased. Despite this increase, hyperglycemia is common, suggesting that peripheral insulin resistance coexists. Consistent with this hypothesis is the finding that peripheral monocytes have been obtained from patients with cirrhosis and shown to have fewer insulin receptors. The specific mechanism responsible for the decreased cellular receptor number and resultant insulin resistance is not known.

Glucose intolerance or diabetes may be a reflection of underlying liver disease associated with diabetes. For example, hemochromatosis is a disorder of iron metabolism that is frequently associated with glucose intolerance. Excess iron is deposited in the liver, pancreatic islets, and other organs. As a result, diabetes and hepatic fibrosis and cirrhosis may be manifestations of progressive disease.

Autoimmune forms of chronic active liver disease are also associated with diabetes characterized by inheritance of specific HLA alleles. The relative risk for diabetes is increased threefold in individuals who carry the HLA-B8 allele and approximately fourfold in those carrying the HLA-Dw3 allele. Both of these alleles are found twice as often in patients with autoimmune chronic active hepatitis.

Liver disease may be evident in the absence of other recognizable hereditary factors. In particular, hepatic steatosis has been reported in 30–80% of diabetic patients. Accumulation of triglycerides may occur by any or a combination of the following factors:

- increased uptake from peripheral fatty acids
- increased fatty triglyceride synthesis (either carbohydrates or nonesterified fatty acids)
- reduced hepatic oxidation of fat
- increased formation of VLDL
- reduced hepatic release of newly formed VLDL

Hepatic steatonecrosis is characterized by large fat-droplet deposition associated with hepatic fibrosis and may lead to cirrhosis in some patients. Progressively more patients with nonalcoholic steatohepatitis are being recognized. Modifiable factors include control of diabetes, lipids, and obesity.

Recent evidence has associated the hepatitis C virus infection with diabetes. Glucose intolerance is particularly common in patients with chronic hepatitis C (60). Testing for hepatitis C infection in diabetic patients with abnormal liver-related enzymes is therefore mandatory. Studies to date have not found particular epidemiological factors for hepatitis C infection in diabetes or a direct role for hepatitis C in the development of diabetes (61).

Diabetic patients are at increased risk for hepatitis not only as a consequence of diabetes but as a consequence of medical management of their disease. Iatrogenic liver disease can occur with oral hypoglycemic agents such as chlorpropamide. This drug may result in a cholestatic or granulomatous liver injury. Similar reactions have been seen with tolbutamide and with troglitazone. Primary hepatocellular injury has also been found with hypolipidemic drugs such as lovastatin.

SMALL INTESTINE

Diarrhea may be evident in 20% of diabetic patients, particularly those with known autonomic neuropathy. Motor disturbances of the small intestine do not entirely explain the pathogenesis of diarrhea. Predisposition of bacterial overgrowth may induce diarrhea. Additionally, because adrenergic nerves stimulate intestinal reabsorption of fluids and electrolytes, decreased adrenergic tone may contribute to pathogenesis. Small-bowel malabsorption of bile salts may induce diarrhea via a colonic stimulatory effect.

There is frequency of the HLA-DR3 genotype in type 1 diabetes, which explains why many patients also have celiac disease. Appropriate recognition of this condition is critical to effect the necessary dietary restriction of gluten. Serological screening with anti-endomysial and anti-gluten antibodies is 95% sensitive and specific for celiac disease. Small-bowel biopsy should be considered for any patient for whom this diagnosis is a possibility (62).

Exocrine pancreatic insufficiency may occur. Diabetic patients have impaired responses to stimulation with duodenal infusion of amino acids or intravenous secretin or cholecystokinin. Pancreatic exocrine insufficiency rarely becomes severe enough to contribute to malabsorption; however, in patients with diarrhea, it is prudent to replace pancreatic enzymes (63).

Autonomic neuropathy may cause diarrhea by its effects on gut motility and/or enterocyte absorption. Although gut dysmotility makes sense and has been the most widely accepted explanation for diabetic diarrhea, motility testing and small-bowel transit studies have produced variable and inconsistent results. Adrenergic nerve dysfunction interferes with normal electrolyte and fluid absorption by the enterocyte (64).

Evaluation of diarrhea in a diabetic patient should begin with a good history. Care should be taken to exclude medication-related diarrhea. Sorbitol may be implicated as an additive to medications and diabetic foods. Biguanides may also be responsible for diarrhea in some patients. The patient should be asked about particular dietary exacerbates (milk products suggesting lactose intolerance). Diarrhea that resolves with fasting suggests an osmotic diarrhea caused by ingested substances. In contrast, diarrhea that continues in the absence of ingestion, as with nocturnal awakening, is more suggestive of a secretory-type process, and neuroendocrine causes should be pursued. Stools should be obtained for occult blood examination for ova and parasites, fecal leukocytes, and qualitative fecal fat.

Patients with large-volume diarrhea and those with positive assessment of qualitative fecal fat should be further studied with a 72-h fecal fat collection. This must be done while ingesting a 100-g fat diet. Screens for malabsorption should be done in patients who have diminished albumin stores or low serum carotene levels. A D-xylose test is a good screen for small-bowel malabsorptive disorders. Serum B12 level should be considered in patients with suspected diarrhea involving the distal small bowel because the primary absorption area is in the ileum. Erythrocyte folate levels are particularly elevated in patients with bacterial overgrowth and should be checked in the appropriate setting. Directed investigation of the small intestine by small-bowel biopsy and/or radiographic studies should be done in patients with protracted symptoms. Pancreatic function testing should be considered in patients with steatorrhea. Proctosigmoidoscopy and possibly full colonoscopy with biopsies of the right and left colon and rectum to exclude microscopic or collagenous colitis or amyloid should also be considered. Empiric therapeutic trials of antibiotics, gluten-free diet, and pancreatic enzymes may less accurately define the diagnosis but can be considered when facilities for detailed study are not available (65).

Evaluation of stool electrolytes is helpful in separating osmotic from secretory-type diarrheas. A calculated osmolality based on 2 (stool Na^+ + K^+) subtracted from the calculated serum osmolality of 290 gives the calculated osmotic gap. Patients with osmotic diarrhea typically have an osmotic gap >50 and more frequently >100. Patients with an osmotic gap of <50 should be considered for secretory diarrheal workup. This includes evaluations for carcinoid, glucagonoma, gastrinoma, VIPoma, and rostaglandin-producing tumors.

Treatment of diabetic diarrhea should address the specific etiology. Celiac sprue and pancreatic insufficiency should be treated with gluten-free diet and pancreatic enzyme supplements, respectively. A trial of antibiotics is appropriate if bacterial overgrowth is found or cannot be ruled out (Table 44.2). Hydrophilic dietary supplements, such as psyllium, may be useful if diarrhea alternates with constipation. Care should be taken, however, in patients with a tendency toward gastric bezoar, which may be aggravated by high-residue diets. Chelation of bile salts with cholestyramine may reduce the bile acid component of diarrhea. Standard synthetic opiates such as diphenoxylate and loperamide are potent, nonaddicting antidiarrheal agents and should be tried early in the course. Care must be exercised not to produce obstipation and impaction.

Because GI adrenergic function is impaired in diabetic autonomic neuropathy, adrenergic agonists should stimulate intestinal reabsorption of fluids and electrolytes (66). Clonidine may reverse adrenergic nerve dysfunction and improve diarrhea. This agent also has potent antimotility effects, which may partly explain symptomatic improvement in some patients. Initial treatment should begin with 0.1 mg two or three times a day, increased to 0.4–0.6 mg titrating up over several days. Because the antihypertensive effects of clonidine are mediated through the central nervous system, diabetic patients with severe autonomic neuropathy may not experience worsening of preexisting postural hypotension, which may actually improve. If the medication is withdrawn, it should be done slowly to avoid rebound hypertension.

Table 44.2 Drug Therapy for Diabetic Diarrhea

Drug	Starting Dose
Psyllium (sugar-free)	1 tsp to 1 Tbsp 1–3 times/day
Kaolin + pectin (mixture)	2 Tbsp 2 times/day
Cholestyramine	1 packet (4 g) 1–6 times/day
Tetracycline	250 mg 4 times/day
Ampicillin	250 mg 4 times/day
Pancreatic enzymes	2–4 tablets or capsules with meals and snacks
Diphenoxylate	2.5 mg 2 times/day
Loperamide	2 mg 2 times/day
Clonidine	0.2 mg 2 times/day
Sandostatin	50–100 µg 3 times/day

The long-acting somatostatin analog octreotide is effective in some refractory patients. Octreotide probably inhibits the release of gastroenteropancreatic endocrine peptides, which may be a pathogenic factor responsible for diarrhea and electrolyte imbalance in diabetic patients (67). Recent studies with this agent in patients with intestinal pseudo-obstruction and bacterial overgrowth suggest that it may increase gut transit and decrease abdominal distention–related complaints. The initial dose is 50–100 µg three to six times a day, as needed. Adverse effects of this agent include pain at the site of injection, which can be reduced by warming the syringe by hand and then injecting slowly over 2–3 min. Additional symptoms include abdominal cramps, bloating, and flatulence. Diabetic diarrhea may be worsened by this agent, usually because of steatorrhea, which may respond to pancreatic enzyme supplements. The drug is expensive and should be reserved for patients with severe refractory symptoms (68).

CONSTIPATION

Constipation is the most common GI complication, affecting nearly 25% of diabetic patients and >50% of individuals with diabetic autonomic neuropathy. Myoelectric studies of the colon have demonstrated diminished motility in response to ingestion of a standard meal (gastrocolonic reflux). Cholinergic agents stimulate colonic motility, suggesting a defect in neural control of the smooth muscle. Colonic smooth muscle is capable of responding to cholinergic stimulation; therefore, neuroprokinetic agents may be effective.

Severe constipation may be complicated by ulceration, perforation, and fecal impaction. Barium studies pose a risk to patients with underlying visceral myopathy, so barium-related impaction must be avoided. Aggressive catharsis should be used in patients undergoing barium studies, such as GI series or enema. Fecal impaction may also cause overflow diarrhea and incontinence and must be considered in the differential underlying constipation of diabetic diarrhea. Long-standing constipation with straining predisposes to stretch injury of the nerves to the anal sphincter, which may lead to fecal incontinence through reduced sphincteric pressure. Precipitous change in bowel habits should prompt colonic evaluation to exclude the possibility of an obstructive lesion such as stricture or neoplasm (69).

Anorectal manometry may be useful in evaluating the rectal anal inhibitory reflex. This test is helpful in distinguishing colonic hypomotility from rectosigmoid dysfunction causing outlet obstructive symptoms. Biofeedback and/or patient training with regard to defecation may be directed with this technique.

Colonic segmental transit time may be derived by mean segmental transit radiopaque markers that are ingested orally. Sequential X-rays on alternate days demonstrate passage of these radiopaque markers through the right and left colon and rectosigmoid area. This provides objective measurement of bowel transit and helps define patient complaints, both at baseline and in response to therapy.

Treatment for constipation should begin with emphasis on good bowel habits, which include regular exercise and maintenance of adequate hydration and fiber consumption. Many constipated patients respond to a high–soluble fiber diet supplemented with daily hydrophilic colloid (1–2 Tbsp psyllium) one to three times a day. This is best given with a meal. The patient should avoid psyllium just before bedtime because its efficacy is compromised. Osmotic agents such as sorbitol or lactulose (1–2 Tbsp three or four times a day) may be helpful. These doses can be titrated to effect. The intermittent use of saline or osmotic laxatives (30 ml milk of magnesia or antacids) may be required for patients with more severe symptoms. Stimulatory laxatives should be avoided because of their tendency to damage the colonic myenteric plexus with long-term use. Magnesium-containing agents must be used with caution if renal insufficiency exists. Metoclopramide, 10–20 mg, 0.5 h before meals may help patients with intractable constipation because of its effects on colonic smooth muscle. Additionally, 200 µg mistoprostil three or four times a day is effective in patients with protracted constipation through its influence on the migrating motor complex (70).

FECAL INCONTINENCE

Fecal incontinence may be associated with severe diabetic diarrhea or constitute an independent disorder of anorectal dysfunction. Incontinent diabetic patients have decreased basal sphincteric pressure, suggesting abnormal internal and external anal sphincter function. The threshold of recognition of rectal distension in incontinent diabetic patients appears to be higher and not related to differential rectal compliance, suggesting impaired afferent function. External sphincteric function is impaired in some cases.

Patients who have had any rectal trauma are at increased risk for fecal incontinence. This mostly occurs in women who may have sustained a rectal tear during childbirth. Rectal foreign-body insertion may further decrease the sphincteric tone.

Assessing the volume of incontinence in diabetic patients is essential. Large-volume diarrhea and incontinence suggest more of a pancolonic or small-bowel cause than an isolated anorectal dysfunction.

Anorectal function can be evaluated by anorectal manometry and a test of continence for solids and liquids. Anorectal manometry profiles the maximum basal sphincter pressure in the maximum "squeeze" sphincter pressure. In addition, the rectal anal inhibitory reflex is measured by inflation of a balloon in the rectum. This causes a reflex relaxation in the internal anal sphincter. Identification of rectal dysfunction allows for therapy, including biofeedback treatment, which attempts to improve rectal distention sensing as well as sphincteric function in patients with an intact rectal sensation.

ABDOMINAL PAIN

Autonomic neuropathy may present with abdominal pain. Consideration should be given to diagnoses of acute cholecystitis, pancreatitis, gastroparesis, and diabetic ketoacidosis. Patients will occasionally present with severe epigastric pain not attributable to any of these conditions. When signs of neuropathy are present, the most likely diagnosis is diabetic abdominal radiculopathy. Symptoms of severe anorexia and weight loss are easily confused with gastroparesis or pancreatic disease such as neoplasia. For unclear reasons, symptoms typically resolve after many months. The diagnosis may be established by an abnormal electromyograph of the anterior abdominal wall muscles compared with an electromyograph of the thoracic paraspinal muscles. Analgesics, antiepileptic drugs (e.g., gabapentin, tegretol), or amitriptyline may help in select patients. Transcutaneous stimulation devices or nerve root injection may also be helpful in intractable cases.

BIBLIOGRAPHY

1. Camilleri M: Gastrointestinal manifestations of diabetes mellitus: overview. *Eur J Gastroenterol Hepatol*, 1995

2. Sninsky CA: Gastrointestinal complications of diabetes mellitus. *Curr Ther Endocrinol Metab* 5:420–425, 1994

3. Locke GR III: Epidemiology of gastrointestinal complications of diabetes mellitus. *Eur J Gastroenterol Hepatol* 7:711–716, 1995

4. Vinik AI, Erbas T: Recognizing and treating diabetic autonomic neuropathy. *Cleve Clin J Med* 68:928–944, 2001

5. Vinik AI, Glowniak JV: Hormonal secretion in diabetic autonomic neuropathy. *N Y State J Med* 82:871–886, 1982

6. Rothstein RD: Gastrointestinal motility disorders in diabetes mellitus. *Am J Gastroenterol* 85:782–785, 1990

7. Jones KL, Horowitz M, Wishart MJ, Maddox AF, Harding PE, Chatterton BE: Relationships between gastric emptying, intragastric meal distribution, and blood glucose concentrations in diabetes mellitus. *J Nucl Med* 36:2220–2228, 1995

8. le Roux CW, Patterson M, Vincent RP, Hunt C, Ghatei MA, Bloom SR: Postprandial plasma ghrelin is suppressed proportional to meal calorie content in normal-weight but not obese subjects. *J Clin Endocrinol Metab* 90:1068–1071, 2005

9. Ariga H, Imai K, Chen C, Mantyh C, Pappas TN, Takahashi T: Does ghrelin explain accelerated gastric emptying in the early stages of diabetes mellitus? *Am J Physiol Regul Integr Comp Physiol* 294:R1807–R1812, 2008

10. Woerle HJ, Szoke E, Meyer C, Dostou JM, Wittlin SD, Gosmanov NR, Welle SL, Gerich JE: Mechanisms for abnormal postprandial glucose metabolism in type 2 diabetes. *Am J Physiol Endocrinol Metab* 290:E67–E77, 2006

11. Frank JW, Saslow SB, Camilleri M, Thomforde GM, Dinneen S, Rizza RA: Mechanism of accelerated gastric emptying of liquids and hyperglycemia in patients with type II diabetes mellitus. *Gastroenterology* 109:755–765, 1995

12. Stacher G: Diabetes and the stomach. *Dig Liver Dis* 32 (Suppl. 3):S253–S254, 2000

13. Bertin E, Schneider N, Abdelli N, Wampach H, Cadiot G, Loboguerrero A, Leutenegger M, Liehn JC, Thiefin G: Gastric emptying is accelerated in obese

type 2 diabetic patients without autonomic neuropathy. *Diabetes Metab* 27:357–364, 2001

14. Kuo P, Rayner CK, Horowitz M: Gastric emptying, diabetes, and aging. *Clin Geriatr Med* 23:785–808, 2007

15. Fehmann HC, Weber V, Goke R, Goke B, Arnold R: Cosecretion of amylin and insulin from isolated rat pancreas. *FEBS Lett* 262:279–281, 1990

16. Young A: Inhibition of gastric emptying. *Adv Pharmacol* 52:99–121, 2005

17. Schmitz O, Brock B, Rungby J: Amylin agonists: a novel approach in the treatment of diabetes. *Diabetes* 53 (Suppl. 3):S233–S238, 2004

18. Schvarcz E, Palmer M, Aman J, Horowitz M, Stridsberg M, Berne C: Physiological hyperglycemia slows gastric emptying in normal subjects and patients with insulin-dependent diabetes mellitus. *Gastroenterology* 113:60–66, 1997

19. Kong MF, King P, Macdonald IA, Blackshaw PE, Perkins AC, Armstrong E, Buchanan KD, Tattersall RB: Effect of euglycemic hyperinsulinaemia on gastric emptying and gastrointestinal hormone responses in normal subjects. *Diabetologia* 41:474–481, 1998

20. Chaikomin R, Rayner CK, Jones KL, Horowitz M: Upper gastrointestinal function and glycemic control in diabetes mellitus. *World J Gastroenterol* 12:5611–5621, 2006

21. Schirra J, Leicht P, Hildebrand P, Beglinger C, Arnold R, Goke B, Katschinski M: Mechanisms of the antidiabetic action of subcutaneous glucagon-like peptide-1(7-36) amide in non-insulin dependent diabetes mellitus. *J Endocrinol* 156:177–186, 1998

22. Schirra J, Katschinski M, Weidmann C, Schafer T, Wank U, Arnold R, Goke B: Gastric emptying and release of incretin hormones after glucose ingestion in humans. *J Clin Invest* 97:92–103, 1996

23. Samsom M, Szarka LA, Camilleri M, Vella A, Zinsmeister AR, Rizza RA: Pramlintide, an amylin analog, selectively delays gastric emptying: potential role of vagal inhibition. *Am J Physiol Gastrointest Liver Physiol* 278:G946–G951, 2000

24. Woerle HJ, Mariuz PR, Meyer C, Reichman RC, Popa EM, Dostou JM, Welle SL, Gerich JE: Mechanisms for the deterioration in glucose tolerance associated with HIV protease inhibitor regimens. *Diabetes* 52:918–925, 2003

25. Horowitz M, O'Donovan D, Jones KL, Feinle C, Rayner CK, Samsom M: Gastric emptying in diabetes: clinical significance and treatment. *Diabet Med* 19:177–194, 2002

26. Camilleri M: Clinical practice: diabetic gastroparesis. *N Engl J Med* 356:820–829, 2007

27. Fraser RJ, Horowitz M, Maddox AF, Harding PE, Chatterton BE, Dent J: Hyperglycemia slows gastric emptying in type 1 (insulin-dependent) diabetes mellitus. *Diabetologia* 33:675–680, 1990

28. Woerle HJ, Albrecht M, Linke R, Zschau S, Neumann C, Nicolaus M, Gerich J, Goke B, Schirra J: Importance of changes in gastric emptying for postprandial plasma glucose fluxes in healthy humans. *Am J Physiol Endocrinol Metab* 294:E103–E109, 2008

29. Farrell FJ, Keeffe EB: Diabetic gastroparesis. *Dig Dis* 3:291–300, 1990

30. Vantyghem MC, Press M: Management strategies for brittle diabetes. *Ann Endocrinol (Paris)* 67:287–296, 2006

31. Pasricha PJ, Pehlivanov ND, Gomez G, Vittal H, Lurken MS, Farrugia G: Changes in the gastric enteric nervous system and muscle: a case report on two patients with diabetic gastroparesis. *BMC Gastroenterol* 8:21, 2008

32. Perdichizzi G, Bottari M, Pallio S, Fera MT, Carbone M, Barresi G: Gastric infection by *Helicobacter pylori* and antral gastritis in hyperglycemic obese and in diabetic subjects. *New Microbiol* 19:149–154, 1996

33. Gillett HR, Ferguson A: Coeliac disease and insulin-dependent diabetes mellitus. *Lancet* 349:1698, 1997

34. Koch KL: Electrogastrography: physiological basis and clinical application in diabetic gastropathy. *Diabetes Technol Ther* 3:51–62, 2001

35. Kara S, Dirgenali F, Okkesim S: Detection of gastric dysrhythmia using WT and ANN in diabetic gastroparesis patients. *Comput Biol Med* 36:276–290, 2006

36. Toporowska-Kowalska E, Wasowska-Krolikowska K, Szadkowska A, Bodalski J: Electrogastrography in children and adolescents with type 1 diabetes: weak correlation with metabolic control parameters. *Acta Paediatr* 95:1439–1445, 2006

37. Toporowska-Kowalska E, Wasowska-Krolikowska K, Szadkowska A, Mlynarski W, Bodalski J: Prevalence of EGG derangement in newly diagnosed type 1 diabetes in childhood. *J Pediatr Gastroenterol Nutr* 43:190–194, 2006

38. Annese V, Lombardi G, Frusciante V, Germani U, Andriulli A, Bassotti G: Cisapride and erythromycin prokinetic effects in gastroparesis due to type 1 (insulin-dependent) diabetes mellitus. *Aliment Pharmacol Ther* 11:599–603, 1997

39. Abell TL, Bernstein RK, Cutts T, Farrugia G, Forster J, Hasler WL, McCallum RW, Olden KW, Parkman HP, Parrish CR, Pasricha PJ, Prather CM, Soffer EE, Twillman R, Vinik AI: Treatment of gastroparesis: a multidisciplinary clinical review. *Neurogastroenterol Motil* 18:263–283, 2006

40. Melga P, Mansi C, Ciuchi E, Giusti R, Sciaba L, Prando R: Chronic administration of levosulpiride and glycemic control in IDDM patients with gastroparesis. *Diabetes Care* 20:55–58, 1997

41. Rosa-e-Silva L, Troncon LE, Oliveira RB, Iazigi N, Gallo L Jr, Foss MC: Treatment of diabetic gastroparesis with oral clonidine. *Aliment Pharmacol Ther* 9:179–183, 1995

42. Lacy B, Yu S: Tegaserod: a new 5-HT4 agonist. *J Clin Gastroenterol* 34:27–33, 2002

43. Gaddipati KV, Simonian HP, Kresge KM, Boden GH, Parkman HP: Abnormal ghrelin and pancreatic polypeptide responses in gastroparesis. *Dig Dis Sci* 51:1339–1346, 2006

44. Murray CD, Martin NM, Patterson M, Taylor SA, Ghatei MA, Kamm MA, Johnston C, Bloom SR, Emmanuel AV: Ghrelin enhances gastric emptying in diabetic gastroparesis: a double blind, placebo controlled, crossover study. *Gut* 54:1693–1698, 2005

45. Patil CS, Singh VP, Jain NK, Kulkarni SK: Inhibitory effect of sildenafil on gastrointestinal smooth muscle: role of NO-cGMP transduction pathway. *Indian J Exp Biol* 43:167–171, 2005

46. Orihata M, Sarna SK: Inhibition of nitric oxide synthase delays gastric emptying of solid meals. *J Pharmacol Exp Ther* 271:660–670, 1994

47. Cho SH, Park H, Kim JH, Ryu YH, Lee SI, Conklin JL: Effect of sildenafil on gastric emptying in healthy adults. *J Gastroenterol Hepatol* 21:222–226, 2006

48. Park MI, Camilleri M: Gastroparesis: clinical update. *Am J Gastroenterol* 101:1129–1139, 2006

49. Schirra J, Nicolaus M, Roggel R, Katschinski M, Storr M, Woerle HJ, Goke B: Endogenous glucagon-like peptide 1 controls endocrine pancreatic secretion and antro-pyloro-duodenal motility in humans. *Gut* 55:243–251, 2006

50. van Bronswijk H, Dubois EA, Pijl H, Cohen AF: New drugs: exenatide and sitagliptin. *Ned Tijdschr Geneeskd* 152:876–879, 2008

51. Heine RJ, Van Gaal LF, Johns D, Mihm MJ, Widel MH, Brodows RG: Exenatide versus insulin glargine in patients with suboptimally controlled type 2 diabetes: a randomized trial. *Ann Intern Med* 143:559–569, 2005

52. Sheffield CA, Kane MP, Busch RS, Bakst G, Abelseth JM, Hamilton RA: Safety and efficacy of exenatide in combination with insulin in patients with type 2 diabetes mellitus. *Endocr Pract* 14:285–292, 2008

53. Ahmad SR, Swann J: Exenatide and rare adverse events. *N Engl J Med* 358:1970–1971, 2008

54. Vinik A: Impaired gastrointestinal motility and glycemic control in patients with type 2 diabetes. *Clin Geriatr* 13:6–45, 2005

55. Patrick A, Epstein O: Review article: gastroparesis. *Aliment Pharmacol Ther* 27:724–740, 2008

56. Jacober S, Vinik A, Narayan A, Strodel W: Jejunostemy feeding in the management of gastroparesis diabeticorum. *Diabetes Care* 18:217–219, 1985

57. Reardon TM, Schnell GA, Smith OJ, Schubert TT: Surgical therapy of diabetic gastroparesis. *J Clin Gastroenterol* 11:204–207, 1989

58. Chapman BA, Wilson IR, Frampton CM, Chisholm RJ, Stewart NR, Eagar GM, Allan RB: Prevalence of gallbladder disease in diabetes mellitus. *Dig Dis Sci* 41:2222–2228, 1996

59. Shpitz B, Sigal A, Kaufman Z, Dinbar A: Acute cholecystitis in diabetic patients. *Am Surg* 61:964–967, 1995

60. Gray H, Wreghitt T, Stratton IM, Alexander GJ, Turner RC, O'Rahilly S: High prevalence of hepatitis C infection in Afro-Caribbean patients with type 2 diabetes and abnormal liver function tests. *Diabet Med* 12:244–249, 1995

61. Grimbert S, Valensi P, Lévy-Marchal C, Perret G, Richardet JP, Raffoux C, Trinchet JC, Beaugrand M: High prevalence of diabetes mellitus in patients with chronic hepatitis C: a case control study. *Gastroenterol Clin Biol* 20:544–548, 1996

62. Saukkonen T, Savilahti E, Reijonen H, Ilonen J, Tuomilehto-Wolf E, Akerblom HK: Coeliac disease: frequent occurrence after clinical onset of insulin-dependent diabetes mellitus. *Diabet Med* 13:464–470, 1996

63. Ogbonnaya KI, Arem R: Diabetic diarrhea: pathophysiology, diagnosis, and management. *Arch Intern Med* 150:262–267, 1990

64. Vinik AI, Maser RE, Mitchell BD, Freeman R: Diabetic autonomic neuropathy. *Diabetes Care* 26:1553–1579, 2003

65. Valdovinos MA, Camilleri M, Zimmerman BR: Chronic diarrhea in diabetes mellitus: mechanisms and an approach to diagnosis and treatment. *Mayo Clin Proc* 687:691–702, 1993

66. Vinik AI, Suwanwalaikorn S: Autonomic neuropathy. In *Current Therapy of Diabetes Mellitus*. DeFronzo RA, Ed. St. Louis, MO, Mosby, 1997, p. 165–176

67. Nakabayashi H, Fujii S, Miwa U, Seta T, Takeda R: Marked improvement of diabetic diarrhea with the somatostatin analogue octreotide. *Arch Intern Med* 154:1863–1867, 1994

68. Virally-Monod ML, Guillausseau PJ, Assayag M, Tielmans D, Ajzenberg C, Vasseur-Mallus S, Imberty C, Warnet A: Variable efficacy of octreotide in diabetic diarrhea. *Diabetes Metab* 22:356–358, 1996

69. Sun WM, Katsinelos P, Horowitz M, Read NW: Disturbances in anorectal function in patients with diabetes mellitus and fecal incontinence. *Eur J Gastroenterol Hepatol* 8:1007–1012, 1996

70. Haines ST: Treating constipation in the patient with diabetes. *Diabetes Educ* 21:223–232, 1995

Dr. Vinik is Professor of Medicine and Neurobiology at the Eastern Virginia Medical School (EVMS) and Director of the Diabetes Research Center, Norfolk, Virginia. Dr. Nakave and Dr. del Pilar Silva Chuecos are fellows in the EVMS Diabetes and Neuroendocrine Units, Norfolk, Virginia. Dr. Johnson is Professor of Medicine at the EVMS, Norfolk, Virginia.

45. Bladder Dysfunction

CAI FRIMODT-MØLLER, MD, DMSc, FEBU

B
ladder disturbances related to diabetes were recognized >40 years ago, but
although much emphasis has been put on this subject, it is still ignored by
many doctors and patients. A major reason for this is the lack of symptoms
for a long period and then suddenly the patient experiences a quick progression of
serious voiding problems.

ETIOLOGY AND PATHOPHYSIOLOGY

Urodynamic and urophysiological investigations have revealed loss of viscero-
sensory innervation of the bladder, thus identifying a connection with peripheral
neuropathy, which for many years has been known as a major symptom complex
in diabetes. The patient loses his or her ability to detect the "desire to void," which
usually occurs at the filling rate of 300–400 ml in healthy subjects. The distension
of the detrusor muscle (i.e., the bladder wall) gradually weakens the contractility
of the detrusor, resulting in the inability to expel the urine contents of the bladder,
which results in the development of urinary retention. From a pathophysiological
point of view, the gradual loss of sensation blocks the viscoelastic and the viscous
properties of the detrusor muscle, which results in a weakening of the bladder wall
stiffness, thereby delaying reflexes to the afferent nerve paths. The viscero-motor
pathways are patent, so the diabetic patient will be able to use his or her detrusor
muscle capacity to expel urine. But when the ongoing stretching of the bladder
wall continuously weakens the muscular filaments of the detrusor, the possibility
of building up tension is lost. The end result will be a steady increase in residual
urine and hypoactivity of the detrusor, and the patient will need to strain to support detrusor function.

CLINICAL FEATURES

Incidence and Prevalence

Incidence and prevalence of neurogenic bladder dysfunction in patients with
diabetes are higher in type 1 diabetic patients (40–50%) than in type 2 diabetic
patients (25%). Among patients with type 1 diabetes, there is a time period of ~10

years from the outbreak of the disease for the neurogenic disorders to develop. This time development is identical with the development of peripheral diabetic neuropathy. Roughly, the prevalence rate of diabetic bladder dysfunction is 1–3 per 1,000 individuals.

Sex and Age Distribution

No difference is seen in male and female populations regarding neurogenic bladder dysfunction. With regard to age, little information is available for children and adolescents. In the elderly population (>65 years old), the prevalence of neurogenic bladder disorders is equal in both sexes, but bladder dysfunction of nonneurogenic origin (for instance, benign prostatic hyperplasia) occurs significantly more frequently in the male population.

Symptoms

Symptoms have an insidious onset with gradual loss of bladder sensation. The patient seldom pays any attention to the growing interval between voidings, and the elderly man is quite happy not to be disturbed by nocturia. Although a number of patients with diabetes experience polyuria, they also report a reduced number of voidings per day (two to three during the day and zero to one during the night). Gradually, the symptoms become more serious as residual urine develops, and the patient will, on careful questioning, report having to strain during voiding, will record an impaired stream force, and will have an interrupted stream and a prolonged voiding act. Finally, he or she will have a feeling of retention or a feeling of lower abdominal distension. It is noteworthy that only ~25% of patients complain of their symptoms.

Clinical Findings

Findings of primary interest are *1*) measurement of residual urine, *2*) voiding-volume chart, and *3*) uroflowmetry. Residual urine is easily measured by ultrasound, which gives a rough estimate of the bladder content, where volumes <100 ml are acceptable but where repeated residual volumes >200 ml are pathological, either of neurogenic or obstructive origin.

An easy test to perform is to let the patient fill in a chart for voidings and voided volumes over 3 days. Important information can thus be obtained regarding the average voided volume, which is normally ~250–350 ml, but in diabetic patients, usually averages 500–600 ml. Flow curves with a bell configuration and a peak flow >20 ml/s are regarded as normal, whereas a prolonged and flat flow curve with a peak flow <15 ml/s should raise suspicion.

Frequently, a mixture of findings occur among the noninvasive tests, and the only method of distinguishing between diabetic cystopathy and other types of bladder dysfunction is to perform a urodynamic investigation measuring the intravesical, abdominal, and detrusor pressures simultaneously with flow recording. An additional cystoscopy is often also required to study the bladder wall, the bladderneck, and the prostatic part of the urethra. Whereas an obstruction of the bladder outlet will result in increasing detrusor tension, which can be seen as trabeculation, the changes of the bladder wall in the patient with diabetes typically result in a flaccid folded bladder wall. Looking at the bladder outlet, the diabetic patient with neurogenic disturbances often presents a stiff narrow bladderneck and no prostatic enlargement. A patient with infravesical obstruction demonstrates either a stiff, closed bladderneck or occluding prostatic adenomas in the prostatic urethra.

DEFINITION

If the noninvasive tests demonstrate residual urine volumes >500 ml, voiding-volume charts show voiding intervals of 6–8 h and voided volumes >600 ml, and flow studies demonstrate bell-shaped flow curves with normal peak flows, a diabetic bladder with sensory loss is predictable. This neurogenic disorder is termed diabetic cystopathy.

DIABETIC CYSTOPATHY AND OTHER DISORDERS IN THE DIABETIC PATIENT

There is a close relationship between diabetic cystopathy and peripheral neuropathy, where ~85% of patients with neurogenic bladder disorders also suffer from peripheral neuropathy and vice versa (Fig. 45.1). It should therefore be kept in mind that a patient presenting with symptoms of peripheral neuropathy (and where, for instance, examination of his or her vibratory threshold shows marked reduction) is at high risk of suffering from concomitant neurogenic dysfunction of the bladder.

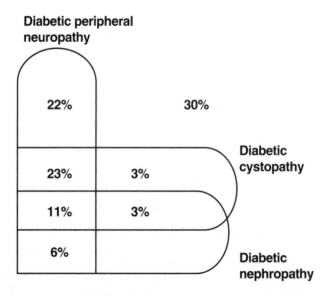

Figure 45.1 Venn diagram illustrating the interrelationship between diabetic peripheral neuropathy, diabetic cystopathy, and diabetic nephropathy in 116 diabetic patients.

Diabetic Nephropathy and Retinopathy

Diabetic nephropathy (in this chapter defined as persistent proteinuria) has a similar high relation to peripheral neuropathy (85%) and a lower but still significant (70%) relation to diabetic cystopathy (Fig. 45.1). Diabetic retinopathy, regardless of severity of illness, did not show any relation to diabetic cystopathy.

TREATMENT

The primary objective in dealing with diabetic cystopathy is to eliminate the high residual volume and to find means of replacing the irreversible sensory loss. Because the loss of sensation is permanent, the treatment must be followed to achieve lifelong control of the bladder.

The principles of nonsurgical management are as follows:

1. Schedule voiding every 3–4 h.
2. Perform triple voiding (i.e., repeated voidings 3–5 min after the primary voiding until no urine can be passed; straining is usually applied).
3. If residual urine exceeds 2–300 ml following the above-mentioned regimens and the uroflowmetry curve is in the lower peak flow level, treatment with α-adrenergic blockers should be administered.
4. If residual urine exceeds 500 ml, clean, intermittent catheterization is recommended one to three times daily, with the frequency of catheterizations depending on the amount of residual urine and whether the patient has symptomatic bacteriuria. In the case of asymptomatic bacteriuria, there is no need for prophylactic chemotherapy. However, if the patient has symptomatic bacteriuria, prophylaxis with a bacteriostatic antibiotic drug is recommended.

If these methods are ineffective, the urologist might have to resort to surgical intervention—bladderneck incision/resection to relieve the patient of any risk of outlet obstruction.

In patients with urodynamically disclosed obstruction, surgery is inevitable. A temporary medical treatment with α-blocking agents should be tried, but long-term medical treatment is not recommendable. Whether transurethral resection or transurethral microwave treatment is used is up to the urologist. Prostatic stents in a diabetic patient with increased risk of bacteriuria should be avoided because a foreign body (e.g., a stent) has a high risk of developing symptomatic bacteriuria.

Earlier recommendations of using bethanecol chloride as a parasympathomimetic drug in the neuropathic bladder are not in effect today, partly because the side effects of the high doses of the drug create a lot of discomfort. Urodynamic investigations have demonstrated an increase in bladderneck tonus, thereby worsening the bladder outlet.

Another earlier recommendation to perform a reduction cystoplasty to reduce the bladder capacity has also been given up. Within a short time, the bladder will regain its former capacity.

TREATMENT RESULTS

The better diabetes is regulated, the greater the chance of avoiding neurological disturbances. The earlier the diabetic cystopathy is recognized, the better the results. A thorough urological investigation as early as possible is recommended, and if no outlet obstruction has been detected, the general practitioner or the diabetologist can proceed with the controls.

For a long period, prophylactic measures, such as voiding around the clock with intervals of 3–4 h, double-triple voiding activities at every micturition, residual urine control by ultrasonography every third month, regular urine culturing to detect bacteriuria every 3 months, and an annual check of renal function by means of S-creatinine, will reduce the risk of developing irreversible bladder dysfunction and probably also prevent end-stage renal disease.

If residual urine exceeds 500 ml at a minimum of two ultrasonic investigations, it is recommended that the patient perform intermittent self-catheterization at least once daily, probably before sleep and again in the morning. If the residual volume increases, despite these measures, the patient will have to rely on catheterization every 4–5 h daily. Whenever any progression of bladder dysfunction is noted, the patient should be referred to the urologist for reinvestigation.

Last, but not least, a close cooperation between the patient, his or her general practitioner, the diabetologist, and the urologist is crucial for success in avoiding or reducing the symptoms of diabetic cystopathy.

BIBLIOGRAPHY

Ellenberg M, Weber H: The incipient asymptomatic diabetic bladder. *Diabetes* 16:331–335, 1967

Faerman I, Maler M, Jadzinsky M, Alvarez E, Fox D, Zilbervarg J, Cibeira JB, Colinas R: Asymptomatic neurogenic bladder in juvenile diabetics. *Diabetologia* 7:168–172, 1971

Frimodt-Møller C: Diabetic cystopathy: a review of the urodynamic and clinical features of neurogenic bladder dysfunction in diabetes mellitus. *Dan Med Bull* 25:49–60, 1978

Kaplan SA, Te AE, Blaivas JG: Urodynamic findings in patients with diabetic cystopathy. *J Urol* 153:342–344, 1995

Sasaki K, Chancellor MB, Phelan MW, Yokoyama T, Fraser MO, Seki S, Kubo K, Kuman H, Groat WC, Yoshimura N: Diabetic cystopathy correlates with a long-term decrease in nerve growth factor levels in the bladder and lumbosacral dorsal root ganglia. *J Urol* 168:1259–1264, 2002

Ueda T, Yoshimura N, Yoshida O: Diabetic cystopathy: relationship to autonomic neuropathy detected by sympathetic skin response. *J Urol* 157:580–584, 1997

Dr. Frimodt-Møller is Chief Urologist at the Erichsen's Private Hospital, Copenhagen, Denmark.

46. Erectile Dysfunction

Kenneth J. Snow, MD

E rectile dysfunction (ED) is a well-known complication of diabetes. Previously, the term "impotence" was used for all aspects of sexual dysfunction, which led to confusion. In 1992, the National Institutes of Health Consensus Conference recommended that the term "erectile dysfunction" be used to describe problems relating to penile erections and defined ED as the inability to achieve or maintain an erection long enough to permit satisfactory sexual intercourse.

PREVALENCE AND PATHOPHYSIOLOGY OF ED

Despite being a common problem in men, especially diabetic men, the medical community has only recently begun to address the extent of sexual problems. The recent Massachusetts Male Aging Study, which evaluated nearly 1,300 men aged 40–70 years, found some degree of erectile difficulty in 52% of these subjects. Studies report the incidence of ED in diabetic men varying from 27.5 to 75%. As the age of the study population increased, the incidence increased, with up to 95% of diabetic men aged >70 years having some degree of ED. In diabetic men aged <30 years, 20% had ED.

For diabetic men, the incidence of ED seems to be related to age, duration of diabetes, the level of glucose control as reflected by an elevated A1C level, and the presence or absence of diabetes complications. Macrovascular risk factors that often accompany diabetes, such as hypercholesterolemia, hypertension, and smoking, also contribute to the risk of ED. For most patients, the etiology of ED is due to multiple factors. Hypogonadism is also common in diabetic men and can contribute to ED.

There are a variety of medications that can affect erectile function. Table 46.1 lists some of the more commonly used medications. Thiazide diuretics and β-blockers have been shown to be associated with ED. Earlier β-blockers caused more difficulties than more recent β-blockers. Even local ophthalmologic β-blockers may affect erections. Many drugs that affect the central nervous system may inhibit sexual function by direct action on the central neurological impulses or by the production of prolactin. Many over-the-counter drugs, such as pseudoephedrine, and certain antihistamines, such as diphenhydramine and chlorpheniramine, can affect ED as well.

Table 46.1 Commonly Used Drugs that Affect Erectile Function

Cardiovascular
  β-Blockers (especially propranolol, metoprolol, penbutolol, pindolol, timolol)
  Certain α-blockers (clonidine, guanfacine)
  α- and β-blockers (labetalol)
  α-Methyldopa
  Thiazide diuretics
  Older antihypertensives (reserpine, guanethidine, hydralazine)
  Spironolactone
  Digoxin
  Calcium channel blockers (fairly low risk)
Central nervous system–acting drugs
  Antidepressants (including tricyclics and SSRIs)
  Antipsychotics
  Tranquilizers
  Anorexiants
Allergy related
  Corticosteroids
  Theophylline
  Bronchodilators
Antifungals
  Fluconazole, ketoconazole, itraconazole
Miscellaneous
  Metoclopramide, flutamide, clofibrate, gemfibrozil
Recreational
  Marijuana
  Alcohol
Nonprescription
  Antihistamines (chlorpheniramine, diphenhydramine, chlotrimeton)
  Decongestants
  Cimetidine

SSRI, selective serotonin reuptake inhibitor.

NORMAL AGING CHANGES

Some men seeking help for ED may only be experiencing changes that are part of the normal aging process. As men age, they lose the ability to achieve spontaneous erections from visual sexual images or sexual fantasy. More direct genital stimulation (foreplay) may still lead to erections. In addition, with aging, distraction and fatigue are more likely to lead to erectile difficulties, and sexual activity needs to be attempted in a place with minimum distractions when the individual is not fatigued.

DIAGNOSTIC EVALUATION

History

As part of the evaluation of ED, a careful history should be performed with an emphasis placed on history of sexual and reproductive functions, as well as pertinent, related medical history (Table 46.2). The first issue that needs to be clarified is what exactly is the problem. Many patients may complain of ED, whereas the primary problem is decreased libido or ejaculatory problems. When dealing with ED, the duration of the problem and its presentation—whether sudden or gradual, with or without progression—provides information to suggest a greater or lesser likelihood of organic disease. The presence of nocturnal or morning erections suggests a psychogenic component to ED, although their absence does not dispute it, because morning erections decrease in frequency as men age.

Because poor blood glucose control increases the likelihood of ED, ascertain the patient's glycemic control as well as the presence of diabetes complications. Concomitant medical illnesses should be identified, with particular attention paid to medications used and the presence of vascular disease.

Psychological Considerations

If possible, the initial interview should be carried out with the sexual partner present. Although this arrangement may not always be possible, it is useful for the health care provider to observe the dynamics between the two individuals. ED can cause, or be caused by, problems in a relationship, and this knowledge can be useful in determining the course of evaluation and/or treatment. Significant numbers of men with ED and diabetes will have psychological problems. Referral to a mental health professional with expertise in sexual counseling is often helpful.

Physical Examination

When performing the physical examination, seek evidence of specific disease states relating to sexual function and carry out a more general screening to assess overall health (Table 46.2). Of particular importance is evidence of the following:

- normal virilization
- anatomical changes, such as Peyronie's disease, hypospadias, or past injury
- testicular abnormalities
- diffuse vascular disease
- diabetic neuropathies

Table 46.2 Evaluation of Men with Diabetes and ED

History	Physical examination
Exact problem	Blood pressure
Onset	Cardiovascular examination
Duration	Neurological examination
Duration and control of diabetes	Breast examination
Diabetes complications	Genital examination
Other medical conditions	
Medications (prescription and	**Diagnostic tests**
nonprescription)	A1C, lipids, creatinine, liver function
Performance anxiety	tests, hemoglobin, testosterone
Social setting	
Relationship problems	
Health of partner	
Other stresses in patient's life	

An adequate evaluation of a man with ED cannot be performed without examination of the penis and testes.

Laboratory Measurements

The list of laboratory tests that are needed for a complete evaluation of ED starts with an assessment of overall health and, in particular for diabetic men, an assessment of glucose control (A1C) and the presence of diabetes-related conditions (Table 46.2).

In nondiabetic patients, testosterone is not routinely measured unless the individual elicits either symptoms or signs of testosterone deficiency. Men with chronic illnesses, such as diabetes, hypertension, and hyperlipidemia, have a higher incidence of low testosterone levels. Recent studies have suggested that the incidence of low testosterone levels in men with metabolic syndrome may exceed 50%. Therefore, in diabetic men, it is useful to screen for testosterone as part of the initial evaluation.

There is some debate on whether total or free testosterone should be measured. Total testosterone depends on the amount of testosterone that is bound to sex hormone–binding globulin (SHBG) as well as to albumin. SHBG increases with age, especially in men aged >55 years, making the total testosterone level less useful in this age-group. Also, testosterone will be affected by any significant change in serum proteins, such as that seen in the nephrotic syndrome. In the past, some have argued to check free testosterone to avoid this issue. Often, though, the free testosterone assay is not accurate. This issue is of particular concern if the free testosterone is not measured using either equilibrium dialysis or bioavailable testosterone. A reasonable approach, especially if there is any concern regarding the reliability of the free testosterone assay, is to measure the total testosterone level. Any low value should be confirmed with a repeat measurement. If there is a question of a protein-binding issue (i.e., if the patient is aged >55 years or has nephrotic syndrome), obtain a direct measurement of SHBG and determine whether there is any significant change in the level that is affecting total testosterone values.

If the testosterone is low, the next step is to measure the leutinizing hormone. An elevated level indicates primary testicular failure, whereas a normal or low level is seen in central hypogonadism. If the testosterone level is normal in a patient with a normal physical examination, no further laboratory evaluation is needed.

Nocturnal Penile Tumescence and Rigidity Monitoring

If the differentiation between organic and psychogenic ED is difficult to determine, measuring nocturnal penile activity may be beneficial. A portable home monitor, the RigiScan, can measure tumescence and rigidity while the patient sleeps in the privacy of his own home. Patients with ED of an organic origin should have an abnormal nocturnal tumescence study. Patients with psychogenic disease may still have nocturnal erections. Thus, the presence of normal nocturnal erections confirms a psychogenic etiology for ED.

Further Testing

Duplex ultrasound after the intracavernosal injection of papaverine or prostaglandin E1 can be used to monitor cavernosal artery pressure. Caution should be taken when interpreting these results, however, because decreased blood flow is seen in diabetic men with normal erections compared with men without diabetes. There is still no substitute for a good history and examination of lower-extremity pulses and femoral bruits for diagnosing vascular disease. The patient's history and physical examination will generally disclose the presence of diabetic neuropathy.

TREATMENT FOR ED

The first goal for a diabetic man with ED is to achieve optimal control of his blood glucose while avoiding hypoglycemia. In addition, if the patient is on a drug that is known to affect erectile function, consider changing the medication to an agent less likely to be a problem. Even if the drug was not the entire cause for the ED, and full function does not resume, the medication may have been contributing along with other factors.

Patients with primary gonadal failure need permanent testosterone replacement. Treatment of testosterone deficiency will help ameliorate the symptoms of gonadal insufficiency—lethargy, depression, muscle weakness, anemia, and osteoporosis. Although men with primary gonadal failure and ED will frequently respond to testosterone therapy, men with other medical problems, such as diabetes and slightly low testosterone levels, will usually not see a reversal of ED by supplementing with testosterone.

The use of testosterone, however, may prove beneficial in conjunction with other therapies. Several studies have now shown that low testosterone levels decrease the efficacy of phosphodiesterase type 5 (PDE-5) therapy and that replacing testosterone improves the response to PDE-5 therapy. Thus, a patient who has previously tried a PDE-5 agent, had an inadequate response, and is then identified as having a low testosterone level may have a significantly improved response if he is treated with testosterone replacement.

Because testosterone may aggravate a preexisting prostate cancer, a digital rectal examination and a prostate-specific antigen (PSA) test should be performed before testosterone treatment. The rectal examination and PSA test should be rechecked after 3–6 months of treatment. An abnormal examination or an increase in the PSA >1.5 ng/ml implies prostatic stimulation that warrants evaluation by a urologist. Hematocrit levels should also be checked regularly because of the risk of polycythemia, especially in smokers. A baseline hematocrit >52% or a rise to >54% is a contraindication to testosterone therapy.

If controlling blood glucose, changing medications, or replacing testosterone does not sufficiently reestablish normal sexual function, other methods should be considered. Because of the variety of therapies available, treatment for ED should be tailored to the patient's complaints, using the therapy most readily accepted by the patient. Patients who have no trouble attaining an adequate erection with foreplay but who lose the erection prematurely before ejaculation are said to have early detumescence or venous leakage. They do not need medications or devices to produce an erection but rather something to prevent detumescence. Rubber constriction devices such as rings of various sizes or adjusting constriction bands are available and are simple, safe, and inexpensive. The vast majority of diabetic patients who have a significant neurovascular component as the cause of their ED should be started with oral therapy.

Oral Medications

Released in early 1998, sildenafil (Viagra) has revolutionized the treatment of ED. Sildenafil inhibits PDE-5. During sexual stimulation, nitric oxide is released in the corpus cavernosum, which activates guanylate cyclase and results in increased levels of cGMP. This causes smooth muscle relaxation in the corpus cavernosum, allowing increased blood flow with tissue expansion. PDE-5 degrades cGMP, which allows the penis to return to its usual flaccid state. Inhibition of PDE-5 by sildenafil causes an increase in cGMP with subsequent increased vaso-dilation.

The drug is rapidly absorbed with peak serum levels 30–120 min after taking it. Therefore, patients should be instructed to take the medication ~1 h before attempting intercourse and should also be informed that sexual stimulation (fore-play) is necessary to attain an erection. Absorption of the drug is delayed with a fatty meal. The recommended starting dose of sildenafil is 50 mg 1 h before sexual activity. The dosage can be increased to 100 mg if needed or decreased to 25 mg if the side effects outlined below occur. A patient should not take more than one dose each day.

Sildenafil has been shown to improve erections in up to 70% of diabetic men with ED. Patients with complete or near-complete loss of erectile function have a lower response rate. The most common side effects include headache, flushing, dyspepsia, and nasal congestion. The drug is contraindicated for patients taking nitrates because of the high likelihood of developing significant hypotension.

Concern has been raised regarding the cardiac safety of sildenafil. Studies have not shown sildenafil to increase the risk of a cardiac event. Physicians need to remember that patients with ED are more likely to have cardiac disease and that several of the risk factors for ED are also risk factors for coronary artery disease. In the diabetic population, this concern needs to be even higher because of the possibility of silent ischemia. If the physician has any concern regarding possible undiagnosed cardiac ischemia, cardiac stress testing should be performed before initiating therapy. A prescription for sildenafil should be considered on par with a prescription for initiation of a new exercise regimen, and appropriate cardiac pre-cautions should be taken.

Tadalafil (Cialis) was approved for use in the U.S. in 2003. This agent also works through inhibition of PDE-5. Its pharmacokinetics are quite different from sildenafil, with a maximal concentration achieved 2 h (0.5–6.0 h) after taking the drug and with a half-life of 24 h. The drug has shown efficacy as long as 36 h after taking it. Thus, the drug is less often used on demand, but rather in anticipation of sexual activity later. The starting dose is 10 mg, with options to increase to 20 mg or to decrease to 5 mg as needed.

Tadalafil has been shown to improve erections in up to 70% of diabetic men with ED. Common side effects include headache, flushing, rhinitis, dyspepsia, and lower back pain. The latter is felt to be due to cross-reactivity with PDE-11 pres-ent in skeletal muscle. The drug is contraindicated with nitrates.

Vardenafil (Levitra) was also approved for use in the U.S. in 2003 and also works by inhibition of PDE-5. The drug reaches maximal concentration in just under 1 h and has a half-life of ~4–6 h; thus, its pharmacokinetics are similar to those of sildenafil. The starting dose is 10 mg, with the option to increase to 20 mg. Dosages of 2.5 and 5 mg are available for patients on antiretroviral therapy or ketoconazole.

Vardenafil has been shown to improve erections in ~70% of diabetic men with ED. Common side effects include headache, flushing, rhinitis, and dyspepsia. The drug is contraindicated for patients taking nitrates.

For patients who do not respond to a PDE-5 inhibitor or who have a contraindication to its use, second-line therapy can involve intracavernosal injection therapy, intraurethral prostaglandin E1 therapy, the use of a vacuum assistance device, or a penile implant.

Intracavernosal Injection Therapy

The effectiveness of intrapenile injection with vasoactive substances was first demonstrated in 1983. Papavarine and phentolamine are used in combination. The addition of prostaglandin E1 was found to improve the results, with up to 90% of patients responding. Recently, the use of prostaglandin E1 alone has increased. It is the only intrapenile drug approved for use by the U.S. Food and Drug Administration. It does not appear to be as effective in diabetic ED (~50% success rate) as the mixtures. Acceptance of this therapy has been limited by the patient's willingness to perform intrapenile injections. Studies have revealed that half of all patients do not continue therapy by the end of 1 year. Penile scarring and priapism are potential complications.

Intraurethral Therapy

Prostaglandin E1 has been formulated into an intraurethral suppository that is absorbed into the corpora spongiosum of the glans penis and migrates rapidly into the corpora cavernosa. In diabetic men, 40–60% will attain adequate erections with this therapy. Penile or scrotum pain and orthostatic hypotension are rare complications.

Vacuum Assistance Devices

Vacuum pumps are plastic cylinders that are placed over the penis. Air is evacuated from the cylinder, creating a negative pressure, and drawing venous blood into the penis. A ring is placed around the base of the penis to retain the erection. Satisfactory erections are obtained in ~75% of patients, and ~50% of patients have long-term satisfaction with the resulting sexual function. This method is safe but quite mechanical. Younger men and those patients who do not have a long-term relationship may find the technique cumbersome and embarrassing. Yet, some couples use the procedure of pumping the device and placement of the ring as a form of foreplay and turn this negative factor into a positive one. Greater involvement of the partner in the decision process will often increase the likelihood for use of a vacuum assistance device.

Penile Implants

Penile implants were the first modern therapy for ED. There are two basic types. The simpler model is the semirigid rod. The second type, an inflatable rod, has more hardware that is placed in the penis and scrotum. Earlier models had a high rate of mechanical failure, but this rate has decreased significantly with engineering improvements. Satisfaction rates among diabetic men and their partners are frequently quite high. With the development of newer therapies, the number of implants performed yearly has substantially decreased.

New Therapies

Apomorphine is now available in Europe and other parts of the world for the treatment of ED. The drug is a D1/D2 dopamine agonist that acts centrally to improve erectile function without effects on libido. Administered sublingually, apomorphine has a rapid onset of action (~15 min). Efficacy is less than that seen with PDE-5 inhibitors. Nausea, yawning, and somnolence are the most common side effects. The drug is not available in the U.S., and there are no plans currently for it to be released here.

Topical alprostadil is also available in many parts of the world. Efficacy is limited, and side effects include burning and the possibility of transference to the sexual partner.

WHEN TO REFER A DIABETIC PATIENT WITH ED

After performing the initial evaluation, therapy may be started if the cause of ED is clear and the physician is comfortable with the use of oral therapy. If the cause is not clear or if therapy with an oral medication is not successful, the patient should be referred to a specialist for further treatment.

BIBLIOGRAPHY

Brant WO, Bella AJ, Lue TF: Treatment options for erectile dysfunction. *Endocrinol Metab Clin North Am* 36:465–479, 2007

Carson, CC: Phosphodiesterase type 5 inhibitors: state of the therapeutic class. *Urol Clin North Am* 34:507–515, 2007

Drugs that cause sexual dysfunction: an update (Review). *Med Lett Drugs Ther* 34:73–78, 1992

Feldman HA, Goldstein I, Hatzichristou DG, Krane RJ, McKinley JB: Impotence and its medical and psychosocial correlates: results of the Massachusetts Male Aging Study. *J Urol* 151:54–61, 1994

Hakim LS, Goldstein I: Diabetic sexual dysfunction. *Endocrinol Metab Clin North Am* 25:379–400, 1996

Lue TF: Erectile dysfunction. *NEJM* 342:1802–1813, 2000

Mulligan T, Frick MF, Zuraw QC, Stemhagen A, McWhirter C: Prevalence of hypogonadism in males aged at least 45 years: the HIM study. *Int J Clin Pract* 60:762–769, 2006

Meuleman E, et al.: Clinical evaluation and the doctor-patient dialogue. In *Erectile Dysfunction*. Plymouth, U.K., Plymbridge Distributors, 2000, p. 115–138

Sharpless J, Snow K: Gender-specific issues. In *Joslin's Diabetes Deskbook*. Boston, MA, Joslin Diabetes Center, 2001, p. 473–550

Snow KJ: Erectile dysfunction: a review and update. *Formulary* 39:261–268, 2004

Dr. Snow is Chief of Adult Diabetes and Director of the Sexual Function Clinic, Joslin Clinic, Joslin Diabetes Center, Boston, Massachusetts.

47. Sexual Dysfunction in Women with Diabetes

Deborah J. Lightner, MD, and Felecia Rittenhouse Fick, CRTT, RPA-C

Diabetes affects the vascular, renal, and neurological systems, secondarily disturbing sexual function in the affected female patient at higher rates than in nondiabetic patients. Whereas many publications address various aspects of erectile dysfunction in men with diabetes, female sexual dysfunction, despite higher prevalence than male sexual dysfunction, remains much less discussed and less studied. Patient modesty, health care provider time, and third-party insurance coverage may limit the evaluation of this important quality-of-life issue. We review herein the available information on this subject so that the female diabetic population might be better served.

GETTING STARTED: THE MEDICAL REVIEW

The key to helping the female diabetic patient is to address her sexual health during the history portion of the clinical visit. Health care providers are increasingly pressured to see more patients and spend less time with each one. This time constraint makes it difficult for providers to ask about a patient's sexual function. Health care providers may not be well versed on the right questions to ask and thereby are unable to establish by history the sexual dysfunction that is bothersome to the patient or the current treatment appropriate for this problem. Concern may exist that the provider is unable to offer help with these sensitive issues, but there are increasingly effective therapies available.

A sexual history should take only a few minutes to complete and can be incorporated into the screening questions for abuse. As routine as it is to ask about the patient's safety, the health care provider can inquire about a patient's sexual function; it is an important component of quality of life. The questions should be specifically aimed at the four types of female sexual dysfunction that occur:

1. hypoactive sexual desire disorder, or decreased libido
2. female sexual arousal disorder
3. female orgasmic disorder
4. female sexual pain disorder

Each disorder occurs separately from the others. For example, a woman may have hypoactive sexual desire disorder but can be stimulated, aroused, and capable of a pleasurable and orgasmic experience. Alternatively, a patient with an arousal disorder, such as failure to lubricate, may be orgasmic if able to supply the lubrication with commercially available water-based lubricants. Specific questions might include, "Have you noticed a decrease in your sexual desire?" and "Do you think about sexual activity less often than you used to?" For arousal disorders, common in diabetic patients, specific questions might include, "Do you have difficulty staying aroused once you become sexually involved?" "Are your vaginal tissues dry during sexual experiences?" "Are you able to have an orgasm?" "Do you have pain with sexual activity?" and "Where does this occur?" Most important, in any sexual history, is the question of how significant this symptom is to the patient. Furthermore, sexuality changes with the life cycle, and decreased sexual desire or responsiveness may be normal during lactation, with certain medications and chemotherapy agents, or with the recent loss of a spouse. It is the patient's own degree of discomfort that should direct further investigation and therapy.

Health care providers may request that a patient return at another time for a longer appointment to fully address sexual concerns. Likewise, referral to another health care provider more conversant in sexual dysfunction may also be appropriate, and the patient should be so advised.

REFERRAL TO A SPECIALIST

The greatest continuity and integration of care comes from the patient's primary care provider. If the primary care recommendations fail to adequately address the patient's sexual health, then a referral to a specialist should be considered. Specialists in female sexual dysfunction may include urologists, gynecologists, psychologists, or psychiatrists. Physician assistants who specialize in this area of medicine can also provide quality health care as well as long-term follow-up, which is important for this patient population. A team approach is especially helpful because sexual dysfunction is a multifaceted reflector of the patient's overall mental, physical, and emotional health.

PATHOPHYSIOLOGY AND RISK FACTORS

The risk of sexual dysfunction in diabetic female patients appears highly correlated to two areas: women with complications of diabetes and those in whom diabetes or other life issues have had an impact on diminishing quality of life. Many studies have shown that premenopausal women with type 1 diabetes do not report higher rates of desire disorder, orgasmic dysfunction, or pain problems compared with a cohort of otherwise healthy women. However, while one questionnaire-based study showed that there was decrease in lubrication in type 1 diabetic women compared with a control group, their risk of sexual dysfunction was significantly increased with the duration of diabetes and degree of diabetes control as measured by A1C.

This low risk, unfortunately, is not seen in type 2 diabetic women. A recent comparison study of older women with type 2 diabetes and healthy age-matched control subjects revealed an increased prevalence of sexual dysfunction in the women with type 2 diabetes across all four diagnostic categories. Perhaps the answer lies in animal studies. A recent animal study in diabetic female rat vaginas demonstrated thinning of vaginal epithelial cell layers (about half as many layers as in normal healthy rats), decreased vaginal submucosal vasculatures, and vaginal tissue fibrosis. This combination of adverse changes, if occurring in the older female patient with type 2 diabetes, might lead to decreased vaginal lubrication, decreased arousal, and secondary dyspareunia. Vaginal lubrication is a transudate of plasma and therefore requires a responsive genital vascular supply. Inability to increase blood flow to the genital organs that produce this normal transudate can result in dyspareunia. A decline in vaginal blood flow, therefore, may be related to sexual arousal disorders. It is unclear whether uncomplicated type 1 diabetic women are at risk for this reduction in blood flow and increase in fibrosis. One study of female subjects with type 1 diabetes demonstrated decreased levels of vaginal pulse amplitude (one measure of the responsiveness of genital blood flow) compared with healthy control subjects. However, other measurements, such as labial temperatures during sexual arousal (another measure of genital blood flow), did not show any difference between female subjects with and without type 1 diabetes.

If the diabetic woman's vagina loses elasticity and she develops a blunted vaso-active responsiveness, thereby reducing lubrication, the effects of diabetes may become more apparent in the aging individual with diabetes. The inherent changes of aging place women at risk for both of these phenomena, so a two-hit risk to the vaginal function may result in the aging diabetic woman, increasing her risk of sexual dysfunction.

There is some literature to suggest that diabetic women are at risk for sexual dysfunction as a result of poorer sensory nerve function; that is, the diabetes complications might include the development of a neuropathy affecting genital sensation, as detected by vibration perception tests. That reduction of genital sensation may or may not secondarily produce sexual dysfunction.

Some suggest that hypoactive sexual desire disorder from a distortion of body image may occur if obesity is associated with type 2 diabetes. Secondary evidence suggests that is not so because there is poor correlation of a diabetic woman's sexual dysfunction with her BMI.

THERAPEUTIC INTERVENTION

If a woman's sexual dysfunction is mild and of brief duration, practical and brief intervention by the health care team may be effective. Supportive therapy for life events can be curative of her distress. Other treatment options might include treatment for disturbed sleep and the multiple somatic manifestations of depression, if found. Multiple drugs are associated with female sexual dysfunction, and they include antihistamines, antihypertensives, anticholinergics, and any drug that causes related side effects or modifications in the central nervous system, including sedatives, hypnotics, pain medications, antiepileptic medications, and antidepressants. In coordination with a knowledgeable health care provider, the cessation or replacement of any of these can also be efficacious. One should never change or discontinue antihypertensives, antiepileptic medications, etc., without professional medical advice.

Estrogen replacement therapy may play a role in the treatment of sexual dysfunction. For example, patients with sexual dysfunction and premature ovarian dysfunction may respond to hormonal supplementation. Arousal disorders secondary to atrophic vaginal tissues and poor vaginal lubrication may respond to low-level estrogen replacement in the form of a pill, a patch, or vaginal cream, with estrogen reversing vaginal atrophy generally within a 6-week treatment period. Vaginal lubricants are helpful in premenopausal women with diabetes and failure of lubrication or in postmenopausal women who have risk factors preventing estrogen replacement.

As one study suggested that androgen therapy might help improve female sexual dysfunction in women failing adequate estrogen replacement after a surgically induced menopause, a placebo-controlled trial of a testosterone patch for postmenopausal women on estrogen therapy and distress secondary to sexual dysfunction was conducted, and it suggested that sexual function improved modestly. However, this was not performed in diabetic subjects, and safe androgen replacement doses have not been established for women. A further caveat is that androgen supplementation is associated with adverse changes in lipid and liver function profiles and, if used in the postmenopausal woman, should be cautiously used, monitored, and stopped if a therapeutic trial is not successful. Currently accepted androgen-estrogen combinations are indicated only for intractable menopausal symptoms. Larger trials of androgenic agents are currently underway and specifically track the complications of testosterone gel in women, including cardiovascular events. Currently, the U.S. Food and Drug Administration (FDA) does not approve the use of androgens for female sexual dysfunction.

Peripherally acting agents, such as sildenafil, vardenafil, and tadenafil, mediate smooth-muscle relaxation and blood engorgement via phosphodiesterase type 5 (PDE-5) inhibition and have been enormously successful in the treatment of male erectile dysfunction. Sildenafil trials in women have demonstrated a similar hemodynamic effect on the genitals. However, this physiological response does not reliably transfer into a subjective feeling of arousal and/or desire, and these trials of these agents have been discontinued. Vasoactive intestinal peptide (VIP) is also a major neurotransmitter found in the vaginal vasculature. However, thus far there has been no clinical data showing that these peripherally acting vasodilators affect either vaginal or clitoral blood flow. Topical prostaglandin acts locally as a mediator of blood flow; topical formulations of Alprostadil (a synthetic analog of prostaglandin E-1) are also being studied.

Centrally acting agents are more promising. Compounds such as melanocortin agonists and dopamine agonists are undergoing evaluation for female sexual dysfunction. As examples, apomorphine, bremelanotide (a melanocortin receptor agonist), and bupropion (an FDA-approved selective serotonin reuptake inhibitor–class antidepressant with dopamine agonist activity) have been investigated in several studies but without clear objective responses. Further clinical trials are clearly called for. Patients should be counseled to avoid naturopathic remedies that are uncontrolled by federal licensure and unproven in scientific studies.

Other therapies appropriate for women with sexual dysfunction may include behavioral modification. To minimize introital localized coitally associated pain occurring with pelvic floor tension myalgia, a patient may find benefit in relaxation exercises for the pubococcygeal muscles of the pelvic floor. Pelvic floor tension myalgia can often be simply diagnosed in the patient with a compatible history by transvaginal palpation of the spastic and poorly relaxing levator muscles, reproducing coital discomfort. Women who have pain on penetration or with thrusting may modify coital positions, giving them more control (i.e., using the female superior position or having both partners lie on their sides). Vaginismus can also be significantly improved with behavioral techniques.

A decrease in orgasmic capacity may result from hypoactive desire, decreased or poorly sustained arousal, or physical discomfort during sex. Therefore, treatment of any of these problems may significantly improve orgasmic capacity. Before assuming that orgasmic disorder is related to diabetic neuropathy, the patient should be carefully asked whether she is still orgasmic with other genital stimulation (i.e., manually, with a vibrator, or by a partner). Many women, particularly with age, have a difficult time reaching orgasm from penile-vaginal thrusting alone. Women with orgasmic difficulty may simply require more adequate and deliberate clitoral stimulation.

Lastly, concerns about infertility may adversely affect a couple's sex life. Fear of pregnancy and sexually transmitted diseases can also interfere with sexual desire and activity and can be addressed specifically.

CONCLUSION

Questions regarding female sexual health should be a routine part of the history taking because female sexual dysfunction is common, yet without direct questioning, it remains largely underreported by patients. Limited studies have shown that women with diabetes may have an increased risk of female sexual dysfunction compared with normal age-matched healthy control subjects. However, that risk appears primarily related to the prevalence of diabetes complications and to any negative impact of the disease on quality of life. The aging woman with diabetes may be subject to a double risk of diabetes complications and her aging vasculature. Her risk of sexual dysfunction may be higher than that of the younger well-controlled diabetic woman. Further research is clearly necessary because the true prevalence of diabetes resulting in female sexual dysfunction is unknown. If female sexual dysfunction is uncovered, the type of dysfunction is used to direct therapy, with appropriate referrals made as necessary. The female diabetic patient will appreciate the attention to this important aspect of her well-being and to the improvement in her quality of life.

BIBLIOGRAPHY

Buster JE, Kingsberg SA, Aguirre O, Brown C, Breaux JG, Buch A, Rodenberg CA, Wekselman K, Casson P: Testosterone patch for low sexual desire in surgically menopausal women: a randomized trial. *Obstet Gynecol* 105:944–952, 2005

Enguehard-Gueiffier C, Gueiffier A: Recent progress in medicinal chemistry of D4 agonists. *Curr Med Chem* 13:2981–2993, 2006

Erol B, Tefekli A, Sanli O, Ziylan O, Armagan A, Kendirci M, Eryasar D, Kadioglu A: Does sexual dysfunction correlate with detrioration of somatic sensory system in diabetic women? *Int J Impot Res* 15:198–202, 2003

Ezlin P, Mathieu C, Van Den Bruel A, Bosteels J, Vanderschueren D, Demyttenaere K: Sexual dysfunction in women with type 1 diabetes. *Diabetes Care* 25:672–677, 2002

Heiman JR, Gittelman M, Costabile R, Guay A, Friedman A, Heard-Davidson A, Peterson C, Dietrich J, Stevens D: Topical alprostadil (PGE1) for the treatment of female sexual arousal disorder: in-clinic evaluation of safety and efficacy. *J Psychosom Obstet Gynaecol* 21:31–41, 2006

Grady D: Postmenopausal hormones: therapy for symptoms only. *N Engl J Med* 348:1835–1837, 2003

Hays J, Ockene J, Brunner RL, Kotchen JM, Manson JE, Patterson RE, Aragaki AK, Shumaker SA, Brzyski RG, LaCroix AZ, Granke IA, Valanis BG: Effects of estrogen plus progestin on health-related quality of life. *N Engl J Med* 348:1839–1854, 2003

Jensen SB: Sexual dysfunction in insulin-treated diabetics: a six-year follow-up study of 101 patients. *Arch Sex Behav* 15:271–283, 1986

Leedom L, Feldman M, Procci W, Zeidler A: Symptoms of sexual dysfunction and depression in diabetic women. *J Diabet Complications* 5:38–41, 1991

Schover LR, Jensen SB: *Sexuality and Chronic Illness: A Comprehensive Approach.* New York, Guilford, 1988

Schreiner-Engel P, Schiavi RC, Vietorisz D, Smith H: The differential impact of diabetes type on female sexuality. *J Psychosom Res* 31:23–33, 1987

Segraves RT, Clayton A, Croft H, Wolf A, Warnock J: Bupropion sustained release for the treatment of hypoactive sexual desire disorder in premenopausal women. *J Clin Psychopharmacol* 24:339–342, 2004

Slob AK, Koster J, Radder JK, van der Werff ten Bosch JJ: Sexuality and psychophysiological functioning in women with diabetes mellitus. *J Sex Marital Ther* 16:59–69, 1990

Spector IP, Leiblum SR, Carey MP, Rosen RC: Diabetes and female sexual function: a critical review. *Ann Behav Med* 15:257–264, 1993

Tyrer G, Steel JM, Ewing DJ, Bancroft J, Warner P, Clarke BF: Sexual responsiveness in diabetic women. *Diabetologia* 24:166–171, 1983

Wincze JP, Albert A, Bansal S: Sexual arousal in diabetic females: physiological and self-report measures. *Arch Sex Behav* 22:587–601, 1993

Dr. Lightner is an Associate Professor of Urology in the Department of Urology, the Mayo Clinic, Rochester, Minnesota. Ms. Fick is a certified physician assistant in the Department of Urology at the Mayo Clinic, Rochester, Minnesota.

48. Postural Hypotension

Italo Biaggioni, MD

Maintenance of upright posture is made possible by instantaneous cardio-vascular adaptation that depends primarily on an intact autonomic nervous system. When this system fails, as may occur in diabetic autonomic neuropathy, orthostatic hypotension ensues. The incapacitating nature of orthostatic hypotension underscores the importance of cardiovascular autonomic reflexes for normal life. The cardiovascular autonomic neuropathy seen in patients with diabetes shares common features with primary autonomic failure. Because the latter has been extensively studied, some of the recommendations in this chapter are derived from our knowledge of this condition. Nonetheless, features pertinent to diabetic autonomic neuropathy are emphasized.

PHYSIOLOGY

When a healthy nondiabetic individual stands, up to 700 ml of blood pools in the legs and lower abdominal veins. Venous return decreases, resulting in a transient decline in cardiac output. The reduction in central blood volume and arterial pressure is sensed by cardiopulmonary volume receptors and arterial baroreceptors. Afferent signals from these receptors reach vasomotor centers in the brain stem. Efferent fibers from these centers reduce parasympathetic output and increase sympathetic outflow. Norepinephrine is released from postganglionic sympathetic nerve terminals at target organs, resulting in an increase in heart rate and cardiac contractility, partial restoration of venous return and diastolic ventricular filling by venoconstriction, and an increase in peripheral resistance by arteriolar vasoconstriction. As a net effect of these adaptive mechanisms, upright cardiac output remains reduced by 10–20% compared with supine, systolic blood pressure is reduced by 5–10 mmHg, diastolic blood pressure increases by 2–5 mmHg, mean blood pressure remains almost unchanged, and heart rate increases by 5–20 beats/min.

PATHOPHYSIOLOGY

Orthostatic hypotension is defined as a sustained reduction of systolic blood pressure of at least 20 mmHg or diastolic blood pressure of 10 mmHg within 3 min of standing or head-up tilt to at least 60° on a tilt table. It is best characterized clinically if the decrease in arterial blood pressure is associated with symptoms such as lightheadedness, blurry vision, and pain in the back of the neck, finally leading to transient loss of consciousness. Symptoms never occur while supine but usually occur shortly after standing and are always relieved immediately on sitting or lying down. Failure to meet these criteria should make us rule out other causes of loss of consciousness that may occur in diabetic patients (e.g., hypoglycemia, arrhythmias, transient ischemic attacks).

DIAGNOSIS

Subclinical cardiovascular autonomic neuropathy is relatively common, but overt orthostatic hypotension usually appears as a late complication. Spectral analysis of heart rate variability appears to be very sensitive in detecting cardiac autonomic impairment, but the diagnosis of cardiovascular autonomic neuropathy also can be done easily with simple measurements of heart rate and blood pressure (Table 48.1).

Table 48.1 Assessment of Autonomic Function: Bedside Physiological Tests

Posture
- Measure BP and HR after patient has been supine 10 min and standing 3 min.
- Express as supine/standing values.
- Normal response: systolic BP = –15 to 0 mmHg, diastolic BP = –5 to 5 mmHg, HR = 0 to 20 bpm

SA ratio
- Have patient breathe deeply six times per minute while monitoring HR in a continuous strip.
- Measure longest R-R interval during expiration (R-R_{exp}) and shortest R-R interval during inspiration (R-R_{insp}). Take an average of six breaths.
- SA ratio = R-R_{exp}/R-R_{insp}.
- Normal response: ≥1.2

Valsalva ratio
- Use a 6- to 12-ml syringe barrel as the mouthpiece connected to the sphygmomanometer.
- Ask patient to blow to 40 mmHg for 15 s while monitoring HR in a continuous strip. Repeat three times. Make sure effort is barred by thorax and not mouth (e.g., by introducing a pin-sized leak in the mouthpiece).
- Measure shortest R-R during strain (R-R_{strain}) and longest R-R after release (R-$R_{release}$).
- Valsalva ratio = R-$R_{release}$/R-R_{strain}.
- Normal response: ≥1.4

Cold pressor test
- Measure baseline BP and HR. Have patient place a hand in ice water for 1 min. Measure BP and HR at the end of the minute.
- Normal response: rise in systolic BP >15 mmHg

BP, blood pressure; HR, heart rate; SA, sinus arrhythmia.

Whereas no single test completely differentiates patients with autonomic failure from age-matched control subjects, taken together, they provide a reliable indicator of the presence and severity of cardiovascular autonomic impairment. Patients with severe autonomic neuropathy lack the compensatory increase in upright heart rate and plasma norepinephrine that should accompany orthostatic hypotension. Autonomic neuropathy, however, is not always the cause of orthostatic hypotension in diabetic patients. The presence of orthostatic tachycardia usually indicates that the orthostatic hypotension may be triggered by potentially reversible factors in patients with borderline autonomic function (e.g., hypovolemia, pharmacological agents) (Table 48.2). Therefore, these autonomic function tests, or even the simple measurement of supine and upright blood pressure and heart rate, can provide important clinical information.

Two additional factors may precipitate hypotension in patients with autonomic failure. *1*) Meals lower blood pressure dramatically in patients with primary autonomic failure and therefore may provoke symptomatic postprandial orthostatic hypotension. *2*) Insulin lowers blood pressure in diabetic patients with autonomic neuropathy and has no effect in individuals without autonomic neuropathy. The frequency and magnitude of these problems may be small in most patients but may be of importance in a given patient.

PROGNOSIS

A mortality rate as high as 25% in 5 years has been reported in patients with diabetes and autonomic neuropathy. Cardiovascular autonomic neuropathy appears to be an independent risk factor for increased mortality. Patients with autonomic neuropathy frequently have other complications of diabetes, and this may also contribute to their poor prognosis. For example, these patients have silent myocardial ischemia and a prolonged QT interval, which may predispose them to sudden death.

TREATMENT

There is no proven specific therapy for preventing or reversing cardiovascular autonomic neuropathy other than tight glycemic control in type 1 diabetes. Trials involving few patients have shown a slight delay in progression of autonomic neu-

Table 48.2 Drugs that May Precipitate or Worsen Orthostatic Hypotension in Patients with Autonomic Failure

- Diuretics
- Tricyclic antidepressants
- Phenothiazides
- Venodilators (nitrates)
- α-Blockers (used for hypertension or benign prostrate hypertrophy)
- Insulin

ropathy in patients receiving experimental treatment with aldose reductase inhibitors or combined therapy with an ACE inhibitor, vitamins C and E, and aspirin. Confirmatory studies in larger patient populations are needed before such therapy can be widely recommended. Data from the Diabetes Control and Complications Trial suggest that intensive insulin therapy may delay the progression of diabetic peripheral neuropathy in type 1 diabetic patients. In type 2 diabetes, tight glycemic control prevents microvascular complications (i.e., nephropathy) but does not appear to prevent cardiovascular disease. It is not known if it prevents progression of autonomic neuropathy. Intensive insulin therapy also produced a slight improvement in results of tests of autonomic function in type 1 diabetes. However, patients with autonomic neuropathy appear to be at a greater risk of developing severe hypoglycemia during insulin treatment, and this risk should be considered before intensive therapy is recommended for them. Conversely, hypoglycemia causes transient autonomic impairment that compromises counterregulatory mechanisms, with worsening subsequent hypoglycemic episodes. It is possible that hypoglycemia-induced autonomic failure may also impair orthostatic tolerance.

In general, a stepwise approach to treatment according to the severity of the symptoms is preferable (Table 48.3). These should be considered general guidelines, and treatment should be individualized. Some recommendations may actually be contraindicated in a given patient.

Nonpharmacological Therapy

In patients with persistent symptoms, conservative nonpharmacological therapy is indicated. The aim is to eliminate aggravating factors, improve intravascular volume, and reduce orthostatic venous pooling. Medical therapy includes the following (Table 48.3):

- Train patients to avoid standing motionless or standing up quickly. Instruct them that orthostatic symptoms tend to be worse early in the

---

Table 48.3 Stepwise Approach to Management of Orthostatic Hypotension

1. Remove aggravating factors
   - Volume depletion
   - Anemia
   - Drugs*
   - Prolonged bed rest/deconditioning
   - Alcohol
2. Medical treatment
   - Liberalize salt intake, salt supplements
   - Head-up tilt during the night
   - Abdominal binder or waist-high support stockings
   - Exercise as tolerated
3. Pharmacological treatment†
   - Fludrocortisone
   - Short-acting pressor agents

*See Table 48.2; †see Table 48.4.

morning, after meals, if arms are raised above heart level, and in hot environments.

- Increase salt intake. Patients with autonomic failure may be unable to conserve sodium, and liberalization of sodium intake is generally recommended.
- Avoid supine diuresis. These patients have exaggerated nocturnal diuresis with relative hypovolemia and worsening of orthostatic hypotension early in the morning. Nocturnal diuresis can be reduced by elevating the head of the bed with 6- to 9-inch blocks.
- Decrease venous pooling. During the day, patients should wear waist-high custom-fitted elastic support stockings that will exert pressure on the legs and reduce venous pooling (some patients find them cumbersome to wear, and sensory neuropathy or vasculopathy may limit their use). Most of the venous pooling occurs in the lower abdomen, so abdominal binders can be tried first.
- Avoid wearing support stockings while supine because they may contribute to diuresis and supine hypertension.

Pharmacological Therapy

Some patients may require pharmacological therapy in addition to nonpharmacological therapy. At this stage, the goal of treatment is to minimize symptoms rather than to normalize an upright blood pressure.

- Fludrocortisone: Therapy is usually initiated with fludrocortisone acetate at a low dose (0.1 mg/day) and increased slowly to 0.3 mg/day if needed. A weight gain of 1–2 kg and mild ankle edema may be desirable in these patients. However, hypokalemia, supine hypertension, and pulmonary edema may occur, and patients must be monitored carefully. Fludrocortisone will not be effective unless it is given in conjunction with increased salt intake (e.g., sodium chloride tablets, 1 g with meals).

Table 48.4 Pharmacological Agents in Treating Orthostatic Hypotension

Drug	Initial Dose	Side Effects	Contraindications
NaCl	2 g/day	Nausea, diarrhea	
Fludrocortisone (Florinef)	0.1–0.3 mg/day	Hypokalemia, supine hypertension	Congestive heart failure
Midodrine (Proamitine)	5–10 mg*	Scalp itching, goose bumps	
Yohimbine (Yocon)	5.4 mg*	Nervousness, tremor	

Refer to more detailed sources for a complete list of side effects and contraindications. *A dose of these short-acting pressor agents, given before exertion, will improve orthostatic symptoms for 2–3 h. In general, administration of more than three doses per day is discouraged to avoid side effects and development of tolerance.

- Pressor agents: The goal in using these drugs is to provide patients with periods when they can remain upright rather than to try to keep severely afflicted patients symptom free throughout the day.

Most of the agents listed in Table 48.4, if effective in a given patient, will increase blood pressure for 2–3 h. In general, these agents are best given before periods of exertion as needed rather than at fixed (e.g., three times per day) intervals. This approach may reduce the likelihood of side effects and the development of tolerance that reduces their long-term efficacy. Patients should also avoid lying down for 4–5 h after taking these drugs to prevent supine hypertension. These drugs have negligible effects in healthy subjects; the increase in blood pressure seen in patients with autonomic failure is a reflection of their extreme hypersensitivity to most pressor and depressor agents. Therefore, treatment should be started at very small doses and should be individualized. This is best done by measuring blood pressure before and 1–2 h after administration of the first dose of each drug. Some of these agents may be contraindicated in patients with other diabetes complications. Octreotide is often recommended for the treatment of orthostatic hypotension in other conditions, but in our experience, however, its use is limited by gastrointestinal side effects in patients with diabetes.

Treatment of Related Conditions

Autonomic failure can be associated with low-production anemia and inappropriately low serum erythropoietin levels. If other causes of anemia are ruled out, patients can be treated with recombinant erythropoietin (25–50 units/kg subcutaneously three times per week). Erythropoietin has been shown to improve upright blood pressure, and its use may be warranted for this reason alone rather than as a treatment for anemia.

Many patients may also have supine hypertension resulting from preexisting essential hypertension or as part of their autonomic failure. In occasional patients, significant hypertension may be present even in the seated position. During the day, supine hypertension is best managed by simply avoiding the supine position. At night, it is often necessary to give vasodilators at bedtime, after which the patient should be advised against getting up during the night without assistance. The following agents have been used with success:

- very low doses of nitrates as transdermal preparations (e.g., 0.1–0.2 mg/h Nitro-Dur applied at bedtime and removed on arising)
- hydralazine hydrochloride (25–100 mg)
- calcium channel blockers (e.g., 30 mg nifedipine)

Patients with angina may also be difficult to manage. Nitrates and other venodilators may produce dramatic hypotension in patients with autonomic failure. Conversely, angina may be precipitated by postural hypotension and relieved by resuming the supine position. β-Blockers may be an alternative treatment in these patients if no contraindication to their use exists. Propranolol (20–60 mg/day) and pindolol (15 mg/day) will probably not worsen orthostatic hypotension and may actually improve symptoms in some patients.

BIBLIOGRAPHY

Biaggioni I: Erythropoietin in autonomic failure, In *Primer on the Autonomic Nervous System*. 2nd ed. Roberton D, Ed. San Diego, California, Elsevier Academic Press, 2004, p. 421–422

Boulton AJ, Vinik AI, Arezzo JC, et al.: Diabetic neuropathies: a statement by the American Diabetes Association. *Diabetes Care* 28:956–962, 2005

Davis SN, Mann S, Galassetti P, et al.: Effects of differing durations of antecedent hypoglycemia on counterregulatory responses to subsequent hypoglycemia in normal humans. *Diabetes* 49:1897–1903, 2000

Hoeldtke RD, Horvath GG, Bryner KD, Hobbs GR: Treatment of orthostatic hypotension with midodrine and octreotide. *J Clin Endocrinol Metab* 83:339–343, 1998

Maser RE, Mitchell BD, Vinik AI, et al.: The association between cardiovascular autonomic neuropathy and mortality in individuals with diabetes: a meta-analysis. *Diabetes Care* 26:1895–1901, 2003

Pagani M: Heart rate variability and autonomic diabetic neuropathy. *Diabetes Nutr Metab* 13:341–346, 2000

Stephenson JM, Kempler P, Perin PC, et al.: Is autonomic neuropathy a risk factor for severe hypoglycaemia? The EURODIAB IDDM Complications Study. *Diabetologia* 39:1372–1376, 1996

Vinik AI, Ziegler D: Diabetic cardiovascular autonomic neuropathy. *Circulation* 115:387–397, 2007

Wright RA, Kaufmann HC, Perera R, et al.: A double-blind, dose-response study of midodrine in neurogenic orthostatic hypotension. *Neurol* 51:120–124, 1998

Dr. Biaggioni is Professor of Medicine and Pharmacology at Vanderbilt University, Nashville, Tennessee.

49. Cardiometabolic Syndrome and the Prevention of Cardiovascular Complications

MARC-ANDRE CORNIER, MD, AND ROBERT H. ECKEL, MD

The cardiometabolic syndrome (CMS), also commonly referred to as the metabolic syndrome (MetS), is a clustering of components that reflect the status of the times, including overnutrition, sedentary lifestyles, and resultant excess adiposity. The primary purpose for identifying the CMS was to identify individuals at high risk for cardiovascular disease (CVD) that is obesity related, extending beyond traditional CVD risk factors, such as LDL cholesterol (1). The CMS includes the clustering of abdominal adiposity, insulin resistance, metabolic dyslipidemia (hypertriglyceridemia, low levels of HDL cholesterol, small dense LDL cholesterol), elevated blood pressure, prothrombotic state, and proinflammatory state (Table 49.1). Because the CMS is a cluster of different conditions, and not a single disease, a clear definition has been more difficult to develop. Nevertheless, in 2008 the CMS is an evolving concept that continues to be data driven and evidence based.

CLINICAL IMPORTANCE

Definitions

Although the MetS has become widely acknowleged since its inclusion in the National Cholesterol Education Program's Adult Treatment Panel III (NCEP ATP III) (1) guidelines of 2001, the concept of "clustering" metabolic disorders and CVD risk factors has been discussed in the scientific literature for many decades. The clinical utility of identifying people with the CMS or MetS has raised concerns from the American Diabetes Association (ADA) and other scientific groups (2,3). Overall, a combination of factors, such as improved methodologies and increased awareness of the comorbidities of cardiovascular and metabolic diseases, has led to the notion that identifying such a syndrome could be a practical clinical tool for identifying high-risk individuals. Although there are divergent criteria for the identification of the MetS, they all tend to agree that the core components include central obesity (waist circumference), insulin resistance, dyslipidemia, and hypertension (2). The CMS, though less well defined, elaborates this clustering by including other components that reflect insulin resistance and CVD and diabetes risk. In general, until more evidence accumulates that elucidates the cause of the CMS and/or MetS and their impact on CVD and type 2

Table 49.1 Components of the CMS

Central obesity
Insulin resistance
Metabolic dyslipidemia
Elevated blood pressure/hypertension
Prothrombotic state
Proinflammatory state
Nonalcoholic fatty liver disease

diabetes incidence and outcomes, these controversies are unlikely to be resolved. However, identification of the multiple components is undeniably an opportunity to encourage patients to make lifestyle changes that will attenuate their chances for CVD and metabolic disease later in life.

Epidemiology

The prevalence of the CMS as identified as the MetS has been examined closely and has been found to be increasing throughout the world. The epidemics of obesity and metabolic disease are not only relevant for the U.S. and the "urbanized" world but have also become significant problems in developing nations (4). Prevalence estimates of the MetS in the U.S. and around the world, however, are dependent on a number of different factors, including the definition that is used to determine inclusion as well as the composition of the population being studied (e.g., sex, age, race, ethnicity, and socioeconomic status). Inclusion or exclusion of type 2 diabetes in these estimates also has an important impact, as the vast majority of type 2 diabetic patients meet the minimum criteria for the CMS or MetS. Although the prevalence of obesity and CMS increases with age, the current literature supports the notion that prevalence of the clustering of metabolic risk factors in youth is also increasing and may be an important predictor of future risk for diabetes and CVD.

Pathophysiology

As previously discussed, the primary purpose of identifying the CMS was to identify a clustering of features that were associated with increased CVD risk. As the term "syndrome" implies, a specific causative etiology to the CMS is not clear, and neither was a common, unifying pathophysiological cause necessarily intended. Nevertheless, abdominal adiposity and insulin resistance appear to be at the core of the pathophysiology of the CMS and its individual components.

A proposed explanation linking increased abdominal adiposity, insulin resistance, and other comorbid conditions is a follows (5). Free fatty acids (FFAs) are released in abundance from an expanded adipose tissue mass. In the liver, FFAs result in increased production of glucose and less suppressability of hepatic glucose output by insulin. Additionally, the excess FFAs lead to increased rates of triglyceride (TG) biosynthesis and secretion of VLDLs. Associated lipid/lipoprotein abnormalities include reductions in HDL cholesterol and increased density of LDL particles. FFAs also reduce insulin sensitivity in muscle by inhibiting insulin-mediated glucose uptake. Associated defects include a reduction in glucose partitioning to glycogen and increased lipid accumulation. Elevated circulating glucose, and to some extent FFAs, increase pancreatic insulin secretion, resulting in hyperinsulinemia. Hyperinsulinemia may result in enhanced sodium reabsoption and increased sympathetic nervous system activity and contribute to hypertension, as might also increased levels of FFA.

Superimposed and contributory to the insulin resistance produced by excessive FFAs is the paracrine and endocrine effect of the proinflammatory state. Produced by a variety of cells in adipose tissue, including adipocytes and monocyte-derived macrophages, the enhanced secretion of interleukin-6 (IL-6) and tumor necrosis factor-α, among others, results in more insulin resistance and lipolysis of adipose tissue TG stores, resulting in increased circulating FFAs. IL-6 and other cytokines also are increased in the circulation and may enhance hepatic glucose production, the production of VLDL by the liver, and insulin resistance in muscle. Cytokines and FFAs also increase the production of fibrinogen and plasminogen activator inhibitor-1 (PAI-1) by the liver, complementing the overproduction of PAI-1 by adipose tissue. This results in a prothrombotic state. A reduction in the production of the anti-inflammatory and insulin-sensitizing cytokine adiponectin is also associated with obesity and insulin resistance.

Risks of the CMS

CVD. One of the primary observations regarding the clustering of metabolic disorders was the association of these features with increased CVD risk. It is well accepted and established that multiple risk factors confer greater risk than a single risk factor. In fact, the findings that led to the development of the Framingham Risk Score (FRS) are based on this observation. The NCEP ATP III emphasized that the risk for CVD can be further reduced by the modification of risk factors beyond LDL lowering (1). Thus, they identified a clustering of factors that further increase the risk for CVD. The vast majority of studies have found that patients with the CMS/MetS have more CVD and are at increased risk for developing CVD. Most studies report an increased CVD risk 1.5- to 3-fold higher when the CMS/MetS is present, and a recent meta-analysis that included 36 different reports found that the overall relative risk for incident CVD events and death for individuals with the MetS was 1.78 (95% CI; 1.58–2.00) (6). This generally holds true even in very-high-risk individuals, such as those with preexisting coronary heart disease (CHD) and diabetes. Furthermore, as one would expect, the more components or features of the CMS/MetS that are present, the greater the CVD risk. A few exceptions to these findings, however, have been noted. Whether the CVD risk in the CMS is greater than the sum of the individual risk has been debated. The Framingham experience has certainly long suggested that multiple risk factors increase CVD risk more than the sum of the individual risk factors, and a recent meta-analysis found that the risk for CVD is still increased in people with the MetS even after controlling for the component risk factors (6). Other studies, however, have shown that the risk of the CMS/MetS is not greater than the sum of its parts (7,8). It is also unclear whether identifying the CMS offers greater prediction of CVD risk than previously established risk assessments such as the FRS. It has also been argued, however, that the identification of the CMS/MetS was never intended to be used as tool for predicting CVD.

Type 2 Diabetes. The CMS/MetS has also been shown to be a strong predictor of type 2 diabetes. The presence of the CMS increases the risk and is highly predictive of new-onset type 2 diabetes. The risk for incident type 2 diabetes is up to five times higher in individuals with the CMS/MetS compared with those without the syndrome. Interestingly, the presence of both the CMS/MetS and insulin resistance has an additive effect, as these patients exhibit a six- to sevenfold increased risk for type 2 diabetes. The effect of varying definitions of insulin resistance on the risk for type 2 diabetes may be significant, because the risk for type 2 diabetes conferred by either impaired fasting glucose (IFG) or impaired glucose tolerance (IGT) is higher than that conferred by other individual components of the syndrome. Further, hyperinsulinemia, IFG, and IGT have been shown to predict the development of diabetes, independent of other components of the CMS. This has led many investigators to question whether the syndrome's ability to predict diabetes is due to a single factor (i.e., insulin resistance) or whether it represents an additive effect of multiple metabolic abnormalities. Again, it must be emphasized that the identification of the CMS was not intended to be a predictive model for type 2 diabetes progression, although it does appear to predict type 2 diabetes better than it predicts CVD.

TREATMENT

A discussion on the therapeutic options for managing the CMS must be prefaced with the understanding that there are no randomized controlled trials published to help guide specific recommendations. In addition, because it is unclear whether there is a unifying pathophysiological mechanism resulting in the CMS, it is unclear whether it can be treated in of itself. The following discussion will therefore center on treating the individual components of the CMS, with the overall goals of reducing the risk for or preventing not only CVD, but also type 2 diabetes, as outlined in Table 49.2. Nevertheless, concentrating therapeutic efforts on treating the excess adiposity and insulin resistance associated with the CMS may provide the most overall success in attaining these goals. In addition, certain therapeutic options may impact more than one component of the CMS.

Lifestyle Modification

It is well established that weight loss is beneficial for treating all of the components of the CMS, including excessive adiposity, dyslipidemia, hypertension, insulin resistance, and hyperglycemia (9), and the magnitude of weight loss need not be drastic. The Finnish Diabetes Prevention Study (10) and the Diabetes Prevention Program (DPP) (11) in the U.S. both showed that lifestyle intervention with increased physical acitivity and reduction in dietary fat/calories, resulting in modest weight loss, significantly reduced the incidence of type 2 diabetes compared with the control groups. Lifestyle intervention was also associated with significant reductions in the incidence of the CMS/MetS in the DPP. In addition, a weight loss of as small as 5–10% of body weight can significantly reduce triglycerides and increase HDL cholesterol as well as improve blood pressure, fasting blood glucose, insulin, and A1C. Notably, the DPP demonstrated that weight loss was the number one predictor of reduction in the incidence of diabetes. In fact, for every kilogram of weight loss, the risk of diabetes development was decreased by 16%.

Table 49.2 Therapy of Metabolic Risk Factors

Therapeutic Target	Goals and Recommendations
Abdominal obesity	5–10% weight loss or weight maintenance Lifestyle modification with diet and increased physical activity • Pharmacologic weight loss therapy • Bariatric surgery
Insulin resistance/ hyperglycemia	Prevention or delay of progression to type 2 diabetes • Lifestyle modification and weight loss as described above • Pharmacotherapy Treatment of diabetes • Appropriate glycemic control
Metabolic dyslipidemia	
Primary target: LDL cholesterol	LDL cholesterol lowering as per NCEP-ATP III goals (see Table 49.3)
Secondary target: Non-HDL cholesterol	If TG ≥200 mg/dl, lower non-HDL cholesterol to <30 mg/dl plus the LDL cholesterol goal and/or lower apoB to <80–90 mg/dl
Tertiary target: HDL cholesterol	If HDL cholesterol <40 mg/dl in men or <50 mg/dl in women, consider therapy for HDL cholesterol raising
Elevated blood pressure	Goal BP is <140/90 mmHg (<130/80 mmHg if diabetes or CKD present)
Prothrombotic state	Consider low-dose aspirin for high-risk patients
Proinflammatory state	No specific goals. Treat all of the above risk factors

Diet. A decrease in caloric intake is an avenue by which to promote a chronic negative energy balance resulting in weight loss. Although the macronutrient classification of the eliminated calories is of lesser importance when addressing overall energy balance, the type of macronutrients habitually consumed can influence the health of the individual with CMS. It is unclear, however, what the best diet recommendation should be for the individual patient with the CMS. Currently, most guidelines recommend a low-fat diet, which is associated with a fairly high carbohydrate intake. Due in part to the recent rise in the popularity of low-carbohydrate diets, there has been interest in the effect of carbohydrate intake on serum lipid levels. Investigations into this question have consistently reported that carbohydrate intake is positively associated with plasma TGs and negatively associated with HDL cholesterol. In addition, lower-carbohydrate diets have been associated with improved carbohydrate metabolism in those with insulin resistance and/or type 2 diabetes. Although weight loss has been shown to be greater with lower carbohydrate diets in the short term, the effects on long-term weight loss have been mixed. A diet high in complex, unrefined carbohydrates with an emphasis on fiber and low in added sugars is recommended for individuals with or at risk for the CMS. This type of diet was recommended for participants in the lifestyle intervention group of the DPP (i.e., high carbohydrate, low fat), which, as previously noted, contributed to weight loss and to a decrease in diabetes incidence.

Although the effects of total fat consumption on insulin sensitivity are variable, evidence points toward the type of fat that is consumed as having an effect on insulin sensitivity, with saturated fat associated with insulin resistance and fasting insulin levels. Because saturated fat also increases LDL cholesterol and CVD risk, it is prudent to recommend a reduction in saturated fat intake (<7% of caloric intake) and an increase in the unsaturated fatty acids, specifically linoleic (5–10% of caloric intake) and α-linolenic (0.7–1.6% of caloric intake), as is promoted by the U.S. Department of Agriculture dietary guidelines. *Trans*-fat consumption also relates to insulin resistance, CVD, and type 2 diabetes; thus the intake of *trans*-fat should be restricted to <1% of total calories. Both serum cholesterol and overall CVD risk have been shown to be improved by type of dietary fat, i.e., a reduction in saturated fat and an increase in unsaturated fat, more so than total fat intake. The Nurses' Health Study reported that a 5% increase in saturated fat intake was associated with a 17% increase in coronary risk, whereas monounsaturated and polyunsaturated fat intakes were inversely related to coronary disease. The degree of insulin resistance may also determine what macronutrient composition is most appropriate to promote weight loss.

In addition to the effects of diet on weight loss, other "diet-related" lifestyle modifications can have a significant impact on blood pressure regulation. A clear positive association has been shown between sodium intake and blood pressure, with excessive sodium intake associated with hypertension. In addition, sodium restriction has been shown to be an important strategy in the prevention and treatment of hypertension and its associated morbidities. The Dietary Approaches to Stop Hypertension (DASH) diet showed that lower sodium intake reduced blood pressure in patients with high-normal blood pressure and mild hypertension (12). Guidelines therefore recommend that daily sodium intake should be restricted to no more than 65–100 mmol. In addition to sodium restriction, increased potassium intake has also been shown to improve blood pressure, especially in the setting of high sodium intake. Guidelines have recommended the intake of foods enriched with potassium, such as fruit and vegetables, with a goal of 3.5–4.7 g (90–120 mmol) of potassium per day.

In summary, dietary intake clearly has an impact on all of the components of the CMS. Although each case should be treated individually, it is prudent to recommend a diet absent or nearly absent in *trans*-fat, low in saturated fat, higher in unsaturated fats, high in complex carbohydrates, and low in sodium.

Physical Activity. A lifestyle intervention designed to increase physical activity and decrease, or possibly maintain, body weight is another important approach for global CVD risk modification. Higher cardiorespiratory fitness and increased self-reported physical activity have been shown to be inversely related to CVD mortality and to the incidence of IGT and type 2 diabetes. Although it is difficult to separate out the effect of exercise, independent of weight loss, increased physical activity appears to reduce CVD risk and incidence of type 2 diabetes. Even in the absence of weight loss, exercise has been shown to reduce visceral adipose tissue (13). Thus, it should not be surprising that physical activity has been shown to predict the incidence of CMS or MetS in a dose-dependent manner. Physical activity and cardiorespiratory fitness likely protect against the development of the CMS through their effects on each of the individual components. Exercise is particularly effective at reducing insulin resistance and has also been shown to improve dyslipidemia and hypertension, albeit to varying degrees. Whether physical activity is accompanied by a change in body weight (particularly abdominal adiposity) is an important mediator in its ability to modify each of the components. Clinically, it may seem more difficult to elicit changes in physical activity in normally sedentary individuals than to prescribe insulin-sensitizing, antihypertensive, and lipid-lowering medications, but exercise may be the best option for addressing each of the components of the CMS concurrently without the added polypharmacy risk. This is particularly important in the pediatric population. As the incidence of obesity and the CMS continues to increase in children and adolescents, nonpharmacological therapeutic approaches will become increasingly important for preventing progression to CVD and type 2 diabetes.

Pharmacological Therapy

Excess Adiposity. Central adiposity is a core component of the CMS and may be one of the key elements in the pathophysiology responsible for the development of the CMS and its components. It therefore seems logical to aggressively target weight loss. As discussed above, lifestyle interventions resulting in modest weight loss can result in significant clinical benefits. Lifestyle modification, however, is too often met with failure and frustration. The National Institutes of Health (NIH) guidelines for the treatment of obesity recommend consideration of pharmaceutical therapy for weight loss for individuals with BMI $\geq$30 kg/m^2 or for those with BMI $\geq$27 kg/m^2 and comorbidities associated with their excess weight. The majority of patients who meet the criteria for the CMS will therefore meet the criteria for considering pharmaceutical weight-loss therapy. It is beyond the scope of this chapter to review the pharmacotherapy for weight loss, and this topic has been recently reviewed elsewhere (14). Currently, only sibutramine and orlistat are FDA approved for long-term use. Studies have shown that pharmacological therapy for weight loss results in improvements in the individual components of the CMS, including a 4-year randomized controlled study of orlistat that showed a significant reduction in the progression to diabetes in high-risk individuals. The long-term benefits of these agents in reducing CVD in those with the CMS, however, have not yet been clearly established. Nevertheless, these agents should be considered as a potential valid treatment option.

Insulin Resistance/Hyperglycemia. Insulin resistance is another core component of the CMS that potentially deserves specific attention when discussing pharmacotherapy. As discussed above, weight loss and lifestyle modification independent of weight loss can lead to clinically meaningful improvements in insulin sensitivity and should be considered the primary therapeutic options for treating insulin resistance. The difficulties and frustrations associated with weight-loss efforts and lifestyle modification have driven the demand for using pharmaceutical agents that target insulin resistance more directly. The exact role of using these agents, however, is less clear. There are now several randomized controlled trials showing that agents that target insulin resistance, such as metformin, acarbose, and the thiazolidinediones, can help prevent the progression to type 2 diabetes in individuals with impaired glucose tolerance. It must be remembered, however, that these studies have not directly targeted individuals with the CMS. It is unclear whether these agents truly prevent the progression to type 2 diabetes or simply treat glucose intolerance or mild hyperglycemia. In addition, it is unclear from these studies whether these agents improve CVD outcomes. Therefore, as with weight-loss medications, the goals for the use of agents targeting insulin resistance must be kept clear.

Dyslipidemia. The "metabolic" dyslipidemia is characterized by elevated concentrations of triglycerides, low levels of HDL cholesterol, and small, dense LDL cholesterol particles. Dyslipidemia, especially elevated LDL cholesterol, is a major modifiable risk factor for CVD, and proper management has been shown to significantly reduce CVD events and deaths. This has prompted the guidelines to recommend reaching appropriate LDL cholesterol concentrations as the primary goal. Although it is necessary to state the importance of implementing therapeutic lifestyle changes in patients with the MetS (e.g., increased physical activity and decrease in *trans-* and saturated fat and cholesterol intake), a portion of MetS patients will require drug therapy to achieve lipid goals.

The NCEP ATP III guidelines have identified elevated LDL cholesterol as the primary target of cholesterol-lowering therapy, after which other components of dyslipidemia should be addressed (1). The recent consensus statement from the ADA and the American College of Cardiology (ACC) has adopted similar goals for patients with the CMS (15). The LDL cholesterol goal is dependent on a person's absolute risk for CHD, meaning the higher the risk, the lower the goal, as outlined in Table 49.3. The majority of CMS patients will be of moderately high to high risk. The NCEP guidelines recommend that LDL cholesterol goals should be set at <130 mg/dl, with the option of targeting <100 mg/dl in moderately high-risk individuals. Target goals should be set at an LDL cholesterol <100 mg/dl in high-risk patients, with the option of aiming for <70 mg/dl in the very-high-risk patient

Table 49.3 Goals for LDL Cholesterol Lowering

Risk Category	LDL Cholesterol Goals	Recommendations
Lower risk: 0–1 major risk factor 10-year risk <10%	<160 mg/dl	Lifestyle modification Consider pharmacotherapy if LDL cholesterol ≥190 mg/dl after lifestyle modification
Moderate risk: ≥2 major risk factors 10-year risk <10%	<130 mg/dl	Lifestyle modification Consider pharmacotherapy if LDL cholesterol ≥160 mg/dl after lifestyle modification
Moderately high risk: ≥2 major risk factors 10-year risk 10–20%	<130 mg/dl Optional <100 mg/dl	Lifestyle modification Consider pharmacotherapy if LDL cholesterol ≥130 mg/dl or, optionally, ≥100 mg/dl after lifestyle modification
High risk: CHD or CHD risk equivalents*	<100 mg/dl Optional <70 mg/dl	Lifestyle modification Consider pharmacotherapy if LDL cholesterol ≥100 mg/dl or, optionally, ≥70 mg/dl after lifestyle modification

(16). The guidelines recommend setting a secondary lipid goal for non-HDL cholesterol and/or apolipoprotein (apo)B. Specifically, for individuals with TGs ≥200 mg/dl, after achieving LDL cholesterol goals, the goal should be to decrease non-HDL cholesterol (LDL cholesterol + VLDL cholesterol). The goal for the non-HDL cholesterol is 30 mg/dl greater than LDL cholesterol (1). According to the ACC/ADA, the apoB goals should be either <90 or <80 mg/dl for high-risk and highest-risk patients, respectively. A primary lipid target to reach this goal will be either further LDL cholesterol lowering or triglyceride lowering. A tertiary lipid goal should be for HDL cholesterol. Although the NCEP ATP III guidelines classify low HDL cholesterol as <40 mg/dl in both men and women, there is no specific target goal for HDL cholesterol because there is insufficient evidence to specify a therapy goal. Similarly, as the guidelines classify hypertriglyceridemia as TG concentrations ≥150 mg/dl, no specific TG goals have been set.

As LDL cholesterol lowering is the primary treatment goal of metabolic dyslipidemia, the use of LDL cholesterol–lowering agents, such as the hydroxymethylglutaryl (HMG)-CoA reductase inhibitors or statins, have become the standard first-line therapy. Due to their minimal drug-drug interactions and side effects, statins are considered to be the most effective and powerful class of drugs for reducing LDL cholesterol concentrations. Non–lipid-lowering or pleiotropic effects of statins have also been implicated in their beneficial effects on inflammation, endothelial function, and CVD events. Statins are highly effective in decreasing CVD mortality and morbidity, but despite the number of primary and secondary prevention trials showing benefits in reducing CVD outcomes with statin therapy, there are no published trials to date that have specifically targeted patients with the CMS. Other LDL cholesterol–lowering agents, such as bile acid sequestrants and cholesterol absorption inhibitors, lower LDL cholesterol more moderately than statins but may be considered for monotherapy in "statin-intolerant" patients or in combination with a statin for more aggressive LDL cholesterol lowering. Secondary lipid targets can be targeted with fibrates, niacin, and/or ω-3 polyunsaturated fatty acids; however, no clinical trials to date have compared statins against the combination of statins plus these other agents on CVD outcomes. The potential benefits of combining these agents must be weighed against the increased risks and costs.

Elevated Blood Pressure/Hypertension. Management of elevated blood pressure and hypertension is another key target in CVD risk reduction in the MetS patient, although there are no clear guidelines for blood pressure management specific to this population. The Seventh Report of the Joint National Committee on Prevention, Detection, Evaluation, and Treatment of High Blood Pressure has recommended that the goal blood pressure in those without diabetes or chronic kidney disease (CKD) should be <140/90 mmHg and <130/80 mmHg for those with diabetes or CKD (17). As with management of dyslipidemia, the primary therapeutic intervention for blood pressure management should be lifestyle modification, as discussed above, but many patients will require pharmacological therapy to reach blood pressure goals. It has been proposed that ACE inhibitors or angiotensin receptor blockers should be the first-line classes of agents in the CMS, especially in the setting of diabetes or CKD. Certainly, these classes of agents have been shown to be effective in reducing the incidence of albuminuria or progression of nephropathy in patients with diabetes. Other classes of antihypertensive therapies, such as thiazide-type diuretics and β-blockers, have also shown benefit. The majority of patients who need antihypertensive therapy will likely need more than one agent for proper blood pressure control.

Prothrombotic State. The CMS is associated with elevated levels of coagulation factors such as fibrinogen and PAI-1. Although low-dose aspirin is frequently recommended to patients with CMS, there are no specific studies of the use of aspirin or other antiplatelet agents for the primary prevention of CVD in individuals with the CMS specifically. Long-term use of aspirin therapy has been advocated in the secondary prevention of CVD, and some have recommended aspirin in high-risk patients with the CMS, especially those with CVD. Until there are more data, however, the use of aspirin in the primary prevention of CVD should remain as an "individual clinical judgment."

Proinflammatory State. The CMS is associated with elevated markers of inflammation. Elevated levels of C-reactive protein (CRP), a systemic marker of inflammation, have been shown to be associated with greater risk for CVD in patients with CMS. There are, however, no currently recommended direct therapies targeting inflammation. Lifestyle modification and weight loss results in reduced CRP concentrations, as does the treatment of the other associated comorbidities, such as dyslipidemia, elevated blood pressure, and insulin resistance/hyperglycemia.

Bariatric Surgery

Perhaps the most promising treatment of multiple risk factors within the CMS in the context of severe obesity lies in bariatric surgery. Multiple guidelines for the treatment of obesity recommend consideration of bariatric surgery for weight loss for individuals with BMI ≥40 kg/m² or for those with BMI ≥35 kg/m² and comorbidities associated with their excess weight. Many patients who meet the criteria for the CMS will therefore meet the criteria for considering bariatric surgery. These surgical procedures can be divided into three categories: malabsorptive, including biliopancreatic diversion and duodenal switch; restrictive, including vertical banded gastroplasty and the laparoscopic adjustable gastric band; and combination procedures, the gold standard of which is the Roux-en-Y gastric bypass. Titles in the literature reflect optimism about its role in resolving many health risk factors and in attenuating at least a portion of the epidemics of obesity, diabetes, and perhaps the CMS. Bariatric surgery has been found to be associated with not only reduced mortality, but also with the improvement and resolution of multiple comorbidities associated with obesity, including hypertension, diabetes, nonalcoholic fatty liver disease, obstructive sleep apnea, cardiopulmonary failure, CVD, arthritis, polycystic ovary syndrome, dyslipidemia, hyperuricemia, and infertility. Thus, bariatric surgery appears to be beneficial on many levels in treating numerous risk factors of the CMS in obese patients who qualify for the surgery and should be considered as a valid treatment option for the CMS patient.

UNANSWERED QUESTIONS

Despite the great interest in the CMS, many unanswered questions remain. There has been much debate and controversy over whether there is a unifying pathogenesis of the CMS. Although abdominal adiposity and insulin resistance appear to be at the core of the development of the CMS, it is still not clear whether all of the components are directly related to these conditions. How should the CMS be best defined is another important question that deserves considerable attention. As is evident from the number of different definitions proposed by different groups, there is not a consensus on how to best define the CMS. This issue is important to resolve for a number of different reasons. Without a consensus definition, it is difficult to perform research on the CMS, and this creates confusion for the clinicians. Should a marker for the prothrombotic state or inflammation be added? In addition, whatever the components, should they all be considered equal in their importance or risk prediction? This is reflected by some definitions requiring some, but not all, components to be present. In addition, whether the CMS should reflect more of a continuum of risk as opposed to a "present" or "absent" situation has also been debated. How should the CMS be best treated? Beyond favorable lifestyle modification, most would agree that treating each of the individual components of the CMS is important. It is less clear, however, what the goals of treatment for the individual components should be for individuals with the CMS. For example, should lipid or blood pressure goals be treated more aggressively than IGT in those with the CMS? It is also unclear whether targeting a more unifying pathophysiological process, such as abdominal adiposity or insulin resistance, should be recommended at this time.

SUMMARY AND CONCLUSIONS

The CMS is a clustering of components or risk factors associated with an increased risk for CVD and type 2 diabetes. A consensus definition of the CMS has been difficult to develop but is an important consideration for the groups involved and continues to be a "work in progress." Although the prevalence of the CMS depends on the definition used and population studied, it has been clearly increasing globally. The CMS is not exclusive to adults. In fact, the prevalence of the CMS in younger populations is increasing in parallel with childhood obesity. This will likely be associated with increased risk for CVD and type 2 diabetes in adulthood. Although not intended to be a risk predictor, most studies show that the CMS is associated with a ~1.5-fold increased CVD risk. The risk for incident type 2 diabetes is more than five times higher in individuals with the CMS compared with those without the syndrome. In addition, the CMS is associated with a number of other comorbidities, such as nonalcoholic fatty liver disease, sleep disorders, reproductive tract disorders, and microvascular disease.

There are no specific guidelines for the treatment of the CMS and/or its components. In addition, because it is unclear whether there is a unifying pathophysiological mechanism resulting in the CMS, it is unclear whether the CMS can be treated in and of itself. Lifestyle modification and weight loss should be at the core of treating or preventing the CMS and its components. It is well established that weight loss with diet and physical activity is beneficial for treating all of the components, including excessive adiposity, dyslipidemia, hypertension, insulin resistance, and hyperglycemia. In addition, there is some consensus on treating the individual components of the CMS with the overall goals of reducing the risk for or preventing CVD and type 2 diabetes. Nevertheless, concentrating therapeutic efforts on treating the excess adiposity and insulin resistance associated with the CMS may provide the most overall success in attaining these goals. In addition, pharmacotherapy and surgery for weight loss also have an important role. Pharmacotherapy targeting a number of the components of the CMS, in addition to aggressive management of LDL cholesterol and therapy for the prothrombotic state, has also been generally accepted as appropriate management of these high-risk patients. There is more controversy over pharmacotherapy targeting insulin resistance and hyperglycemia. Although insulin resistance appears to be a core component of the CMS, the exact role of using agents such as metformin or thiazolidinediones is less clear. Finally, a number of unanswered questions regarding the CMS remain, including questions regarding the definition, pathogenesis, and treatment of the CMS.

BIBLIOGRAPHY

1. Expert Panel on Detection, Evaluation, and Treatment of High Blood Cholesterol in Adults: Executive Summary of the Third Report of The National Cholesterol Education Program (NCEP) Expert Panel on Detection, Evaluation, and Treatment of High Blood Cholesterol in Adults (Adult Treatment Panel III). *JAMA* 285:2486–2497, 2001

2. Alberti KG, Zimmet P, Shaw J: Metabolic syndrome--a new world-wide definition: a consensus statement from the International Diabetes Federation. *Diabet Med* 23:469–480, 2006

3. Kahn R, Buse J, Ferrannini E, Stern M: The metabolic syndrome: time for a critical appraisal: joint statement from the American Diabetes Association and the European Association for the Study of Diabetes. *Diabetes Care* 28:2289–2304, 2005

4. Grundy SM: Metabolic syndrome pandemic. *Arterioscler Thromb Vasc Biol* 28:629–636, 2008

5. Eckel RH, Grundy SM, Zimmet PZ: The metabolic syndrome. *Lancet* 365:1415–1428, 2005

6. Gami AS, Witt BJ, Howard DE, Erwin PJ, Gami LA, Somers VK, Montori VM: Metabolic syndrome and risk of incident cardiovascular events and death: a systematic review and meta-analysis of longitudinal studies. *J Am Coll Cardiol* 49:403–414, 2007

7. McNeill AM, Rosamond WD, Girman CJ, Golden SH, Schmidt MI, East HE, Ballantyne CM, Heiss G: The metabolic syndrome and 11-year risk of incident cardiovascular disease in the Atherosclerosis Risk in Communities study. *Diabetes Care* 28:385–390, 2005

8. Dekker JM, Girman C, Rhodes T, Nijpels G, Stehouwer CD, Bouter LM, Heine RJ: Metabolic syndrome and 10-year cardiovascular disease risk in the Hoorn Study. *Circulation* 112:666–673, 2005

9. Pasanisi F, Contaldo F, de Simone G, Mancini M: Benefits of sustained moderate weight loss in obesity. *Nutr Metab Cardiovasc Dis* 11:401–406, 2001

10. Ilanne-Parikka P, Eriksson JG, Lindstrom J, Hamalainen H, Keinanen-Kiukaanniemi S, Laakso M, Louheranta A, Mannelin M, Rastas M, Salminen V, Aunola S, Sundvall J, Valle T, Lahtela J, Uusitupa M, Tuomilehto J: Prevalence of the metabolic syndrome and its components: findings from a Finnish general population sample and the Diabetes Prevention Study cohort. *Diabetes Care* 27:2135–2140, 2004

11. Knowler WC, Barrett-Connor E, Fowler SE, Hamman RF, Lachin JM, Walker EA, Nathan DM: Reduction in the incidence of type 2 diabetes with lifestyle intervention or metformin. *N Engl J Med* 346:393–403, 2002

12. Sacks FM, Svetkey LP, Vollmer WM, Appel LJ, Bray GA, Harsha D, Obarzanek E, Conlin PR, Miller ER 3rd, Simons-Morton DG, Karanja N, Lin PH: Effects on blood pressure of reduced dietary sodium and the Dietary Approaches to Stop Hypertension (DASH) diet: DASH-Sodium Collaborative Research Group. *N Engl J Med* 344:3–10, 2001

13. Ohkawara K, Tanaka S, Miyachi M, Ishikawa-Takata K, Tabata I: A dose-response relation between aerobic exercise and visceral fat reduction: systematic review of clinical trials. *Int J Obes (Lond)* 31:1786–1797, 2007

14. Eckel RH: Clinical practice: nonsurgical management of obesity in adults. *N Engl J Med* 358:1941–1950, 2008

15. Brunzell JD, Davidson M, Furberg CD, Goldberg RB, Howard BV, Stein JH, Witztum JL: Lipoprotein management in patients with cardiometabolic risk: consensus statement from the American Diabetes Association and the American College of Cardiology Foundation. *Diabetes Care* 31:811–822, 2008

16. Grundy SM, Cleeman JI, Merz CN, Brewer HB Jr, Clark LT, Hunninghake DB, Pasternak RC, Smith SC Jr, Stone NJ: Implications of recent clinical trials for the National Cholesterol Education Program Adult Treatment Panel III guidelines. *Circulation* 110:227–239, 2004

17. Chobanian AV, Bakris GL, Black HR, Cushman WC, Green LA, Izzo JL Jr, Jones DW, Materson BJ, Oparil S, Wright JT Jr, Roccella EJ: The Seventh Report of the Joint National Committee on Prevention, Detection, Evaluation, and Treatment of High Blood Pressure: the JNC 7 report. *JAMA* 289:2560–2572, 2003

Drs. Cornier and Eckel are from the Division of Endocrinology, Metabolism, and Diabetes, University of Colorado Denver, Aurora, Colorado.

50. Primary and Secondary Prevention: Lipid Outcome Studies in Diabetes

CRAIG WILLIAMS, PHARMD, AND STEVEN HAFFNER, MD

DIABETES AND CORONARY HEART DISEASE: EXTENT OF DISEASE

Type 2 diabetes is associated with a two- to fourfold increased risk of cardiovascular disease. In addition, diabetic patients have an increased rate of mortality after a myocardial infarction. In the general population, the incidence of coronary heart disease (CHD) in diabetic subjects without preexisting cardiovascular disease is similar to the incidence of cardiovascular disease in nondiabetic subjects with previous cardiovascular disease. Nevertheless, there is heterogeneity of risk for CHD among subjects with diabetes. Traditional risk factors such as smoking and hypertension remain important determinants of CHD risk in this population. Duration of diabetes is also a strong risk factor. Thus, newly discovered diabetic individuals without other traditional risk factors do not have the same CHD risk as individuals with long-standing diabetes or multiple comorbidities. In the U.K. Prospective Diabetes Study (UKPDS) 23, the baseline predictors of cardiovascular disease in order of entry into a Cox proportional hazards model were as follows: *1)* LDL cholesterol, *2)* low HDL cholesterol, *3)* A1C, *4)* systolic blood pressure, and *5)* cigarette smoking.

LIPOPROTEINS IN TYPE 2 DIABETES AND CLINICAL TRIALS

In the normal hepatocyte, insulin stimulates the production of fatty acids and the degradation of apolipoprotein B100 (apoB). ApoB is the primary protein constituent of VLDL, intermediate-density lipoprotein, and LDL. Because hepatocytes do not develop resistance to insulin-stimulated fatty acid production, the higher circulating insulin levels in type 2 diabetes results in an increased hepatic production in fatty acids. This occurs simultaneously with an increase in apoB secretion due to the loss of insulin-stimulated intracellular degradation of apoB. These changes, along with the increased secretion of fatty acids from adipocytes, substantially contribute to the alterations in the lipid profile that are seen in patients with type 2 diabetes.

Compared with nondiabetic subjects, patients with diabetes have higher triglyceride (TG) levels, lower HDL cholesterol, and higher apoB but a relatively "normal" LDL cholesterol. Based on that observation of relatively normal LDL cholesterol levels but higher TG and lower HDL cholesterol, focus in the past had been on fibrate and niacin therapy for diabetic dyslipidemia. Indeed, gemfibrozil has been shown to reduce CHD in diabetic subjects in the Helsinki Heart Study and the Veterans Affairs High-Density Lipoprotein Cholesterol Intervention Trial (VA-HIT), and fenofibrate reduced CHD in the newer Fenofibrate Intervention and Event Lowering in Diabetes (FIELD) trial. Niacin reduced CHD in patients with elevated fasting blood glucose in the 3,908-patient Coronary Drug Project trial, and an impressive reduction in events was seen with niacin plus simvastatin in the HDL-Atherosclerosis Treatment Study (HATS), but that study was small and did not include a group on simvastatin monotherapy for comparison. The transition from the view of fibric acid or niacin as initial therapy to the current approach of statin-based LDL lowering as initial therapy came from analyses of newer trials coupled with an increased understanding of the role of the different lipoproteins in the pathogenesis of diabetic vascular disease.

The lipoprotein changes described above result in a larger number of small LDL particles in the patient with diabetic dyslipidemia. Although TG is elevated and HDL cholesterol is reduced, it is unclear what etiologic role these changes play in the macrovascular disease characterized by type 2 diabetes. Because dyslipidemia is uncommon in type 1 diabetes, the increased macrovascular risk seen in these patients suggests a susceptibility of the diabetic arterial wall to circulating LDL particles independent of alterations in TG or HDL. Indeed, pharmacological therapy aimed at raising HDL cholesterol by inhibiting the cholesteryl ester transfer protein enzyme not only failed to reduce clinical events in the 15,067-patient ILLUMINATE trial but actually increased the combined end point of nonfatal myocardial infarction and cardiovascular death by 20%. In that trial, 45% of participants had diabetes at baseline. The outcome of ILLUMINATE illustrates how much we still have to learn about the function of HDL particles before we widely adopt HDL cholesterol as a target of therapy. Conversely, analyses of LDL cholesterol–lowering trials have revealed a disproportionately greater benefit from LDL cholesterol lowering in diabetic patients with low HDL cholesterol and high TG. When analyzed by presence of diabetes, diabetic patients have greater benefit from the same degree of LDL cholesterol–lowering therapy compared with nondiabetic patients (Table 50.1). Additionally, higher-risk diabetic subjects (i.e., longer duration of diabetes, preexisting cardiovascular disease, older age, etc.) have greater benefit from LDL cholesterol lowering compared with lower-risk diabetic subjects (Table 50.1).

In support of this clinical approach of lowering LDL cholesterol first was the finding in the FIELD trial of a substantially greater benefit of statins as compared to fenofibrate to reduce CHD end points in patients with diabetes. FIELD was designed as a placebo-controlled study of fenofibrate in 9,795 patients with diabetes. Because the trial design allowed for use of non-study lipid-lowering therapy, there was a relatively high rate of statin drop-in (nearly 40% of placebo patients by study end). Because fenofibrate modestly lowers LDL cholesterol (12% in trial), there was a lower drop-in rate of statin usage in the patients randomized to fenofibrate (~20%). Although this difference in the use of statins complicated the analysis of the trial, it allowed the authors to analyze outcomes for patients receiving statin therapy compared to fenofibrate. It was subsequently reported that fenofibrate lowered CHD events by 19% compared to a 49% reduction for statins.

Table 50.1 Reduction in 10-Year Risk of Major Cardiovascular Disease End Points (CHD Death/Nonfatal Myocardial Infarction) in Major Statin Trials, or Substudies of Major Trials, in Diabetic Subjects (*n* = 16,032)

Study	CVD prevention	Statin dose and comparator	Risk reduction (%)	Relative risk reduction (%)	Absolute risk reduction (%)	LDL cholesterol reduction
4S-DM	2°	Simvastatin 20–40 mg vs. placebo	85.7 to 43.2	50	42.5	186 to 119 mg/dl (36%)
ASPEN 2°	2°	Atorvastatin 10 mg vs. placebo	39.5 to 24.5	34	12.7	112 to 79 mg/dl (29%)
HPS-DM	2°	Simvastatin 40 mg vs. placebo	43.8 to 36.3	17	7.5	123 to 84 mg/dl (31%)
CARE-DM	2°	Pravastatin 40 mg vs. placebo	40.8 to 35.4	13	5.4	136 to 99 mg/dl (27%)
TNT-DM	2°	Atorvastatin 80 mg vs. 10 mg	26.3 to 21.6	18	4.7	99 to 77 mg/dl (22%)
HPS-DM	1°	Simvastatin 40 mg vs. placebo	17.5 to 11.5	34	6.0	124 to 86 mg/dl (31%)
CARDS	1°	Atorvastatin 10 mg vs. placebo	11.5 to 7.5	35	4	118 to 71 mg/dl (40%)
ASPEN	1°	Atorvastatin 10 mg vs. placebo	9.8 to 7.9	19	1.9	114 to 80 mg/dl (30%)
ASCOT-DM	1°	Atorvastatin 10 mg vs. placebo	11.1 to 10.2	8	0.9	125 to 82 mg/dl (34%)

Studies were of differing lengths (3.3–5.4 years) and used somewhat different outcomes, but all reported rates of cardiovascular disease death and nonfatal myocardial infarction. In this tabulation, results of the statin on 10-year risk of major cardiovascular disease end points (CHD death/nonfatal myocardial infarction) are listed for comparison between studies. Correlation between 10-year cardiovascular disease risk of the control group and the absolute risk reduction with statin therapy is highly significant (*P* = 0.0007). Analyses provided by Craig Williams, PharmD, Oregon Health & Science University, 2007. From American Diabetes Association (2009).

This finding from FIELD, along with the LDL cholesterol–lowering trials, complements the understanding of atherosclerosis as a disease of apoB lipoprotein retention and inflammation in the vascular wall. Although TG-rich VLDL remnant lipoproteins are elevated in diabetes and do contribute to atherosclerosis, the increased LDL particle count and mildly elevated LDL cholesterol in diabetic dyslipidemia remains the proven target of pharmacological therapy. Whether therapy aimed at lowering TG and raising HDL cholesterol with fibrates or niacin will provide additional benefit when added to statin-based LDL lowering remains to be proven and is being tested in the ongoing Action to Control Cardiovascular Risk in Diabetes (ACCORD) and AIM-HIGH trials. Additional LDL cholesterol lowering with ezetimibe added to statins is being tested in the ongoing IMPROVE-IT trial.

CURRENT AMERICAN DIABETES ASSOCIATION AND NATIONAL CHOLESTEROL EDUCATION PROGRAM GUIDELINES

The American Diabetes Association (ADA) focuses as a matter of priority on LDL cholesterol, followed by HDL cholesterol and TG levels (Table 50.2). This order of priorities was initially based on observational data from the UKPDS and is now supported by the newer trial data just discussed. The secondary goals for the ADA and the National Cholesterol Education Program (NCEP) guidelines are slightly different.

In the NCEP guidelines, if subjects have a TG level >200 mg/dl after meeting LDL cholesterol goals, the secondary goal is non-HDL cholesterol (total cholesterol minus HDL cholesterol), which is 30 mg/dl above the LDL cholesterol goal. Conversely, the ADA guidelines state that while TG <150 mg/dl and HDL cholesterol >40 mg/dl (>50 mg/dl in women) is desirable, the only lipoprotein target for pharmacological therapy is LDL cholesterol. Rather than focus on establishing a secondary lipoprotein goal, the ADA guidelines discuss the option of adding niacin or a fibrate once LDL cholesterol is at goal with a statin. This approach has

---

Table 50.2 Primary Goal and Priorities of Treatment from NCEP and ADA Guidelines

ADA

Primary goal: Lifestyle modification for all patients with diabetes and metabolic syndrome. Statin-based therapy for 1) all patients with diabetes and CVD or 2) those with diabetes aged >40 years with one additional cardiac risk factor.*

First priority: Relative LDL cholesterol reduction ~40% from pretreatment baseline. Absolute LDL cholesterol goal <100 mg/dl in all patients and <70 mg/dl in diabetic patients with CVD.

Second priority: Fibrate or niacin combination therapy can be considered in patients with high TG (>150 mg/dl) and/or low HDL cholesterol (<40 mg/dl in men and <50 mg/dl in women).

NCEP

Primary goal: Lifestyle modification for all patients with diabetes and metabolic syndrome. LDL cholesterol–lowering therapy, with statin-based regimen for all patients with diabetes aged >20 years.

First priority: Achieve absolute LDL cholesterol <100 mg/dl in all patients with diabetes and <70 mg/dl in diabetic patients with CVD.

Second priority: After LDL cholesterol goal is reached, consider intensification of pharmacotherapy† in patients with TG >200 mg/dl to reach a non-HDL cholesterol goal (total cholesterol minus HDL cholesterol), which is 30 mg/dl above the LDL cholesterol goal (e.g., if LDL cholesterol goal is <70 mg/dl, then non-HDL cholesterol goal is <100 mg/dl).

---

*Includes 1) cigarette smoking, 2) hypertension (blood pressure ≥140/90 mmHg), 3) family history of premature cardiovascular disease (primary cardiac event in first-degree male relative <55 years of age or first-degree female relative <65 years of age), and 4) age (men aged ≥45 years, women aged ≥55 years). †Intensification of pharmacotherapy can include fibrate or niacin therapy or greater LDL cholesterol lowering to reach non-HDL cholesterol goal. Data from NCEP (Grundy et al. 2004) and ADA (2009).

the strength of using agents that have proven outcomes benefit in monotherapy trials, but, as clearly stated by the ADA, adding these agents in addition to LDL cholesterol–lowering therapy has not yet been proven to further reduce CHD.

Although the ADA and NCEP present slightly different secondary approaches, they agree on the primary approach of lowering LDL cholesterol. Consistent with that approach and the finding of increased benefit of LDL cholesterol lowering in higher-risk patients (Table 50.1), both the ADA and NCEP agree that in patients with diabetes and CHD, the goal LDL cholesterol is <70 mg/dl. It is worth noting that in the diabetic subanalysis of the Scandinavian Simvastatin Survival Study (4S; a study with high baseline LDL cholesterol), the patients who received placebo had a 10-year Framingham CHD event rate of nearly 90% (Table 50.1).

Initiation of statin therapy in patients with diabetes and CHD should be irrespective of baseline LDL cholesterol, with a goal LDL cholesterol reduction of 40% from baseline as well as <70 mg/dl. There is a broader range of options for diabetic subjects without CHD if baseline LDL cholesterol is not elevated. In the NCEP guidelines, if LDL cholesterol is already <100 mg/dl, then additional lowering is optional. The ADA guidelines on this topic were greatly informed by the findings of the Heart Protection Study (HPS) from 2002.

In HPS, the 5,963 diabetic subjects benefited from LDL cholesterol lowering with 40 mg simvastatin regardless of baseline LDL cholesterol. Patients with baseline LDL cholesterol <100 mg/dl (and even <80 mg/dl) experienced similar relative reductions in CHD events as patients with elevated baseline LDL cholesterol. A degree of caution is warranted in applying these findings to primary prevention in diabetic subjects because 50% of the diabetic patients in HPS had CHD at study entry. However, on post hoc analysis, the diabetic subjects without baseline CHD experienced a similar absolute risk reduction in CHD events compared with the diabetic subjects with baseline CHD. This finding underlies the recommendation from ADA that statin therapy should be added to lifestyle therapy for any diabetic patient aged >40 years irrespective of baseline LDL cholesterol. This recommendation is supported by more recent studies in diabetic subjects, including the Treating to New Targets (TNT) study and Collaborative Atorvastatin Diabetes Study (CARDS).

COMBINATION THERAPY

The current recommendation of the ADA acknowledges the potential benefit of combination therapy but does not make definitive recommendations about its use. This is because of the absence of evidence-based medicine from clinical trials as well as safety concerns, particularly about adding fibrate therapy to statin therapy. Currently, no clinical outcomes trials have been completed on diabetic subjects using a combination of statin and fibric acid or statin and nicotinic acid. The HATS regression trial data, which report on subjects with familial combined hyperlipidemia (Brown et al. 2001), suggest that low-dose simvastatin (10–20 mg) plus high-dose nicotinic acid (3–4 g/day) reduced CHD by ~80% and slowed progression of atherosclerosis in a small group of 150 patients. Both subjects with diabetes and subjects with the metabolic syndrome were included in this population. More definitive information on combination therapy may come from the

ACCORD trial, in which ~5,000 subjects with type 2 diabetes who are being treated with 20 mg simvastatin are then being randomized to placebo or 200 mg micronized fenofibrate.

Traditionally, providers have been concerned about the use of combination therapy because of the increased risk of myositis and rhabdomyolysis. However, the risk of rhabdomyolysis with nicotinic acid in combination with statins is very low. The risk with fibrates is higher and was highlighted by the increased mortality seen in subjects on gemfibrozil and cervistatin (Baycol) before cerivastatin was removed from the worldwide market. Due to differences in metabolism, the risk of combination therapy is higher when gemfibrozil is added to a statin compared to other fibrates. However, a component of the risk of statin plus fibrate is pharmacodynamic and is unrelated to kinetics and metabolism. Therefore, any fibrate added to any statin carries a greater risk of rhabdomyolysis compared to statin monotherapy. Of note, fibrate monotherapy causes rhabdomyolysis about six times as commonly as statin monotherapy. Other clinical factors that increase risk and should be considered before this combination is used include renal dysfunction and hypothyroidism. Additional concerns with nicotinic acid relate to its possible effect on insulin resistance and increasing glucose intolerance. Older studies have suggested marked rises in A1C in subjects treated with 4 g nicotinic acid per day. However, more recent studies with smaller doses of nicotinic acid and careful attention to monitoring glycemic control have shown much smaller effects on A1C. Additionally, a reanalysis of the original Lipid Research Clinics study found that the benefit of niacin was actually greater in patients with an elevated fasting glucose at baseline. Therefore, it is likely that patients with diabetes or impaired fasting glucose derive disproportionately greater CHD benefit from niacin, despite a small worsening of glycemic control in some individuals.

THE METABOLIC SYNDROME AND ApoB

According to the National Health and Nutrition Examination Survey (NHANES) dataset, there are ~60% more patients in the U.S. with metabolic syndrome than with diabetes. The use of the term "metabolic syndrome" has recently been controversial due to disagreements over both its definition and etiology. The term describes the clustering of cardiovascular risk factors (hypertension, glucose intolerance, and dyslipidemia) that often accompany obesity. Many patients who are medically obese (BMI >30 kg/m^2), however, do not have the metabolic syndrome. This individual discordance, despite the strong population association, underlies the ongoing controversy regarding the appropriate clinical use of the term. It is worth noting that in 2007, the World Health Organization (WHO) declined to recognize the metabolic syndrome as a distinct clinical entity in their 10th revision of the International Classification of Diseases (ICD-10) manual, despite offering criteria for its definition in 1999. Despite this, and despite the controversy, the term "metabolic syndrome" does provide a meaningful context for both the clinician and the patient regarding the global cardiometabolic risk that is often found in obese subjects with or without diabetes.

The NCEP III Adult Treatment Panel defines the metabolic syndrome as the presence of three of five risk factors, including waist circumference, high TG, low

HDL cholesterol, hypertension, and a fasting glucose ≥110 mg/dl (Table 50.3). The prevalence of the metabolic syndrome in subjects with type 2 diabetes has been examined in several populations and appears to be ~80%. Although it is possible that the remaining diabetic subjects without the metabolic syndrome are at lower risk of CHD, this aspect requires further study, and the substantial risk of CHD in type 1 diabetes is a reminder that obesity does not have to be present for diabetes to pose a substantial CHD risk. The CHD risk of type 1 diabetes was recently and nicely reviewed by Retnakaran et al. (2008).

The NCEP nicely discusses that the primary therapy for metabolic syndrome is behavioral (i.e., weight loss and increased physical activity). As recently shown by Jensen et al. (2008), obesity carries increased CHD risk independent of other lifestyle factors, including poor diet and smoking. Although aggressive targeting of lipids in obese patients without the metabolic syndrome is not currently advocated, the risk of CHD is clearly elevated in nondiabetic subjects with the metabolic syndrome. Although the ADA Standards of Medical Care has recommendations for the treatment of impaired glucose tolerance (IGT) to prevent diabetes, it does not use the term "metabolic syndrome" or discuss pharmacological interventions for CHD risk reduction in patients with IGT. However, in 2007 the ADA, in association with the American College of Cardiology (ACC), convened a consensus development conference to address lipoprotein management in patients with insulin resistance and multiple cardiometabolic risk factors (hyperglycemia, dyslipidemia, and hypertension). Although the term "metabolic syndrome" is not used in the document, the population being discussed is the same. The resulting consensus statement, published in 2008, appropriately reiterates LDL as the primary lipoprotein driving the development of atherosclerosis in this insulin-resistant population. The treatment targets are less clear cut.

Consistent with the NCEP update from 2004, the statement calls for a goal LDL cholesterol <70 mg/dl in diabetic patients with CHD. However, in those with cardiometabolic risk factors but without diabetes, they call for an LDL cholesterol goal of <100 mg/dl as long as two out of the three following risk fac-

Table 50.3 NCEP ATP III: the Metabolic Syndrome*

Risk Factor	Defining Level
Abdominal obesity (waist circumference)	
Men	>102 cm (>40 inches)
Women	>88 cm (>35 inches)
Triglycerides	≥150 mg/dl
HDL cholesterol	
Men	<40 mg/dl
Women	<50 mg/dl
Blood pressure	≥130/85 mmHg
Fasting glucose	≥110 mg/dl

*Diagnosis is established when three or more of these risk factors are present. From the Expert Panel on Detection, Evaluation, and Treatment of High Blood Cholesterol in Adults (2001).

tors are present: smoking, hypertension, or early family history of CHD (Table 50.4).

In addition, while the statement appropriately identifies non-HDL cholesterol as a target of therapy, it also introduces apoB as a goal of therapy and fails to identify any of those three targets (LDL cholesterol, non-HDL cholesterol, and apoB) as a primary goal of therapy (Table 50.4). Although apoB makes sense as a potential goal of therapy in patients with diabetes or the metabolic syndrome, it has yet to be used as a primary treatment target in a large outcomes trial. When the available outcomes studies with LDL cholesterol–lowering therapy are examined post hoc, the results for the predictability of apoB compared to LDL cholesterol and non-HDL cholesterol are mixed. The largest of those analyses, by Kastelein et al. (2008), analyzed the Incremental Decrease in End Points through Aggressive Lipid Lowering (IDEAL) and TNT trials together for a total of 18,889 patients and concluded that non-HDL cholesterol and apoB were similarly predictive for CHD event reduction. Approximately 15% of the patients in those trials had diabetes, with an unknown but certainly higher percentage having the metabolic syndrome.

The larger issue with using apoB as a secondary target is the question of what to do with the patient who is at their LDL cholesterol goal but not at their apoB goal. Although an elevated apoB could offer the opportunity to reinforce lifestyle counseling, the questions surrounding the role of combination lipid therapy that were previously discussed leave open the question of what therapeutic approach to take to lower apoB when LDL cholesterol is already appropriately at goal. It is also not clear how often apoB would be found to be elevated if diabetic patients are strictly complying with the newer LDL cholesterol goals of <70 mg/dl and <100 mg/dl. Unpublished data from one of the authors (C. Williams) suggests that number to be ~1 in 20 in patients with an LDL cholesterol goal of <70 mg/dl.

Table 50.4 Suggested Treatment Goals in Patients with Cardiometabolic Risk Factors and Lipoprotein Abnormalities

	Goals		
	LDL cholesterol (mg/dl)	Non-HDL cholesterol (mg/dl)	ApoB (mg/dl)
Highest-risk patients, including those with *1)* known CVD or *2)* diabetes plus one or more additional major CVD risk factor	<70	<100	<80
High-risk patients, including those with *1)* no diabetes or known clinical CVD but two or more additional major CVD risk factors or *2)* diabetes but no other major CVD risk factors	<100	<130	<90

Other major risk factors (beyond dyslipoproteinemia) include smoking, hypertension, and family history of premature CHD.

Due to these unanswered questions about apoB and the established role of LDL cholesterol in patients with metabolic syndrome and diabetes, the goals outlined in the ADA/ACC consensus statement for LDL cholesterol and non-HDL cholesterol should be followed while we await further outcomes for combination therapy before adopting apoB as a routine secondary target in general practice.

SUMMARY

Type 2 diabetic subjects have a marked increase in CHD. For establishing cholesterol treatment goals, both the ADA and the NCEP ATP III guidelines consider diabetes to be a CHD risk equivalent. The primary goal for both of these organizations is the reduction of LDL cholesterol to <100 mg/dl, with a goal of <70 mg/dl in diabetic patients with CHD. For secondary goal targeting and therapy, NCEP recommends lowering non-HDL cholesterol in subjects who have a TG level >200 mg/dl to a goal that is 30 mg/dl above the LDL goal. The ADA comments on the possible benefit of combination therapy with niacin or fibrates in patients with TG >150 mg/dl and HDL <40 mg/dl (<50 mg/dl in women) but emphasizes the lack of outcomes data in this area. These differences are relatively minor, and the clear message from both organizations is for aggressive LDL cholesterol lowering in patients with diabetes. Recent attention on the metabolic syndrome is appropriate, given the worldwide epidemic of obesity and CHD. Although the focus of therapy remains behavior and lifestyle intervention, pharmacological therapy should be used achieve the target values of specific risk factors. Because these patients have multiple risk factors for CHD by definition, an LDL cholesterol goal of <100 mg/dl is appropriate in these patients as well.

BIBLIOGRAPHY

American Diabetes Association: Standards of medical care in diabetes—2009. *Diabetes Care* 32 (Suppl. 1):S13–S62, 2009

American Diabetes Association/American College of Cardiology: Foundation Consensus Statement: lipoprotein management in patients with cardiometabolic risk. *Diabetes Care* 31:811–822, 2008

Brown BG, Zhao X-Q, Chait A, Fisher LD, Cheung MC, Morse JS, Dowdy AA, Marino EK, Bolson EL, Alaupovic P, Frohlich J, Serafini L, Huss-Frechette E, Wang S, DeAngelis D, Dodek A, Albers JJ: Simvastatin and niacin, antioxidant vitamins, or the combination for the prevention of coronary disease. *N Engl J Med* 345:1583–1592, 2001

Expert Panel on Detection, Evaluation and Treatment of High Blood Cholesterol in Adults: Executive summary of the Third Report of the National Cholesterol Education Program (NCEP) Expert Panel on Detection, Evaluation and Treatment of High Blood Cholesterol in Adults (Adult Treatment Panel III). *JAMA* 285:2486–2497, 2001

Grundy SM, Cleeman JI, Merz CN, Brewer HB Jr, Clark LT, Hunninghake DB, Pasternak RC, Smith SC Jr, Stone NJ; National Heart, Lung, and Blood Institute; American College of Cardiology Foundation; American Heart Association: Implications of recent clinical trials for the National Cholesterol Education Program Adult Treatment Panel III Guidelines. *Circulation* 110:227–239, 2004

Haffner SM, Lehto S, Ronnemaa T, Pyorala K, Laakso M: Mortality from coronary heart disease in subjects with type 2 diabetes and in nondiabetic subjects with and without prior myocardial infarction. *N Engl J Med* 339:229–234, 1998

Heart Protection Study Collaborative Group (HPS): MRC/BHF Heart Protection Study of cholesterol-lowering with simvastatin in 5963 people with diabetes: a randomized placebo-controlled trial. *Lancet* 361:2005–2016, 2003

Jensen MK, Chiuve SE, Rimm EB, Dethlesfsen C, Tjonneland A, Joensen AM, Overvad K: Obesity, behavioral lifestyle factors, and risk of acute coronary events. *Circulation* 117:3062–3069, 2008

Kastelein JJ, van der Steeg WA, Holme I, Gaffney M, Cater NB, Barter P, Deedwania P, Olsson AG, Boekholdt SM, Demicco DA, Szarek M, LaRosa JC, Pedersen TR, Grundy SM, TNT Study Group, IDEAL Study Group: Lipids, apolipoproteins, and their ratios in relation to cardiovascular events with statin treatment. *Circulation* 117:3002–3009, 2008

Keech A, Simes RJ, Barter P, Best J, Scott R, Taskinen MR, Forder P, Pillai A, Davis T, Glasziou P, Drury P, Kesäniemi YA, Sullivan D, Hunt D, Colman P, d'Emden M, Whiting M, Ehnholm C, Laakso M, FIELD study investigators: Effects of long-term fenofibrate therapy on cardiovascular events in 9795 people with type 2 diabetes mellitus (the FIELD study): randomized controlled trial. *Lancet* 366:1849–1861, 2005

Reaven GM: Insulin resistance and its consequences: non-insulin-dependent diabetes mellitus and coronary heart disease. In *Diabetes Mellitus: A Fundamental and Clinical Text.* LeRoith D, Ed. Philadelphia, PA, Lippincott-Raven, 1996, p. 509–519

Retnakaran R, Zinman B: Type 1 diabetes, hyperglycemia and the heart. *Lancet* 371:1790–1799, 2008

Turner RC, Millns H, Neil HA, Stratton IM, Manley SE, Matthews DR, Holman RR: Risk factors for coronary artery disease in non-insulin dependent diabetes mellitus (UKPDS 23). *BMJ* 316:823–828, 1998

Dr. Williams is Associate Professor, Departments of Pharmacy and Medicine, Oregon Health and Science University, Portland, Oregon. Dr. Haffner is Professor, Department of Medicine, University of Texas Health Science Center, San Antonio, Texas.

51. Noninvasive Cardiac Testing

Josh Todd, MD, Jeff P. Steinhoff, MD, Venu Menon, MD, and Sidney C. Smith, Jr., MD

Diabetes quadruples the risk of developing atherosclerotic coronary heart disease (CHD), which is the leading cause of death in the diabetic population. Diabetes is currently estimated to affect >200 million people worldwide. Of the estimated 18 million Americans with diabetes, ~20% (or 3.6 million) are asymptomatic. In addition to presenting with premature CHD, patients with diabetes have markedly worse short- and long-term prognosis than their nondiabetic counterparts. The 7-year mortality rate for diabetic patients without prior myocardial infarction (MI) (20%) is similar to that of nondiabetic patients with a prior MI (19%). People with diabetes also have worse in-hospital mortality with MI, worse outcomes after treatment with thrombolysis, and worse prognosis after the development of cardiogenic shock. The likelihood of restenosis after percutaneous coronary intervention is increased in patients with diabetes, even when coronary stents are used. The presence of diabetes is particularly detrimental in women and negates the protective effect of female sex in the premenopausal period. Women with diabetes also display higher 28-day and 1-year mortality after MI than their nondiabetic counterparts.

The American Diabetes Association (ADA) recommends noninvasive cardiac testing for patients with *1)* typical or atypical cardiac symptoms and *2)* an abnormal resting electrocardiogram (ECG). Additional guidelines from the American College of Cardiology Foundation (ACCF)/American Society of Nuclear Cardiology (ASNC) recommend noninvasive stress testing in the following asymptomatic diabetic populations: *1)* high risk of congestive heart failure (CHF) using the Framingham risk criteria, *2)* intermediate or high risk of CHD with new-onset atrial fibrillation, and *3)* new-onset left ventricular dysfunction with or without clinical signs of CHF.

The following discussion will review the results of tests specifically designed to evaluate the heart. Tests such as the ankle-brachial index and the carotid Doppler ultrasound, which can identify the presence of peripheral arterial disease, a known marker for CHD, will not be covered in this section.

RESTING ELECTROCARDIOGRAM

The resting 12-lead ECG is a safe, inexpensive, and easily available test. It may reveal diagnostic Q waves that indicate silent MI in this population. The rates of silent MI as diagnosed by a surface ECG in the Framingham study 30-year follow-up were 28% for men and 35% for women; however, diabetes has not conclusively emerged as an independent predictor of silent MI. In addition, there is considerable debate as to whether strict glucose control will prevent MI or cardiovascular events. Though insensitive, the presence of ECG criteria for left ventricular hypertrophy is a relatively specific indicator for increased left ventricular mass in the adult population. Left ventricular hypertrophy is an adverse risk marker for future cardiovascular complications.

In patients being evaluated for an acute coronary syndrome, the presence of diagnostic ST elevation on the ECG is a marker for an occluded infarct-related artery. These subjects require emergent consideration for primary reperfusion therapy with thrombolysis or primary percutaneous intervention. Patients with dynamic ST segment changes or resting ST depression on their ECG are also at high risk for subsequent death or MI or may require urgent revascularization.

RESTING ECHOCARDIOGRAM

The echocardiogram is a safe, noninvasive ultrasound evaluation of the heart that provides useful information in the diabetic patient with suspected CHD. It can diagnose the presence of left ventricular contractile dysfunction, a powerful predictor of future cardiovascular risk. Patients with occult or manifest CHD may have wall-motion abnormalities on this study, which are diagnostic for prior MI or consistent with ischemia in the territory of a coronary artery. Other forms of cardiomyopathy secondary to hypertension or microvascular disease may also become apparent. In addition, the echocardiogram provides invaluable information about valvular function and right ventricular function and provides an accurate estimate of pulmonary artery pressures.

EXERCISE TREADMILL TESTING

The standard exercise treadmill test (ETT) uses periodically increasing workloads such as treadmill speed and elevation to increase a patient's heart rate. The target heart is ≥85% of the age-predicted maximum heart rate. The age-predicted maximal heart rate in beats per minute is calculated as 220 minus the age of the patient in years. An ischemic response is often defined as ≥1 mm horizontal or downsloping ST depression at 60–80 ms after the J-point occurring during exercise or recovery. High-risk end points that warrant termination of the test include the following: ≥2 mm of ST segment depression, ST elevation in leads without prior Q waves, a drop in systolic blood pressure or inability to increase systolic blood pressure from baseline, severe limiting angina, multifocal premature ventricular beats, or ischemic changes within the first 3 min of the test.

Lee et al. (2001) evaluated the accuracy of ETT in 190 patients with diabetes. A total of 73 patients (38%) had ischemic findings. Subsequent coronary angiography revealed a sensitivity of 47%, a specificity of 81%, a positive predictive value of 85%, and a negative predictive value of 41%. Subjects with left ventricular hypertrophy and female subjects were at high risk to develop false-positive

ECGs. The stress ECG is also not interpretable in patients with left bundle branch block and pre-excitation. These patients should have concomitant imaging studies as part of their diagnostic evaluation. A significant proportion of patients with diabetes have morbid obesity, peripheral vascular disease, or peripheral neuropathy, which impede performance of exercise. A pharmacological stress study using adenosine, dipyridamole, or dobutamine should be considered in this subset. Furthermore, Ho et al. (2008) have demonstrated that patients who can exercise but cannot increase their heart rate appropriately, likely due to autonomic dysfunction from neuropathy, have higher rates of MI, CHF, cardiac revascularization, and all-cause mortality.

STRESS ECHOCARDIOGRAPHY

Stress echocardiography combines ECG monitoring with echocardiographic evaluation of wall motion. It is often added to a standard ETT to increase the sensitivity and specificity and add incremental prognostic information. Inducible wall-motion abnormalities precede symptoms in the classic ischemic cascade. This is especially true in diabetic patients who may not have typical angina symptoms with exercise. Dobutamine stress echocardiography (DSE) can be used as an alternative to exercise, and the safety of this modality has been established. The response of the normal myocardial segment to exercise is to increase contractility, which is manifested by increased wall thickening of the segment. A biphasic response or a failure to augment contractility in a vascular territory is strongly suggestive of an underlying ischemic substrate. The extent of wall-motion abnormality and the inability of the ventricular cavity size to diminish are markers for high-risk anatomy. In addition, DSE is also able to distinguish between hibernating, stunned, and infarcted myocardial segments.

Kamalesh et al. (2002) looked at mortality in 233 patients (98% male) with normal stress echocardiograms, of which 89 (37%) had diabetes. A high MI and cardiovascular death rate in diabetic patients with normal stress echocardiograms compared with nondiabetic subjects (6.0 vs. 2.7% per year) was reported. Marwick et al. (2002) prospectively evaluated a larger cohort of 937 diabetic patients after stress echocardiography. This cohort was 57% male, with a mean age of 59 ± 13 years. Although a normal stress echocardiogram was associated with a better prognosis, patients who had a normal exercise echocardiogram had markedly better outcomes (4% 2-year mortality) compared with those patients with normal dobutamine echocardiograms (17% 2-year mortality). In fact, the inability to exercise was the strongest prognostic factor for cardiovascular death and MI. In a cohort of 396 diabetic patients, Sozzi et al. (2003) found the event rate for death or MI was lower but not inconsequential in subjects with a normal DSE, with 5, 8, and 10% at 1, 3, and 5 years, respectively. This evidence underscores the importance of aggressive risk factor treatment in all diabetic patients, regardless of a "negative" stress echocardiogram. People with diabetes who have an abnormal DSE result represent a subgroup at very high risk. The likelihood of cardiac death or MI with an abnormal DSE (fixed or ischemic response) resulted in a 7, 18, and 23% event rate at 1, 3, and 5 years, respectively. Similarly, Marwick et al.'s (2002) data in diabetic patients with established CHD showed 10, 22, and 38% mortality at 1, 3, and 5 years, respectively, with a DSE demonstrating ischemia.

MYOCARDIAL PERFUSION IMAGING

Single-Photon Emission Computed Tomography

Single-photon emission computed tomography (SPECT) myocardial perfusion imaging (MPI) uses radioisotopes, such as thallium, technetium sestamibi, and technetium tetrofosmin, as flow tracers. In this modality, exercise and dobutamine are used to increase to target heart rate, or adenosine, dipyridamole, and recently approved regadenoson are administered for vasodilation. Under stress, myocardium supplied by normal or nonsignificantly diseased coronary arteries will receive adequate blood flow, and tracer uptake will be uniform. Diseased coronary arteries are unable to increase blood flow to meet the increased demand. The myocardium beyond these diseased segments will have diminished tracer uptake and demonstrate a "perfusion defect."

There have been numerous studies reporting the prognostic value of SPECT MPI. De Lorenzo et al. (2002) evaluated 180 asymptomatic diabetic patients with exercise or dipyridamole technetium-99m sestamibi. In addition to finding silent ischemia in 21%, the study revealed a 2% annual death and MI rate for normal and a 9% rate for abnormal SPECT MPI studies. The worst prognosis was seen in patients with "mixed" defects, indicating a combination of myocardial scar from a prior silent MI and ischemic tissue.

Berman et al. (2003) found a similarly higher event rate in patients with diabetes compared with nondiabetic subjects. In a study that compared 1,222 diabetic patients with 4,111 nondiabetic patients, a higher annual mortality rate in type 1 diabetic patients versus type 2 diabetic patients versus nondiabetic patients of 2.5, 1.8, and 0.6%, respectively, was reported for normal SPECT MPI studies. Higher cardiac mortality was also seen in abnormal scans, with a 9% annual mortality for patients with type 1 diabetes compared with 4.6 and 4.7% annual mortality for nondiabetic and type 2 diabetic patients, respectively. In this cohort, type 1 diabetic patients were more likely to be younger, have had a prior MI, have undergone prior angioplasty and coronary artery bypass grafting surgery, and be diagnosed with hypertension.

For patients who cannot tolerate adenosine or dipyridamole infusion because of bronchospasm, allergy, or marked bradycardia, regadenoson or dobutamine stress SPECT MPI is a useful option with prognostic value in patients with diabetes. Regadenoson had been reported to have better tolerability and less incidence of bronchospasm in patients with chronic obstructive pulmonary disease. Schinkel et al. (2002) followed a cohort of 207 diabetic patients who underwent dobutamine stress SPECT MPI with technetium-99m sestamibi or tetrofosmin. This population had a higher degree of abnormal scans (64%) than other studies. Nevertheless, this cohort demonstrated a similar poor prognosis in patients with abnormal results, with a death or MI rate of ~10, 22, and 28% at 1, 3, and 5 years, respectively. The event rate was similarly low for normal perfusion studies and was

~0–1, 3, and 5% at 1, 3, and 5 years, respectively. As with other studies, prognosis was also correlated with the extent of ischemia.

Vanzetto et al. (1999) evaluated 158 high-risk diabetic patients who were defined as having two or more risk factors (age >65 years, hypertension, tobacco abuse, peripheral vascular disease, microalbuminuria, elevated cholesterol, or abnormal resting ECG). These patients underwent exercise or dipyridamole thallium SPECT MPI. Although a low overall annual event rate (1.5%) was observed in patients with normal perfusion or ≤22% of myocardium with perfusion defects, a marked difference was again demonstrated between patients who could and could not exercise. The annual mortality was 0.7% for patients who could exercise and demonstrated normal or ≤22% abnormal perfusion area compared with 4.6% in patients unable to exercise with similar perfusion. The annual rate for cardiac death was 11.6% for patients with >22% of myocardium with ischemia and 23.3% for combined cardiac death and MI. Giri et al. (2002) evaluated 929 diabetic patients and also found multivessel ischemia to be a powerful predictor for adverse outcomes. Women with diabetes are at higher risk for adverse events after abnormal SPECT MPI studies. In the cohort examined by Berman et al. (2003), female diabetic subjects had statistically higher annual mortality for all perfusion abnormalities compared with their male counterparts. Hachamovitch et al. (2003) also demonstrated higher mortality in female diabetic subjects compared with male subjects for any given ischemic burden, regardless of therapy. Furthermore, it also appeared that despite the >50% reduction in mortality observed with revascularization in both sexes, women still had higher mortality.

Positron Emission Tomography

Cardiac positron emission tomography (PET) MPI utilizes different radioisotopes than that of SPECT imaging. Agents used include rubidium-82 (Rb-82) and 13N-ammonia, which require production on site. The utility of PET over traditional SPECT imaging is in obese patients in whom the attenuation correction is a factor. Additionally, due to higher energy tracers, PET offers better spatial, contrast, and temporal resolution. In patients with diabetes and metabolic syndrome, the often excessive adiposity often creates artifacts that can reduce the sensitivity and specificity of the imaging study.

When comparing the diagnostic accuracy of Rb-82 PET MPI to 99m-Tc-sestamibi MPI in 224 patients, the interpretations were classified as definitely normal or abnormal in 96% of PET studies compared to 81% of SPECT studies. Diagnostic accuracy was also higher in the PET for stenosis severity of >70% (89 vs. 79%, $P = 0.001$). Another study of 64 consecutive patients (which included 36% diabetic patients) undergoing PET MPI with subsequent angiograms demonstrated a sensitivity of 92% for stenosis >70% on angiogram. In obese patients (BMI >30 kg/m^2), the sensitivity of PET in 32 patients was 100%. Specificity of the test when compared to angiographic data was 83%. However, because the amount of data for PET MPI is limited, current guidelines from the American College of Cardiology/American Heart Association (AHA)/ASNC in 2003 recommend that PET MPI be utilized in patients with equivocal SPECT MPI results or as an alternative initial test in patients who cannot exercise.

ELECTRON BEAM COMPUTED TOMOGRAPHY

CHD manifests with a significant amount of atherosclerotic plaque before the arterial lumen is compromised. This plaque, which is associated with the arterial intima, may calcify as a result of age, ongoing inflammation, or other unrecognized factors. Electron beam computed tomography (EBCT) quantitates the calcium level in the coronary arteries. Unfortunately, the arteries of patients with diabetes often have independent calcification of the arterial media (Monckeberg's calcinosis), which cannot be distinguished by EBCT. Although EBCT has prognostic value in certain populations and age-groups as a marker of atherosclerotic burden and subclinical CHD, it is not currently recommended by the American Heart Association for diagnosis or prognosis in patients with diabetes.

Multislice Computed Tomography Coronary Angiography

Many studies have begun to demonstrate the accuracy of computed tomography (CT)-assisted coronary angiography, also known as multislice CT (MSCT) coronary angiography, in low- and moderate-risk patients. It is fast, noninvasive, and becoming more available in many centers. Essentially, this allows coronary angiography to be performed in patients undergoing a CT of the chest. It also allows evaluation of pulmonary parenchyma and the great vessels. Its limitations, in the general population, are need for IV contrast with the potential for renal injury, the weight limitations of CT scanning, the need for breath-holding for 6–25 s (depending on the resolution of the scanner), and the need for normal sinus rhythm.

There are unfortunately few published studies evaluating patients with diabetes using MSCT. This is likely due in part to the higher risk profile of patients with diabetes as well as the higher levels of arterial calcification, which can hinder imaging of the coronary lumen using CT. Pundziute et al. (2007) evaluated a cohort of 86 patients with diabetes and 129 without diabetes with symptoms concerning for angina using MSCT. Not surprisingly, more patients with diabetes had coronary artery disease as well as more severe coronary artery disease. Compared with patients without diabetes, patients with diabetes demonstrated more calcified and noncalcified plaques but fewer mixed-composition atherosclerotic plaques.

Because the strength of MSCT is the exclusion ability of obstructive coronary artery disease over other stress modalities, the higher risk features of diabetic patients may not allow routine testing in such a population. Nevertheless, much of the data for MSCT have a better sensitivity than that of MPI and similar specificity. In a large systematic review published in 2007 that included >45 studies, the top-tier studies (as determined by the authors) demonstrated a sensitivity of 98% and specificity of 88% for finding a stenosis >50%. Based on anatomic distribution, the left circumflex had the lowest sensitivity (88%) and any distal vessel (80%) when compared to other coronary segments. The negative predictive value in the above study was 96%. The 2008 AHA guidelines suggest the following role for MSCT: that noninvasive coronary angiography is reasonable for symptomatic patients who are at intermediate risk for coronary artery disease after initial risk stratification, including patients with equivocal stress test results.

INVASIVE TESTING

The limitations of coronary angiography have been shown by the use of intravascular ultrasound. Despite this, coronary angiography remains the gold standard for diagnosis and evaluation as well as clinical decision making in current practice. Angiography is recommended for patients with noninvasive studies demonstrating multivessel disease or other high-risk findings. Subjects with symptoms and signs suggestive of a high pretest likelihood of disease should proceed to coronary angiography directly. Coronary angiography does have a small incidence of adverse events, such as renal failure, stroke, MI, vascular access site injury, bleeding, and infection. The role of newer modalities, such as magnetic resonance angiography, is currently being explored.

BIBLIOGRAPHY

American Diabetes Association: Standards of medical care in diabetes—2009 (Position Statement). *Diabetes Care* 32:S13–S62, 2009

American Diabetes Association/American College of Cardiology: Coronary heart disease in women with diabetes [article online]. *Diabetes & Cardiovascular Disease Review* Issue 5:1–8, 2003. Available from http://www.diabetes.org/uedocuments/Issue5.women.diabetes.cvd.pdf. Accessed 7 March 2009

Bateman TM, Heller GV, McGhie AI, et al.: Diagnostic accuracy of rest/stress ECG-gated Rb-82 myocardial perfusion PET: comparison with ECG-gated Tc-99m sestamibi SPECT. *J Nucl Cardiol* 13:24–33, 2006

Berman DS, Kang X, Hayes SW, Friedman JD, Cohen I, Abidov A, Shaw LJ, Amanullah AM, Germano G, Hachamovitch R: Adenosine myocardial perfusion single-photon emission computed tomography in women compared with men: impact of diabetes mellitus on incremental prognostic value and effect on patient management. *J Am Coll Cardiol* 41:1125–1133, 2003

Brindis RG, Douglas PS, Hendel RC, et al.: ACCF/ASNC appropriateness criteria for single-photon emission computed tomography myocardial perfusion imaging (SPECT MPI): a report of the American College of Cardiology Foundation Quality Strategic Directions Committee Appropriateness Criteria Working Group and the American Society of Nuclear Cardiology endorsed by the American Heart Association. *J Am Coll Cardiol* 46:1587–1605, 2005

De Lorenzo A, Lima RSL, Siqueira-Filho AG, Pantoja MR: Prevalence and prognostic value of perfusion defects detected by stress technetium-99m sestamibi myocardial perfusion single-photon emission computed tomography in asymptomatic patients with diabetes mellitus and no known coronary artery disease. *Am J Cardiol* 90:827–832, 2002

Douglas PS, Khandheria B, Stainback RF, et al.: ACCF/ASE/ACEP/AHA/ASNC/SCAI/SCCT/SCMR 2008 appropriateness criteria for stress echocardiography: a report of the American College of Cardiology Foundation Appropriateness Criteria Task Force, American Society of Echocardiography, American

College of Emergency Physicians, American Heart Association, American Society of Nuclear Cardiology, Society for Cardiovascular Angiography and Interventions, Society of Cardiovascular Computed Tomography, and Society for Cardiovascular Magnetic Resonance endorsed by the Heart Rhythm Society and the Society of Critical Care Medicine. *J Am Coll Cardiol* 51:1127–1147, 2008

Giri S, Shaw LJ, Murthy DR, Travin MI, Miller DD, Hachamovitch R, Borges-Neto S, Berman DS, Waters DD, Heller GV: Impact of diabetes on the risk stratification using stress single-photon emission computed tomography myocardial perfusion imaging in patients with symptoms suggestive of coronary artery disease. *Circulation* 105:32–40, 2002

Hachamovitch R, Hayes SW, Friedman JD, Cohen I, Berman DS: Comparison of the short-term survival benefit associated with revascularization compared with medical therapy in patients with no prior coronary artery disease undergoing stress myocardial perfusion single photon emission computed tomography. *Circulation* 107:2900–2906, 2003

Ho PM, Rumsfeld JS, Maddox TM, Magid DJ, Ross C: Impaired chronotropic response to exercise stress testing in patients with diabetes predicts future cardiovascular events. *Diabetes Care* 31:1531–1533, 2008

Kamalesh M, Matorin R, Sawada S: Prognostic value of a negative stress echocardiographic study in diabetic patients. *Am Heart J* 143:163–168, 2002

Klocke FJ, Baird MG, Lorell BH, et al.: ACC/AHA/ASNC guidelines for the clinical use of cardiac radionuclide imaging--executive summary: a report of the American College of Cardiology/American Heart Association Task Force on Practice Guidelines (ACC/AHA/ASNC Committee to Revise the 1995 Guidelines for the Clinical Use of Cardiac Radionuclide Imaging). *J Am Coll Cardiol* 42:1318–1333, 2003

Lee CD, Folsom AR, Pankow JS, Brancati FL, Atherosclerosis Risk in Communities (ARIC) Study Investigators: Cardiovascular events in diabetic and non-diabetic adults with or without history of myocardial infarction. *Circulation* 109:855–860, 2004

Lee DP, Fearon WF, Froelicher VF: Clinical utility of the exercise ECG in patients with diabetes and chest pain. *Chest* 119:1576–1581, 2001

Marwick TH, Case C, Sawada S, Vasey C, Short L, Lauer M: Use of stress echocardiography to predict mortality in patients with diabetes and known or suspected coronary artery disease. *Diabetes Care* 25:1042–1048, 2002

Pundziute G, Scholte AJHA, Schuijf JD, Kroft LJM, Jukema JW, van der Wall EE, et al.: Noninvasive assessment of plaque characteristics with multislice computed tomography coronary angiography in symptomatic diabetic patients. *Diabetes Care* 30:1113–1119, 2007

Redberg RF, Greenland P, Fuster V, Pyorala K, Blair SN, Folsom AR, Newman AB, O'Leary DH, Orchard TJ, Psaty B, Schwartz JS, Starke R, Wilson PW: Prevention Conference VI: Diabetes and Cardiovascular Disease Writing

Group III: risk assessment in persons with diabetes. *Circulation* 105:e144–e152, 2002

Schinkel AFL, Elhendy A, van Domburg RT, Bax JJ, Vourouri EC, Sozzi FB, Valkema R, Roelandt JRTC, Poldermans D: Prognostic value of dobutamine-atropine stress myocardial perfusion imaging in patients with diabetes. *Diabetes Care* 25:1637–1643, 2002

Sampson UK, Dorbala S, Limaye A, Kwong R, Di Carli MF: Diagnostic accuracy of rubidium-82 myocardial perfusion imaging with hybrid positron emission tomography/computed tomography in the detection of coronary artery disease. *J Am Coll Cardiol* 49:1052–1058, 2007

Sozzi FB, Elhendy A, Roelandt JR, van Domburg RT, Schinkel AF, Vourvouri EC, Bax JJ, De Sutter J, Borghetti A, Poldermans D: Prognostic value of dobutamine stress echocardiography in patients with diabetes. *Diabetes Care* 26:1074–1078, 2003

Stein PD, Yaekoub AY, Matta F, Sostman HD: 64-slice CT for diagnosis of coronary artery disease: a systematic review. *Am J Med* 121:715–725, 2008

Vanzetto G, Halimi S, Hammoud T, Fagret D, Benhamou PY, Gordonnier D, Bernard D, Machecourt J: Prediction of cardiovascular events in clinically selected high-risk NIDDM patients. *Diabetes Care* 22:19–26, 1999

Dr. Todd is a Cardiology Fellow at University of North Carolina, Chapel Hill, Chapel Hill, North Carolina. Dr. Steinhoff is a Cardiologist at the Heart and Vascular Institute of Florida, Safety Harbor, Florida. Dr. Menon is a staff cardiologist in the Section of Cardiovascular Imaging, the Robert and Suzanne Tomsich Department of Cardiovascular Medicine, at the Sydell and Arnold Miller Family Heart & Vascular Institute, Cleveland Clinic, Cleveland, Ohio. Dr. Smith is Professor of Medicine and Director, Center for Cardiovascular Science and Medicine, Division of Cardiology, University of North Carolina at Chapel Hill, Chapel Hill, North Carolina.

52. Acute Coronary Syndrome and Myocardial Infarction in the Diabetic Patient

Josh Todd, MD, Eron D. Crouch, MD, Venu Menon, MD, and Sidney C. Smith, Jr., MD

Although there has been a decline in the overall age-adjusted mortality rate among patients with known atherosclerotic coronary heart disease (CHD), there has been an increase in the mortality rate of diabetic patients with CHD. Currently, CHD accounts for 75% of all deaths in patients with diabetes. In addition, the incidence of death from cardiovascular causes in patients with diabetes and no history of CHD is similar to that observed in patients with known CHD and no diabetes. These observations highlight the prevalence of undiagnosed CHD in patients with diabetes and the gravity of myocardial infarction (MI) in this population.

FACTORS COMPLICATING MI IN PATIENTS WITH DIABETES

In general, diabetic patients with acute MI (AMI) have a poorer prognosis than their nondiabetic counterparts. Studies have shown that the in-hospital death rate after admission for AMI is ~1.5–2.0 times higher in patients with diabetes than in nondiabetic individuals. Likewise, patients with diabetes who survive MI have a 40% higher risk of death after 6 years. AMI in diabetic patients may be complicated by several factors that contribute to this poorer short- and long-term prognosis.

Accelerated Atherosclerosis

Several large autopsy registries have demonstrated increased coronary atherosclerotic burden in subjects with diabetes compared with their nondiabetic counterparts. Long-standing hyperglycemia, and subsequent hyperinsulinemia, leads to the development of microvascular disease, endothelial dysfunction, and increased transmigration of macrophages and other inflammatory cells into the subendothelium. Macrophages ingest modified LDL cholesterol molecules, giving rise to foam cells, the hallmark of atherosclerosis. For uncertain reasons among patients with diabetes, these atherosclerotic coronary arteries tend to remodel inwardly, further accelerating lumen occlusion. Subsequently, patients with diabetes have more pronounced and often multivessel coronary disease (including left main).

Prothrombotic State

Studies have also shown that diabetic patients with acute coronary syndrome (ACS) are more likely than nondiabetic subjects to present with intracoronary thrombi (94 vs. 55%, respectively). These findings are probably related to the increased incidence of ulcerated intracoronary plaques (94 vs. 61%, respectively) seen in diabetic patients with ACS. In addition, the platelets of diabetic patients have an increased number of glycoprotein (GP) IIb/IIIa receptors and aggregate more readily than the platelets of nondiabetic patients. Furthermore, patients with diabetes have been shown to have increased levels of plasma fibrinogen and factor VII, which correlate with an increased risk of MI and sudden death.

Larger MI Zone

Diabetic patients tend to have larger MIs than nondiabetic subjects. This is primarily because of more diffuse macrovascular and microvascular disease among patients with diabetes, which also contributes to more significant peri-infarct zone ischemia. Silent infarctions also plague up to 20–30% of all individuals with diabetes, leading to a significant number of delayed or missed diagnoses. A substudy of the Coronary Artery Surgery Study registry suggested that diabetic patients with silent ischemia had significantly lower survival than nondiabetic subjects with silent ischemia (59 vs. 82%, respectively) at 6 years.

Autonomic Dysfunction

Autonomic dysfunction is an independent predictor of major cardiac events. It affects up to 50% of patients with diabetes and may contribute to lowering the threshold for a life-threatening arrhythmia by causing an imbalance in sympathovagal tone. Autonomic dysfunction also increases the risk of hemodynamic instability.

STRATEGIES TO PREVENT MI IN PATIENTS WITH DIABETES

As previously mentioned, studies indicate that patients with diabetes, but no history of CHD, have a risk of cardiovascular death similar to nondiabetic patients with known CHD. As a result, the current American Heart Association (AHA) guidelines, American Diabetes Association (ADA) guidelines, and recommendations from the Adult Treatment Panel III of the National Cholesterol Education Program all suggest that risk factors in diabetic patients with no history of CHD should be modified as intensively as in nondiabetic subjects with known CHD. The major modifiable risk factors are discussed below.

Glycemic Control

Although controlled clinical trials have not fully established the role of good glycemic control in preventing macrovascular disease, they have confirmed the benefit of good glycemic control in patients with type 1 and type 2 diabetes for the prevention of microvascular disease. The goal for glycemic therapy is to achieve a fasting glucose level between 90 and 130 mg/dl (5.0 and 7.2 mmol/l) and an A1C level of <7%. Postprandial hyperglycemia may be an independent risk factor for CHD; however, there are currently no universally accepted guidelines to address this issue. The ADA recommends a 2-h postprandial glucose level of <180 mg/dl (<10 mmol/l).

Weight Reduction

The majority of type 2 diabetic patients are overweight (BMI 25–29.9 kg/m^2) or obese (BMI ≥30 kg/m^2). Excess body fat raises insulin resistance and may accelerate a decline in insulin secretion. Studies have shown that weight reduction can reduce insulin resistance and perhaps mitigate the metabolic risk factors associated with diabetes. For the optimal chance of maintaining weight loss, the goal should be to lose 10% of initial body weight gradually over 12 months.

Physical Activity

Physical inactivity contributes to the development of obesity; however, even patients with diabetes who are not obese can benefit from physical activity. Physical activity can improve insulin sensitivity; lower total cholesterol, LDL cholesterol, and triglycerides; raise HDL cholesterol; and further decrease the risk for CHD by improving overall cardiovascular fitness and function. Patients should receive a physical activity prescription based on the clinical judgment of the physician. The usually recommended prescription is ~30 min of moderate-intensity exercise daily, although additional physical activity may be beneficial, if tolerable to the patient. The AHA provides an exercise prescription that can be recommended for clinical practice.

Lipid Control

The principle of managing patients with diabetes and no known CHD using treatment goals that are similar to those for the nondiabetic patient with known CHD can be extended to lipid management. Guidelines set by the National Cholesterol Education Program recommend that patients with diabetes maintain an LDL cholesterol of <100 mg/dl (<5.6 mmol/l) with an optional goal of <70 mg/dl (3.9 mmol/l), which is also supported by the ADA. For patients with triglyceride levels >200 mg/dl (>11.1 mmol/l), the target goal is a non-HDL cholesterol level (total cholesterol minus HDL cholesterol) of ≤130 mg/dl (≤7.2 mmol/l). It is also desirable to maintain an HDL cholesterol level >40 mg/dl (>2.2 mmol/l) for men and >50 mg/dl (>2.8 mmol/l) for women. These recommendations are supported by the Heart Protection Study (HPS), which demonstrated benefit from statin therapy among patients with diabetes and LDL cholesterol levels <100 mg/dl (<5.6 mmol/l). In this study, 20,536 patients with CHD, stroke, peripheral vascular disease, or diabetes were randomized to receive either 40 mg simvastatin daily or placebo for 5 years. Among the subgroup of patients with diabetes and known CHD, the event rate was 33% for the group treated with simvastatin versus 38% for the placebo group. In diabetic patients with no prior history of CHD, the event rate was 9 versus 14%, respectively. Overall, the mean LDL cholesterol level of the simvastatin-treated group was 77 mg/dl (4.3 mmol/l). The Pravastatin or Atorvastatin Evaluation and Infection Therapy (PROVE IT) trial enrolled 4,162 patients, including >700 patients with diabetes who had been hospitalized for an ACS, and compared 40 mg pravastatin daily (standard therapy) with 80 mg atorvastatin daily (intensive therapy). At 2 years, the PROVE IT trial demonstrated a significant reduction in events from using high-dose atorvastatin in patients with diabetes, which achieved a mean LDL cholesterol of 62 mg/dl (3.4 mmol/l), compared with using standard-dose pravastatin, which achieved a mean LDL cholesterol of 95 mg/dl (5.3 mmol/l; 28.8 vs. 34.6%, respectively). Thus, current guidelines state that it is reasonable to prescribe statin therapy for high-risk patients, such as those with diabetes, even when the LDL cholesterol level is between 70 mg/dl (3.9 mmol/l) and 100 mg/dl (5.6 mmol/l).

Blood Pressure Control

Several controlled clinical trials have indicated that the risk of cardiovascular events and diabetes-associated death increases with increases in blood pressure and that lowering the blood pressure of patients with diabetes can significantly reduce this risk. The U.K. Prospective Diabetes Study illustrated that even modest blood pressure reduction in diabetic patients (10 mmHg systolic and 5 mmHg diastolic) can reduce the risk of developing congestive heart failure by 56%. The Heart Outcomes Prevention Evaluation (HOPE) trial randomized >9,000 patients with evidence of vascular disease or diabetes plus one other cardiovascular risk factor to the ACE inhibitor ramipril versus placebo. Overall, ramipril significantly reduced the composite end point of MI, stroke, or cardiovascular mortality to 14%, compared with 17.8% in the placebo group. In addition, the Microalbuminuria, Cardiovascular, and Renal Outcomes-HOPE (MICRO-HOPE) trial of 3,577 diabetic patients was terminated 6 months early because ramipril was shown to reduce the incidence of MI by 22%, stroke by 33%, cardiovascular death by 37%, and all-cause mortality by 24% compared with placebo. For these reasons, the AHA recommends that in the absence of contraindications, ACE inhibitors be administered to all diabetic patients. The Joint National Committee-7 on Prevention, Detection, Evaluation, and Treatment of High Blood Pressure; the ADA; and the National Kidney Foundation (NKF) all recommend that all patients with diabetes maintain a blood pressure of <130/80 mmHg. The NKF also recommends that diabetic patients with proteinuria >1 g/day lower their blood pressure goal to <125/75 mmHg. Several studies have emphasized the importance of blood pressure control, especially in long-standing diabetic patients, who are more likely to have already developed macro- and microvascular disease. In these patients, blood pressure control appears to be a more important factor for prevention of cardiovascular events than glucose control.

Smoking Cessation

Because smoking is an independent risk factor for developing CHD, complete cessation should be the primary goal for all smokers, but especially those with diabetes. Counseling or referral to smoking-cessation programs should be offered to all diabetic smokers at every office visit. There are a variety of pharmacological therapeutic options (i.e., bupropion and nicotine-replacement products). Importantly, these options have been shown to be more effective when used in conjunction with a high-quality smoking cessation program. Bupropion should be used with precaution in patients with known or suspected ACS or heart failure because of its proarrhythmic potential. Patients who choose to quit without the help of a smoking-cessation program should have a follow-up within 2 weeks of their scheduled quit date and another after 1 month of abstinence.

INITIAL MANAGEMENT OF MI IN PATIENTS WITH DIABETES

Diagnosis

Up to one-third of patients with diabetes who present with AMI have symptoms other than the classic substernal chest pressure radiating into the left arm, or they have no symptoms at all until the development of congestive heart failure. Atypical presentations, such as jaw or neck pain, epigastric pain associated with vomiting, isolated shortness of breath, and diabetic ketoacidosis, are common. Often, a high index of suspicion is needed to make the diagnosis. Up to 35% will not have characteristic electrocardiogram (ECG) ST elevations or Q waves indicating myocardial injury or infarction, respectively. In addition, diabetic patients often have renal insufficiency, which may falsely elevate cardiac markers. The Joint European Society of Cardiology/American College of Cardiology (ACC) Foundation/AHA/ World Heart Foundation Task Force has defined the following to assist in the diagnosis of AMI: detection of a rise and/or fall in cardiac biomarkers (preferably troponin with at least one value above the upper reference limit) and at least one of the following: *1*) symptoms of ischemia, *2*) ECG changes indicative of new ischemia, *3*) development of pathological Q waves on the ECG, and *4*) imaging evidence of a new loss of viable myocardium or new regional wall motion abnormality.

Management Strategies in ST Segment Elevation MI

Emergent target-vessel reperfusion with fibrinolytic therapy or primary percutaneous intervention (PCI) is the standard of care for the management of ST segment elevation MI (STEMI). Although several large, randomized, clinical trials have demonstrated a survival benefit in using fibrinolytic therapy for STEMI, none have been specifically designed to evaluate its efficacy in patients with diabetes. A meta-analysis of nine large, randomized, clinical trials evaluating the use of fibrinolytic therapy for STEMI reviewed 58,600 patients, of whom 4,529 (7.7%) had diabetes. In the subgroup of diabetic patients, fibrinolytic therapy significantly reduced overall mortality (13.6%) compared with the control group (17.3%) at 35 days. A slightly higher incidence of stroke was observed in the group receiving fibrinolytic therapy (1.9%) versus the control group (1.3%). Alteplase and reteplase should be used with adjunctive heparin, whereas the nonspecific fibrinolytic agents (such as streptokinase and urokinase) can be used without heparin. Additionally, adjunctive aspirin has demonstrated a 42% reduction in vascular mortality compared with streptokinase or aspirin alone (25%). However, current guidelines suggest that for all patients presenting with STEMI symptoms of >3 h duration, when transfer to a PCI center is possible within 60 min of presentation, a reperfusion strategy using PCI is more beneficial than fibrinolytic therapy.

A review of 11 clinical trials comparing primary PCI and fibrinolytic therapy in patients presenting with STEMI showed an overall decrease in the combined end point of mortality or nonfatal reinfarction at 30 days (7.0 vs. 12.9%, respectively.) This benefit was more evident in the subgroup analysis of patients with diabetes, where a 30-day mortality or nonfatal reinfarction rate of 9.2% was observed for individuals who underwent primary PCI versus 19.3% for individuals treated with fibrinolytic therapy.

In diabetic patients presenting with STEMI, PCI with coronary stenting is preferred over PCI alone. The Controlled Abciximab and Device Investigation to Lower Late Angioplasty Complications (CADILLAC) trial demonstrated that PCI with coronary stenting reduced the composite end point of death, reinfarction, disabling stroke, and need for revascularization compared with PCI alone (10.5 vs. 18.0%, respectively) and was particularly beneficial in diabetic patients (9.2 vs. 19.3%, respectively).

In the setting of an AMI, there have been a limited number of trials comparing primary PCI with bare metal stents (BMSs) and drug-eluting stents (DESs). Because of this, there have been few recommendations about stent choice in patients presenting with STEMI. In a recent meta-analysis comparing BMS and DES (evaluating 2,746 patients in eight randomized controlled trials, with ~10% of subjects having diabetes), there were lower rates of repeat revascularization (hazard ratio 0.38, $P < 0.001$) and nonstatistically significant (but trend towards benefit) in death, acute stent thrombosis, and recurrent MI.

Medical management of patients presenting with STEMI should include immediate therapy with aspirin (325 mg) and unfractionated heparin (UFH) or low–molecular weight heparin (LMWH). Based on current ACC/AHA guidelines, clopidogrel is reasonable as a 300-mg oral loading dose for patients who have received fibrinolytic therapy or have not received reperfusion therapy, and clopidogrel is recommended as a 600-mg oral loading dose for patients undergoing PCI. Data from the COMMIT-CCS-2 trial and CLARITY-TIMI 28 have demonstrated that the loading of 300 mg clopidogrel does have a combined end point benefit in both strategies of revascularization. GP IIb/IIIa receptor antagonists can be given en route or in the catheterization laboratory.

Management Strategies in Non–ST Segment Elevation MI

The initial management of non–ST segment elevation MI (NSTEMI) is different from that of STEMI, owing to different pathophysiology. The target vessel in patients with NSTEMI is usually not completely occluded or supplies a small territory. The cornerstone of therapy is rapid platelet inhibition and plaque stabilization, followed by medical management among low-risk patients and an early invasive strategy for high-risk patients. Hemodynamically unstable patients with NSTEMI should receive emergent primary PCI. In the absence of contraindication, all patients with NSTEMI should receive either UFH or LMWH, although LMWH may be slightly more efficacious. The Efficacy and Safety of Subcutaneous Enoxaparin in Non–Q wave Coronary Events (ESSENCE) trial showed that enoxaparin significantly reduced the incidence of death, recurrent MI, and angina at 30 days when compared to UFH (16.6 vs. 19.8%, respectively). The use of GP IIb/IIIa receptor inhibitors in the conservative management of patients with NSTEMI is controversial; however, there is evidence to support their use in patients in whom an early invasive strategy is planned. A meta-analysis of six large-scale clinical trials enrolling a total of 23,072 patients admitted for NSTEMI/unstable angina, including 6,458 diabetic patients, found that 30-day mortality was significantly lower in diabetic patients using GP IIb/IIIa receptor inhibitors than in placebo subgroups (4.6 vs. 6.2%, respectively). In addition, the 1-year mortality in patients with diabetes undergoing an early invasive strategy was significantly decreased by the use of abciximab from 4.5 to 2.5%.

In a recent meta-analysis comparing BMS and DES (evaluating 2,749 patients in eight randomized, controlled trials, with ~10% of subjects having diabetes), there were lower rates of repeat revascularization (hazard ratio 0.38, $P < 0.001$) and a nonstatistically significant difference in death, acute stent thrombosis, and recurrent MI between the groups, but there was a trend toward benefit. The randomized, controlled SIRIUS trial compared BMS to sirolimus-eluting stents in diabetic subjects in a subgroup analysis. In 279 diabetic patients, target lesion revascularization was reduced with sirolimus-eluting stents when compared to

BMS (6.9 vs. 22.3%, $P < 0.001$). Additionally, the SIRIUS trial demonstrated a benefit in major adverse cardiac events that favored sirolimus-eluting stents over BMS (9.2 vs. 25%, $P < 0.001$). Other trials comparing different stents (SCORPIUS and DIABETES) have shown similar results for target lesion revascularization and major adverse cardiac event rates.

Surgical Revascularization

No clinical trials have evaluated outcomes of emergent coronary artery bypass graft (CABG) in the setting of AMI; however, an accumulating body of evidence points toward CABG as the preferred revascularization strategy in diabetic patients with unstable angina and multivessel coronary disease. The Bypass Angioplasty Revascularization Investigation (BARI) trial enrolled 1,829 patients, including 353 diabetic patients with angiographically documented multivessel coronary artery disease and either clinically severe angina or objective evidence of marked myocardial ischemia requiring revascularization. At 5 years, there was significantly increased all-cause mortality (35 vs. 19%) and cardiac mortality (20.6 vs. 5.8%) with multivessel PCI compared with surgical revascularization. The results of two other randomized trials comparing multivessel angioplasty to CABG are consistent with the BARI findings. These results raised concern about selection of angioplasty as a revascularization method in diabetic patients with multivessel coronary artery disease. Subsequent reports from the BARI investigators suggested that the survival benefit of CABG was limited to the 81% of diabetic patients receiving internal mammary grafts. Cardiac mortality was 2.9% when internal mammary grafts were used versus 18.2% when only saphenous vein graft conduits were used. The latter rate was similar to that of patients receiving percutaneous transluminal coronary angioplasty (20.6%). Some of the lingering questions regarding revascularization in diabetic patients with multivessel disease will be addressed in the ongoing BARI 2D study.

Glycemic Control

The role of tight glycemic control for diabetic patients in the setting of AMI is proven but infrequently practiced. The Diabetes Mellitus, Insulin, Glucose Infusion in Acute Myocardial Infarction (DIGAMI) study investigators randomized 620 patients with diabetes (83% with type 2 diabetes) with MI in 19 hospitals across Sweden to an experimental strategy of initial insulin glucose infusion followed by multidose insulin treatment for 3 months and compared that to a control strategy of insulin supplementation only if clinically indicated. The experimental treatment resulted in a dramatic reduction in mortality at 1 year (19 vs. 26%, $P < 0.027$). This 30% reduction in mortality was maintained at 3.4 years of follow-up (33 vs. 44%) and translated into a treatment effect of one life saved for every nine patients treated. On subgroup analysis, the maximum benefit was realized in low-risk patients without prior exposure to insulin, with an absolute mortality reduction of 15%. The role of both high- and low-dose glucose-insulin potassium infusions has been studied, with mixed results in the universe of patients presenting with AMI. The recent Glucose-Insulin-Potassium Study (GIPS) randomized 940 patients receiving primary PCI for an STEMI to metabolic modulation with glucose-insulin-potassium (GIK) versus control. Whereas treatment with GIK did not decrease overall mortality in the trial, mortality among diabetic patients receiving GIK therapy ($n = 49$) was 4%, compared with 12% among control subjects with diabetes ($n = 50$). Based on the above data, the 2007 ACC/AHA guidelines for NSTEMI recommend that in acute glucose management (in the first 3 days) to keep preprandial glucose <110 mg/dl (6.1 mmol/l) and maximal glucose <180 mg/dl (10 mmol/l).

PERI-INFARCTION AND LONG-TERM MANAGEMENT GUIDELINES

Patients with diabetes surviving MI have higher late mortality than their counterparts without diabetes. Late mortality is mainly related to recurrent MI and the development of heart failure. Peri-infarction and long-term management of diabetic patients consist of *1*) intensive modification of risk factors (discussed in the previous section), *2*) optimizing medical therapy, *3*) appropriate postinfarction stress testing, and *4*) cardiac rehabilitation.

Aspirin

The AHA recommends (class I), in the absence of contraindications, a chewed 325-mg aspirin be administered as soon as possible after presentation and 162–325 mg to be continued for at least 1 month for patients with BMS and 3–6 months for patients receiving DES, depending on the type of stent. Then, patients can be continued indefinitely at 75–162 mg/day of aspirin.

Clopidogrel

The AHA recommends (class I) that 75 mg/day clopidogrel be administered to hospitalized patients who are unable to take aspirin because of hypersensitivity or major gastrointestinal intolerance. In hospitalized patients with NSTEMI in whom a conservative approach is planned, clopidogrel should be added to aspirin as soon as possible on admission and administered for at least 12 months. In patients for whom a PCI is planned, clopidogrel should be taken a minimum of 1 month (and ideally up to 12 months) for BMS and 12 months for drug-eluting stents and should be continued for at least 12 months in patients who are not at high risk for bleeding. In patients taking clopidogrel in whom elective CABG is planned, the drug should be withheld for 5–7 days.

UFH and LMWH

The AHA recommends (class I) that anticoagulation with subcutaneous LMWH or intravenous UFH be added to antiplatelet therapy with aspirin and/or clopidogrel throughout the remainder of the hospitalization or for 7 days, whichever occurs first. The AHA also acknowledges (class IIb) that the majority of the literature suggests that enoxaparin is superior to UFH as an anticoagulant in patients with unstable angina or NSTEMI, unless CABG is planned within 24 h.

GP IIb/IIIa Antagonists

The AHA recommends (class I) that a platelet GP IIb/IIIa antagonist be administered, in addition to acetylsalicylic acid (ASA; aspirin) and heparin, to patients in whom catheterization and PCI are planned. The GP IIb/IIIa antagonist may also be administered just before PCI. The AHA also acknowledges (class IIb) that the majority of the literature suggests that eptifibatide or tirofiban can be administered, in addition to ASA and LMWH or UFH, to patients with continuing ischemia, with an elevated troponin, or with other high-risk features for which an invasive management strategy is not planned. In addition, the platelet GP IIb/

IIIa antagonist can be administered to patients already receiving heparin, ASA, and clopidogrel in whom catheterization and PCI are planned. The GP IIb/IIIa antagonist may also be administered just before PCI.

β-Blockers

The AHA recommends (class I) that in the absence of contraindications, oral β-blockers be administered to all patients. They discourage the acute use of intravenous β-blockers in patients with the potential for severe heart failure, cardiogenic shock, or high-degree atrioventricular block. In the absence of the above, intravenous β-blockers can be used acutely in patients with hypertension or tachyarrhythmias (class IIa).

ACE Inhibitors

The AHA recommends (class I) that in the absence of contraindications, ACE inhibitors be administered to all patients with diabetes.

Statins and Other Lipid-Lowering Agents

The AHA recommends (class I) lipid-lowering agents and diet in all post-ACS patients, including postrevascularization patients, treating to a target LDL cholesterol level <100 mg/dl (<5.6 mmol/l). As noted earlier in this chapter, HPS and PROVE IT demonstrated benefit for patients treated with statin therapy whose LDL cholesterol levels were <100 mg/dl (<5.6 mmol/l). The AHA also acknowledges (class IIb) that the majority of literature suggests that a fibrate should be administered if HDL cholesterol is <40 mg/dl (<2.2 mmol/l), occurring as an isolated finding or in combination with other lipid abnormalities. In addition, fibrate therapy may be given to patients with HDL cholesterol <40 mg/dl (<2.2 mmol/l) and triglycerides of >200 mg/dl (11.1 mmol/l). Last, hydroxymethylglutaryl-CoA reductase inhibitors and diet should begin 24–96 h after admission and continued after hospital discharge for all patients with LDL cholesterol >100 mg/dl (>5.6 mmol/l).

Nitroglycerin

The AHA recommends (class I) that anginal discomfort lasting >2 or 3 min should prompt the patient to discontinue the activity or remove himself or herself from the stressful event. If pain does not subside immediately, the patient should be instructed to take nitroglycerin. If the first tablet or spray does not provide relief within 5 min, this should prompt the patient to seek immediate medical attention by calling 9-1-1 and going to the nearest hospital emergency department, preferably via ambulance or the quickest available alternative.

Other Agents

Angiotensin receptor blockers (ARBs) are an appropriate alternative in patients with MI complicated by systolic left ventricular dysfunction who cannot tolerate ACE inhibitors. The use of an ARB in combination with an ACE inhibitor, in the peri-infarction setting, has not found widespread acceptance due to the results of the Valsartan in Acute Myocardial Infarction Trial (VALIANT), which concluded that the combination of valsartan and captopril increased adverse events and did not improve survival. In the setting of chronic heart failure, this combination is sometimes used, due in part to the Candesartan in Heart Failure Assessment in Reduction of Mortality (CHARM) Trial, which found a reduction in cardiovascular deaths and hospital admissions for heart failure, independent of ejection fraction or baseline treatment.

The selective aldosterone receptor blocker eplerenone is sometimes used in patients with AMI complicated by systolic left ventricular dysfunction and either heart failure or diabetes. It is usually used in patients who are already receiving therapeutic doses of β-blocker and ACE inhibition because this strategy was shown in the Eplerenone Post-AMI Heart Failure Efficacy and Survival Study (EPHESUS) to reduce morbidity and mortality more than β-blockade with ACE inhibition alone. The Randomized Aldactone Evaluation Study (RALES) also concluded a mortality benefit for aldosterone receptor blockade; however, this study was not performed in the setting of AMI.

Cardiac Rehabilitation

The AHA recommends (class I) the referral of postinfarction patients to an outpatient cardiac rehabilitation program.

SUMMARY

Patients with diabetes and underlying CHD have a more complex pathophysiology and worse prognosis. Optimal management of these patients begins with intensive prevention strategies. In the setting of STEMI, emergent PCI is preferable over fibrinolysis, especially for those patients beyond the first 3 h of symptoms. Most diabetic patients with NSTEMI will undergo coronary angiography and possibly primary PCI within the first 48 h of presentation. No clinical trials have evaluated outcomes of emergent CABG in the setting of AMI; however, an accumulating body of evidence suggests that CABG (with left internal mammary artery grafting) is superior to multivessel PCI in diabetic patients with unstable angina. Peri-infarction and long-term management of these patients requires aggressive risk factor modification, optimization of medical therapy, appropriate postinfarction stress testing, and cardiac rehabilitation. Because of their higher morbidity and mortality after MI, managing diabetic patients is challenging, and it is imperative that the clinician use a comprehensive medical strategy for this population.

BIBLIOGRAPHY

American Heart Association: American Heart Association Prevention Conference VI: Writing Groups I-V: diabetes and cardiovascular disease. *Circulation* 105:e132–e169, 2002

Anderson JL, Adams CD, Antman EM, et al.: ACC/AHA 2007 guidelines for the management of patients with unstable angina/non-ST-Elevation myocardial infarction: a report of the American College of Cardiology/American Heart Association Task Force on Practice Guidelines (Writing Committee to Revise the 2002 Guidelines for the Management of Patients With Unstable Angina/Non-ST-Elevation Myocardial Infarction) developed in collaboration with the American College of Emergency Physicians, the Society for Cardiovascular Angiography and Interventions, and the Society of Thoracic Surgeons endorsed by the American Association of Cardiovascular and Pulmonary Rehabilitation and the Society for Academic Emergency Medicine. *J Am Coll Cardiol* 50:e1–e157, 2007

Antman EM, Hand M, Armstrong PW, et al.: 2007 Focused update of the ACC/AHA 2004 Guidelines for the Management of Patients with ST-Elevation

Myocardial Infarction: a report of the American College of Cardiology/American Heart Association Task Force on Practice Guidelines: developed in collaboration with the Canadian Cardiovascular Society endorsed by the American Academy of Family Physicians: 2007 Writing Group to Review New Evidence and Update the ACC/AHA 2004 Guidelines for the Management of Patients With ST-Elevation Myocardial Infarction, Writing on Behalf of the 2004 Writing Committee. *Circulation* 117:296–329, 2008

Aronson D, Rayfield E: Diabetes. In *The Textbook of Cardiovascular Medicine*. 2nd ed. Philadelphia, PA, Lippincott, Williams & Wilkins, 2002

Baumgart D, Klauss V, Baer F, et al.: One-year results of the SCORPIUS study: a German multicenter investigation on the effectiveness of sirolimus-eluting stents in diabetic patients. *J Am Coll Cardiol* 50:1627–1634, 2007

Bypass Angioplasty Revascularization Investigation (BARI) Investigators: Influence of diabetes on 5-year mortality and morbidity in a randomized trial comparing CABG and PTCA in patients with multi-vessel disease. *Circulation* 96:1761–1779, 1997

Cannon CP, Braunwald E, McCabe CH, Rader DJ, Rouleau JL, Belder R, Joyal SV, Hill KA, Pfeffer MA, Skene AM, Pravastatin or Atorvastatin Evaluation and Infection Therapy-Thrombolysis in Myocardial Infarction 22 Investigators: Intensive versus moderate lipid lowering with statins after acute coronary syndromes. *N Engl J Med* 350:1495–1504, 2004

CASS Principal Investigators: Myocardial infarction and mortality in the Coronary Artery Surgery Study (CASS) randomized trial. *N Engl J Med* 310:750–758, 1984

Collins R, Armitage J, Parish S, Sleigh P, Peto R, Heart Protection Study Collaborative Group: MRC/BHF Heart Protection Study of cholesterol-lowering with simvastatin in 5963 people with diabetes: a randomised placebo-controlled trial. *Lancet* 361:2005–2016, 2003

Grundy SM, Howard B, Smith S Jr, Eckel R, Redberg R, Bonow RO: American Heart Association Prevention Conference VI: Diabetes and Cardiovascular Disease: executive summary: conference proceeding for healthcare professionals from a special writing group of the American Heart Association. *Circulation* 105:2231–2239, 2002

HOPE Investigators: Effect of ramipril on cardiovascular and microvascular outcomes in people with diabetes mellitus: results of the HOPE study and MICRO-HOPE substudy. *Lancet* 355:253–259, 2000

Jimenez-Quevedo P, Sabate M, Angiolillo DJ, et al.: Long-term clinical benefit of sirolimus-eluting stent implantation in diabetic patients with de novo coronary stenoses: long-term results of the DIABETES trial. *Eur Heart J* 28:1946–1952, 2007

Kastrati A, Dibra A, Spaulding C, et al.: Meta-analysis of randomized trials on drug-eluting stents vs. bare-metal stents in patients with acute myocardial infarction. *Eur Heart J* 28:2706–2713, 2007

King SB 3rd, Smith SC Jr, Hirshfeld JW Jr, et al.: 2007 Focused update of the ACC/AHA/SCAI 2005 guideline update for percutaneous coronary intervention: a report of the American College of Cardiology/American Heart Association Task Force on Practice guidelines. *J Am Coll Cardiol* 51:172–209, 2008

Klein L, Gheorghiade M: Management of the patient with diabetes mellitus and myocardial infarction: clinical trial update. *Am J Med* 116:47S–63S, 2004

Malmberg K: Prospective randomized study of intensive insulin treatment on long-term survival after acute myocardial infarction in patients with diabetes mellitus. *BMJ* 314:1512–1515, 1997

Mooradian AD: Cardiovascular disease in type 2 diabetes mellitus: current management guidelines. *Arch Intern Med* 163:33–40, 2003

Moussa I, Leon MB, Baim DS, et al.: Impact of sirolimus-eluting stents on outcome in diabetic patients: a SIRIUS (SIRolImUS-coated Bx Velocity balloon-expandable stent in the treatment of patients with de novo coronary artery lesions) substudy. *Circulation* 109:2273–2278, 2004

Nesto RW: Treatment of acute myocardial infarction in diabetes mellitus. Available from www.uptodate.com. Version 17.1. Accessed February 2009

Pitt B, Remme W, Zannad F, Neaton J, Martinez F, Roniker B, Bittman R, Hurley S, Kleiman J, Gatlin M, Eplerenone Post-Acute Myocardial Infarction Heart Failure Efficacy and Survival Study Investigators: Eplerenone, a selective aldosterone blocker, in patients with left ventricular dysfunction after myocardial infarction. *N Engl J Med* 348:1309–1321, 2003

Pitt B, Zannad F, Remme W, Cody R, Castaigne A, Perez A, Palensky J, Wittes J: The effect of spironolactone on morbidity and mortality in patients with severe heart failure: Randomized Aldactone Evaluation Study Investigators. *N Engl J Med* 341:709–717, 1999

Thygesen K, Alpert JS, White HD, et al.: Universal definition of myocardial infarction. *J Am Coll Cardiol* 50:2173–2195, 2007

Yusuf S, Sleight P, Pogue J, Bosch J, Davies R, Dagenais G: Effects of an angiotensin-converting-enzyme inhibitor, ramipril, on cardiovascular events in high-risk patients: the Heart Outcomes Prevention Evaluation Study Investigators. *N Engl J Med* 342:145–153, 2000

Dr. Todd is a Cardiology Fellow at the University of North Carolina at Chapel Hill, Chapel Hill, North Carolina. Dr. Crouch is an Active Staff Cardiologist and Co-director of the Cardiac Rehabilitation Program, Trinity Mother Frances Hospital, Tyler, Texas, and of the Trinity Clinic, Corsicana, Texas. Dr. Menon is a staff cardiologist in the Section of Cardiovascular Imaging, the Robert and Suzanne Tomsich Department of Cardiovascular Medicine, Sydell and Arnold Miller Family Heart & Vascular Institute, Cleveland Clinic, Cleveland, Ohio. Dr. Smith is Professor of Medicine and Director, Center for Cardiovascular Science and Medicine, in the Division of Cardiology, University of North Carolina at Chapel Hill, Chapel Hill, North Carolina.

53. ACE Inhibitors and Angiotensin II Receptor Antagonists as Reducers of Vascular Complications

Sarah Capes, MD, MSc, FRCPC, and Hertzel Gerstein, MD, MSc, FRCPC

Angiotensin-converting enzyme (ACE) inhibitors and angiotensin II receptor (A2) antagonists are drugs that have two main effects: promoting potentially beneficial metabolic changes in the vasculature and lowering blood pressure. The metabolic changes associated with both classes of drugs include reducing the effects of angiotensin II on target tissue, thereby decreasing vasoconstriction and decreasing stimulation of vascular smooth muscle growth. ACE inhibitors have the added effect of increasing levels of bradykinins (which promote vasodilation and increase insulin sensitivity), lowering levels of plasminogen activator inhibitor, and decreasing platelet aggregation. Equally important, the blood pressure–lowering effect of these and other classes of drugs has been shown in numerous clinical trials to translate into an improved cardiovascular prognosis for patients with diabetes. This chapter will summarize the evidence regarding the vascular benefits of ACE inhibitors and A2 antagonists in patients with diabetes.

METABOLIC EFFECTS OF ACE INHIBITORS AND A2 ANTAGONISTS

ACE Inhibitors Prevent Cardiovascular Events Independent of Their Blood Pressure–Lowering Effect

Cardiovascular disease affects >50% of all people with diabetes and is the major cause of death. At least four recent studies have explored the cardioprotective effects of ACE inhibitors in participants with either a history of cardiovascular disease or diabetes. The largest of these studies was the Heart Outcome Prevention Evaluation (HOPE) study. In the HOPE study, 3,577 people with diabetes were randomly assigned to treatment with 10 mg/day ramipril, versus placebo, in addition to their usual medications. Ramipril reduced the risk of the combined outcome of myocardial infarction (MI), stroke, or cardiovascular death by 25% over 4.5 years of follow-up (Table 53.1). About half of the diabetic patients had a diagnosis of hypertension at the time of randomization, and in those patients, the study drug (ramipril or placebo) was added to their usual antihypertensive medication (β-blocker in 28%, diuretic in 20%, and calcium channel blocker in 44%). Ramipril had only a modest blood pressure–lowering effect, and the reduced morbidity and mortality that was observed in patients treated with ramipril was shown to be inde-

Table 53.1 Results of the HOPE Study in Patients with Diabetes

Outcome	Placebo Rate (%)	Relative Risk Reduction [% (95% CI)]	P
MI, stroke, or CV death	19.8	25 (12–36)	0.0004
MI	12.9	22 (6–36)	0.01
Stroke	6.1	33 (10–50)	0.0074
CV death	9.7	37 (21–51)	0.0001
Total death	14.0	24 (8–37)	0.004

CV, cardiovascular.

pendent of the change in blood pressure. Thus, the HOPE study clearly shows that ACE inhibitors have a cardioprotective effect over and above any antihypertensive effect. On the basis of this study, 22 high-risk, middle-aged people with diabetes would have to be treated with ramipril for 4.5 years to prevent one MI, stroke, or cardiovascular death. ACE inhibitors also improve outcome for patients with chronic congestive heart failure. Indeed, in the Studies of Left Ventricular Dysfunction (SOLVD) trial, enalapril reduced mortality and hospitalization for heart failure by 26% compared with placebo in patients with chronic congestive heart failure and reduced ejection fraction.

Although ACE inhibitors differ in structure and pharmacokinetic properties, all members of the class are likely to have similar cardioprotective effects. Notwithstanding this assumption, neither the optimal cardioprotective dose nor the comparable doses of each of the members of this class have been established. It is important to note, however, that higher doses of ACE inhibitors may be required for optimal cardioprotection. For example, in the Study to Evaluate Carotid Ultrasound Changes in Patients Treated with Ramipril and Vitamin E (SECURE) substudy of the HOPE study, there was evidence of a dose-response effect with slower progression of carotid atherosclerosis in patients treated with higher doses of ramipril (10 mg/day vs. 0 or 2.5 mg/day).

A2 Antagonists May Prevent Cardiovascular Events in Patients with Diabetes

The cardioprotective effects of A2 antagonists have been studied in select groups of individuals, and emerging evidence suggests that A2 antagonists may also have beneficial vascular metabolic effects. Studies in which patients with type 2 diabetes were treated with A2 antagonists are summarized in Table 53.2. Only one study has clearly demonstrated a reduction in cardiovascular events in diabetic patients using an A2 antagonist. This study, the Losartan Intervention for Endpoint Reduction in Hypertension (LIFE) study, only included people with significant hypertension and left ventricular hypertrophy. It showed the benefit of losartan over atenolol within the group as a whole and the diabetes subgroup. Patients who were treated with 50–100 mg losartan had a significant 24% lower

Table 53.2 A2 Antagonists in Type 2 Diabetes

Study	n	% with Diabetes	Mean Age (yr)	Drug/Dose	Outcome	Results (A2 Antagonist vs. Comparator)	P
LIFE (diabetes, ↑BP, and left ventricular hypertrophy)	1,195	100	67	50–100 mg losartan vs. 50–100 mg atenolol	CV death, stroke, or MI	RRR = 0.24 (95% CI 0.02–0.42)	0.031
RENAAL study (diabetic nephropathy)	1,513	100	60	50–100 mg losartan vs. placebo	Doubling of serum creatinine, ESRD, or death	RRR = 0.16	0.02
					Fatal or nonfatal CV event	RRR = 0.1	0.26
					MI	RRR = 0.28	0.08
					First hospitalization for coronary heart failure	RRR = 0.32	0.005
CALM study (diabetes, ↑BP, and microalbuminuria)	199	100	60	16 mg candesartan vs. 20 mg lisinopril vs. combination of both drugs	Systolic and diastolic blood pressure, ACR	Combination reduced systolic and diastolic BP and urine ACR more than either drug alone	<0.05
IDNT study (diabetic nephropathy)	1,715	100	58–59	300 mg irbesartan vs. 10 mg amlodipine vs. placebo	Doubling of serum creatinine, ESRD, or death	RRR = 0.23 (vs. amlodipine) and 0.2 (vs. placebo)	0.006 / 0.02
IRMA study (diabetes and microalbuminuria)	590	100	58	150–300 mg irbesartan vs. placebo	Time to onset of diabetic nephropathy	RRR = 0.7 (95% CI 0.39–0.86) for 300 mg irbesartan	<0.001
						RRR = 0.39 (95% CI–0.08–0.66) for 150 mg irbesartan	0.08

ACR, albumin-to-creatinine ratio; BP, blood pressure; ↑BP, increased blood pressure (hypertension); CV, cardiovascular; CALM, Candesartan and Lisinopril Microalbuminuria; ESRD, end-stage renal disease; IDNT, Irbesartan Diabetic Nephropathy Trial; IRMA, Irbesartan in Patients with Type 2 Diabetes and Microalbuminuria; RRR, relative risk reduction.

risk of cardiovascular death, stroke, or MI than those who were treated with 50–100 mg atenolol, despite equal lowering of blood pressure in both groups.

Other studies confined to patients with overt diabetic nephropathy have shown an improvement in renal outcomes, and some of these studies have also shown a trend toward improved cardiovascular prognosis. For example, in the Reduction of Endpoints in NIDDM with the Angiotensin II Antagonist Losartan (RENAAL) study, treatment with 50–100 mg losartan led to a significant 16% reduction in the primary end point of doubling of serum creatinine, end-stage renal failure, or death compared with placebo. The RENAAL study also showed a lower risk of first hospitalization for congestive heart failure and a trend toward reduced risk of fatal and nonfatal cardiovascular events in losartan-treated patients.

CARDIOPROTECTIVE EFFECTS OF BLOOD PRESSURE LOWERING

Systematic reviews and meta-analyses of the effects of various blood pressure–lowering agents have shown that lowering blood pressure by 10–12 mmHg systolic and 5–6 mmHg diastolic leads to as much as a 16% reduction in the risk of coronary artery disease and a 38% reduction in stroke risk. The beneficial effect of blood pressure lowering with ACE inhibitors was demonstrated in a meta-analysis performed by the Blood Pressure Lowering Treatment Trialists' Collaboration, which combined individual patient data from the HOPE study and three smaller studies in which ACE inhibitors were compared with placebo. The meta-analysis showed that high-risk patients (including those with diabetes) who were treated with an ACE inhibitor, compared with placebo, had significant 20–30% reductions in risk of stroke, coronary heart disease, major cardiovascular events, and cardiovascular death, as well as a reduction in total mortality (Fig. 53.1).

An overview of trials comparing blood pressure–lowering regimens based on different drugs did not find significant differences in cardiovascular outcomes among hypertensive patients treated with ACE inhibitors versus those treated with diuretic, β-blocker, or calcium antagonist–based regimens. The results of this overview were confirmed by the Antihypertensive and Lipid Lowering Treatment to Prevent Heart Attack Trial (ALLHAT). ALLHAT enrolled 42,418 hypertensive patients (about one-third of whom had diabetes) who were randomized to blood pressure regimens based on chlorthalidone, lisinopril, or amlodipine. All three regimens were equally effective in lowering the rate of the primary outcome of fatal coronary heart disease or nonfatal MI. Patients treated with chlorthalidone also had a lower risk of heart failure than individuals in the other two groups.

These studies reinforce the primary importance of good control of hypertension to prevent cardiovascular events in patients with diabetes. It is important to note that most hypertensive patients with diabetes will require more than one drug to adequately control their blood pressure. Indeed, in the U.K. Prospective Diabetes Study, 63% of patients required two or more antihypertensive agents to achieve optimal blood pressure control. The results of ALLHAT and the overview performed by the Blood Pressure Lowering Treatment Trialists' Collaboration suggest that first treatment with a diuretic, ACE inhibitor, β-blocker, or calcium

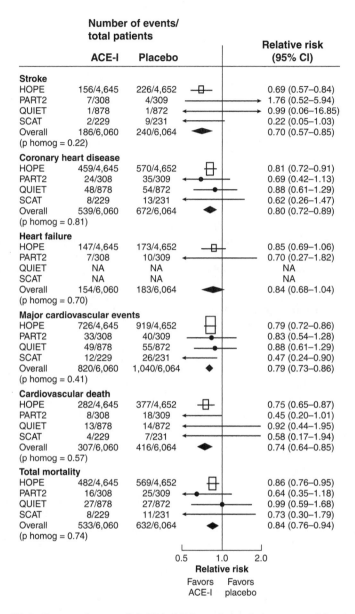

Figure 53.1 Comparisons of ACE inhibitor–based therapy with placebo. Boxes and horizontal lines represent relative risk and 95% CI for each trial. Size of boxes is proportional to inverse of variance of that trial result. Diamonds represent the 95% CI for pooled estimates of effect and are centered on pooled relative risk. ACE-I, ACE inhibitor; NA, data not available; PART2, Prevention of Atherosclerosis with Ramipril Trial; p homog, *P* value from the χ^2 text for homogeneity; QUIET, Quinapril Ischemic Event Trial; SCAT, Simvastatin/Enalapril Coronary Atherosclerosis Trial.

antagonist is appropriate (unless there is a specific indication for the use of one of these classes, such as ACE inhibitors for diabetic patients with microalbuminuria). For the majority of diabetic patients who require more than one drug to control their blood pressure, the results of the HOPE study strongly support the inclusion of an ACE inhibitor in the blood pressure–lowering regimen.

CONCLUSION

Blood pressure lowering is key to the prevention of cardiovascular events in hypertensive patients with diabetes. Diuretics, ACE inhibitors, β-blockers, and calcium antagonists provide similar benefits when used as initial blood pressure–lowering therapy. The large reduction in cardiovascular events in the face of a small reduction in blood pressure that was noted in the HOPE study suggests that ACE inhibitors have beneficial vascular effects that extend beyond their blood pressure–lowering effect. Although early data are suggestive, A2 antagonists have not yet clearly been proven to provide similar cardioprotection, and there is no evidence to support the combination of an ACE inhibitor and A2 antagonist at this time. The ADA currently recommends that

- pharmacological therapy for patients with diabetes and hypertension should be with a regimen that includes either an ACE inhibitor or an angiotensin receptor blocker
- ACE inhibitors should also be considered in the treatment of normotensive individuals with diabetes at high risk of cardiovascular disease to lower the risk of cardiovascular events.

BIBLIOGRAPHY

ALLHAT Officers and Coordinators for the ALLHAT Collaborative Research Group: Major outcomes in high-risk hypertensive patients randomized to angiotensin-converting enzyme inhibitor or calcium channel blocker vs diuretic: the Antihypertensive and Lipid-Lowering Treatment to Prevent Heart Attack Trial (ALLHAT). *JAMA* 288:2981–2997, 2002

American Diabetes Association, Standards of medical care in diabetes—2009. Diabetes Care 32:S13–S62, 2009.

Blood Pressure Lowering Treatment Trialists' Collaboration: Effects of ACE inhibitors, calcium antagonists, and other blood-pressure-lowering drugs: results of prospectively designed overviews of randomised trials. *Lancet* 356:1955–1964, 2000

Brenner BM, Cooper ME, de Zeeuw D, Keane WF, Mitch WE, Parving HH, Remuzzi G, Snapinn SM, Zhang Z, Shahinfar S, for the RENAAL Study Investigators: Effects of losartan on renal and cardiovascular outcomes in patients with type 2 diabetes and nephropathy. *N Engl J Med* 345:861–869, 2001

Heart Outcome Prevention Evaluation (HOPE) Study Investigators: Effects of ramipril on cardiovascular and microvascular outcomes in people with diabetes mellitus: results of the HOPE study and the MICRO HOPE substudy. *Lancet* 355:253–259, 2000

Lindholm LH, Ibsen H, Dahlof B, Devereux RB, Beevers G, de Faire U, Fyhrquist F, Julius S, Kjeldsen SE, Kristiansson K, Lederballe-Pedersen O, Nieminen MS, Omvik P, Oparil S, Wedel H, Aurup P, Edelman J, Snapinn S: Cardiovascular morbidity and mortality in patients with diabetes in the Losartan Intervention for Endpoint Reduction in Hypertension Study (LIFE): a randomised trial against atenolol. *Lancet* 359:1004–1010, 2002

Dr. Capes is Assistant Professor, Department of Medicine, McMaster University, Hamilton, Ontario, Canada. Dr. Gerstein is Professor, Department of Medicine, McMaster University, Hamilton, Ontario, Canada. Dr. Gerstein holds the McMaster University Population Health Institute Chair in Diabetes Research (sponsored by Aventis).

54. Foot Ulcers, Peripheral Arterial Disease, and Risk Classification

Peter Sheehan, MD

FOOT ULCERS

Epidemiology and Impact

Diabetic foot ulcerations are a disturbing complication of diabetes that often result in a diminished quality of life. Of people with diabetes, 15% develop ulcers, 15% of ulcers develop osteomyelitis, and 15% of ulcers result in amputation. Foot ulcers are costly, with a 2-year cost of nearly $30,000, and account for ~20% of hospital inpatient days for patients with diabetes. This is striking when one considers that >33% of U.S. government health care spending (Centers for Medicare and Medicaid Services) is for people with diabetes, and 60% of these costs are for inpatient care. Thus, the economic impact is staggering.

When the outcome is amputation, costs soar to nearly $60,000. There is a profound emotional loss for the patient who submits to amputation, similar to bereavement. Unfortunately, amputation is not the end to the story: ~50% will have a contralateral amputation within 3 years, and 50% will die within 5 years. Although it is agreed that these patients are quite moribund and carry a high cardiovascular risk, the psychosocial upheaval of an amputation may contribute in part to their demise.

Currently, we have >100,000 nontraumatic amputations yearly in the U.S. Although the amputation rate as expressed per 1,000 individuals with diabetes may have plateaued or fallen slightly—as the denominator has increased so much in the past decade—it is still disturbing that more advances have not been made relative to other cardiovascular events, such as myocardial infarction and stroke.

Pathogenesis of Foot Ulcers in Diabetes

As characterized by a component model, Pecoraro et al. (1990) delineated the "causal pathway" to amputation by a landmark analysis of individual clinical factors in patients with diabetes. No factor alone was "sufficient" but rather required a concert of several to result in amputation. Nearly 75% of amputations had the following component pathway:

- peripheral neuropathy, a sine qua non
- trauma, usually the simple repetitive trauma of daily ambulation
- ulceration, typically of the plantar skin, and faulty healing

With the faulty healing of diabetes, the wound becomes chronic and adds risks of infection and amputation.

Chronic wounds differ greatly from acute wounds in the lack of orderly progression to healing. Chronic wounds such as foot ulcers are stuck in the inflammatory phase of wound healing and cannot progress to the proliferative phase of new vessel growth (angiogenesis) and wound healing. A more difficult issue is whether a diabetic foot ulcer is unique as a chronic wound in its pathogenesis and pathophysiology. The following characteristics are more unique to foot ulcers in diabetes: neuropathy, macrovascular disease, microvascular disease, and cellular/inflammatory pathways.

Neuropathy. Clearly, the most important contributing factor to the development of foot ulcers and the faulty healing observed is the presence of peripheral neuropathy and, more specifically, loss of protective sensation (LOPS). This permits the recurrent mechanical injury sustained in daily ambulation to build into a crescendo of inflammatory activity that leads to tissue strain and injury, all without detection by the neuropathic host. In fact, the initial lesion of an ulceration is a "hot spot" over an area of high pressure that is detectable with dermal thermography. In addition, patients with neuropathy have limited joint mobility and bony deformities, which contribute to higher plantar foot pressures, thus the unfortunate coexistence of high foot pressures with an inability to feel them. Finally, there is coincident autonomic neuropathy impairing the ability of the skin to maintain sweating and oil production, leading to excessive dryness and fissuring, potential portals for infection.

Macrovascular Disease. Part of the faulty healing seen in diabetes can be attributed to wound hypoxia on the basis of both macrovascular and microvascular disease. Diabetes is a cardiovascular disease equivalent, with a relative risk of peripheral arterial disease (PAD) of 4–5. PAD risk increases even before the onset of hyperglycemia in type 2 diabetes, implicating the pre-diabetic state in its pathogenesis. This state is characterized by insulin resistance, oxidative stress, and altered free fatty acid metabolism. This milieu leads to endothelial dysfunction with impaired nitric oxide signaling and vasoreactivity, the results of complex mechanisms in vasoconstriction, inflammation, and hypercoaguability. This may account for the powerful risk of vascular disease seen in diabetes.

Diabetes is unique as a risk factor not only for its power, but also for its predilection to involve the small arteries below the knee, the tibial vessels. Here, the disease is typically diffuse and distal, but it spares the arteries of the foot. In addition, the PAD is strongly associated with neuropathy, which allows the vascular disease to slowly worsen without sensory feedback. Thus, a patient with diabetes may have severe PAD and ischemia with little or no symptoms (see PAD discussion later).

Microvascular Disease. Patients with diabetes and neuropathy also have a significant microvascular defects. Hyperglycemia is associated with a ubiquitous involvement of the microvasculature that is manifested by capillary sclerosis and dropout, particularly in people with type 1 diabetes. This can be seen with capillaroscopy and measurement of elevated capillary pressures. In type 2 diabetic patients with neuropathy, functional microvascular abnormalities can be seen, specifically endothelial dysfunction and impaired vasoreactivity. These abnormalities are best demonstrated by laser Doppler imaging of the microcirculation with defective vasodilatory response to heat (generalized defect), acetylcholine (endothelial defect), and sodium nitroprusside (vascular smooth muscle defect). In addition, neuropathy affects the neuroinflammatory microvascular vasodilatation in response to injury or noxious stimuli, the Lewis triple flare.

Impaired angiogenesis is seen in diabetes. Among the many inputs into angiogenesis are neural mediators, such as acetylcholine, substance P, and neuropeptide Y. Deficiencies in these substances result in the impaired neuroinflammatory response. It is interesting to speculate that the presence of peripheral neuropathy itself and its loss of neuropeptides may contribute to impaired angiogenesis and wound healing on a cellular basis.

Cellular/Inflammatory Pathways. Diabetes is known to affect cellular and inflammatory pathways that are involved in wound healing. Hyperglycemia, primarily through a hyperosmotic effect, may slow neutrophil chemotaxis. In vitro studies of fibroblasts taken from subjects with diabetes show altered function and response to stimulatory challenges.

Diabetes can be viewed as a state of chronic vascular inflammation. There is now a vast body of literature that altered glucose and free fatty acid metabolism results in oxidative stress, endothelial dysfunction, and activation of inflammatory cytokines, in particular those regulated by nuclear factor-κB (NFκB). In diabetes, one can demonstrate increased expression of tumor necrosis factor-α, transforming growth factor-β, interleukin-6, and other inflammatory factors. These factors are also overexpressed in chronic wounds, and there is likely an amplification of the expression in the inflammatory milieu seen in diabetes.

NFκB has several parallel signaling pathways in the skin. Activation may result from physical injury, from toll-like receptors that bind bacterial cell wall components, and from activation from cytokines. Thus, in a diabetic foot ulcer, the inflammation seen in the wound is sustained by several pathways that ultimately amplify and augment the response.

In addition, there exists a tonic stimulation (i.e., perpetual, sustained) of inflammatory signaling maintained by the accumulation of advanced glycosylation end products (AGEs) and activation of their receptors (RAGEs). The RAGE pathway also ultimately activates NFκB. It has been shown that feeding diabetic mice a high-AGE diet results in impaired wound healing. One can see that the interplay of these separate signaling pathways results in an unfortunate synergy in the production and maintenance of inflammation that characterizes a nonhealing chronic wound. In addition, inflammation leads to increased fibrosis, and the limited joint mobility seen in the diabetic foot is likely to be a result of inflammatory excess rather than the commonly held notion of collagen cross-linking and tendon shortening.

It is in the area of inflammation where there is a possibility that systemic interventions, in addition to good foot ulcer care, may have an impact. By controlling hyperglycemia, oxidative stress, endothelial dysfunction, AGE formation, or other metabolic consequences of diabetes, one can hope to help subside inflammatory activity generally and its contribution to the excess inflammation seen in diabetic foot ulcers specifically.

Finally, new concepts in wound healing and tissue repair highlight the fact that a substantial portion of the endothelial cells and fibroblasts that repopulate the wound are derived from circulating precursor cells that originate from bone marrow stem cells. This pathway has been found to be impaired in animal models of diabetes. In addition, patients with diabetes and/or cardiovascular risk factors with endothelial dysfunction have fewer circulating precursor cells than normal control subjects, a fact that may contribute to failure of vascular repair and impaired wound healing.

In conclusion, the most common pathway to amputation is one that occurs in people with diabetes and neuropathy who develop a foot ulcer, usually from the recurrent mechanical trauma of daily ambulation. Then there is faulty healing, which ultimately results in the loss of the limb. Faulty healing is seen in all chronic wounds, by definition, and the defect is seen as a lack of progression through the hierarchical stages of healing. The chronic wound is stuck in the inflammatory phase.

Assessment and Evaluation

In the initial evaluation of a foot with an ulceration, the two most important assessments are for infection and ischemia. The vascular evaluation need not be extensive and would initially consist of determining the presence or absence of pedal pulses (dorsalis pedis and posterior tibial). Further evaluation, including the ankle-brachial index (ABI), will be discussed later.

Clinical assessment would include a measurement of area and depth, both being predictors of healing. The presence of infection remains largely a clinical diagnosis, with signs consisting of erythema, warmth, odor, and drainage. The presence of bone infection is a common and crucial diagnosis in determining outcomes. It is suspected if there is a coexisting exposed bone or joint, sinus tracts, or deep abscess. All ulcers should be evaluated with a probe to determine underlying infection. There is a positive predictive value of osteomyelitis if one is able to guide a probe (usually a cotton-tipped applicator) to touch bone. Noninvasive evaluation should include an X-ray and, if osteomyelitis is still suspected, magnetic resonance imaging. Bone scans are of little utility and low specificity. In a stable patient, a simple repeat X-ray in 2 weeks will help exclude the presence of osteomyelitis.

Cultures of the ulcer are restricted to those that are clinically infected. Cultures of noninfected wounds are not helpful and often lead to unnecessary treatment. When cultures are performed, they should sample deep tissues by aspiration or curettage. Swab cultures are not useful. Although the initial antibiotic treatment is empiric, culture results may later influence the choice of antibiotics.

Treatments

In a Consensus Development Conference on diabetic wound care, the American Diabetes Association cited six established treatment modalities that have evidence-based support (Table 54.1). The standard of care for noninfected nonischemic ulcers is comprised largely of three modalities: off-loading of mechanical stress, sharp debridement, and dressings providing a moist wound environment.

The most effective and extensively studied method of off-loading is the total contact cast. This is a highly effective "low-tech" modality that yields consistent healing results for >75% of ulcers. It requires technical skill and experience, however, and must be applied serially every 1–2 weeks. The alternatives would be felt reliefs and/or short leg walker braces. The removable braces may be more effec-

Table 54.1 Established Treatment Modalities for Foot Ulcers

- Off-loading
- Debridement
- Moist wound dressings
- Treatment of infection
- Revascularization
- Amputation

tive when rendered irremovable by shrouding with plaster or adhesives, enforcing patient compliance in wearing the device at all times. Bed rest is not adequate off-loading, as brief episodes of activity will negate hours of bed rest.

Debridement should be sharp, usually with a scalpel, and should be performed early and often. Most noninfected ulcers are safely debrided in an outpatient setting. At a minimum, the wound should be "saucerized," removing all necrotic and overriding tissue and callus. More extensive debridement and the use of debridement devices, such as ultrasound and shearing hydrocurrent, may stimulate the wound-healing cascade.

A moist wound environment has been shown to enhance the migration of keratinocytes and promote wound healing. There are myriad dressings available to provide this beneficial effect. There is currently no clear evidence that any specific dressing type is superior to others. The dressing should, in addition, minimize trauma and infection. The choices include saline-moistened gauze, xeroform gauze, hydrocolloids, hydrogels, alginates, foams, and collagens. The choice of the dressings is determined by the wound characteristics, such as drainage, exudates or dryness, and the state of the surrounding tissue. Increasingly, the ease and frequency of dressing change and the costs of the dressing and nursing care are factors that influence decision making because most patients are managed in the home-care setting.

The importance of treating infections should be underscored because uncontrolled infection is a frequent cause of worsened tissue loss and limb loss. Uninfected wounds, in contrast, need no specific concern, and antibiotic treatment does have its costs, does present some risk of adverse events, and may lead to bacterial resistance. When present, infection is classified as mild, moderate, or severe, as described by the Infectious Disease Society of America. A mild infection is characterized by cellulitis extending <2 cm from the margins of the ulcer; for a moderate infection, the cellulitis extends >2 cm or presents with a deep abscess or osteomyelitis. An infection becomes severe when there are signs of systemic involvement, such as fever, hypotension, or metabolic instability and hyperglycemia.

Treatment and outcomes for mild infections and for those involving superficial infection, usually with gram-positive bacteria, can generally be controlled with commonly available oral antibiotics. Examples would be clindamycin and amoxicillin/clavulanic acid. Oral linezolid has been shown to be superior and should be used if infection with methicillin-resistant staphylococci is suspected. Moderate and severe infections are considered limb threatening and require more aggressive management. In general, the wound requires thorough debridement and incision and drainage of any deep infection. Deep cultures should be obtained, and the patient placed on parenteral antibiotic. The U.S. Food and Drug Administration (FDA) has approved ertepenam and piperacillin/tazobactam for moderate infections and, if severe, imipenem/cilastatin. When there is suspicion of methicillin-resistant *Staphylococcus aureus*, linezolid or vancomycin should be added, not substituted. Treatment duration is generally 7–14 days and can be delivered in the home-care setting once the patient is stable. In addition, complex surgical wounds can have staged closure at a later time, with the wound and patient safely managed with negative-pressure wound therapy and a visiting nurse.

Osteomyelitis is a common and troublesome consequence of a local spread of infection from a contiguous ulcer. Although aggressive surgical ablation is usually not necessary, medical therapy with antibiotics alone is too often unsuccessful. A combination of conservative surgery, usually using bore debridement and drainage of infection, combined with 4–6 weeks of parenteral therapy, will achieve higher cure rates, approaching 80–90%. The most frequent cause of failure of treatment is neglect of standard wound care, especially inadequate off-loading technique.

For the noninfected nonischemic ulcer, more advanced modalities are available for those ulcers that have not healed with standard of care. These include becaplermin (recombinant platelet-derived growth factor), Apligraf (bilayered human skin equivalent), and Dermagraph (human dermal replacement therapy). These modalities are safe and effective and have FDA approval; however, they are more costly. When to use these modalities relies on clinical judgment of the healing potential of the ulcer.

Recently, change in ulcer area in as early as a month has been shown to be a predictor of complete healing later. Many clinicians are using the failure of the ulcer area to diminish by 50% at 4 weeks as an indication to utilize more advanced, but more expensive, modalities.

PAD

Epidemiology and Natural History of PAD in Diabetes

Diabetes as a Risk Factor for PAD. PAD is a manifestation of atherosclerosis characterized by occlusive disease of the lower extremities that may or may not have symptoms and is a marker for atherothrombotic disease in other vascular beds, i.e., coronary and cerebral. PAD affects ~12 million people in the U.S.

Although there are other well-known risk factors, such as advanced age, hypertension, and hyperlipidemia, diabetes and smoking are the strongest risk factors for PAD. Moreover, in at least one analysis, diabetes was the most strongly associated risk factor for PAD, with a relative risk of >4. It has also become clear that the risk of PAD may precede the development of overt diabetes and hyperglycemia. This underscores the cardiovascular impact of the "pre-diabetes" of glucose intolerance, insulin resistance, and endothelial dysfunction.

For people with diabetes, the risk of PAD is further increased by age and duration of diabetes. There a strong association of PAD with diabetic peripheral neuropathy. As will be discussed, this association and the coincidence of PAD and neuropathy have implications for the clinical presentation and progression of disease.

In patients with diabetes, race is also a significant associated factor for PAD. African Americans and Hispanics with diabetes have a higher prevalence of PAD than non-Hispanic whites, even after adjustment for other known risk factors and the excess prevalence of diabetes. Amputation incidence is also increased in African Americans and Hispanics, although this may also reflect reduced access to medical care.

It is important to note that diabetes as a PAD risk factor is unique in its pattern of disease expression. Diabetes is most strongly associated with popliteal and tibial (below-the-knee) PAD, whereas other risk factors (e.g., smoking and hypertension) are associated with more proximal disease.

Thus, as a risk factor for PAD, diabetes stands alone—not only is it the most powerfully associated risk factor, but it also uniquely involves the distal territories of the peripheral vasculature, a characteristic that proves crucial to understanding its clinical manifestations.

Prevalence and Impact of PAD in Diabetes. The true prevalence of PAD in people with diabetes has been difficult to determine because most patients are asymptomatic or because the symptoms are atypical, and many patients do not report them. Furthermore, pain perception may be blunted by the frequent presence of peripheral neuropathy. In addition, screening modalities have not been uniformly agreed upon or validated. Although amputation has been used by some as a measure of PAD prevalence, medical care and local indications for amputation versus revascularization of the patient with critical limb ischemia vary widely. The nationwide age-adjusted amputation rate in diabetes is ~8 per 1,000 patient-years, with a prevalence of ~3%. However, there is great variability because of the non-uniformity of care. The best screening tool is the ABI, and in a large survey of patients with diabetes aged >50 years by general practitioners using the ABI, the prevalence of PAD was 29%.

The clinical impact of PAD can be assessed by two perspectives: *1*) its progression and the onset or worsening of symptoms and *2*) the excess risk of cardiovascular events associated with systemic atherosclerosis. As far as disease progression, most patients with PAD remain stable in their symptoms. However, although the majority of patients remain stable in their lower-limb symptoms, there is systemic atherosclerosis with a striking excess in cardiovascular event rates over the same 5-year time period, wherein 20% of PAD patients sustain nonfatal events (e.g., myocardial infarction, stroke) and 30% die. The outcomes and prognoses for more diseased patients with critical limb ischemia are predictably worse. Within 6 months of presentation, 30% will have amputations, and 20% will die.

As previously mentioned, the presence of neuropathy strongly influences the clinical presentation. The presence of neuropathy blunts pain perception and makes symptoms such as claudication less common, allowing a later presentation with more severe lesions than in the nondiabetic patient. In a vicious cycle, the presence of PAD increases nerve ischemia and hypoxia, resulting in worsened sensory neuropathy. Accordingly, diabetic patients with PAD are more likely to present with advanced disease compared with nondiabetic patients, often with an ulcer and critical limb ischemia as a presenting symptom.

The Pathophysiology of PAD in Diabetes

The association of diabetes and cardiovascular disease is well established and beyond the scope of this chapter. However, endothelial dysfunction, insulin resistance, and inflammation need to be underscored.

Most patients with diabetes, including those with PAD, demonstrate abnormalities of endothelial function and vascular regulation. The mediators of endothelial cell dysfunction in diabetes are numerous, but an important final common pathway is derangement of nitric oxide bioavailability. Nitric oxide is a potent stimulus for vasodilatation and limits inflammation. Furthermore, nitric oxide inhibits vascular smooth muscle cell migration and proliferation and limits platelet activation. Therefore, the loss of normal nitric oxide homeostasis can result in the risk of a cascade of events in the vasculature, leading to atherosclerosis and its consequent complications. Several mechanisms contribute to the endothelial dysfunction, including hyperglycemia, free fatty acid production, and, most importantly, insulin resistance.

Inflammation has been established as both a risk marker and perhaps a risk factor for cardiovascular disease, including PAD. Elevated levels of C-reactive protein are strongly associated with the development of PAD. In addition, levels of C-reactive protein are known to be elevated in patients with impaired glucose regulation syndromes, including obesity, pre-diabetes, and diabetes.

Clinical Manifestations and Presentation of PAD in Diabetes

The most common symptom of PAD is intermittent claudication (from the Latin *claudio*, "to limp"), classically defined as pain, cramping, or aching in the calves, thighs, or buttocks, which appears reproducibly with walking and is relieved by rest. More extreme presentations of PAD include rest pain, tissue loss, or gangrene. These limb-threatening manifestations of PAD are collectively termed critical limb ischemia. Most patients with PAD are asymptomatic. It has been reported that of those with PAD, >50% are asymptomatic or have atypical symptoms, about one-third have claudication, and a small percentage have more severe forms of the disease.

It is important for the clinician to understand that the presentation of people with diabetes and PAD differs distinctly from those with PAD from other risk factors, such as smoking and hypertension. Although diabetes is an important risk factor for claudication, in patients with diabetes, PAD is often more subtle in its presentation than in those without diabetes. This is related to the pattern of disease distribution and the association with neuropathy. In contrast to the focal and proximal atherosclerotic lesions of PAD typically found in other high-risk patients, in patients with diabetes, the lesions are more likely to be more diffuse and distal. Importantly, PAD in individuals with diabetes is usually accompanied by peripheral neuropathy with impaired sensory feedback, enabling the silent progression of occlusive disease.

A patient with diabetes and asymptomatic PAD could also have a "pivotal event" that leads acutely to an ischemic ulcer and a limb-threatening situation. A typical story would be a man with PAD and neuropathy who wore a tight-fitting dress shoe to a wedding, and he then develops an ulcer at the day-long affair. In contrast to the plantar location of neuropathic ulcers, ischemic ulcers are commonly seen around the edges of the foot, including the apices of the toes and the back of the heel. Thus, an asymptomatic, usually undiagnosed, patient lapses abruptly into critical limb ischemia. Clearly, by identifying a patient with subclinical disease and instituting preventive measures, it may be possible to avoid acute, limb-threatening ischemia.

As mentioned, PAD is also a major risk factor for lower-extremity amputation, especially in the patient with diabetes. Moreover, even for the asymptomatic patient, PAD is a marker for systemic vascular disease involving coronary, cerebral, and renal vessels, leading to an elevated risk of events such as myocardial infarction, stroke, and death. In a study that compared patients with PAD with and without diabetes, those with diabetes had more severe disease below the knee, had a fivefold higher amputation rate, and had double the mortality of the nondiabetic patients.

Perhaps most importantly, it should be appreciated that PAD in diabetes also adversely affects quality of life, contributing to long-term disability and functional impairment that is often severe. Of patients with PAD, those with diabetes have worse function, even in the absence of claudication. This may lead to a "cycle of disability," with progressive deconditioning and loss of function. Too often, this initiates a downward spiral to an overall psychological and social decline for the patient.

Evaluation and Assessment of PAD in Diabetes

Diagnosing PAD is of clinical importance for two reasons. The first is to identify a patient who has a high risk of subsequent myocardial infarction or stroke, regardless of whether symptoms of PAD are present. The National Cholesterol Education Program Adult Treatment Panel III stated that PAD be considered a "coronary disease equivalent." The second is to elicit and treat symptoms of PAD, which may be associated with functional disability and risk of limb loss, and attempt to prevent progression of disease.

The initial assessment of PAD in patients with diabetes should begin with a thorough medical history and physical examination. A thorough walking history may elicit classic claudication symptoms, although more patients may have atypical symptoms, and most are asymptomatic.

Two important components of the physical examination are visual inspection of the foot and palpation of peripheral pulses. Dependent rubor, pallor on elevation, absence of hair growth, dystrophic toenails, and cool, dry, fissured skin are signs of vascular insufficiency and should be noted. Palpation of peripheral pulses should be a routine component of the physical exam. The absence of both pedal pulses, when assessed by a person experienced in this technique, strongly suggests the presence of vascular disease.

Noninvasive Evaluation for PAD: ABI. The ABI is a reproducible and reasonably accurate noninvasive measurement for the detection of PAD and the determination of disease severity. The ABI is defined as the ratio of the highest systolic blood pressure in the ankle divided by the highest systolic blood pressure at the arm. The only tools required to perform the ABI measurement include a handheld 5- to 10-MHz Doppler probe and a blood pressure cuff (Fig. 54.1). An ABI ≤0.90 is diagnostic of PAD. An ABI value >1.3 suggests poorly compressible arteries at the ankle level due to the presence of medial arterial calcification, an issue not uncommon in the diabetic population.

Because of the high estimated prevalence of PAD in patients with diabetes and because most patients are asymptomatic, a Consensus Statement of the American Diabetes Association has recommended that ABI screening should be performed in patients >50 years of age who have diabetes. If normal, the test should be repeated every 5 years. A screening ABI should be considered in diabetic patients <50 years of age who have other PAD risk factors (e.g., smoking, hypertension,

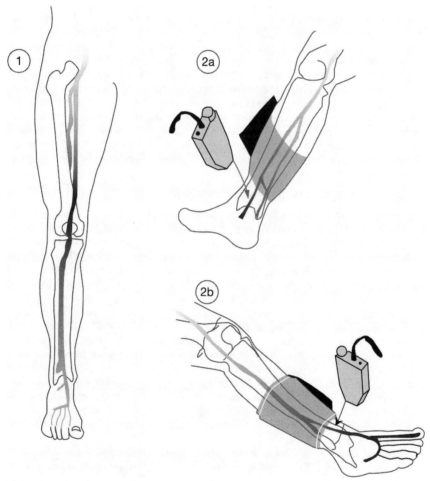

Figure 54.1 Methodology for assessment of ABI. *1*: Anterior view, right lower limb, normal aterial anatomy. *2*: ABI. Place blood pressure cuff above pulse. Place Doppler probe over arterial pulse. *2a*: Posterior tibial artery, ankle systolic pressure. *2b*: Dorsalis pedis artery. ABI calculation: divide systolic leg blood pressure by systolic arm blood pressure. (ABI >0.9 is normal.) Adapted from Boulton et al. (2008).

hyperlipidemia, or duration of diabetes >10 years). Certainly, a diagnostic ABI should be performed in any patient with symptoms of PAD.

Vascular Lab Evaluation: Segmental Pressures and Pulse Volume Recordings. In the patient with a confirmed diagnosis of PAD in whom assessment of the location and severity is desired, the next step should be a vascular laboratory evaluation for segmental pressures and pulse volume recordings (PVRs). These tests should also be considered for patients with poorly compressible vessels or those with a normal ABI in whom there is high suspicion of PAD. Segmental pressures and PVRs are determined at the toe, ankle, calf, low thigh, and high thigh. Segmental pressures help with localization of the stenosis or occlusion, whereas PVRs provide segmental plethysmographic wave form analysis, a qualitative assessment of blood flow.

Anatomical Studies: Duplex Sonography and Magnetic Resonance Angiogram. For those patients in whom revascularization is considered and anatomical localization of stenoses or occlusions is important, an evaluation with a duplex ultrasound or a magnetic resonance angiogram may be valuable. Duplex ultrasound can directly visualize vessels. Magnetic resonance angiogram is noninvasive, with minimal risk of renal insult. It may give images that are comparable to conventional X-ray angiography, especially in occult pedal vessels, and may be used for anatomical diagnosis.

Treatment of PAD in Patients with Diabetes

Diabetes is now recognized as a cardiovascular equivalent and as such compels the clinician to place the patient with diabetes into primary risk factor interventions. The presence of PAD further increases the risk of cardiovascular events and as such suggests considerations for secondary risk interventions. Thus, patients with diabetes should be managed by current guidelines; those with PAD as well may benefit from more aggressive interventions, especially for hypertension, lipid management, and antiplatelet therapy.

Intermittent Claudication. Medical therapy for intermittent claudication includes exercise rehabilitation as the cornerstone therapy, as well as the adjunctive use of pharmacological agents. Exercise programs call for ≥3 months of intermittent treadmill walking three times per week. Exercise therapy has minimal associated morbidity and is likely to improve the cardiovascular risk factor profile. Of note, however, is that it is most effective when performed under supervision. Cilostazol is the drug of choice if pharmacological therapy is necessary for the management of PAD in patients with diabetes. It is an oral phosphodiesterase type III inhibitor. Its main mechanism of action is probably as a vasodilator, acting on vascular smooth muscle.

Critical Limb Ischemia and Revascularization. The indications for limb revascularization are *1*) disabling claudication or *2*) critical limb ischemia (rest pain or tissue loss) refractive to conservative therapy. Disabling claudication is a relative, not absolute, indication and requires significant patient consultation.

One must weigh existing symptoms against the risk of the procedure and its expected effect and durability. Although most ischemic limbs can be revascularized, some cannot. Lack of a target vessel, unavailability of autogenous vein, or irreversible gangrene beyond the midfoot may preclude revascularization. In some patients, a choice must be made between prolonged medical therapy and primary amputation.

Two general techniques of revascularization exist: open surgical procedures and endovascular interventions, such as angioplasty and stenting. The two approaches are not mutually exclusive and may be combined, such as iliac angioplasty combined with a below-knee saphenous vein bypass. The risks, expected benefit, and durability of each must be considered. In either approach, appropriate patient preparation, intraprocedure monitoring, and postprocedure care will minimize complications.

Endovascular intervention is more appropriate in patients with focal disease, especially stenosis of larger, more proximal vessels, and when the procedure is performed for claudication. Open procedures have been successfully carried out for all lesions and tend to have greater durability. However, open procedures are associated with a small but consistent morbidity and mortality. The choice between the two modalities in an individual patient is a complex decision and requires team consultation.

Bypass to the tibial or pedal vessels with autologous vein has a long track record in limb salvage and remains the most predictable method of improving blood flow to the threatened limb. The procedure is safe, durable, and effective. Below-the-knee bypass accounts for 75% of lower-limb procedures in patients with diabetes, with the anterior tibial/dorsalis pedis artery the most common target vessel. Tibial angioplasty is less preferred because of poor long-term patency and durability. Nonetheless, in selected patients, especially high-risk or moribund individuals, tibial angioplasty and stenting may serve as a maneuver to "buy time" to resolve an episode of critical limb ischemia. In addition, there is also some new, promising experience with endovascular atherectomy.

Major amputation in the ischemic foot is necessary and indicated only when there is overwhelming infection that threatens the patient's life, when rest pain cannot be controlled, or when extensive necrosis secondary to a major arterial occlusion has destroyed the function of the foot. Using these criteria, the number of major limb amputations should be limited.

Most amputations can be prevented and limbs salvaged through a multi-armed treatment of antibiotics, debridement, revascularization, and staged wound closure. However, amputation may offer an expedient return to a useful quality of life, especially if a prolonged course of treatment is anticipated, with little likelihood of healing. Decisions should be made on an individual basis, with rehabilitative and quality-of-life issues considered highly. Diabetic patients should have full and active rehabilitation following amputation.

FOOT EXAM AND RISK ASSESSMENT

Musculoskeletal Assessment

The musculoskeletal assessment should include evaluation for any gross deformity. Rigid deformities are defined as any contractures that cannot easily be manually reduced and are most frequently found in the digits. Common forefoot deformities that are known to increase plantar pressures and are associated with skin breakdown include claw toe and hammer toe. An example of this deformity is shown in Fig. 54.2.

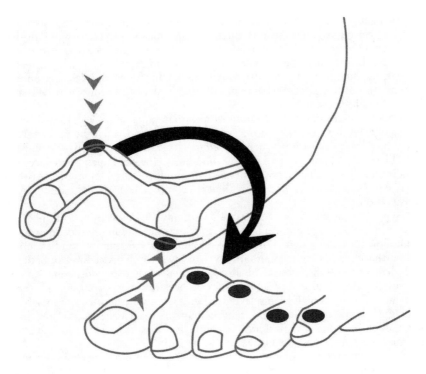

Figure 54.2 Claw toes.

An important and often overlooked or misdiagnosed condition is Charcot arthropathy (Fig. 54.3). This occurs in the neuropathic foot and most often affects the midfoot. This may present as a unilateral red, hot, swollen, flat foot with profound deformity.

Neurological Assessment

Peripheral neuropathy is the most common component cause in the pathway to diabetic foot ulceration. The clinical exam that is recommended, however, is designed to identify LOPS rather than early neuropathy. The clinical examination to identify LOPS is simple and requires no expensive equipment. It should be regularly performed in the screening exam and will normally comprise the 10-g monofilament and vibration.

Ten-gram monofilaments. Monofilaments, sometimes known as Semmes-Weinstein monofilaments, were originally used to diagnose sensory loss in leprosy. Nylon monofilaments are designed to buckle when a 10-g force is applied. Loss of the ability to detect this pressure at one or more anatomical sites on the plantar surface of the foot has been associated with loss of large-fiber nerve function and LOPS. It is recommended that four sites (first, third, and fifth metatarsal heads and plantar surface of distal hallux) be tested on each foot.

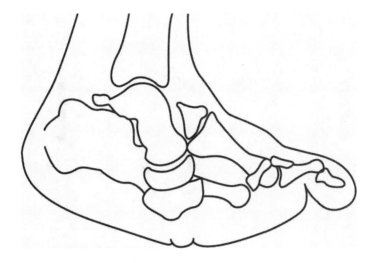

Figure 54.3 Charcot foot.

The technique for testing pressure perception with the 10-g monofilament is illustrated in Fig 54.4. Patients should close their eyes while being tested. The sites of the foot may then be examined by telling the patient to respond "yes" or "no" when asked if they believe that the monofilament is being applied to a particular site. The patient should be able to recognize the pressure as well as identify the correct site of pressure. Areas of callus should always be avoided when testing for pressure perception.

128-hz tuning fork. The tuning fork is widely used in clinical practice and provides an easy and inexpensive test of vibratory sensation. This should be tested over the tip of the great toe bilaterally, and an abnormal response can be defined as when the patient loses vibratory sensation and the examiner still perceives it whilst holding the fork on the tip of the toe.

Vascular Assessment

PAD is a component cause in approximately one-third of foot ulcers and is often a significant risk factor associated with recurrent wounds. Therefore, its assessment is important in defining the overall lower-extremity risk status. Vascular examination should include palpation of the posterior tibial and dorsalis pedis pulses. These should be characterized as either "present" or "absent." If PAD is suspected in a patient with palpable pulses, an ABI evaluation will give more sensitivity.

Risk Assessment

With these three components of the foot exam (i.e., musculoskeletal, neurological, and vascular), a risk assessment can be performed, and a treatment plan and follow–up frequency can be offered (Table 54.2). This risk classification has been validated as a useful predictor of ulceration, hospitalization, and amputation

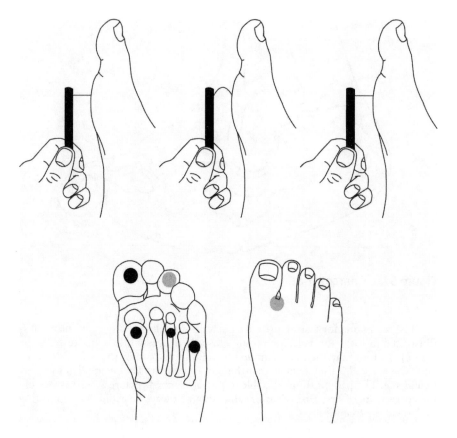

Figure 54.4 Neurological assessment using the 10-g monofilament.

and is a safe, noninvasive bedside exam. As clinicians become more confident in their ability to perform a comprehensive foot exam, more preventative measures should be used, and clinical outcomes should improve for patients with diabetes.

REFERENCES

American Diabetes Association: Consensus Development Conference on diabetic foot wound care: 7–8 April 1999, Boston, Massachusetts. *Diabetes Care* 22:1354–1360, 1999

American Diabetes Association: Peripheral arterial disease in people with diabetes. *Diabetes Care* 26:3333–3341, 2003

Boulton AJ, Armstrong DG, Albert SF, Frykberg RG, Hellman R, Kirkman MS, Lavery LA, Lemaster JW, Mills JL Sr, Mueller MJ, Sheehan P, Wukich DK,

Table 54.2 Risk Classification Based on the Comprehensive Foot Examination

Risk Category	Definition	Treatment Recommendations	Suggested Follow-up
0	No LOPS, no PAD, no deformity	• Patient education, including advice on appropriate footwear	Annually (by generalist and/or specialist)
1	LOPS ± deformity	• Consider prescriptive or accommodative footwear • Consider prophylactic surgery if deformity is not able to be safely accommodated in shoes. Continue patient education.	Every 3–6 months (by generalist or specialist)
2	PAD ± LOPS	• Consider prescriptive or accommodative footwear • Consider vascular consultation for combined follow-up	Every 2–3 months (by specialist)
3	History of ulcer or amputation	• Consider prescriptive or accommodative footwear • Consider vascular consultation for combined follow-up if PAD is present	Every 1–2 months (by specialist)

American Diabetes Association, American Association of Clinical Endocrinologists: Comprehensive foot examination and risk assessment: a report of the Task Force of the Foot Care Interest Group of the American Diabetes Association, with endorsement by the American Association of Clinical Endocrinologists. *Diabetes Care* 31:1679–1685, 2008

Brem H, Sheehan P, Rosenberg HJ, Schneider JS, Boulton AJ: Evidence-based protocol for diabetic foot ulcers. *Plast Reconstr Surg* 117 (7 Suppl.):193S–209S, 2006

Norgren L, Hiatt WR, Dormandy JA, Nehler MR, Harris KA, Fowkes FG, TASC II Working Group, Bell K, Caporusso J, Durand-Zaleski I, Komori K, Lammer J, Liapis C, Novo S, Razavi M, Robbs J, Schaper N, Shigematsu H, Sapoval M, White C, White J, Clement D, Creager M, Jaff M, Mohler E 3rd, Rutherford RB, Sheehan P, Sillesen H, Rosenfield K: Inter-Society Consensus for the Management of Peripheral Arterial Disease (TASC II). *Eur J Vasc Endovasc Surg* 33 (Suppl. 1):S1–S75, 2007

Pecoraro RE, Reiber GE, Burgess EM: Pathways to diabetic limb amputation: basis for prevention. *Diabetes Care* 13:513–521, 1990

Sheehan P, Jones P, Caselli A, Giurini JM, Veves A: Percent change in wound area of diabetic foot ulcers over a 4-week period is a robust predictor of complete healing in a 12-week prospective trial. *Diabetes Care* 26:1879–1882, 2003

Steed DL, Attinger C, Brem H, Colaizzi T, Crossland M, Franz M, Harkless L, Johnson A, Moosa H, Robson M, Serena T, Sheehan P, Veves A, Wiersma-Bryant L: Guidelines for the prevention of diabetic ulcers. *Wound Repair Regen* 16:169–174, 2008

Steed DL, Attinger C, Colaizzi T, Crossland M, Franz M, Harkless L, Johnson A, Moosa H, Robson M, Serena T, Sheehan P, Veves A, Wiersma-Bryant L: Guidelines for the treatment of diabetic ulcers. *Wound Repair Regen* 14:680–692, 2006

Dr. Sheehan is a member of the Senior Faculty at Mount Sinai School of Medicine, New York, New York.

Index

continuous subcutaneous insulin
infusion (CSII) pumps, 322–
330
coronary angiography, 614
coronary artery disease (CAD). *See also*
acute coronary syndrome
azotemic diabetic patients, 510
blood pressure, 632.
See also coronary heart disease
(CHD)
cardiac testing, 613
cholesterol, 505–507
erectile dysfunction (ED), 568
exercise, 365
pregnancy, 39–40
studies/trials, 203
surgery, 352
surgical revascularization, 623
coronary heart disease (CHD), 209,
402, 412–413, 587, 598–606,
608–614, 617–619, 632, 633*t*
cortisol, 398
counterregulatory hormones, 76,
124–125, 230, 350, 371, 395
cytokines, 480

D

depression, 116, 119–120, 122
dermopathy, 438, 439*f*
development delay and epilepsy
(DEND syndrome), 11
diabetes. *See also* under individual types
classification, 8
complications, 345–346
cost, 2*t*
diagnosis, 6
prevention trials, 205*t*
treatment goals, 1–3
diabetes self-management education
(DSME), 137–141, 175
diabetes self-management support
(DSMS), 137–141
diabetic cystopathy, 560–562
diabetic gastroenteropathy, 50–51
diabetic ketoacidosis (DKA), 38, 46,
75–84, 114, 124–134, 149, 155,
192, 449

diabetic kidney disease (DKD),
474–477. *See also* chronic
kidney disease (CKD); diabetic
nephropathy (DN)
diabetic macular edema (DME),
458–461, 465–467
diabetic monoradiculopathy/
amyoradiculopathy, 522–530
diabetic nephropathy (DN), 38, 49–50,
116, 195, 422–431, 474–491,
560*f*–561. *See also* chronic
kidney disease (CKD); diabetic
kidney disease (DKD)
diabetic neuropathy
bladder dysfunction, 559
diabetic monoradiculopathy/
amyoradiculopathy, 525–527
erectile dysfunction (ED), 567
exercise, 195
extremity, lower, 516–520
gastrointestinal (GI) disturbances,
532–533
impaired glucose tolerance (IGT),
202
pregnancy, 34
sexual dysfunction in women, 576
diabetic proximal neuropathy (DPN),
526–530
diabetic retinopathy (DR), 39, 46–48,
116, 194–195, 458–461, 561
diabetic sensorimotor polyneuropathy,
527
diabetic thoracoabdominal neuropathy,
524–525
dialysis, 39, 296, 299, 347, 475, 481,
490, 503, 566
diet, 92–93, 489. *See also* medical
nutrition therapy (MNT)
diethylpropion, 190
dietitian, 175*t*–176*t*, 177
distal symmetric polyneuropathy
(DSPN), 522
diuretics, 429, 488–489
dobutamine stress echocardiography
(DSE), 610–611
domeperidone, 541
Down's syndrome, 75

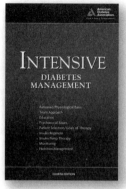

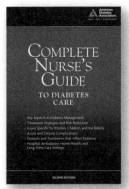
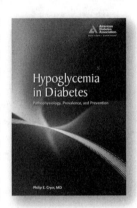
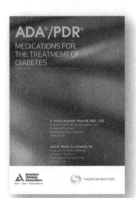
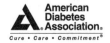

Guide Your Patients to Health with These New Titles

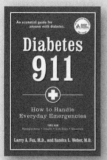

Diabetes 911: How to Handle Everyday Emergencies
by Larry A. Fox, MD, and Sandra L. Weber, MD
When it comes to a condition as serious as diabetes, the best way to solve problems is to prevent them from ever happening. Do you know what to do in case of an emergency? With _Diabetes 911_, you will learn the necessary skills to handle hypoglycemia, insulin pump malfunctions, natural disasters, travel, depression, and sick days.
Order no. 4887-01; Price $12.95

Real-Life Guide to Diabetes
by Hope S. Warshaw, MMSc, RD, CDE, BC-ADM,
and Joy Pape, RN, BSC, CDE, WOCN, CFCN
Real-Life Guide puts everything you need to know about diabetes into a one-of-a-kind book packed with the information you won't find anywhere else. Learn to prevent long-term complications, understand the ins and outs of health insurance, work physical activity into your daily life, and control your blood glucose, cholesterol, and blood pressure. Bring a realistic approach to your diabetes care plan.
Order no. 4893-01; Price $19.95

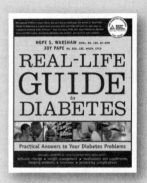

To order these or other titles from the American Diabetes Association, call
1-800-232-6733
or log on to **http://store.diabetes.org.**

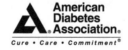

American Diabetes Association
Cure • Care • Commitment